Study Guide and Solutions Manual

*i*GENETICS

A Molecular Approach

THIRD EDITION

Peter J. Russell

Reed College

Bruce Chase

University of Nebraska at Omaha

Benjamin Cummings

San Francisco   Boston   New York
Cape Town   Hong Kong   London   Madrid   Mexico City
Montreal   Munich   Paris   Singapore   Sydney   Tokyo   Toronto

Editor-in-Chief: Beth Wilbur
Executive Director of Development: Deborah Gale
Acquisitions Editor: Gary Carlson
Executive Marketing Manager: Lauren Harp
Associate Project Editor: Rebecca Johnson
Managing Editor, Production: Michael Early
Production Supervisor: Jane Brundage
Production Supervisor, Media: James Bruce
Production Management/Composition: Linda Kern, Progressive Publishing Alternatives
Image Rights and Permissions Manager: Zina Arabia
Manufacturing Buyer: Michael Penne

Cover Photo Credit: Martin Krzywinski, Canada's Michael Smith Genome Sciences Center.

Benjamin Cummings
is an imprint of

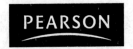

www.pearsonhighered.com

ISBN 10: 0-321-58101-6; ISBN 13: 978-0-321-58101-3

Manufactured in the United States of America.

CONTENTS

PREFACE

Genetics is a fascinating subject. That findings from genetics-based research routinely capture the attention of news media reflects the ongoing impact of genetics in many areas of everyday life. Its fundamental principles and applications are now used throughout the life sciences and in areas as diverse as forensics, disease diagnosis and the management of endangered species. What is not apparent in news stories about genetics are the challenges faced in obtaining a solid understanding of genetic principles and applications. I have written this guide to help students overcome these challenges and to provide multiple, productive strategies for gaining a solid understanding of genetics.

Each chapter of the guide contains a set of features that will help students acquire a well-rounded, thorough understanding of genetic principles and their applications. First, I provide an outline of the text for an organizational overview. Second, I group key terms contextually to challenge the reader to use and distinguish between related terms by developing concept maps. Third, I present suggestions for analytical approaches and strategies for problem solving. Fourth, I offer a set of multiple-choice questions—some designed to stimulate recall of text material, others designed to stimulate clearer thinking and to probe for a deeper understanding. Fifth, I offer a set of thought questions for the text and accompanying media that ask the reader to garner evidence, argue for a viewpoint, and generate hypotheses. Sixth, I provide complete solutions to all of the text questions and problems. I have written these solutions to anticipate student questions and present the logic behind multiple approaches. Students who arrive at a correct answer, but without a clear explanation of how they achieved this, are encouraged to consult these solutions. It is not just the answer but also the logic leading to the answer that is important for understanding genetic principles. Moreover, it is imperative that students realize that just reading the solutions without independently attempting to solve the problems—using the guide primarily as an answer key—does not provide a shortcut to understanding. Students who want to gain a solid understanding of genetics will find no substitute for independent and systematic problem solving efforts. Indeed, I intend this guide as a resource to facilitate and enhance these efforts.

I am indebted to Peter Russell for providing exceptionally clear, well organized, and thoughtful material with which to work. I would like to thank users of previous editions of this guide for their feedback. I would also like to express my gratitude to Rebecca Johnson, project editor for the Study Guide at Benjamin Cummings, as well as Crystal Clifton and the copy editors at Progressive Publishing Alternatives, for their comments, diligence, care, and support during the preparation of this guide. Finally, I welcome comments and suggestions from the users of the guide.

Bruce Chase, University of Nebraska at Omaha
bchase@unomaha.edu

1

Genetics: An Introduction

Chapter Outline

Classical and Modern Genetics

Geneticists and Genetic Research
The Subdisciplines of Genetics
Basic and Applied Research
Genetic Databases and Maps
Organisms for Genetics Research

Review of Key Terms, Symbols, and Concepts

In your own words, write a brief, precise definition of each term in the groups below. Check your definitions using the text. Then develop a concept map using the terms in each list.

1	2	3
classical genetics	genetic database	eukaryote
modern genetics	Entrez	prokaryote
principles of heredity	GenBank	Bacteria
mutation	OMIM	Archaea
recombination	NCBI	model organism
genomics	BLAST	nucleus
hypothetico-deductive	PubMed	plasma membrane
investigation	Nucleotide (database)	nuclear envelope
genetic cross	Protein (database)	endoplasmic reticulum (ER)
transmission genetics	Structure (database)	ribosome
molecular genetics	Genome (database)	mitochondrion
population genetics	RefSeq	chloroplast
quantitative genetics	PopSet	translation
recombinant DNA technology	genetic map	messenger RNA
polymerase chain reaction (PCR)	map unit	centriole
basic research	gene locus	*Saccharomyces cerevisiae*
applied research	frequency of recombination	*Drosophila melanogaster*
DNA cloning		*Caenorhabditis elegans*
DNA fingerprinting		*Arabidopsis thaliana*
genome analysis		*Mus musculus*
regulation of gene expression		*Homo sapiens*
		Neurospora crassa
		Paramecium
		Chlamydomonas reinhardtii
		Pisum sativum
		Zea mays
		Danio rerio
		Escherichia coli

Building Concept Maps Using Genetics Terms

Every chapter of the text introduces new terms used in the "language of genetics." Like new words of a foreign language, each term has a precise meaning and contextual use. To help develop your ability to "speak" the language of genetics, each chapter of this guide will provide lists of key terms, symbols, and concepts. After reading a chapter in the text, review the lists. Without consulting the text and in your own words, write a brief, precise definition of each term. Check your definition against that in the text. Then visualize the relationships between the terms by constructing a concept map using the terms in each list.

What is a concept map? A concept map is a visual image that depicts the relationships between ideas. Terms are arranged on a page, and related terms are connected with lines. A word or phrase that explains the relationship of the concepts is placed next to the lines. Different concept maps can be constructed from the same list of terms, depending on how the relationships between the concepts are viewed. Here is a sample concept map illustrating relationships between ancestral canines and modern dogs.

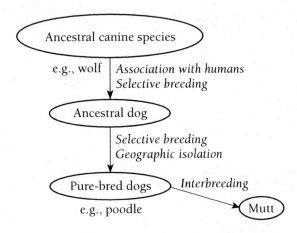

Here are some hints to help you build concept maps using the provided lists of terms:

1. Write each term on a small piece of paper. In some lists, some terms describe broad concepts or categories while others are specific examples of that concept or category. For example, in this chapter, one list contains "genetic material," "DNA," and "RNA." DNA and RNA could be considered examples of genetic material. Identify these types of differences, and group the examples separately from the broad concepts and categories.

2. Arrange the terms on a larger sheet of paper, with the broadest or most abstract ideas at the top and the most specific ideas at the bottom.

3. Arrange the concepts so that two related ideas are placed near (e.g., under) each other.

4. Draw lines between related concepts, rearranging the pieces of paper as needed.

5. On the connecting lines, write words or phrases that explain the relationship between the concepts. Be as precise and succinct as you can. This is challenging, so be patient.

6. Put examples under the concepts they belong with. Connect examples to a concept using an explanatory phrase, such as "e.g." or "specifically."

7. Copy the results onto a single sheet of paper. Draw circles around the concepts, but not the examples.

Questions for Practice

Multiple-Choice Questions

1. Transmission genetics is primarily concerned with
   a. the distribution and behavior of genes in populations.
   b. the passing of genes from generation to generation and their recombination.
   c. the structure and function of genes at the molecular level.
   d. the means by which mutations are retained in nature.

2. Which one of the following is *not* generally a criterion used in selecting an organism for genetic experimentation?
   a. The organism should be able to be used in applied research.
   b. The organism should be easy to handle.
   c. The organism should exhibit genetic variation.
   d. The organism should have a relatively short life cycle.

3. Which one of the following eukaryotic cell structures does *not* contain DNA?
   a. a nucleus
   b. a mitochondrion
   c. the endoplasmic reticulum
   d. a chloroplast

4. Which one of the following is *not* an accurate description of a chromosome?
   a. It is a structure localized in the nucleus.
   b. It is a protein and nucleic acid complex.

    c. It is the cellular structure that contains the genetic material.

    d. In eukaryotes, it is composed of many DNA molecules attached end to end.

5. How does Entrez differ from the PubMed, Nucleotide, Genbank, and OMIM databases?

    a. Entrez is not available at NCBI, while the other databases are.

    b. Unlike the others, Entrez is a system for searching several linked NCBI databases.

    c. Only by searching in Entrez can you identify links to information in the other databases.

    d. Entrez is a portal through which you must pass to search the other databases.

6. A eukaryotic organism is one that

    a. is multicellular.

    b. has a plasma membrane.

    c. has genetic material encapsulated in a nuclear membrane.

    d. all of the above

7. A centriole is an organelle that is

    a. present in the center of a cell's cytoplasm.

    b. composed of microtubules and important for organizing the spindle fibers.

    c. surrounded by a membrane.

    d. part of a chromosome.

8. The rough endoplasmic reticulum is

    a. an intracellular double-membrane system to which ribosomes are attached.

    b. an intracellular membrane that is studded with microtubular structures.

    c. a membranous structure found within mitochondria.

    d. found only in prokaryotic cells.

9. Which one of the following is available at the NCBI website and is a search tool that is useful to compare a nucleotide sequence with other nucleotide sequences in a database?

    a. PubMed

    b. BLAST

    c. OMIM

    d. GenBank

    e. PCR

10. Two geneticists are interested in understanding different aspects of inherited disease. A population geneticist is analyzing its frequency in different human populations while a molecular geneticist is analyzing how defects in the regulation of one gene lead to the disease. Which database is likely to be used more often by the population geneticist?

    a. PubMed

    b. Protein

    c. RefSeq

    d. PopSet

    e. OMIM

Answers: 1b, 2a, 3c, 4d, 5b, 6c, 7b, 8a, 9b, 10d

Thought Questions

1. Why is it difficult to draw a sharp boundary between molecular genetics, transmission genetics, population genetics, and quantitative genetics?

2. Geneticists use the hypothetico-deductive method of investigation. How does this rational approach still allow research projects to go in exciting, unpredictable directions?

3. How are basic and applied research interrelated in the following research areas?

    a. studies of mutations that affect the production of alcohol (ethanol) in yeast

    b. studies of mutations that result in pesticide resistance in *Drosophila melanogaster*

    c. studies of mutations affecting the timing of seed ripening in *Arabidopsis*

    d. studies of transposons in corn

4. What features make an organism well suited for genetic experimentation?

5. How does the information stored in the RefSeq database compare to that stored in the Nucleotide, Genome, and Protein databases? What are the differences between these two databases?

6. What is a gene?

7. What different types of analyses can be made using genetic databases?

8. How are genetic maps used?

9. What hopes and concerns are associated with the field of genomics?

10. How has recombinant DNA technology led to advances in both basic and applied research?

2

DNA: The Genetic Material

Chapter Outline

The Search for the Genetic Material
Griffith's Transformation Experiment
Avery's Transformation Experiment
Hershey and Chase's Bacteriophage Experiment
RNA as Viral Genetic Material

The Composition and Structure of DNA and RNA
The DNA Double Helix
Different DNA Structures
DNA in the Cell
RNA Structure

The Organization of DNA in Chromosomes
Viral Chromosomes
Prokaryotic Chromosomes
Eukaryotic Chromosomes
Unique-Sequence and Repetitive-Sequence DNA

Review of Key Terms, Symbols, and Concepts

In your own words, write a brief, precise definition of each term in the groups below and on the following page. Check your definitions using the text. Then develop a concept map using the terms in each list.

1	2	3
viral genome	histones	C-value paradox
prokaryotic genome	nonhistones	unique-sequence DNA
mitochondrial genome	H1, H2A, H2B, H3, H4	moderately repetitive DNA
chloroplast genome	linker DNA	highly repetitive DNA
plasmid	nucleosome	dispersed repeated DNA
single-, double-stranded	"beads-on-a-string"	interspersed repeated DNA
circular chromosome	solenoid model	tandemly repeated DNA
linear chromosome	karyotype	LINEs
T-even phage	haploid	SINEs
λ, ΦX174	diploid	transposons
nucleoid	C-value	
negative, positive, supercoiling	chromatin	
topoisomerases	10-nm chromatin fiber	
looped domains	30-nm chromatin fiber	
	euchromatin	
	heterochromatin	
	facultative heterochromatin	
	constitutive heterochromatin	
	centromere	
	CEN sequences	
	chromosome scaffold	
	scaffold-associated regions (SARs)	
	telomere	
	simple telomeric sequences	
	telomere-associated sequences	

4	5	6
macromolecule	genetic material	Chargaff's rules
chromosome	DNA	%GC
genome	RNA	X-ray diffraction
nucleic acid	mutation	angstrom unit
DNA, RNA	transformation	3'-OH, 5'-P
ribose, deoxyribose	transforming principle	polarity
phosphodiester bond	nuclease	antiparallel strands
nucleotide	ribonuclease (RNase)	complementary base pair
nucleoside	deoxyribonuclease (DNase)	double helix
polynucleotide	Avery's experiment	major groove
nitrogenous base	Griffith's experiment	minor groove
adenine, guanine	Hershey and Chase's experiment	right-handed helix
cytosine, thymine	Type *IIS, IIR, IIIS, IIIR*, bacteria	left-handed helix
uracil	T2, MS2, Qβ bacteriophage	A-, B-, Z-DNA
purine	phage lysate	oligomer, oligo
pyrimidine	lytic cycle	polarity
	^{32}P, ^{35}S	Watson–Crick model
	HIV, TMV, poliovirus	

Thinking Analytically

This chapter presents a large amount of complex, related information, so its information and problems require attention to detail. To comprehend and retain this information, organize it and develop strategies to place it in context. In addition to concept maps, it will help to construct labeled diagrams that display information contextually. Using the text figure as a guide, sketch labeled diagrams of nucleic acid structure, chromosome packaging, and sequence organization of chromosomes.

This chapter starts with a presentation of the key experimental evidence for the nature and structure of the genetic material. These insightful experiments resolved fundamental questions in biology. To organize this information and place it in context, pay close attention to the subtleties of the experiments presented, and strive to see *how* they provided evidence for or against a particular hypothesis.

It is essential to know the chemical structures of nucleic acids to fully understand the material in upcoming chapters. Start by drawing out the structures using paper and pencil. Copy the component parts of a nucleotide (the sugar, the bases, the phosphodiester linkages) from the text figures, paying close attention to their polarity. Practice them for a few days in a row so that you can draw them easily from memory.

Having a good sense of the dimensions involved in nucleic acid structure and chromosomal packaging is helpful in grasping a mental image of these physical processes. For this reason, it is important to learn (or review) units of measurement and to be able to make conversions between different dimension units. In solving problems, it is helpful to convert values presented in many different units to a smaller set of units. Particularly important unit conversions are:

UNIT/CONVERSION	EXAMPLE
1 Å = 1 angstrom = 1×10^{-10} meter	distance between 2 protons in H_2 = 0.74 Å
1 nm = 1 nanometer = 1×10^{-9} meter	width of a DNA double helix = 2 nm
1 μm = 1 micrometer = 1×10^{-6} meter	typical red blood cell diameter = 7 μm
1 dalton (unit of mass) = 1.66×10^{-24} gram	1 H atom = 1 dalton

The chromosomal organization and packaging of DNA varies in different organisms. Consequently, while there are general principles underlying DNA packaging, there are also organism-specific requirements. As you study this chapter, first identify the general principles used to organize and package genetic material. Then relate these principles to specific examples of organization and packaging in viruses, prokaryotes, and eukaryotes.

DNA packaging occurs in three dimensions, and so it helps to visualize DNA packaging by making sketches. You do not have to be a great artist; the point is to convey the different strategies that organisms use to fit a DNA molecule—that, if left unpackaged, would be larger than most cells—into a cell and have it remain functional.

Not everyone visualizes well in three dimensions, and it can be especially challenging to visualize supercoiling in a circular DNA molecule. If you can locate a spiral telephone cord, the following exercise should help: Take the cord and hold the ends together to form a circle. Sequentially introduce one, two, three, or four additional twists that *tighten* the spirals. For each complete twist you make, a supercoil is added. Since the twist tightens the spiral, it introduces a positive supercoil. If you let the cord "relax" and then make additional twists that *loosen* the spirals, you will be introducing negative supercoils. To determine whether your phone cord is a right- or left-handed helix, wrap your right hand around the spiral, and trace the direction of the spiral with your right index finger. If, while you hold the spiral with your right hand, your index finger traces up the spiral in the same direction that your right thumb points, you are holding a right-handed helix. If it traces down the spiral in an opposite direction, you are holding a left-handed helix. Notice that the orientation of the helix remains the same regardless of whether your right thumb points up or down.

Questions for Practice

Multiple-Choice Questions

1. DNA and RNA are polymers of
   a. nucleosides.
   b. nucleotides.
   c. pentose sugars connected by phosphodiester bonds.
   d. ribonucleotides.

2. A molecule consisting of ribose covalently bonded to a purine or pyrimidine base is a
   a. ribonucleoside.
   b. ribonucleotide.
   c. nuclease.
   d. deoxyribonucleotide.

3. The transforming principle was found to be
   a. a cellular material that could alter a cell's heritable characteristics.
   b. a substance derived from killed viruses.
   c. modified RNA that could change a living cell.
   d. a transmissible substance that revives dead cells.

4. When Griffith injected mice with a mixture of live *R* pneumococcus derived from a *IIS* strain and heat-killed *IIIS* bacteria,
   a. the mice survived, and he recovered live type *IIIR* organisms.
   b. the mice died, but he recovered live type *IIIR* cells.
   c. the mice died, but he recovered live type *IIS* cells.
   d. the mice died, but he recovered live type *IIIS* cells.

5. In the Hershey–Chase experiment, T2 phage were radioactively labeled with either ^{35}S or ^{32}P, and allowed to infect *E. coli*. What results proved that DNA was the genetic material?
   a. The ^{35}S was found in progeny phage, and the ^{32}P was found in phage ghosts.
   b. The ^{35}S was found in phage ghosts, and the ^{32}P was found in progeny phage.
   c. The ^{35}S was found in both progeny phage and in phage ghosts.
   d. The ^{32}P was found in both progeny phage and in phage ghosts.

6. Analysis of the bases of a sample of nucleic acid yielded these percentages: A, 20%; G, 30%; C, 20%; T, 30%. The sample must be
   a. double-stranded RNA.
   b. single-stranded RNA.
   c. double-stranded DNA.
   d. single-stranded DNA.

7. Which of the following is *not* true about a linear molecule of double-stranded DNA?
    a. It is a double helix composed of antiparallel strands.
    b. Bases are paired via hydrogen bonds.
    c. At one end, two 5′ phosphate groups can be found.
    d. Pentose sugars are linked via covalent phosphodiester bonds.

8. Which kind of DNA is *not* likely to be found in cells?
    a. A-form DNA
    b. B-form DNA
    c. Z-form DNA
    d. none of the above

9. Two double-stranded 25-base-pair DNA fragments are heated in solution. Fragment A has 60% GC, and fragment B has 40% GC. Which observation(s) might be made as the solution temperature increases?
    a. At a low enough temperature, both fragments will remain double-stranded.
    b. A will separate into single strands at a lower temperature than B.
    c. B will separate into single strands at a lower temperature than A.
    d. At a high enough temperature, both A and B will separate into single strands.
    e. a, c, and d

10. The chromosome of *E. coli* is packaged in the nucleoid region in a
    a. nuclear membrane.
    b. semicircular form.
    c. relaxed form.
    d. supercoiled form.

11. Topoisomerases are enzymes that do all of the following except
    a. untwist relaxed DNA.
    b. introduce negative supercoils into relaxed DNA.
    c. introduce positive supercoils into relaxed DNA.
    d. change the topological form of the DNA, but not the DNA sequence.

12. The total amount of DNA in the haploid genome of any organism is
    a. its karyotype.
    b. its C-value.
    c. twice its GC content.
    d. an indication of its organizational and structural complexity.

13. Facultative heterochromatin
    a. is always inactive.
    b. is inactive only in certain cells.
    c. contains only moderately repetitive DNA.
    d. can contain unique-sequence DNA.
    e. both b and d
    f. both a and c

14. Which of the following is *not* true about both centromeres and telomeres?
    a. They are characteristically heterochromatic.
    b. They are associated with consensus sequence elements.
    c. They are essential for eukaryotic chromosome function.
    d. They contain a short, species-specific sequence that is repeated hundreds to thousands of times.

15. The fundamental unit of chromatin packaging in eukaryotes is
    a. a histone protein.
    b. a nucleosome.
    c. a 30-nm chromatin fiber.
    d. a looped domain.

16. Examples of tandemly repeated DNA sequences include all of the following except
    a. genes for ribosomal RNA.
    b. LINEs.
    c. genes for histones.
    d. simple telomeric sequences.

17. Which type of chromatin contains expressed genes?
    a. constitutive heterochromatin
    b. facultative heterochromatin
    c. euchromatin
    d. Barr bodies

Answers: 1b, 2a, 3a, 4d, 5b, 6d, 7c, 8a, 9e, 10d, 11c, 12b, 13e, 14d, 15b, 16b, 17c

Thought Questions

1. The histones, H1, H2A, H2B, H3, and H4, are the most highly conserved of all proteins. It has been proposed that they serve a basic function in all eukaryotes. What are the implications of this assertion for evolutionary theory?

2. The histones are highly basic proteins that interact with DNA (specifically, with the acidic sugar–phosphate backbone). What kinds of proteins are the nonhistones? How might they differ from the histones in their interactions with DNA?

3. How do you account for the presence of both unique and repetitive sequences in the genomes of eukaryotes? Why are the latter mostly lacking in prokaryotes?

4. An amphibian that lives in a swamp has 30-fold more DNA than a human who lives on the 48th floor of a luxury apartment complex. In what way is the amphibian richer?

5. Summarize the structure, composition, and organization of chromosomes in eukaryotic cells. How does the structure, composition, and organization of viral and prokaryotic chromosomes differ?

6. Describe the logic behind the series of experiments that conclusively demonstrated that DNA was the genetic material in some cells. Is DNA the only nucleic acid that can serve as genetic material?

7. Describe the various forms of DNA (A, B, Z) that have been identified. What are their most significant differences? Are any of these differences likely to have functional significance? If so, what are they?

8. Watson and Crick reputedly deduced the structure of DNA by applying observations made by others to molecular models, without any direct experimental observations of their own. Is this legitimate scientific procedure? If so, why? If not, why not?

9. Draw out the chemical structure of a double-stranded DNA molecule so that one strand has the sequence 5'-ATG-3'. Indicate the polarity of each strand, the location and the kinds of bonds that exist, and the approximate dimensions of the molecule.

10. Double-stranded DNA molecules have negatively charged sugar–phosphate backbones and a major and minor groove into which the chemical groups of the bases project. Some proteins that interact with DNA do so in a highly sequence-specific manner, while others interact in a largely sequence-nonspecific manner. What different features of the DNA molecule might these two classes of protein be recognizing?

Thought Questions for Media

After reviewing the media on the *iGenetics* website, try to answer these questions.

1. In the animation depicting Avery's transformation experiment, how did Avery and his colleagues show that polysaccharides were not the transforming principle?

2. In the animation depicting Hershey and Chase's bacteriophage experiment, how were the T2 phage initially labeled with either ^{35}S or ^{32}P?

3. The T2 phage labeled with ^{32}P had only their DNA labeled. Why doesn't this information, by itself, provide evidence that DNA is the genetic material of T2?

4. What experiment provided evidence that DNA is the genetic material?

5. In the animation depicting how the *E. coli* chromosome is supercoiled, is the DNA of *E. coli* compacted by adding negative or positive supercoils?

6. Which enzyme is responsible for adding negative supercoils?

7. Which enzyme is responsible for removing negative supercoils?

1. We now know that the genetic material of viruses can be either RNA or DNA and that it can be either single- or double-stranded. Why is it still important to determine the type of nucleic acid associated with a new virus?

2. Once you determine the type of nucleic acid of a new virus, how can you determine which one of several known viruses is most closely related to it?

Solving Genetics Problems

In this and each subsequent chapter is a set of end-of-chapter problems organized to follow the general presentation of text material. Working through them independently will help you develop a practical and thorough understanding of genetics. Solving a problem requires effort and often is successful only after a few tries using alternate approaches. Indeed, there are multiple "right" approaches to many problems. The effort problem solving requires is worthwhile, as pursuing the various "right" approaches provides an opportunity for learning. It reinforces your understanding of genetic principles and helps you gain a deeper understanding of the relationships between the terms, ideas, and facts that are presented in the text.

Although there are multiple "right" approaches, there is one unproductive approach. In it, you scan through the problem and then check to see if you can understand the answer presented in this guide. Why is this approach ill-advised? Simply put, because it fools you into thinking that you have understood the material. When you read a solution to a problem that you have not yourself devised, you have not developed the skills to analyze the situation, evaluate and apply your knowledge of genetic principles, and identify a productive path leading to a solution. You may feel you understand the answer, but the purpose of doing the problems—to gain a deeper understanding of genetic principles—will have been thwarted. Since you have not developed the skills needed to solve a similar problem, on an exam you will be stuck.

Taking a "right" approach will help you develop a deeper understanding. It's not the same thing as finding *the* correct answer, usually because there is more than one approach to solving the problem. Here are some pointers:

1. Read the problem straight through without pausing. Get the sense of what it is about.
2. Then read it again, slowly and critically. This time,
   a. Jot down pertinent information.
   b. Assign descriptive gene symbols if they are needed.
   c. Scan the problem from start to finish and then from the end to the beginning, and carefully analyze the *terms* used in the problem. Geneticists use very precise language, so clues to the answer often can be found in the way the problem is stated.
3. If you are unsure how to continue, ask yourself, "What are the options here?"
   a. Write down all the options you perceive.
   b. Carefully analyze whether a particular option will provide a solution.
4. When you think you have a solution, read through the problem once more to ensure that your analysis is consistent with *all* the data in the problem. Try to see if there is a more general principle behind the solution or, for that matter, a clearer or more straightforward solution.
5. If you do get stuck (and everyone does!), DO NOT GO IMMEDIATELY TO THE ANSWER KEY. This will give you only the *illusion* of having solved the problem. On an exam, or in real life, an answer key will not be available. Learn to control the temptation "to just know the answer." Instead, go on to another problem. Come back to this one another time, perhaps the next day. You may be able to sort through some loose ends given a bit of time.
6. If you cannot solve the problem after coming back to it a second time, read through the answer key. Then close the answer key and try the problem once more. The next day, try it a third time without the answer key.

Solutions to Text Questions and Problems

2.1   *Answer:* c

2.2   *Answer:*
   a. lived
   b. died
   c. lived
   d. died (DNA from the *IIIS* bacteria transformed the *IIR* bacteria to a virulent form.)

2.3   *Answer:*
   a. When DNA from the heat-killed *IIIS* bacteria transformed the living *IIR* bacteria, *IIIS* bacteria were recovered. Two characteristics of the living bacteria were transformed: a type II coat was transformed to a type III coat and an *R*-type cell was transformed to an *S*-type cell.
   b. If DNA from *IIS* transformed type *IIIR* bacteria, *IIS* bacteria would be recovered.
   c. Using dead *IIIS* bacteria allowed Griffith to follow two traits: the trait for type II versus type III coats and the trait for *R*- versus *S*-type cells. This was essential for him to distinguish between spontaneous mutation and transformation, as spontaneous mutation of *R*-type bacteria can produce *S*-type bacteria. Since *IIIS* but not *IIS* bacteria were recovered after type *IIIS* bacteria were mixed with living *IIR* bacteria, Griffith could be certain that transformation and not spontaneous mutation had occurred.

2.4   *Answer:*
   a. Avery, MacLeod, and McCarty made extracts from *IIIS* bacteria and showed that exposing living *IIR* bacteria to these extracts could transform *IIR* bacteria into *IIIS* bacteria. The extracts contained different cellular macromolecules, such as lipids, polysaccharides, proteins, and nucleic acids. They first showed that nucleic acids were the only macromolecular component that could transform the *IIR* cells. Then, by treating the nucleic acid component with either ribonuclease or deoxyribonuclease, they showed that the transforming principle copurified with DNA. This strongly suggested that the genetic material was DNA. Although the work suggested that the genetic material was DNA, it could be criticized because the nucleic acids were contaminated by proteins.
   b. Enzymes were used to destroy one of the two components of the nucleic acid mixture. This served to identify which of two nucleic acids was the genetic material. Ribonuclease did not destroy the transforming principle, but deoxyribonuclease did abolish transforming activity. This result supported the hypothesis that DNA was the genetic material.
   c. Their work affirmed and extended Griffith's work in that it identified the probable nature of Griffith's transforming principle as being DNA.

2.5   *Answer:*
   a. In each case, phage ghosts and progeny would be labeled with isotope. Both amino acids and nucleic acids have C, N, and H, so parental phage labeled with isotopes of C, N, or H will have labeled protein coats and DNA. Isotope would be recovered in the DNA of the progeny phage as well as in the phage ghosts left behind in the supernatant after phage infection.
   b. Isotopes of phosphorus selectively label DNA, while isotopes of sulfur selectively label protein. The selective labels allowed Hershey and Chase to track the protein and nucleic acid components of the phage as they reproduced. By selectively labeling DNA and protein, Hershey and Chase could distinguish between DNA and protein as the genetic material.

2.6   *Answer:*
   a. b. and **c.**: All known cellular organisms use double-stranded DNA, so newly discovered multi-cellular or unicellular organisms are expected to have double-stranded DNA genomes. In con-

trast, a variety of bacteriophage and viral genomes are known. They can be single- or double-stranded DNA or RNA.

d. These answers do not offer insight into the nature of the earliest cell-like organisms—these may not have had double-stranded DNA genomes. However, because all cellular organisms have double-stranded DNA genomes, we can infer that cells with the ability to store, replicate, and transcribe genetic information as double-stranded DNA had significant evolutionary advantages.

One can speculate why this might be the case. Both DNA and RNA have the capacity to store information as a sequence of nucleotides. Why then would double-stranded DNA be preferred as the storage molecule for cellular organisms? One possibility is that as the amount of stored information increases, double-stranded DNA is more suitable as a stable information-storage molecule. We know that it has chemical features that allow it to be packaged efficiently within a cell even as its information can remain accessible to cellular proteins. Perhaps the evolution of proteins that could stably package double-stranded DNA was highly advantageous to early organisms as it allowed these organisms to increase their genome size and carry out more functions. If so, it would have been selected for during evolution. A second possibility is that its double-stranded nature allows for its reliable and efficient replication (see Chapter 3). The evolution of proteins (or RNAs) able to assist in DNA replication could have provided a selective advantage for early organisms with double-stranded DNA genomes. A third possibility is that double-stranded DNA is more stable and less reactive than RNA—some RNAs have catalytic properties (see Chapter 5). An information-storage molecule with increased stability could also have been a selective advantage for early organisms.

2.7 *Answer:* To evaluate whether the bacteriophage has a DNA genome, infect the bacteriophage into *E. coli* in medium containing radioactively labeled nucleotide precursor that is selectively incorporated into DNA, such as radioactively labeled dTTP in which the thymine base has been labeled with ^{3}H or ^{14}C. Collect progeny phage and see if they are radioactively labeled. To evaluate whether the bacteriophage has an RNA genome, perform the same type of experiment using radioactively labeled UTP instead of dTTP. One approach to determining if the bacteriophage has single-stranded or double-stranded nucleic acid is to determine its base composition and evaluate whether the molar ratios of adenine and thymine (or adenine and uracil for an RNA genome) are equal, and whether the molar ratios of cytosine and guanine are equal. These are expected to be equal in a double-stranded genome and unequal in a single-stranded genome.

2.8 *Answer:* a

2.9 *Answer:* Two different lines of evidence support the view that a base pair is composed of one purine and one pyrimidine.

1. When the chemical components of double-stranded DNA from a wide variety of organisms were analyzed quantitatively by Chargaff, it was found that the amount of purines equaled the amount of pyrimidines. More specifically, it was found that the amount of adenine equaled the amount of thymine and that the amount of cytosine equaled the amount of guanine. The simplest hypothesis to explain these observations was the existence of complementary base pairing: A on one strand paired with T on the other strand, and G paired with C.

2. More direct physical evidence was provided by X-ray diffraction studies. These established the dimensions of the DNA double helix and allowed for comparison with the known sizes of the bases. The diameter of the double helix is constant throughout its length at 2 nm. This is the right size to accommodate a purine paired with a pyrimidine, but too small for a purine-purine pair and too large for a pyrimidine-pyrimidine pair.

2.10 *Answer:* A deoxynucleotide consists of 2′-deoxyribose plus a phosphate group (PO_4^{-2}) attached to its 5′-carbon, plus a nitrogenous base attached to its 1′-carbon. Since there are four different nitrogenous bases in DNA—adenine (A), thymine (T), guanine (G), and cytosine (C)—there are four different nucleotides. In a DNA molecule, one finds monophosphate nucleotides, so that there is deoxyadenosine monophosphate (dAMP), thymidine monophosphate (TMP), deoxyguanosine monophosphate (dGMP), and deoxycytidine monophosphate (dCMP). Along the sides of the "ladder," the 5′-carbon of one deoxyribose is connected by a covalent phosphodiester (O–P–O) bond to the 3′-carbon of another. A phosphate group is found at the 5′ end of a DNA polynucleotide chain, and a hydroxyl (OH) group is found at the 3′ end of a DNA polynucleotide chain. Weaker hydrogen bonds between complementary A–T and G–C bases hold the complementary strands together. A–T pairs have two hydrogen bonds, while G–C pairs have three hydrogen bonds (see text Figure 2.13, p. 19).

Although A–C and G–T pairs would be purine-pyrimidine base pairs, they do not form because of their inability to pair using hydrogen bonding. Note that A–T base pairs have two hydrogen bonds, while G–C base pairs have three hydrogen bonds. This is consistent with the evidence provided by Chargaff. Quantitative measurements of the four bases in double-stranded DNA isolated from a wide variety of organisms indicated that in all cases, the amount of A equaled the amount of T, and the amount of G equaled the amount of C. Moreover, different DNAs exhibited different base ratios so that while (A) = (T) and (G) = (C), in most organisms (A + T) ≠ (G + C). Put another way, the %GC content of different DNA samples varies. The simplest hypothesis is that there are two base pairs in DNA, A–T and G–C, and the proportion of the two base pairs varies from organism to organism.

2.11   *Answer:* In the question statement, the sequences are given 5′ to 3′, so when the complementary sequence is obtained by pairing A with T, and G with C, the resulting sequences (due to the antiparallel nature of DNA) are obtained with a 3′ to 5′ polarity. Therefore, obtain the complementary sequence and then reverse the order. The following are the complementary sequences given 5′ to 3′.

   a. 3′-TCAATGGACTACCAT-5′ (or 5′-TACCATCAGGTAACT-3′).

   b. 3′-AAGAGTTCTTAAGGT-5′ (or 5′-TGGAATTCTTGAGAA-3′).

2.12   *Answer:* In solving this problem, it is essential to keep track of the 5′ and 3′ ends of the strands, and ensure that when two strands are "reattached," the 5′ end of one strand is always placed next to the 3′ end of the other strand. With this in mind, if you approach the problem solution by trial and error, you will discover that when an 8-bp sequence is broken into two 4-bp sequences and these are reattached, the number of possible sequences depends on whether the bases in the original 8-bp sequence are arranged symmetrically.

   a.   5′-TTAACCGG-3′   (or the equivalent,   5′-CCGGTTAA-3′)
            3′-AATTGGCC-5′   3′-GGCCAATT-5′

   b.   5′-TTCCAAGG-3′ 5′-AAGGTTCC-3′ 5′-CCTTTTCC-3′ and 5′-TTCCCCTT-3′
            3′-AAGGTTCC-5′ 3′-TTCCAAGG-5′ 3′-GGAAAAGG-5′   3′-AAGGGGAA-5′

   c.   5′-AGCTAGCT-3′
            3′-TCGATCGA-5′

   d.   5′-AGCTTCGA-3′   (or the equivalent,   5′-TCGAAGCT-3′)
            3′-TCGAAGCT-5′   3′-AGCTTCGA-5′

2.13   *Answer:* The A–T base pair has two hydrogen bonds, while the G–C base pair has three hydrogen bonds. Thus, the G–C base pair requires more energy to break apart and so is harder to break apart.

2.14   *Answer:*

   a. The double-helix model of DNA suggested by Watson and Crick had to incorporate existing information about its chemical composition and physical structure. In terms of its chemical composition, it was known that DNA is composed of polynucleotides, that (A) = (T) and (G) = (C) (Chargaff's rules), and that while the %GC varies between organisms, the A/T and G/C ratios do not.

   b. The structure and molecular dimensions of the component molecules (the bases, sugars, and phosphates) were known. It was also known from studies of Franklin and Wilkins that the molecule is organized in a highly ordered, helical structure, and that there are two distinctive regularities at 0.34 and 3.4 nm along the molecule's axis.

2.15   *Answer:* Since (G) = (C) and (A) = (T), it follows that (G + A) = (C + T) and (G + T) = (A + C). Thus, b, c, and d are all equal to 1.

2.16   *Answer:* More information is needed. That (A + T) / (G + C) = 1 indicates only that (A + T) = (G + C). If the DNA were double stranded, (G) = (C), and (A) = (T). For the observed ratio, there would need to be 25% A, 25% T, 25% C, and 25% G. However, if the DNA were single stranded, one could still observe this ratio. In single-stranded DNA, there are no restrictions on the relative amounts of the different bases. There are many ways in which one could observe (A + T) / (G + C) = 1. For example, suppose there were 35% A, 15% T, 20% G, and 30% C.

2.17   *Answer:* In double-stranded DNA, if (C) = 17%, then (G) = 17%. This means that the DNA has 34% G–C, and 66% A–T base pairs. Hence, the DNA will have (66/2)(100%) = 33% A.

2.18   *Answer:* Since the DNA molecule is double-stranded, (A) = (T) and (G) = (C). If there are 80 T residues, there must be 80 A residues. If there are 110 G residues, there must be 110 C residues. The molecule has (110 + 110 + 80 + 80) = 380 nucleotides, or 190 base pairs.

2.19   *Answer:* First, notice that (A) ≠ (T) and (G) ≠ (C). Thus, the DNA is not double-stranded. The bacterial virus appears to have a single-stranded DNA genome.

2.20   *Answer:* G–C base pairs have three hydrogen bonds, whereas A–T base pairs have two. Consequently, G–C base pairs are stronger than A–T base pairs. If a double-stranded molecule in solution is heated, the thermal energy "melts" the hydrogen bonds, denaturing the double-stranded molecule into single strands. Double-stranded molecules with more G–C base pairs require more thermal energy to break the hydrogen bonds, so they dissociate into single strands at higher temperatures. Put another way, the higher the GC content of a double-stranded DNA molecule, the higher its melting temperature. Reordering the molecules from lowest to highest %GC, the melting order is (b) 69°, then (a) 73°, (d) 78°, (e) 82°, and (c) 84°.

2.21   *Answer:*
  a. The single-stranded DNA genomes of the ΦX174 and B19 viruses will have A, T, G, and C bases, but unlike double-stranded DNA genomes, A may not equal T and G may not equal C.
  b. If Chargaff had analyzed only ΦX174 and parvovirus B19, he would not have seen a regular pattern of base equalities, and so would have not concluded that 50% of the bases were purines and 50% were pyrimidines, or that G = C and A = T. If these were the *only* genomes he had analyzed, he would have obtained a skewed view of genome composition. He might have concluded that genomes are composed of variable amounts of the four types of nucleotides.
  c. He would have concluded that at least some viral genomes are fundamentally different from those of cellular organisms and that some phage and viral genomes are not constrained by the requirements of a double-stranded structure.

2.22   *Answer:*
  a. Both A-DNA and B-DNA are right-handed double helices, while Z-DNA is a left-handed double helix. The A-DNA double helix has 11 base pairs per complete helical turn and a diameter of 2.2 nm. It has a narrow, very deep major groove and a wide, shallow minor groove. The B-DNA double helix has 10 base pairs per turn and a diameter of 2.0 nm. It is thinner and longer for the same number of base pairs than is A-DNA. It has a wide major groove and a narrow minor groove; both grooves have similar depths. Z-DNA has 12 base pairs per turn and a diameter of 1.8 nm. It is thinner and more elongated than either A-DNA or B-DNA. It has a deep minor groove and a major groove that is very near the surface of the helix, so it is not distinct.
  b. Most of the DNA found in living cells is closest in form to B-DNA, which forms under conditions of high humidity. DNA in cells is in solution, so this DNA has a different state than the purified, crystallized DNA used in X-ray crystallography experiments. DNA in solution has 10.5 base pairs per turn, which is a little less twisted than B-DNA.

    c. DNA can assume the A-DNA structure in certain DNA–protein complexes. As you learned in this chapter, DNA is bound by proteins when it is packaged within cells. As you will see in later chapters, proteins also bind DNA to replicate it and to control which segments of DNA are transcribed into RNA. DNA segments that form an A-DNA structure might be important for any of these processes. There is debate whether Z-DNA exists in cells and what its physiological significance might be.

2.23 *Answer:* With 10 base pairs per complete 360° turn of a B-form double-stranded DNA molecule, there are 200,000/10 = 20,000 complete turns in the viral DNA.

2.24 *Answer:*

    a. Each base pair has two nucleotides, so the molecule has 200,000 nucleotides.

    b. There are 10 base pairs per complete 360° turn, so there will be 100,000/10 = 10,000 complete turns in the molecule.

    c. There is 0.34 nm between the centers of adjacent base pairs. There will be 100,000 × 0.34 nm = 3.4×10^4 nm = 34 μm.

2.25 *Answer:*

    a. Since there are 0.34 nm between the centers of adjacent base pairs, the length of the molecule is 168,900 × 0.34 nm = $5.74x \times 10^4$ nm.

    b. From text Figure 2.4, p. 12, the outer dimensions of the T2 capsid head are 100 × 65 nm. With a 10-nm thick capsid, the internal dimensions would be about 80 × 45 nm. If we model the internal cavity as a modified cylinder with a height of 80 nm, and imagine that the DNA is a long, thin thread that is folded as it is packaged into the cylinder, the DNA would have to be folded after every 80 nm of its length, or about 5.74×10^4 nm/80 nm = 717.5 times.

2.26 *Answer:*

    a. For *E. coli*, the length is $(4.6 \times 10^6 \text{ bp}) \times (0.34 \text{ nm/bp}) = 1.6 \times 10^6$ nm = 1,600 μm (microns). Since *E. coli* has a circular chromosome, this would be a chromosome with a diameter of about 510 μm. For yeast, the average chromosome length is (12,057,500 bp/16 chromosomes) × (0.34 nm/bp) = 2.56×10^5 nm = 256 μm. For humans, the average chromosome length is $(2.75 \times 10^9 \text{ bp}/23 \text{ chromosomes}) \times (0.34 \text{ nm/bp}) = 4.07 \times 10^7$ nm = 40,700 μm.

    b. For B-DNA, there are 10 bp per helical turn. Therefore, the *E. coli* chromosome would have $(4.6 \times 10^6 \text{ bp/chromosome}) \times (1 \text{ turn}/10 \text{ bp}) = 4.6 \times 10^5$ turns. The average yeast chromosome would have (12,057,500 bp/16 chromosomes) × (1 turn/10 bp) = 7.54×10^4 turns. The average human chromosome would have $(2.75 \times 10^9 \text{ bp}/23 \text{ chromosomes}) \times (1 \text{ turn}/10 \text{ bp}) = 1.2 \times 10^7$ turns.

    c. While Z-DNA and B-DNA differ in the distance between successive base pairs and the number of base pairs per turn, these are not large compared to chromosome length. Thus, the answers to (a) and (b) will not be very different.

        Z-DNA has more space between successive base pairs, as there is about 0.57 nm between successive base pairs instead of the 0.34 nm found in B-DNA. Thus, if 20% of each chromosome, were Z-DNA, each chromosome would be 20% × [(0.57 − 0.34)/0.34] = 13.5% longer. A full turn of the double helix in Z-DNA utilizes more base pairs, as there are 12 bp/turn in Z-DNA instead of the 10 bp/turn in B-DNA. Thus, if 20% of each chromosome were Z-DNA, each chromosome would have 20% × [(12 − 10)/12] = 3.33% fewer turns.

    d. These answers point out the need for DNA to be flexible so that it can be packaged and "fit" into a cell. Other forms of DNA, including Z-DNA, do not necessarily shorten a chromosome, but they can affect its flexibility. In the examples considered in this problem, the cells are hundreds to tens of thousands of times smaller than the length of their (average) chromosome. *E. coli* is about 2 μm × 0.5 μm, with a 510-μm diameter chromosome; a yeast cell is about 20 μm wide, with 16 chromosomes that average 256 μm; and a "typical" human cell is about 10 μm wide, with 46 chromosomes that average 40,700 μm. Thus, chromosomes cannot remain as unpackaged molecules inside cells.

2.27 *Answer:* The chance of finding the sequence 5′-GUUA-3′ is $(0.30 \times 0.25 \times 0.25 \times 0.20) = 0.00375$. In a molecule 10^6 nucleotides long, there are nearly 10^6 groups of four bases: The first group of four is bases 1, 2, 3, and 4, the second group is bases 2, 3, 4, and 5, etc. Thus, the number of times this sequence is expected to appear is $0.00375 \times 10^6 = 3,750$.

2.28 *Answer:*

a. The sequence C G A G G in molecule 2 is complementary to the sequence G C T C C in molecule 3. When these pair up, one has:

③ ————— G C T C C T A ⟶

② ⟵ A T C G A G G —————

Each strand has two unpaired bases sticking out. These bases are complementary to each other, so that if the molecule bends, one has:

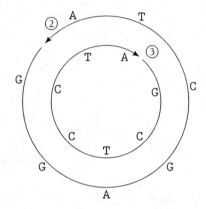

b. The sequence in molecule 3 is complementary to the sequence in molecule 4. It also has opposite polarity, so that the two strands can pair up. One has:

③ ——— G   C   T   C   C   T   A ⟶

⟵ C   G   A   G   G   A   T ——— ④

2.29 *Answer:* Topoisomerases are a class of enzymes that convert one topological form of DNA to another. Topoisomerases untwist relaxed DNA to produce negative supercoils or twist negatively supercoiled DNA to convert it to a more relaxed state. These enzymes allow DNA to be converted between negatively supercoiled, compact DNA and a more relaxed, less compact state.

2.30 *Answer:* Paradoxically, there is no simple relationship between the haploid DNA content of a cell and its structural or organizational complexity. This is the "C-value paradox." While organisms in some taxa show little variation, organisms in other taxa show as much as tenfold variation in their C-values. In addition, organisms do not have C-values corresponding to their organizational or structural complexity. At least one reason for this is the considerable variation in the amount of repetitive-sequence DNA in the genome.

2.31 *Answer:* The genome of *Amoeba proteus* is unlikely to have a hundredfold more genes than have been found in the human genome. There is a general increase in gene number with complexity, so we expect humans to have more genes than does a single-celled organism such as an amoeba. Increases in genome size are driven more by the repetitive DNA content than by gene number. Therefore, the amoeba genome likely has a great deal more repetitive DNA than does the human genome. If we sequenced its genome, we would discover what types of repetitive DNA sequences it has and how they were organized relative to the location of genes.

2.32   *Answer:* c

2.33   *Answer:*

    a. Only eukaryotic chromosomes have centromeres, the sections of the chromosome found near the point of attachment of mitotic or meiotic spindle fibers. In some organisms, such as *Saccharomyces cerevisiae,* they are associated with specific *CEN* sequences. In other organisms, they have a more complex repetitive structure.

    b. Eukaryotic and bacterial chromosomes contain the same pentose sugar, deoxyribose.

    c. Amino acids are found in proteins that are involved in chromosome compaction, such as the proteins that hold the ends of looped domains in prokaryotic chromosomes and the histone and nonhistone proteins in eukaryotic chromatin.

    d. Eukaryotic and bacterial chromosomes share the trait of supercoiling.

    e. Telomeres are found only at the ends of eukaryotic chromosomes and are required for replication and chromosome stability. They are associated with specific types of sequences: simple telomeric sequences and telomere-associated sequences.

    f. Nonhistone proteins are found only in eukaryotic chromosomes and have structural (higher-order packaging) and possibly other functions.

    g. DNA is found in both bacterial and eukaryotic chromosomes. (Some viral chromosomes have RNA as their genetic material.)

    h. Nucleosomes are the fundamental unit of packaging of DNA in eukaryotic chromosomes and are not found in bacterial chromosomes.

    i. Though most bacterial species have circular chromosomes, some have linear chromosomes. In eukaryotes, nuclear chromosomes are linear, while chromosomes of subcellular organelles (mitochondria and chloroplasts) are circular.

    j. Looping is found in both eukaryotic and bacterial chromosomes. In eukaryotic chromosomes, the 30-nm nucleofilament is packed into looped domains by nonhistone chromosomal proteins. In bacterial chromosomes, such as that of *E. coli,* there are about 400 looped domains, each containing about 40 kilobases of supercoiled DNA.

2.34   *Answer:* Nucleosomes are the fundamental unit of DNA packaging in eukaryotic chromosomes. In a nucleosome core particle, a short segment of DNA is wrapped about one-and-three-quarters times around a protein core. This protein core is an octamer consisting of two copies of each of four histone proteins: H2A, H2B, H3, H4. The nucleosome core particle packs the DNA into a flattened disk about 5.7 × 11 nm. Packaging into nucleosomes effectively condenses the DNA by a factor of about seven. The interactions between the histones and the DNA are not sequence specific, but rather are based on the basic, positively charged histone proteins interacting with the acidic, negatively charged sugar–phosphate backbone of the DNA.

    Nucleosome core particles serve to package double-stranded DNA at regular intervals, with short stretches of linker DNA between particles. At this level of packaging, DNA is packed into a "beads-on-a-string" form of chromatin known as the 10-nm nucleofilament. This condensation of DNA also forms the basis for subsequent packaging, first through associations between nucleosomes and then by associations with nonhistone chromosomal proteins. Associations between nucleosomes result in further compaction of the 10-nm nucleofilament, producing a 30-nm chromatin fiber that condenses the DNA another sixfold. Histone H1 plays an important role in this coiling. The 30-nm chromatin fiber is further condensed into looped domains, with each loop containing between 10 and hundreds of kilobases of DNA. The looped domains are anchored inside the nuclear envelope to a filamentous structural framework of protein, the nuclear matrix.

2.35   *Answer:* The evolutionary conservation of histone amino acid sequences indicates that histones perform the same basic role in organizing and packaging DNA in the chromosomes of all eukaryotes. When the five histones form nucleosome complexes on DNA, the histones interact with all types of DNA sequences—they do not physically interact with DNA in a sequence-specific manner. This means that histones must be able to interact with each other and form a complex that recognizes DNA features common to all double-stranded DNA molecules—the periodicities within the DNA double helix such as the spacing of nucleotides and location and charge distributions on sugar and phosphate residues. They also must be able to complex with DNA in a manner that allows it to form orderly structures that compact the DNA and enables themselves to carry out further packaging through interactions with the nonhistone scaffold. These functional properties are likely to limit their amino acid sequence diversity.

2.36 *Answer:*

a. The belt forms a right-handed helix. Although you wrapped the belt around the can axis in a counterclockwise direction from your orientation (looking down at the can), the belt was winding up and around the side of the can in a clockwise direction from its orientation. While the belt is wrapped around the can, curve the fingers of your right hand over the belt, and use your index finger to trace the direction of the belt's spiral. Your right index finger will trace the spiral upward, the same direction your thumb points when you wrap your hand around the can. Therefore, the belt has formed a right-handed helix. If you do this with your left hand, your thumb will point away from the direction the helix twists, indicating that it has not formed a left-handed helix.

b. Three turns were present.

c. Three turns were present. The number of helical turns is unchanged, although the twist in the belt is.

d. The belt appears more twisted because the pitch of the helix was altered, and the edges of the belt (positioned much like the complementary base pairs of a double helix) are twisted more tightly.

e. While twisted around the can, the length of the belt decreases by about 70 to 80%, depending on the initial length of the belt and the belt diameter.

f. Yes. As the DNA of linear chromosomes is wrapped around histones to form the 10-nm microfilament, it becomes supercoiled. In much the same way that you must add twists to the belt for it to lie flat on the surface of the can, supercoils must be introduced into the DNA for it to wrap around the histones.

g. Topoisomerases increase or reduce the level of negative supercoiling in DNA. For linear DNA to be packaged, negative supercoils must be added to it.

2.37 *Answer:* All 16 *Saccharomyces cerevisiae* centromeres have similar, but not identical DNA sequences called *CEN* sequences. Each is 112–120-bp long and contains three sequence domains, called centromere DNA elements (CDEs). CDEII, a 76–86-bp region that is >90% AT, is flanked by CDEI, a conserved RTCACRTG sequence (R = A or G), and CDEIII, a 26-bp AT-rich conserved domain. The CDEs are used to define where kinetochores will form during mitosis and meiosis. The centromeres of other yeast species are quite different. For example, those of the fission yeast *Schizosaccharomyces pombe* are 40 to 80 kb long. They contain complex rearrangements of repeated sequences. Nonetheless, all centromeres provide the same function: They ensure accurate chromosome segregation during mitosis and meiosis.

2.38 *Answer:* Telomeres are characteristically heterochromatic sequences found at the ends of a linear, eukaryotic chromosome. For most organisms, the telomeric sequences at the extreme end of a chromosome are simple, highly repeated, and species specific. Nearby, but not at the very end of a chromosome, are telomere-associated sequences. These are repeated, complex sequences and extend for thousands of bases from the simple telomeric sequences. These sequences are replicated, along with other chromosomal DNA sequences, by a set of enzymes that include DNA polymerases. Telomere organization is quite different in some organisms. In organisms such as *Drosophila*, telomeres consist of transposons belonging to the LINE family of repeated sequences. Telomeres function in DNA replication and provide chromosome stability.

2.39 *Answer:* You would find most protein-coding genes in unique-sequence DNA, as most protein-coding genes exist only in one copy per haploid genome.

2.40   *Answer:*

    a. The five histones (H1, H2A, H2B, H3, and H4) are small, basic, positively charged proteins that are rich in arginine and lysine. Histones H2A, H2B, H3, and H4 are among the most highly conserved of all proteins. In contrast to the small number of histones, there are many types of nonhistones. They are variable in size and are usually negatively charged, acidic proteins.

    b. The five histones are present in all cells of all eukaryotic organisms. Relative to the total amount of DNA, they are present in fairly constant amounts. In contrast, nonhistones differ in number and type between cell types in an organism, at different times in the same cell type, and from organism to organism. As a class, nonhistones may be between 50 and 100% of the mass of DNA.

    c. Histones are positively charged and mostly interact with the negatively charged sugar–phosphate backbone of DNA. Nonhistones are typically negatively charged and can interact with the positively charged histones or with DNA. The HMG class of nonhistones binds to the minor groove of the DNA and causes DNA bending.

    d. The histones H2A, H2B, H3, and H4 are fundamental to packaging DNA into nucleosome core particles and the formation of the 10-nm nucleofilament. Histone H1 is involved in compacting this nucleofilament to produce a 30-nm chromatin fiber. Nonhistones are important in higher-order packaging of DNA and act to determine the degree of chromosome condensation. They form the protein scaffold that anchors looped domains of the 30-nm chromatin fiber, with each loop containing 30–90-kb of DNA. Within the DNA, SARs, or scaffold-associated regions, bind to the nonhistone proteins to determine the boundaries of the loops.

2.41   *Answer:*

    a. Centromeres of higher eukaryotes are associated with hundreds of thousands of copies of simple, short tandemly repeated sequences. These highly repetitive DNA sequences can constitute a significant percentage of a eukaryote's genome. For example, they constitute about 5 to 10% of the human genome, and about 50% of the kangaroo rat genome.

    b. Centromeric regions contain constitutive heterochromatin. The highly repetitive DNA described in part **(a)** is packaged into constitutive heterochromatin.

    c. Genes within euchromatin are typically actively transcribed, while genes within heterochromatin are usually transcriptionally inactive. DNA packaged as euchromatin in one cell or at one developmental stage and packaged as heterochromatin in another cell is considered facultative heterochromatin. An example is a Barr body, an inactivated X chromosome in the somatic cells of XX mammalian females. A Barr body is composed of facultative heterochromatin because a female may have the same X chromosome inactivated in each of her somatic cells. Unlike facultative heterochromatin, constitutive heterochromatin is always heterochromatic. It is present in all cells at identical positions on both members of a pair of homologous chromosomes, and it is composed of mostly repetitive DNA sequences. The highly repetitive sequences associated with telomeres and centeromeres are packaged into constitutive heterochromatin. Therefore, unique-sequence DNA is found mostly in euchromatin and facultative heterochromatin, but not in constitutive heterochromatin.

2.42   *Answer:*

    a. LINEs are 1,000 to 7,000 bp long, while SINEs are 100 to 400 bp long.

    b. Though all eukaryotes have LINEs and SINEs, their relative proportions vary widely between organisms. Some organisms have more LINEs (e.g., *Drosophila*, birds), while others have more SINEs (e.g., humans, frogs). Together, they represent a significant proportion of the moderately repetitive DNA in the genome. LINEs and SINEs are grouped into families of sequences with related characteristics. Often, small numbers of families have very high copy numbers and make up most of the dispersed repeated sequences in the genome. For example, in mammals, the LINE-1 family of LINE elements is present in 500,000 copies and constitutes about 15% of the genome; in primates, the *Alu* family of SINE elements is present in about 1 million copies and makes up about 9% of the genome.

    c. Some but not all LINE elements are transposons. For example, full-length LINE-1 elements that are 6 to 7 kb long encode the enzymes needed for transposition, while truncated LINE-1 elements that are 1 to 2 kb long are unable to transpose. SINEs do not encode enzymes needed for transposition, but they can move if an active LINE transposon supplies the required enzymes.

d. SINEs and LINEs are interspersed repetitive elements, and so they are interspersed with unique-sequence DNA throughout the genome. Some are quite frequent—an *Alu* repeat is located every 5,000 bp in primate genomes, on average.

2.43 *Answer*

a.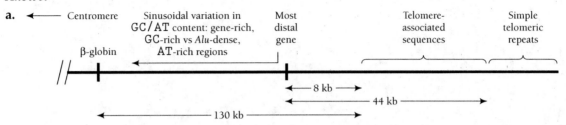

These findings support the view that telomeres are specialized chromosome structures with two distinct structural components: simple telomeric sequences, and telomere-associated sequences. They show that functional genes do not reside in the telomeric region, consistent with the view that telomeres are heterochromatic and have special protective functions in chromosomes. They add significantly to our knowledge of the structure of telomeric and near-telomeric regions. For example, they document the considerable distance over which the telomere-associated sequences are found (about 36 kb), and give a sense of the number, size, and density of genes in the region near this telomere.

b. At least in this region, *Alu* sequences are found more often in AT-rich areas. These areas are not as gene rich as adjacent GC-rich areas. Thus, this class of moderately repetitive sequences and the genes in this area appear to have a nonrandom distribution.

3

DNA Replication

Chapter Outline

Semiconservative DNA Replication
The Meselson–Stahl Experiment

DNA Polymerases, the DNA Replicating Enzymes
DNA Polymerase I
Roles of DNA Polymerases

Molecular Model of DNA Replication
Initiation of Replication
Semidiscontinuous DNA Replication
Rolling Circle Replication

DNA Replication in Eukaryotes
Replicons
Initiation of Replication
Eukaryotic Replication Enzymes
Replicating the Ends of Chromosomes
Assembling Newly Replicated DNA into Nucleosomes

Review of Key Terms, Symbols, and Concepts

In your own words, write a brief, precise definition of each term in the groups below. Check your definitions using the text. Then develop a concept map using the terms in each list.

1	2	3
semiconservative DNA replication	semidiscontinuous DNA replication	semidiscontinuous DNA replication
conservative DNA replication	origin of replication (*oriC*)	rolling circle replication
dispersive DNA replication	replicator sequence	λ phage
Meselson–Stahl experiment	replication bubble	"sticky" ends
CsCl equilibrium gradient	initiator protein (DnaA)	*cos* site
equilibrium density gradient centrifugation	DNA helicase (DnaB)	concatamer
^{15}N, ^{14}N	DNA helicase loader proteins (DnaC)	*ter*
buoyant density	primase (DnaG)	leading strand
DNA polymerase I, II, III, IV, V	primosome	lagging strand
dNTP, dNMP, Mg^{2+}	replisome	
Kornberg enzyme	RNA primer	
template strand	template	
primer	SSB protein	
DNA repair	reannealing	
	replication fork	
	Okazaki fragments	
	bidirectional replication	
	DNA polymerase I (*polA* gene)	
	DNA polymerase III holoenzyme	
	DNA polymerase III	
	dnaE, dnaQ, dnaX, dnaN, dnaD, holA to E genes	
	5'-to-3' synthesis	
	proofreading	
	3'-to-5' , 5'-to-3' exonuclease	
	leading, lagging strand	
	DNA gyrase	
	tension	
	polA1, polA1ex1 mutants	
	temperature-sensitive mutant	

4		
cell cycle	prereplicative complexes	reverse transcription
cyclins	proofreading ability	reverse transcriptase, *TERT*
Cdk	replicator selection	*TLC1, EST1, TEL1, TEL2* genes
DNA polymerase α, δ, ε	replicon	H3-H4 tetramer
DNA replication	telomere	H2A-H2B dimer
DNA repair	telomerase	histone chaperone
origin recognition complex		

Thinking Analytically

Because of its fundamental importance in genetics and in treating diseases such as cancer, there has been a considerable interest in understanding the mechanism of DNA replication. At this point, we understand the mechanism of DNA replication in considerable detail. Not only do we know that DNA replicates semiconservatively, but we know the nature of the complex set of proteins and enzymes that act in a sequential, coordinated fashion to replicate DNA. The best way to understand and retain the details of this complex process is to develop a contextual understanding of them. Start by developing a general understanding of the steps of DNA replication. Ask yourself: What must happen first? How is this accomplished? What happens next? How is that accomplished? Then focus on understanding the activities of each of the enzymes and proteins used in each step. To help develop a contextual understanding and establish a mental image of each of the steps, refer to the text figures that summarize the key events of DNA replication.

After reading each section of the text, assess your understanding and retention of the material by closing the text and sketching out the aspect of DNA replication that has just been presented. Then relate the figure you have sketched to the earlier steps of DNA replication. This will force you to confront unclear concepts and help you identify details you might have missed.

Questions for Practice

Multiple-Choice Questions

1. Consider the Meselson–Stahl experiment where *E. coli* were grown in ^{15}N medium. Which model of DNA replication is eliminated by analyzing DNA after exactly one round of replication in ^{14}N medium?
   a. semiconservative
   b. dispersive
   c. conservative

2. The enzymes most directly concerned with catalyzing DNA synthesis are DNA
   a. ligases.
   b. exonucleases.
   c. polymerases.
   d. primases.

3. Which of the following is *not* essential for the *in vitro* synthesis of DNA?
   a. magnesium ions
   b. DNA polymerase I
   c. DNA primase
   d. a DNA fragment

4. Which enzyme untwists the parent strands of DNA during replication?
   a. DNA primase
   b. DNA helicase
   c. DNA gyrase
   d. DNA ligase

5. Which of the following do *not* provide evidence for semiconservative DNA replication?
   a. the Meselson–Stahl experiment
   b. harlequin chromosomes
   c. the existence of ARS elements
   d. Okazaki fragments

6. Which of the following *E. coli* enzymes have proofreading activity?
   a. DNA polymerase I
   b. DNA ligase
   c. DNA primase
   d. DNA polymerase III

7. DNA replication in certain viruses, such as phage λ, is achieved
   a. using a rolling circle model and semidiscontinuous DNA replication.
   b. using a rolling circle model and continuous DNA replication.
   c. without using an origin of replication.
   d. using DNA fragmentation.

8. During chromosome replication, new histones are translated during
   a. G_1 and S, and nucleosomes are re-formed using new and old histones.
   b. G_1 and S, and new nucleosomes are formed with only these new histones.
   c. S, and nucleosomes are re-formed using new and old histones.
   d. S, and new nucleosomes are formed with only these new histones.

9. Which of the following is *not* associated with the initiation of DNA replication in yeast?
   a. The initiation of DNA replication takes place in a specific stage of the cell cycle.
   b. Replicator selection occurs during G_1 when the replicator is recognized by the multi-subunit origin recognition complex (ORC).
   c. Replication initiation requires activation of prereplicative complexes by cyclin-dependent kinases during S.
   d. DNA is immediately unwound after it is bound by the initiator.

10. What is the function of the enzyme telomerase in mammals?
   a. to replicate telomeres in all cell types
   b. to replicate and expand simple telomeric repeats in germ cells and tumor cells
   c. to expand the length of simple telomeric repeats in brain cells
   d. to replicate telomere-associated sequences and simple telomeric repeats in all cells

Answers: 1c, 2c, 3c, 4b, 5c, 6a, d, 7a, 8c, 9d, 10b

Thought Questions

1. Describe the mechanism of semidiscontinuous DNA replication.

2. In his investigation of the requirements for *in vitro* synthesis of DNA, Kornberg found that an absolute minimum of four components was necessary. What were these components, and why in particular were each and all necessary? Also, what limitations did his *in vitro* method have as compared to *in vivo* synthesis, which involves other components, such as helicase, primase, and ligase?

3. Describe how eukaryotic DNA is assembled into nucleosomes after DNA replication. Where do the new nucleosomes come from?

4. What phenotype would you expect to see in a mutant in the *E. coli polA* gene that showed heat-sensitive 3'-to-5' exonuclease activity, but normal 5'-to-3' exonuclease activity at all temperatures?

5. In humans, how are simple telomeric repeats replicated in a fast-dividing population of cells such as epithelial cells? Are all of them replicated at each cell division?

6. The text describes evidence that telomere length is under genetic control and that in mammals, only immortal cells (e.g., tumor cells, germ cells) have telomerase activity. Why might this be important? In particular, why might it be important for some cells *not* to have telomerase activity?

7. How might you identify the DNA elements used as origins of replication in *S. pombe*? Could you use the same methods to identify such DNA elements in human cells grown in culture? (Hint: Consider how replication origins were identified in *Saccharomyces cerevisiae*.)

Thought Questions for Media

After reviewing the media on the *iGenetics* website, try to answer these questions.

1. In the animation of the experiment by Meselson and Stahl that showed that DNA replication was semiconservative, how did they initially label DNA with ^{15}N?

2. In the animation of DNA synthesis using DNA polymerase, when proofreading occurs, what type of molecule is released?

3. In the animation of the semidiscontinuous model of DNA replication, in which direction is DNA synthesis on the lagging strand, and which direction is this relative to the movement of the replication fork?

1. How can you experimentally determine if a replication fork proceeds bidirectionally or unidirectionally?

2. How can you experimentally determine whether DNA primase randomly starts synthesizing an RNA primer or whether it primes DNA synthesis only at specific sites?

3. In the text, the function of *E. coli* DNA polymerase II was not described. Based on the iActivity, what genetic analysis could you perform to demonstrate that it is involved in DNA repair?

Solutions to Text Questions and Problems

3.1 *Answer:* Bacterial DNA was uniformly labeled with heavy nitrogen by growing *E. coli* for many generations in media containing "heavy" nitrogen, ^{15}N. Such ^{15}N DNA has a greater buoyant density than ^{14}N DNA and can be differentiated from ^{14}N DNA by its banding position in a CsCl density gradient. Semiconservative DNA replication was demonstrated by placing *E. coli* with ^{15}N DNA into ^{14}N media, and following the density of the DNA that was present in cells after growth proceeded through each of several successive generations. If DNA replication were conservative, after one cell division and one round of DNA replication one would expect to see two distinct, equally dense bands, one corresponding to ^{14}N DNA and one corresponding to ^{15}N DNA. This was not seen. If DNA replication were either semiconservative or dispersive, after one cell division and one round of DNA replication one would expect to see one band consisting of DNA with a density halfway between ^{14}N DNA and ^{15}N DNA. This was seen. To further distinguish between semiconservative and dispersive replication, the consequences of another round of cell division and DNA replication were examined. In semiconservative replication, one would expect two bands, one of density halfway between ^{14}N DNA and ^{15}N DNA, and one having ^{14}N DNA density. In dispersive replication, only DNA with both ^{14}N DNA and ^{15}N DNA would be seen. The density of the two bands seen (one at the level of ^{14}N DNA and one at the level of half ^{14}N DNA and half ^{15}N DNA) supported the semiconservative model. See text Figure 3.2, p. 38.

3.2 *Answer:* Key: ^{15}N–^{15}N DNA = HH; ^{15}N–^{14}N DNA = HL; ^{14}N–^{14}N DNA = LL.

   a. Generation 1: all HL; 2: ½ HL, ½ LL; 3: ¼ HL, ¾ LL; 4: ⅛ HL, ⅞ LL; 6: ¹⁄₃₂ HL, ³¹⁄₃₂ LL; 8: ¹⁄₁₂₈ HL, ¹²⁷⁄₁₂₈ LL.

   b. Generation 1: ½ HH, ½ LL; 2: ¼ HH, ¾ LL; 3: ⅛ HH, ⅞ LL; 4: ¹⁄₁₆ HH, ¹⁵⁄₁₆ LL; 6: ¹⁄₆₄ HH, ⁶³⁄₆₄ LL; 8: ¹⁄₂₅₆ HH, ²⁵⁵⁄₂₅₆ LL.

3.3 *Answer:* The CsCl centrifugation result eliminates the possibility of the conservative model of replication, but is still consistent with either semiconservative or dispersive models of DNA replication. To distinguish between these two possibilities using the same sample and the technique of CsCl centrifugation, you could denature the DNA and then subject the single-stranded sample to CsCl centrifugation. This could be done in practice by using an alkaline CsCl gradient, as the two DNA strands will denature at high pH. The expected results are shown below.

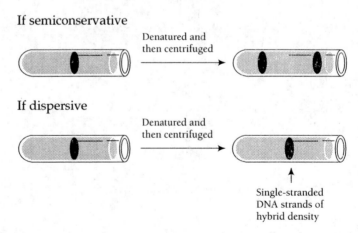

3.4 *Answer:*

   a. Establishing that DNA replication is semiconservative *does not* ensure that it is semidiscontinuous. For example, if DNA polymerase were able to synthesize DNA in both the 3′-to-5′ and 5′-to-3′ directions, DNA replication could proceed continuously on both DNA strands while still being semiconservative. Alternatively, if each of the two old strands were completely (or even substantially) unwound, and replication were initiated from the 3′ end (or 3′ region) of each, it could proceed continuously (or mostly continuously) in a 5′-to-3′ direction along each strand.

   b. Establishing that DNA replication is semidiscontinuous *does* ensure that it is semiconservative. In the semidiscontinuous model, each old, separated strand serves as a template for a new strand. This is the essence of the semiconservative model.

c. Semiconservative DNA replication is ensured by two enzymatic properties of DNA polymerase: it synthesizes just one new strand from each "old" single-stranded template, and it can synthesize new DNA in only one direction (5′ to 3′).

3.5 *Answer:* DNA can be synthesized *in vitro* using the Kornberg enzyme (DNA polymerase I), all four dNTPs (dATP, dGTP, dCTP, dTTP), magnesium ions (Mg^{2+}), and a fragment of double-stranded DNA that will serve as a template.

3.6 *Answer:* In all parts of this question, the 5′-ATG-3′ primer will anneal to each of the templates only at the 3′-TAC-5′ sequence present at each of their 3′ ends. Consequently, all of the reaction products will have the same length. The answers to parts **(a)–(c)** differ because of the way new phosphodiester bonds form during the synthesis of a nascent DNA strand. When a nucleotide is added to a growing polynucleotide chain, a new phosphodiester bond is formed by incorporating the α phosphorus (the phosphorus closest to the 5′-carbon) of the dNTP (see text Figure 3.3, p. 41). Thus, different results will be obtained depending on whether that or another phosphorus is radioactively labeled.

3.7 *Answer:* The primary evidence that the Kornberg enzyme is not the main enzyme for DNA synthesis *in vivo* stems from an analysis of the growth and biochemical phenotypes of two mutants affecting DNA polymerase I: *polA1* and *polAex1*. The mutant *polA1* lacks 99% of polymerase activity but is nonetheless able to grow, replicate its DNA, and divide. The conditional mutant *polAex1* retains most of the polymerizing activity at the restrictive temperature of 42°C but is still unable to replicate its chromosomes and divide (it has lost the enzyme's 5′-to-3′ exonuclease activity). In this way, the analysis of the *polA1* and *polAex1* mutants indicated that there must be other DNA-polymerizing enzymes in the cell.

3.8 *Answer:* The 5′-to-3′ exonuclease activity of DNA polymerase I is essential for DNA replication because a lack of this activity in the conditional mutant *polAex1* (at the restrictive temperature of 42°C) results in the failure of DNA replication. DNA polymerase I functions to remove the RNA primer synthesized during the initiation of DNA replication and replace this RNA with DNA. When DNA polymerase III, the main synthetic enzyme for DNA polymerization, reaches an RNA primer, it dissociates from the DNA. DNA polymerase I functions to continue synthesis of the DNA in a 5′-to-3′ direction. It simultaneously removes the RNA primer using its 5′-to-3′ exonuclease activity and replaces the RNA with DNA nucleotides.

3.9 *Answer:* The deoxyribonucleotides have a triphosphate group at the 5′ end of the molecule and a hydroxyl group at the 3′ end of the molecule. This information establishes the polarity of each of the deoxyribonucleotides (dATP, dGTP, dTTP, and dCTP). Since the phosphodiester bond will form between the 5′ and 3′ ends of adjacent nucleotides, the 5′-to-3′ bonding of the TATCA oligonucleotide can be represented as:

The complementary strand will base-pair with antiparallel orientation:

3.10   *Answer:*

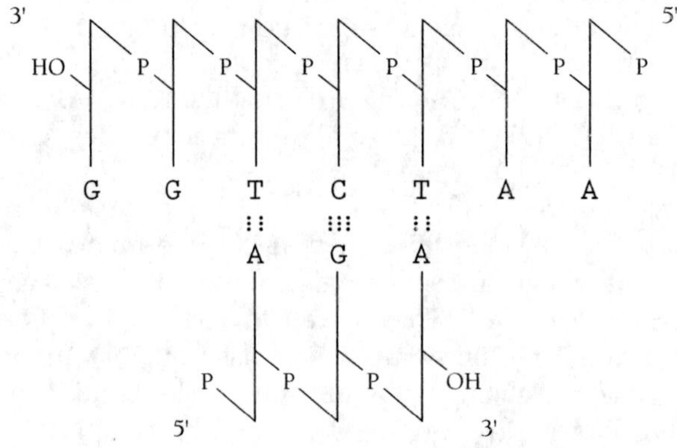

a. The 5′ ends will have either a monophosphate or a triphosphate group; the 3′ ends will have hydroxyl groups.
b. Two dTTPs.
c. The ester bond immediately after the phosphorus closest to the 5′ carbon in dTTP is a high-energy bond. DNA polymerase cleaves this bond and uses the energy obtained from it to catalyze the formation a new bond between the same phosphorus and the 3′ oxygen of the A nucleotide in the primer strand.
d. Two Cs, presumably dCTPs.
e. The alien DNA polymerase could not catalyze the formation of a new phosphodiester bond in the same way, because it must form a bond between a 3′-OH of the dCTP and the 5′-monophosphate of the primer. The high-energy bond of the dCTP is attached to its 5′-carbon, so if this were the source of energy for the new phosphodiester bond, it would have to be used in a very different way. DNA ligase joins a 3′-OH to a 5′-monophosphate using ATP as an energy source. So, a conceivable alternative is that the alien DNA polymerase uses dAMP, dCMP, dGMP and TMP as substrates and ATP as an energy source.
f. There are multiple potential reasons why Earth DNA polymerases synthesize DNA only in the 5′-to-3′ direction. First, the 3′-to-5′ reaction could be slow and inefficient or inaccurate. Second, the 3′-to-5′ reaction might require a different energy source or a different way to use the same energy source. Third, if one enzyme could accomplish synthesis in both directions, one enzyme would need to have two very different enzymatic activities. If one activity is more efficient than the other, that activity might be selected for and the other one might be lost during evolution. Fourth, DNA synthesis on Earth occurs within a replisome. It could be that the efficiency and accuracy of synthesizing DNA using this complex outweighs any advantages that might be gained by being able to synthesize DNA in the 3′-to-5′ direction.

3.11   *Answer:*

a. Semiconservative DNA replication requires that a new double-stranded DNA molecule consist of one old and one newly synthesized strand. The direction of synthesis, how synthesis is initiated, and the exonuclease properties of DNA polymerases do not dictate that DNA replication must be semiconservative. It is synthesis by DNA polymerase of a new strand using an old strand as a template that leads to semiconservative DNA replication.
b. Semidiscontinous DNA replication occurs because 5′-to-3′ DNA synthesis is continuous on one strand (the strand that goes 3′-to-5′ in the same direction as replisome movement), but discontinuous on the other strand. Since DNA polymerase synthesizes DNA only going 5′ to 3′ from a template that goes 3′ to 5′, DNA synthesis must be reinitiated on the strand that goes 3′ to 5′ in the direction opposite to replisome movement. Therefore, the requirement that all DNA polymerases replicate DNA only in the 5′-to-3′ direction results in semidiscontinuous DNA synthesis. The use of an RNA primer to initiate DNA synthesis and the 5′-to-3′ exonuclease activity of some DNA polymerases, which is used later to excise the RNA primer, do not dictate that DNA replication must be semidiscontinuous.

3.12 *Answer:* None are analogs of adenine, B and D are analogs of thymine, C is an analog of cytosine, and A is an analog of guanine.

3.13 *Answer:* Since DNA replication is known to be semidiscontinuous, it is helpful to first consider the details of this model. As the other models are constructed, reference to the semidiscontinuous model can identify the problems associated with them.

a. A *semidiscontinuous model* is shown in text Figures 3.4, p. 43 and 3.5, p. 44. Its main features are that:

i. DNA replication proceeds only in the 5'-to-3' direction.

ii. Because DNA replication proceeds only in one direction, it is continuous on the 3'-to-5' template strand (the leading strand), while it is discontinuous on the 5'-to-3' template strand (the lagging strand). This is why it is *semi*discontinuous.

iii. Replication initiates at a replication origin, where a complex of proteins and enzymes forms at a replication fork. Initially, helicase untwists the DNA and SSBs (single-strand binding proteins) bind the single-stranded DNA to protect it from nuclease attack and keep it unwound.

iv. Since DNA polymerase can polymerize DNA only if a 3'-OH is provided, an RNA primer must be synthesized by a primase–enzyme complex (the primosome). The primosome binds to the single-stranded DNA and synthesizes a short RNA primer in the 5'-to-3' direction.

v. Once an RNA primer is synthesized, DNA polymerase III (a complex of proteins) adds nucleotides onto the 3'-OH in the 5'-to-3' direction, using the unwound DNA as a template. The newly synthesized DNA is thus synthesized onto an RNA primer. This is referred to as an Okazaki fragment. On the lagging strand, synthesis moves "away" from the fork, and synthesis must be reinitiated frequently. On the leading strand, synthesis proceeds "into" the fork. The proteins involved in replication are associated into a replisome, so that the DNA polymerase III of the lagging strand is complexed with DNA polymerase III on the leading strand. The replisome that forms at a replication fork moves as a unit along the DNA, enabling new DNA to be synthesized efficiently on both the leading and lagging strands.

vi. On the lagging strand, DNA polymerase III will (after about 1,000 to 2,000 bp) encounter the 5' end of an RNA primer of the previously synthesized Okazaki fragment. At this point, it dissociates and is replaced by DNA polymerase I, which uses its 5'-to-3' exonuclease activity to excise the RNA primer and replace it with DNA.

vii. Once the RNA primer is replaced with DNA, the gap between adjacent DNA fragments is sealed by DNA ligase.

A *continuous model* would need to consider what we know about the semiconservative nature of DNA replication, as well as the enzymes known to be involved in DNA replication. In particular, the model would have to

- produce new double helices that each have one old and one new strand.
- use DNA polymerases that synthesize DNA only in the 5'-to-3' direction.
- use DNA polymerases requiring a 3'-to-5' template.
- use DNA polymerases that need a primer to initiate replication.

One problem to be solved by any model of continuous-only DNA replication is to ensure that the DNA is completely replicated. For example, if DNA replication starts in the middle of a linear chromosome, and proceeds continuously in only a 5'-to-3' direction using a 3'-to-5' template strand, half of that template strand will remain unreplicated. This problem might be overcome in different ways, depending on whether the chromosome is circular or linear. Each solution, however, presents additional problems.

Suppose DNA replication occurs in a circular chromosome. As in the semidiscontinuous model, a protein or set of proteins would recognize an origin-of-replication site within the DNA molecule. To create a site for initiation of DNA synthesis, an endonuclease would nick one strand. Helicase would then bind the free 5' end and start unwinding it. DNA primase would not be needed, as the free 3'-OH would serve as the end of a "primer." The complementary (3'-to-5') strand would be used as a template for new DNA synthesis. A protein such as SSB would bind to the unwound, nontemplate strand (the strand with an exposed 5′ end) to keep it separate from the template strand. In some unknown manner, this strand would need to be kept separate and perhaps unwound throughout the replication of the template strand. This raises a first problem, as this might be a daunting task given the size of a chromosome compared to the size of a cell. Since DNA replication is semiconservative, this strand (which lacks a priming site) would also need to be replicated. The mechanism by which this would occur is unknown and raises a second problem. In a replication fork proceeding down the length of the template strand, DNA polymerase III would add nucleotides based on the sequence of the 3′-to-5′ template strand, continuously until the site of the origin was reached. Some mechanism would be needed to mark this site so that DNA polymerase III would stop synthesis. A ligation reaction would be needed to join the two ends of the newly synthesized DNA. There are multiple approaches to solving the two problems posed by this model, but in reality, neither problem occurs due to the semidiscontinuous nature of DNA replication.

For linear eukaryotic chromosomes, it would be difficult to initiate DNA synthesis at the very ends of chromosomes. But this would not always be required, as in germ-line cells of eukaryotes, the simple telomeric repeats at the very ends of chromosomes are replicated by telomerase. However, in somatic cells, a distinct mechanism would be needed to identify origin-of-replication sites very near to, but not at, the ends of the chromosomes. After an endonuclease made a nick near the end of a linear chromosome, a DNA polymerase III–like enzyme could add nucleotides 5′ to 3′ based on the sequence of the 3′-to-5′ template strand. A replication fork would proceed down the length of the template strand, replicating just one of the strands. Presumably, the other strand would be bound by an SSB-like protein as it was unwound. (Recall the first problem above.) At the other end of a linear chromosome, a similar process would occur.

In both of these models of continuous DNA replication, no DNA primase was required, and no RNA primer was used. Certainly, other models of continuous DNA replication might be devised that use DNA primase and RNA primers. However, there is then the question of how to remove the primers, and so a DNA polymerase I–like enzyme must be used. One significant problem with these models is that they require one of the two strands of the parental DNA molecule to remain separate from the template strand until it is replicated. Given the sizes of chromosomes in prokaryotes and eukaryotes relative to their cell sizes, this is a considerable problem. It is a problem that is solved by having a replication fork synthesize DNA semidiscontinuously, so that there are only very short stretches of unwound, SSB-bound DNA.

A *discontinuous model* of DNA replication would be nearly identical to the semidiscontinuous model, except that DNA replication would be discontinuous not only on the lagging strand but also on the leading strand. Presumably, DNA polymerase III would "fall off" the leading-strand template periodically and then come back "on board" to continue synthesizing DNA. No new priming would be required, as there would be a free 3′-OH available for DNA polymerase III onto which to add deoxyribonucleotides.

b. Reiji Okazaki provided the primary evidence that DNA synthesis must be discontinuous on at least one strand. He demonstrated the existence of Okazaki fragments, short segments of DNA that have short RNA primers at their 5′ ends. Their existence indicated that DNA synthesis must be periodically re-primed on the lagging strand and therefore that it must be discontinuous on that strand. (Also see the answer to Question 3.20.)

3.14   *Answer:* **a.** C   **h.** H
             b. F   **i.** A
             c. D   **j.** A, B
             d. A, B   **k.** E
             e. A   **l.** A, B, (D, after the first two bases of the RNA
             f. B   primer are positioned)
             g. A, B, D   **m.** G

3.15   *Answer:* Helicase and topoisomerase both act on DNA, but helicase untwists the two strands to separate them while topoisomerase alters the tension in a double-stranded DNA molecule introduced by supercoiling. When helicase untwists the two strands of a double-stranded DNA molecule during DNA replication, tension is produced ahead of the replication fork due to supercoiling of the double-stranded DNA in that region. Topoisomerases add or remove negative supercoils from cellular DNA. During DNA replication, the topoisomerase DNA gyrase relaxes the tension ahead of the replication fork.

3.16   *Answer:* In *E. coli*, replication proceeds bidirectionally from the replication origin (*oriC*). Thus, each replication fork proceeds halfway down the length of the circular *E. coli* chromosome, at which point the replication forks meet and replication is complete. Thus, it will take

$$\frac{4.2 \times 10^6 \text{ bp}}{2 \text{ replication forks}} \times \frac{1 \text{ second}}{1,000 \text{ bp}} \times \frac{1 \text{ minute}}{60 \text{ seconds}} = 35 \text{ minutes}$$

3.17   *Answer:* Since a replication fork moves at a rate of 10^4 bp per minute and each replicon has two replication forks moving in opposite directions, in one replicon, replication would be occurring at a rate of 2×10^4 bp/minute. Since all of the organism's DNA is replicated in 3 minutes, the number of replicons in the diploid genome is

$$\frac{4.5 \times 10^8 \text{ bp}}{3 \text{ minutes}} \times \frac{1 \text{ replicon}}{2 \times 10^4 \text{ bp/minute}} = 7,500$$

3.18   *Answer:* DNA ligase catalyzes the formation of a phosphodiester bond between the 3'-OH and the 5' monophosphate groups on either side of a single-strand DNA gap, sealing the gap (see text Figure 3.6, p. 45). Temperature-sensitive ligase mutants would be unable to seal such gaps at the restrictive (high) temperature, leading to fragmented lagging strands and presumably cell death. If a biochemical analysis were performed on DNA synthesized after *E. coli* were shifted to a restrictive temperature, there would be an accumulation of DNA fragments the size of Okazaki fragments. This would provide additional evidence that DNA replication must be discontinuous on one strand.

3.19   *Answer:* Assume the amount of a gene's product is directly proportional to the number of copies of the gene present in the *E. coli* cell. Assay the enzymatic activity of genes at various positions in the *E. coli* chromosome during the replication period. Then some genes (those immediately adjacent to the origin) will double their activity very shortly after replication begins. Relate the map position of genes having doubled activity to the amount of time that has transpired since replication was initiated. If replication is bidirectional, there should be a doubling of the gene products both clockwise and counterclockwise from the origin.

3.20   *Answer:* Reiji Okazaki and his colleagues added a pulse of radioactive DNA precursor, ^{3}H-thymidine, to cultures of *E. coli* for a small fraction of its generation time (0.5%). To prevent the further incorporation of additional radioactive precursor into the DNA after this period, they chased this pulse with a large amount of nonradioactive thymidine. They then sampled the bacterial DNA at successive intervals as DNA replication continued. When DNA was sampled soon after the labeling period, most of the radioactivity was found in DNA with very low molecular weights, in DNA fragments between 100 and 1,000 nucleotides long. When DNA was sampled at longer intervals, the radioactivity was found in DNA with much higher molecular weight, in much longer DNA fragments. The short DNA fragments seen in the early samplings indicate that DNA replication normally involves the synthesis of short DNA segments—the Okazaki fragments—that are then linked together. This provided evidence that DNA replication occurs in a discontinuous fashion on the lagging strand.

3.21   *Answer:* Clearly, DNA replication in the Jovian specimen does not occur as it does in *E. coli*. Assuming that the double-stranded DNA is antiparallel as it is in *E. coli*, the Jovian DNA polymerases must be able to synthesize DNA in the 5'-to-3' direction (on the leading strand) as well as in the 3'-to-5' direction (on the lagging strand). This is unlike any DNA polymerase on Earth.

3.22   *Answer:*

a. From the question statement, it appears that after the double-stranded DNA is unwound at the origin of replication, fragments of DNA bind to each strand and serve as primers. This is unlike initiation of DNA replication on Earth, where DNA replication is initiated using RNA primers synthesized by DNA primase. Where do the DNA primers used by the alien organism come from? Several hypotheses can be generated to address this question. The simplest is that the single DNA polymerase in the alien organism initiates DNA synthesis by itself. That is, since the alien organism has only a single DNA polymerase, its DNA polymerase synthesizes "DNA primers" as well elongates DNA synthesis from them. For the alien DNA polymerase, the DNA primers are simply the first few nucleotides that are synthesized. Under this hypothesis, the key difference between DNA replication in the alien organism and in *E. coli* is that the alien organism initiates DNA replication without RNA priming.

Consider the implications of this hypothesis. If DNA synthesis is initiated just once and proceeds in just one direction, say 5' to 3' as occurs on Earth, then replication from a central site would produce a newly synthesized DNA strand over only half the length of each parental template strand, and the parental molecule would not be fully replicated. In *E. coli*, DNA synthesis is initiated at one origin of replication, but new RNA primers are synthesized as the replication fork progresses to allow the reinitiation of DNA synthesis on the lagging strand. The alien organism could fully replicate the parental molecules if it reinitiated DNA synthesis on the lagging strand by synthesizing and then extending a DNA "primer."

Two more complex hypotheses could also explain these observations. The first is that the DNA sequences serving as primers somehow are drawn from previously synthesized DNA sequences. One could imagine that they were synthesized during a previous round of replication as part of a larger DNA chromosome, enzymatically cleaved from it, and then stored for use as primers in the next round of DNA replication. In this case, the DNA polymerase would not need the ability to initiate DNA replication without a primer—it would use stored DNA primers. A second complex hypothesis is that DNA synthesis is initiated at just one site (using a primer synthesized during initiation of DNA replication by the DNA polymerase or taken from storage), and the reinitiation of DNA synthesis is unnecessary because this primer is extended at both ends. For this to occur, the alien DNA polymerase would have to have both 5'-to-3' and 3'-to-5' polymerase activity.

b. In *E. coli*, none of the three DNA polymerases can initiate DNA replication without priming. RNA primers are synthesized at the origin of replication by DNA primase, a 5'-to-3' RNA polymerase, and are extended in the 5'-to-3' direction by DNA polymerase III. In the alien organism, DNA primase is not used, because its DNA polymerase does not extend RNA primers. In *E. coli*, DNA polymerase I excises RNA primers using its 5'-to-3' exonuclease activity. Since RNA primers are not used in the alien organism, a DNA polymerase with 5'-to-3' exonuclease activity is not needed. Perhaps this is why only one DNA polymerase is present in the alien organism.

3.23   *Answer:*

a. Concatamers are multiple copies of a chromosome linked end to end, produced by rolling circle replication.

b. Rolling circle replication initiates differently from the bidirectional replication used by *E. coli*. In rolling circle replication, a nick is made in one strand of a double-stranded circle, and the 5' end is displaced. This creates a replication fork, leaving a single-stranded stretch of DNA that serves as a template for the addition of dNTPs to the free 3' end by DNA polymerase III. Unlike initiation in *E. coli*, initiator protein is not used. Once a replication fork and a replisome are formed, the intact circular DNA acts as a leading-strand template. New DNA synthesis occurs continuously as the 5' cut end is displaced from the circular molecule. The displaced strand serves as the lagging-strand template on which DNA synthesis occurs discontinuously. As leading-strand synthesis using the parental DNA circle continues, a concatamer is formed. The concatamer is cleaved into unit-length chromosomes before being packaged in phage particles. This is also unlike DNA replication in *E. coli*, where no concatamer is formed.

3.24 *Answer:*

a. The DNA endonuclease encoded by the *ter* gene recognizes sequences at *cos* sites appearing just once within a λ genome. It makes a staggered cut at these sites to produce the unit-length linear DNA molecules that are packaged.

b. The *ter* enzyme produces complementary ("sticky") 12-base-long, single-stranded ends. After λ infects *E. coli*, these ends pair, and gaps in the phosphodiester backbone are sealed by DNA ligase to produce a closed circular molecule. This molecule recombines into the *E. coli* chromosome if the lysogenic pathway is followed, or replicates using rolling circle replication if a lytic pathway is followed.

3.25 *Answer:*

a. Since M13 has a closed circular genome with $(A) \neq (T)$ and $(G) \neq (T)$, it must have a single-stranded DNA genome. Bidirectional replication would require the initial synthesis of a complementary strand. To produce many phage, many rounds of bidirectional replication would be necessary. However, upon completion of replication and before packaging, the nongenomic strand of the resulting double-stranded molecules would need to be selectively degraded.

b. To produce single-stranded molecules with the same sequence and base composition as the packaged M13 genome, rolling circle replication must use a complementary template. Therefore, DNA polymerase must initially synthesize the genome's complementary strand to make a double-stranded molecule. Then, a nuclease could nick the genomic strand to create a displacement fork. Continuous rolling circle replication using the intact complementary strand as the leading-strand template and without discontinuous replication on the displaced genomic strand will generate single-stranded M13 genomes. To prevent concatamer formation, the newly replicated DNA must be cleaved by an endonuclease after exactly one genome has been replicated. To form a closed circle, the molecule's ends would need to be ligated to each other.

3.26 *Answer:* Multiple DNA polymerases have been identified in all cells; there are 5 in prokaryotes and 15 or more in eukaryotes. All DNA polymerases synthesize DNA from a primed strand in the 5'-to-3' direction using a template. In both eukaryotes and prokaryotes, certain DNA polymerases are used for replication, while others are used for repair. Prokaryotes and eukaryotes differ in how many polymerases they use, and how they use them, in each of these processes.

In *E. coli*, DNA polymerase I and III function in DNA replication. Both have 3'-to-5' exonuclease activity that is used in proofreading. DNA polymerase III is the main synthetic enzyme and can exist as a core enzyme with three polypeptides or as a holoenzyme with an additional six different polypeptides. DNA polymerase I consists of one polypeptide. Unlike DNA polymerase III, it has the 5'-to-3' exonuclease activity needed to excise RNA from the 5' end of Okazaki fragments. DNA polymerases II, IV, and V function in DNA repair.

In eukaryotes, nuclear DNA replication requires three DNA polymerases: Pol α/primase, Pol δ, and Pol ε. After primase initiates new strands in replication by making about 10 nucleotides of an RNA primer, Pol α extends them by adding about 30 nucleotides of DNA. The RNA/DNA primers are extended by Pol δ and Pol ε on the leading and lagging strand. However, it is not clear which enzyme synthesizes which strand. Other DNA polymerases function in DNA repair and mitochondrial DNA replication.

3.27 *Answer:* Chromosomes are prevented from replicating more than once by ensuring that no origin of replication is used a second time in a cell cycle. This is accomplished by initiating DNA replication in two temporally separate steps. The first step occurs in G_1 and involves replicator selection. Prereplicative complexes form on each replicator, but replication initiation does not occur at this time. Only after passage of the cell from G_1 phase to S phase can the second step, replication initiation, occur. Replication initiation occurs only once per origin because after a cell enters S phase, new prereplicative complexes can no longer form.

Replication initiation is limited to S phase by cyclin-dependent kinases. Their activity is needed to activate the prereplicative complexes to initiate replication, but new prereplicative complexes cannot form when their activity is present. Active cyclin-dependent kinases are not present in G_1, so the prereplicative complexes can form in G_1. They cannot initiate replication until S, when active cyclin-dependent kinases are present. Chromosomes are prevented from replicating more than once per cell cycle because once a cell is in S phase, active cyclin-dependent kinases prevent new prereplicative complexes from forming.

3.28   *Answer:* Replicator selection occurs only in G_1 because licensing factors are available to initiate this process during G_1. Licensing factors are the first proteins that bind to origin recognition complexes (ORCs) to form prereplicative complexes (pre-RCs). After they are synthesized in G1, they move to the nucleus and are the first proteins to bind to ORCs to form pre-RCs. Once other proteins are recruited and the entire complex begins to untwist the double-stranded DNA, the licensing factors are released from the complexes and inactivated, either by being degraded or by being exported from the nucleus. If they were not inactivated and remained available in the nucleus to bind to ORCs and form pre-RCs, replication could conceivably be initiated twice at the same spot during the S stage. This will produce chromosomal regions that are doubly replicated. That is, an origin that has already been activated could be activated again, and that region of the chromosome would be replicated again. Consequently, some parts of one chromosome will be present in four copies at the end of S phase instead of the normal two copies.

3.29   *Answer:* Assuming cells spend 4 hours in G_2, there are 4.5 hours from the last 30 minutes of S to metaphase in M. Late-replicating chromosomal regions can be identified by adding ^3H thymidine to the medium, waiting 4.5 hours, and then preparing a slide of metaphase chromosomes. Chromosomal regions displaying silver grains are late replicating, as cells that were at earlier stages of S when the ^3H was added will be unable to reach metaphase in 4.5 hours.

3.30   *Answer:*

    a. Assuming that the fibroblast culture is completely asynchronous, and that cells are distributed in all stages of the cell cycle, $^{10}/24$ of the cells would be in G_1, $^9/24$ in S, $^4/24$ in G_2, and $^1/24$ in M. Only cells in S are replicating their DNA, so only $^9/24$ of the cells are capable of incorporating ^3H-thymidine into their DNA. $(^9/24)(100\%) = 37.5\%$.

    b. If a cell in the very last stages of S phase incorporated ^3H-thymidine into its DNA, it would have to proceed through G_2 (4 hours) before entering M. Not until M are metaphase chromosomes seen. Therefore, you would wait a little over 4 hours to see labeled metaphase chromosomes.

    c. DNA replication is semiconservative, meaning that each of the two double strands is used as a template for the synthesis of a new, complementary strand. When ^3H-thymidine is incorporated into the newly synthesized DNA, it will be incorporated into each new complementary strand, and so be in each chromatid that is synthesized.

    d. Cells that took up ^3H-thymidine into their DNA at the beginning of S phase would need to complete the S stage and then go through G_2 and mitotic prophase before label could be seen in metaphase chromosomes. This would take a little over 13 hours.

        The experiment outlined in this problem provides an elegant means to determine which chromosomal region replicates early in S phase and which chromosomal region replicates late in S phase. Proceed by systematically collecting cells at various times after the ^3H-thymidine pulse. Spread their chromosomes on slides; cover the chromosomes with a photographic emulsion that can detect decay of ^3H particles. After a period of time, develop the emulsion to detect sites on chromosomes that were replicating at a given time during S phase. This kind of experimentation supported a view that there are early- and late-replicating regions of eukaryotic chromosomes. The late-replicating regions are characteristically heterochromatic and include centromeric regions.

3.31   *Answer:*

    a. Sixteen hours is longer than any single stage of the cell cycle. In particular, a cell that just entered G_2 at the beginning of the labeling period would, at the end of a 16-hour labeling period, be in early S phase. Therefore, it would be labeled. Indeed, every cell would be labeled.

    b. Labeled metaphase chromosomes would already be present by the time the ^3H-thymidine was removed, as some of the cells in G_1 at the beginning of the labeling period would go through S and G_2, and be in M after 16 hours.

c. Both chromatids would be labeled, as in a 5-minute pulse of ^{3}H-thymidine.

d. Consider what would happen if metaphase chromosomes were examined in cells collected periodically after the radioactive medium was washed out. Start with cells sampled immediately after the radioactive medium is washed out. Since these cells were left in the radioactive medium for 16 hours, and there is only a little over 13 hours between the beginning of S phase and metaphase of mitosis, the previous S phase of these cells was spent entirely in the presence of ^{3}H-thymidine. Any metaphase chromosomes seen at this time would be labeled in their entirety, so these chromosomes would not be useful to identify regions replicated at a particular time during the S stage. Suppose instead that cells were sampled after about 6 hours in nonradioactive medium. These cells would have been in the first part of G_1 when the radioactive medium was added and spent about the first 8 hours of their S stage in the radioactive medium. All of their chromosomal regions would be labeled except for the regions that replicated late in the S stage. By sampling cells over increasing lengths of time, and comparing the results of different samplings, chromosomal regions that replicated at successively earlier stages could be identified. Finally, consider the cell sample taken after 13 hours in nonradioactive medium. These cells would have just entered the S stage when the nonradioactive medium had been washed out. Since they have only spent the beginning of their S phase in radioactive medium, chromosomal regions that replicated early in S phase would be labeled. However, since the culture was left in radioactive medium for 16 hours, the parents of these cells spent about the last hour of their S phase in the presence of ^{3}H-thymidine. Thus, these cells would have chromosomes that were labeled both at the beginning and at the end of the S stage. Only by comparing this sample to samples obtained earlier might these regions be distinguished.

3.32 *Answer:* While all nuclear eukaryotic DNA is replicated during S phase, heterochromatic DNA often replicates later than the rest of the DNA (see Chapter 2, p. 27). Hence, the telomeric and centromeric regions of chromosomes generally will replicate later than the euchromatic regions within chromosome arms.

3.33 *Answer:* During DNA replication, small RNA-primed DNA fragments (Okazaki fragments) are generated. Radioactivity associated with small DNA fragments would be associated with these Okazaki fragments while radioactivity associated with larger DNA fragments would be associated with DNA fragments that have had their RNA primers excised and replaced with DNA by DNA polymerase I.

a and d. U is present in RNA and not DNA, so radioactivity will be found only in RNA-primed DNA strands (small Okazaki fragments). The α-^{32}P of UTP will be incorporated into the phosphodiester backbone of the RNA primed strand, as will the tritium label if UTP is uniformly labeled with tritium. Therefore, after both time points, radioactivity will be in small fragments (as RNA-primed DNA strands). Since RNA primers are excised by DNA polymerase I, radioactivity will not be found at either time point in large DNA fragments.

b and c. Okazaki fragments are RNA-primed DNA strands, so they contain DNA nucleotides as well as RNA nucleotides. Therefore, for the same reasons described in the answer for parts **(a)** and **(d)**, radioactivity will be in small fragments after both time points. After 30 minutes, it will also be in large fragments, since these are composed of DNA nucleotides.

e. Radioactivity will not be found in small or large fragments after either time point, since the γ-^{32}P is not incorporated into the growing nucleotide chain.

3.34 *Answer:*

a. Most new histone synthesis occurs during the S stage of the cell cycle and is coordinated with DNA replication.

b. New nucleosomes are not replicated semiconservatively. Nucleosomes disassemble from DNA as the replication fork passes a replicating DNA region and then are reassembled on the two DNA double helices past the replication fork using components of both old and new histones. Histone chaperone proteins direct the process of nucleosome assembly.

Each parental histone core of a nucleosome separates into an H3–H4 tetramer (two copies each of H3 and H4) and two copies of an H2A–H2B dimer. The H3–H4 tetramer is transferred directly to one of the two replicated DNA double helices past the replication fork, where it begins nucleosome assembly. The H2A–H2B dimers are released and added to a pool of newly synthesized H2A–H2B dimers. A pool of new H3–H4 tetramers is also present, and one of these tetramers initiates nucleosome assembly on the other DNA double helix past the replication fork. The remaining part of that new nucleosome is assembled by drawing from the pool of parental and new H2A–H2B dimers. Thus, a new nucleosome will have either a parental or new H3–H4 tetramer and a pair of H2A–H2B dimers that may be parental–parental, parental–new, or new–new.

3.35   *Answer:* Telomerase synthesizes the simple-sequence telomeric repeats at the ends of chromosomes. The enzyme is made up of both protein and RNA, and the RNA component has a base sequence that is complementary to the telomere repeat unit. The RNA component is used as a template for the telomere repeat, so that if the RNA component were to be altered, the telomere repeat would be as well. Thus, the mutant in this question is likely to have an altered RNA component.

3.36   *Answer:* Evidence that telomere length is regulated in cells has come from the analysis of mutations of the yeast *TEL1* and *TEL2* genes, which cause cells to maintain their telomeres at a new, shorter-than-wild-type length. These analyses demonstrate that the telomere length is under genetic control. Insights into the consequences of misregulation of telomere length have also come from the analysis of yeast mutants. Analysis of mutations that affect telomerase function (e.g., *TLC1*) and telomere length (*EST1*) have shown that telomerase activity is necessary for long-term cell viability.

These inferences are also supported by observation that mammalian somatic cells lack telomerase, but cells that are "immortal," such as germ cells and cancer cells, do not. Cells that lack telomerase activity will have progressively shorter telomeres as the cells proceed through repeated cycles of mitosis because of the failure to replicate those ends. Cells without telomerase are able to divide only a finite number of times before they become inviable due to the eventual loss of their telomeric sequences.

4

Gene Function

Chapter Outline

Review of Key Terms, Symbols, and Concepts

In your own words, write a brief definition of each term in the groups below. Check your definitions using the text. Then develop a concept map using the terms in each list.

1	2
inborn error of metabolism	enzyme
metabolic pathway	nonenzymatic protein
biochemical pathway	Kartagener syndrome
nutritional mutant	dextrocardia
auxotroph	dynein motor
prototroph	cystic fibrosis (CF)
ascus, asci, ascospore, conidia	transmembrane conductance regulator
mutagen	active transport
Neurospora crassa, mycelium	sickle-cell anemia, sickle-cell trait
minimal, complete medium	hemoglobin
mating type	α, β polypeptide
one-gene–one-enzyme hypothesis	electrophoresis
one-gene–one-polypeptide hypothesis	amino acid substitution
amino acid	hydrophilic
polypeptide	multiple alleles
protein	autosome
N, C terminus	autosomal recessive mutation
pleiotropic	heterozygote
alkaptonuria (AKU)	carrier
phenylketonuria (PKU)	genetic counseling
albinism	pedigree analysis
Tay–Sachs disease	carrier detection
recessive trait	fetal analysis
OMIM	amniocentesis
	chorionic villus sampling

Thinking Analytically

The problems in this chapter require you to make multiple connections. You need to:

1. Relate the genetic properties of a mutation to its visible phenotype.
2. Relate the visible phenotype to a biochemical deficit (a "biochemical phenotype").
3. Relate the biochemical deficit of a mutation back to its genetic properties.

As you make these connections, layers of complexity will unfold in a problem. Clues at one level (genetic properties of the mutations, mutant phenotypes, biochemical abnormalities found in the mutant) can be used to infer what might be happening at another level. Approach the problems systematically, attempting to connect these levels wherever possible.

To relate biochemical pathways to mutant phenotypes, diagram as much of the biochemical pathway as you can, and then try to understand how specific phenotypic consequences arise when a particular step is blocked. Go slowly and be thorough. It is essential to remember that mutations in different steps of a biochemical pathway do not always cause identical mutant phenotypes. In addition, mutations affecting a particular step can have multiple consequences. They may lead to the absence of the final product and cause one phenotype. They may also lead to the accumulation of intermediate metabolites of the pathway and cause a different phenotype. Furthermore, mutations at different steps of a pathway may be able to be "rescued" if different biochemical intermediates are provided to the mutant.

Questions for Practice

Multiple-Choice Questions

1. An inborn error of metabolism is
   a. any biochemical abnormality that results from taking a drug.
   b. any heritable biochemical abnormality.
   c. any recessive mutation.
   d. any dominant mutation.

2. Why was the one-gene–one-enzyme hypothesis recast as the one-gene–one-polypeptide hypothesis?
   a. Genes can encode proteins that are not enzymes.
   b. Some enzymes are not polypeptides.
   c. Some enzymes have more than one polypeptide subunit.
   d. Some polypeptides are not enzymes.

3. Suppose an individual was diagnosed with PKU as a child and was successfully treated. If that individual and a normal, noncarrier (pku^+/pku^+) partner have children, what is the probability that they will have offspring that are carriers for PKU?
   a. 0.00
   b. 0.25
   c. 0.50
   d. 1.00

4. In individuals affected with AKU,
   a. a block in the pathway leads to the accumulation of homogentisic acid.
   b. if homogentisic acid is provided, the pathway can be completed.
   c. a block in the pathway leads to the accumulation of phenylalanine.
   d. if phenylalanine is provided, the pathway can be completed.

5. Two *Neurospora* auxotrophs are unable to grow on minimal medium but are able to grow on minimal medium supplemented with arginine. When each is tested, only one can grow on minimal medium supplemented with ornithine, a biochemical precursor to arginine. Which statement(s) below are supported by these findings?
   a. The auxotrophs are blocked in different biochemical steps.
   b. At least one auxotroph is blocked in a step before ornithine is made.
   c. Both of the auxotrophs are blocked in a step before ornithine is made.
   d. Both of the auxotrophs accumulate ornithine.
   e. both a and b

6. In complex metabolic pathways such as the phenylalanine-tyrosine metabolic pathway,
   a. blocks at different steps always result in the same phenotype.
   b. a block at one step results solely in the accumulation of the biochemical made just before that step.
   c. blocks at different steps can lead to very different phenotypes.
   d. a block at one step can lead to the accumulation of potentially toxic derivatives of biochemicals synthesized before that step.
   e. both a and b
   f. both c and d

7. What is the difference between sickle-cell anemia and sickle-cell trait?
   a. None; they refer to individuals equally affected with the same disease.
   b. Individuals with sickle-cell anemia have severe disease and have two abnormal alleles; individuals with the sickle-cell trait have a less severe form of the disease, as they are heterozygotes with one disease allele and one normal allele.
   c. Individuals with sickle-cell anemia have severe disease; the term "sickle-cell trait" refers to the disease allele present in their families, and not to symptomatic status.
   d. Individuals with sickle-cell anemia have severe disease and are homozygous for a severe disease allele; individuals with sickle-cell trait have mild disease and are homozygous for a less severe disease allele.

8. Both Tay–Sachs disease and Kartagener syndrome are examples of human diseases that are
   a. pleiotropic.
   b. caused by a deficiency in one enzyme activity.
   c. recessive.
   d. both a and c

9. An example of a heritable disease that results from a biochemical defect in a nonenzymatic protein is
   a. PKU.
   b. AKU.
   c. sickle-cell anemia.
   d. Tay–Sachs disease.

10. Which of the following is *not* true about both amniocentesis and chorionic villus sampling?
   a. Both can be performed with an acceptably low risk as early as the eighth week of pregnancy.
   b. Each procedure has a risk of fetal loss.
   c. One is more likely than the other to provide an accurate diagnosis.
   d. Both are valid, useful procedures in genetic counseling.

Answers: 1b, 2c, 3d, 4a, 5e, 6f, 7b, 8d, 9c, 10a

Thought Questions

1. If you were a genetic counselor, how would you counsel the following couple who are contemplating having children? The prospective father is apparently normal, except for a nervous twitch of his nose, but his maternal uncle had PKU as a child and his brother, who plays in a heavy metal band, is hard of hearing. The prospective mother also appears normal, but her father also was diagnosed with PKU as a child and her brother, who plays in the same band as her brother-in-law, is also hard of hearing. You know that PKU and sometimes deafness are autosomal recessive.

2. Distinguish between the procedures of amniocentesis and chorionic villus sampling. How is each useful in genetic counseling? What reasons are there for or against choosing each procedure?

3. All states currently require testing for PKU in infants. Do you expect the frequency of PKU to decline or increase over time? Justify your answer.

4. In the United States, the frequency of PKU is about 1 in 16,000 newborns. The frequency of cystic fibrosis is about 1 in 4,000 newborns. While all states currently require testing for PKU in infants, not all states require testing for cystic fibrosis. Both are autosomal recessive disorders. What are the risks associated with screening for an inherited disease? What reasons might there be not to do so? What reasons might there be to routinely test for PKU (or cystic fibrosis) in newborns?

5. Over 200 hemoglobin mutants have been detected. Explain why some hemoglobin mutations lead to less severe sickle-cell anemia phenotypes than others do.

6. Some alleles of sickle-cell anemia, when heterozygous with a normal allele, confer some resistance to malarial infection. What consequences might this have on selection for this allele in different human populations?

7. Keep in mind your answers to questions 5 and 6 as you respond to the following question. Suppose you have the ability to make point mutations in a gene that encodes an enzyme, and you are able to determine the percentage of normal enzyme activity that remains in the mutant enzyme. What effects would you expect to see if you systematically mutate the gene for the enzyme, changing only one amino acid at a time?

8. Different diseases are more prevalent in different ethnic groups. For example, within the U.S. population, Tay–Sachs disease is more prevalent in individuals of Ashkenazi Jewish descent, while certain types of sickle-cell anemia are more prevalent in some individuals of Hispanic, Native-American, and African-American descent. Given this situation, and the documented history of discrimination based on ethnicity in the United States, what concerns must be addressed if genetic testing is to be used for carrier testing and prenatal diagnosis with the aim of improving the quality of health care?

9. As you have seen in the study of PKU, Tay–Sachs disease, Kartagener syndrome, and sickle-cell anemia, mutations that result in the blockage of a single enzymatic step or the function of a single protein can have pleiotropic phenotypes. Generate a hypothesis about a general principle from these data.

10. What functions do (should) genetic counseling services provide? What do they look for, how do they proceed, what do they recommend, and what, if any, advice do (should) they give?

11. In the United States, legislation has been developed to address the use and privacy of information obtained from genetic testing (see http://www.genome.gov/10002335). What specific protections can be legislated for genetic testing to be performed without fears of stigmatization and discrimination? Under what circumstances, if any, should genetic testing be allowed for diseases for which there is no treatment or cure? For some diseases with very similar symptoms, genetic tests may be useful to distinguish between diseases and improve therapy. Should laws governing the use of genetic tests as diagnostic tests (in symptomatic individuals) differ from laws governing the use of genetic tests as tests for predicting risk (in asymptomatic individuals)?

12. What is meant by "obtaining informed consent" prior to undergoing a genetic test? What information is needed to give informed consent prior to undergoing a genetic test?

Thought Questions for Media

After reviewing the media on the *iGenetics* website, try to answer these questions.

1. In the animation depicting the experiments by Beadle and Tatum, how can *Neurospora* be propagated asexually?
2. How did Beadle and Tatum obtain nutritional mutations?
3. Why did Beadle and Tatum use two rounds of screening for auxotrophs?

1. Why is the arginine pathway present in *Neurospora* also present in humans?
2. Suppose a block is made in a single enzymatic step of the arginine pathway in either humans or *Neurospora*. What is the consequence to the level of the precursor compound synthesized before the blocked enzymatic step?
3. How might citrullinemia, argininosuccinic aciduria, or OTC deficiency lead to ammonia buildup? How might you implement effective therapeutic treatments?

Solutions to Text Questions and Problems

4.1   *Answer:* Enzymes are macromolecules that catalyze chemical reactions. These reactions can be quite simple, such as the addition of a hydroxyl (-OH) group onto a simple compound, or they can be exceedingly complex, such as the replication of an entire chromosome. Enzymes are essential to biological systems because they provide catalytic power and usually increase reaction rates (the rate of production of the product of the chemical reaction) by at least a million-fold. Nearly all of the chemical transformations made in the body proceed at very low rates in the absence of enzymes. Enzymes enable cells to efficiently process nutrients, synthesize essential biochemicals such as amino acids, and synthesize and degrade proteins, nucleic acids, lipids, and other cellular macromolecules. Therefore, enzymes are necessary to catalyze reactions that produce needed compounds and perform essential processes.

4.2   *Answer:* Garrod's work provided the first evidence of a specific relationship between genes and enzymes. By studying families with alkaptonuria, Garrod and Bateson inferred that enzyme deficiencies are genetically controlled traits. Garrod then demonstrated that the position of a block in a metabolic pathway can be determined by the accumulation of the chemical compound that precedes the blocked step. One likely reason that his contemporaries did not appreciate the significance of his work was that, in 1902, when Garrod studied alkaptonuria, there was not a wide understanding of Mendelian principles (the rediscovery of Mendel's work occurred just a few years earlier). Consequently, the concept that genes control traits was not established, and there was no understanding that genes make protein products.

4.3   *Answer:* a

4.4   *Answer:* A double homozygote should have PKU, but not AKU. The PKU block should prevent most homogentisic acid from being formed, so it could not accumulate to high levels and cause AKU.

4.5   *Answer:* The block in PKU leads to decreased tyrosine levels and so should lead to a decrease in melanin formation and pigmentation. However, some tyrosine will be obtained from food, and so the block in the pathway can be partially circumvented in this way. It has been reported that PKU patients are sometimes lighter in pigmentation than their normal relatives.

Since the block in AKU patients lies after (downstream from) the formation of melanin, pigmentation should not be affected in AKU patients. However, the levels of the products of an enzymatic reaction can affect the efficiency with which that reaction proceeds. If the products of an enzymatic reaction accumulate, the reaction may be inhibited. This in turn can lead to the accumulation of the substrates of the reaction. In this case, the accumulation of homogentisic acid in AKU individuals may ultimately lead to elevation of tyrosine levels. This tyrosine might be available for conversion to melanin. Hence, if AKU has any effect, it may be to increase pigmentation levels.

Using the same logic as in Question 4.4, an individual with both PKU and AKU will show symptoms of PKU, but not AKU. Therefore, it is likely that there will be decreased tyrosine levels and a decrease in melanin formation and pigmentation.

4.6   *Answer:* Autosomes are chromosomes that are found in two copies in both males and females. That is, an autosome is any chromosome except the X and Y chromosomes. Since individuals have two of each type of autosome, they have two copies of each gene on an autosome. The alleles—alternative forms of a gene—of the two copies can be the same or different. Individuals have either two normal alleles (homozygous for the normal allele), one normal allele and one mutant allele (heterozygous for the normal and mutant alleles), or two mutant alleles (homozygous for the mutant allele). A recessive mutation is one that exhibits a phenotype only when it is homozygous. Therefore, an autosomal recessive mutation is a mutation that occurs on any chromosome except the X or Y and that causes a phenotype only when homozygous. Heterozygotes exhibit a normal phenotype.

Of the diseases discussed in this chapter, many are autosomal recessive. For example, phenylketonuria, albinism, Tay–Sachs disease, and cystic fibrosis are autosomal recessive diseases.

Heterozygotes for the disease allele are normal, but homozygotes with the disease allele are affected. For phenylketonuria and albinism, homozygotes are affected because they lack a required enzymatic function. In these cases, heterozygotes have a normal phenotype because their single normal allele provides sufficient enzyme function.

Parents contribute one of their two autosomes to their gametes, so that each offspring of a couple receives an autosome from each parent. If in a particular conception each of two heterozygous parents contributes a chromosome with the normal allele, the offspring will be homozygous for the normal allele and be normal. If in a particular conception one of the two heterozygous parents contributes a chromosome with the normal allele and the other parent contributes a chromosome with the mutant allele, the offspring will be heterozygous but be normal. If in a particular conception each parent contributes the chromosome with the mutant allele, the offspring will be homozygous for the mutant allele and develop the disease. Therefore, heterozygous parents can have both normal and affected children. Since each conception is independent, two heterozygous parents can have all normal, all affected, or any mix of normal and affected children.

4.7   *Answer:* A genetic disease such as sickle-cell anemia is caused by a change in DNA that alters levels or forms of one or more gene products. This leads to changes in cellular functions, resulting in a disease state. The examples given in this chapter demonstrate that genetic diseases can be associated with mutations in single genes that affect their protein products. For example, sickle-cell anemia is caused by mutations in the gene for β-globin. Mutations lead to amino acid substitutions that cause the β-globin polypeptide to fold incorrectly. This in turn leads to sickled red blood cells and anemia. Since the environment significantly affects disease severity, many genetic diseases are treatable. For example, PKU can be treated by altering diet. Unlike diseases caused by an invading microorganism or other external agent that are subject to the defenses of the human immune system and that generally have short-lived clinical symptoms and treatments, genetic diseases are caused by heritable changes in DNA that are associated with chronically altered levels or forms of one or more gene products.

4.8   *Answer:* One method is to testcross the male to a retinal atrophic female. Retinal atrophic pups (expected half of the time) would indicate that the male is heterozygous. If the retinal atrophy is associated with a known biochemical phenotype (e.g., an altered enzyme activity), a preferred method is to take a tissue biopsy or blood sample from the male and assess whether normal levels of enzyme activity are present in the male. Recessive mutations in genes for many enzymes, when heterozygous with a normal allele, lead to reduced levels of enzyme activity even though no visible phenotype is observed.

4.9   *Answer:* Beadle and Tatum discovered that one gene specified one enzyme when they showed that nutritional mutations (auxotrophs) in *Neurospora* were associated with defects in specific steps of a biochemical pathway. Mutations in different steps were unable to grow but accumulated the biochemical intermediate made before the enzymatic block. However, they could be grown by adding biochemical intermediate made after the enzymatic block. This genetic analysis indicated that the normal gene specified an enzyme in the pathway that converted one biochemical intermediate to another.

The one-gene–one-enzyme concept does not apply in situations where an enzyme is composed of more than one polypeptide subunit, and different polypeptide subunits are encoded by separate genes. In such cases, multiple genes encode one enzyme. If two genes encode different polypeptide subunits that form one enzyme, then mutations in each gene can result in the same phenotype. That is, mutations in either of the two genes will result in the same enzyme deficiency and the accumulation of the same precursor product. This discovery led to the more accurate hypothesis that one gene encodes one polypeptide.

4.10   *Answer:* Wild-type T4 will produce progeny phages at all three temperatures. Consider what will happen under each model if *E. coli* is infected with a doubly mutant phage (one step is cold sensitive, one step is heat sensitive), and the growth temperature is shifted between 17° and 42° during phage growth.

Suppose model (1) is correct and cells infected with the double mutant are first incubated at 17° and then shifted to 42°. Progeny phages will be produced and the cells will lyse, as each step of the pathway can be completed in the correct order. In model (1), the first step, *A* to *B*, is controlled by a gene whose product is heat sensitive but not cold sensitive. At 17°, the enzyme works, and A will be converted to B. While phage are at 17°, the second, cold-sensitive step of the pathway prevents the production of mature phage. However, when the temperature is shifted to 42°, the accumulated B product can be used to make mature phage, so that lysis will occur.

Under model (1), a temperature shift performed in the reverse direction does not allow for growth. When *E. coli* cells are infected with a doubly mutant phage and placed at 42°, the heat-sensitive first step precludes the accumulation of B. When the culture is shifted to 17°, B can accumulate; but now the second step cannot occur, so no progeny phage can be produced. Therefore, if model (1) is correct, lysis will be seen only in a temperature shift from 17° to 42°. If model (2) is correct, growth will be seen only in a temperature shift from 42° to 17°. Hence, the correct model can be deduced by performing a temperature shift experiment in each direction and observing which direction allows progeny phage to be produced.

4.11 *Answer:* A strain blocked at a later step in the pathway accumulates a metabolic intermediate that can "feed" a strain blocked at an earlier step. It secretes the metabolic intermediate into the medium, thereby providing a nutrient to bypass the earlier block of another strain. Consequently, a strain that feeds all others (but itself) is blocked in the last step of the pathway, while a strain that feeds no others is blocked in the first step of the pathway. Mutant *a* is blocked in the earliest step in the pathway because it cannot feed any of the others. Mutant *c* is next because it can supply the substance *a* needs but cannot feed *b* or *d*. Mutant *d* is next, and mutant *b* is last in the pathway because it can feed all the others. The pathway is *a*→*c*→*d*→*b*.

4.12 *Answer:* Since both mutations cause rose-colored eyes, one possibility is that each mutation affects an enzymatic step in the synthesis of dark-red eye pigment. Two mutations that are independently isolated may affect the same or different steps. Here, we can infer that they do not affect the same step, because the two mutants respond differently when fed artificial medium mixed with ground up adult animals. Therefore, hypothesize that the normal alleles at the *rose-1* and *rose-2* genes produce enzymes lying in a linear biochemical pathway leading to the production of dark-red eye color. Two alternative pathways are possible:

Pathway 1:   rose-colored precursor A $\xrightarrow{rose-1}$ rose-colored precursor B $\xrightarrow{rose-2}$ dark-red pigment

Pathway 2:   rose-colored precursor A $\xrightarrow{rose-2}$ rose-colored precursor B $\xrightarrow{rose-1}$ dark-red pigment

In pathway 1, *rose-1* mutants are blocked at the first step, so they accumulate precursor A. The *rose-2* mutants are blocked at the second step, so they accumulate precursor B. If extracts from *rose-2* mutants are fed to *rose-1* mutants, the *rose-1* mutants will obtain precursor B. This circumvents the block in their pathway: They can complete the pathway and produce dark-red pigment. However, if extracts from *rose-1* mutants are fed to *rose-2* mutants, the *rose-2* mutants will obtain precursor A. They can convert this to precursor B, but they still cannot complete the pathway and are unable to produce dark-red pigment. In pathway 2, the steps of the pathway affected by the mutants are reversed. In this situation, if extracts from *rose-1* mutants are fed to *rose-2* mutants, the *rose-2* mutants will obtain precursor B. This circumvents the block in their pathway so they will be able to produce dark-red pigment. Feeding extracts from *rose-2* mutants to *rose-1* mutants will not allow *rose-1* mutants to complete pathway 2, so the *rose-2* mutants will still have rose-colored eyes. The data are consistent with the mutants affecting the steps shown in pathway 2.

4.13 *Answer:* One approach to this problem is to try to fit the data to each pathway sequentially, as if each were correct. Check where each mutant *could* be blocked (remember, each mutant carries only one mutation), whether the mutant would be able to grow if supplemented with the *single* nutrient that is listed, and whether the mutant would not be able to grow if supplemented with the "no growth" intermediate. It will not be possible to fit the data for mutant 4 to pathway (a), the data for mutants 1 and 4 to pathway (b), or data for mutants 3 and 4 to pathway (c). The data for all mutants can be fit only to pathway (d). Thus, (d) must be the correct pathway.

A second approach to this problem is to realize that in any linear segment of a biochemical pathway (a segment without a branch), a block early in the segment can be circumvented by *any* metabolites that normally appear later in the same segment. Consequently, if two (or more) intermediates can support growth of a mutant, they normally are made after the blocked step in the same linear segment of a pathway. From the data given, compounds D and E both circumvent the single block in mutant 4. This means that compounds D and E lie after the block in mutant 4 on a linear segment of the metabolic pathway. The only pathway where D and E lie in an unbranched linear segment is pathway (d). Mutant 4 could be blocked between A and E in this pathway. Mutant 4 cannot be fit to a *single* block in any of the other pathways that are shown, so the correct pathway is (d).

4.14   *Answer:* If the enzyme that catalyzes the d→e reaction is missing, the mutant strain should accumulate d and be able to grow on minimal medium to which e is added. In addition, it should not be able to grow on minimal medium or on minimal medium to which X, c, or d is added but should grow if Y is added. Therefore, plate the strain on these media and test which intermediates allow for growth of the mutant strain and which intermediate is accumulated if the strain is plated on minimal medium.

4.15   *Answer:*

   a. Start by inducing mutations in *Neurospora crassa* by treating conidia with X-rays. Then, prepare a large set of mutagenized strains by crossing the mutagenized spores with a prototrophic (wild-type) strain of the opposite mating type, collecting asci from the crosses, and germinating one spore from each ascus in a nutritionally complete medium (minimal medium supplemented with all of the amino acids, including lysine, as well as purines, pyrimidines, and vitamins). Crossing the mutagenized spores to the wild-type ensures that any lysine auxotrophs that are recovered are heritable and have a genetic basis. Now identify which of the mutagenized strains are auxotrophs by testing each culture for growth on minimal medium. Those unable to grow are auxotrophs and require a supplement. Finally, identify which of the auxotrophic strains are lysine auxotrophs by testing each auxotrophic strain for its ability to grow on minimal medium supplemented with lysine. Those able to grow on this medium are lysine auxotrophs.

   b. If a strain were blocked in just one of the two lysine biosynthetic pathways, then the other pathway would presumably be sufficient to allow at least some growth. Therefore, a lysine auxotroph must be unable to synthesize lysine using either biosynthetic pathway. It is blocked at one or more points in the pathway that uses aspartate as an initial precursor as well as in the pathway that uses α-ketoglutarate as an initial precursor.

   c. If we assume that the biosynthetic pathway that uses α-ketoglutarate as an initial precursor is a linear pathway, mutants that are blocked at just one step in this pathway will be able to grow on minimal media supplemented with any intermediate synthesized after that step. (Such mutants are also blocked in the lysine biosynthetic pathway that uses aspartate as an initial precursor, but this does not affect our analysis here.) Therefore, for each lysine auxotroph that is recovered, test it for its ability to grow on minimal medium supplemented with α-aminoadipate, homocitrate, α-aminoadipate semialdehyde, or saccharopine. Some mutants will be unable to grow on any of these media, some will be able to grow on just one type of media, and some will be able to grow on two, three, or all four types of media. Mutants unable to grow on any of these media are blocked in the very last step of the pathway, the step that results in the synthesis of lysine. Mutants able to grow on just one of these types of media are blocked in the penultimate step of the pathway: if a mutant is blocked in the penultimate step of the pathway, it will grow only on minimal medium supplemented with the compound synthesized immediately before the synthesis of lysine. Therefore, the compound that is added to minimal media for these mutants is the compound that is synthesized immediately before lysine. Mutants able to grow on two types of media are blocked in the enzymatic step that comes two steps before the synthesis of lysine. They can grow on minimal media supplemented either with lysine, the compound that is synthesized immediately before lysine, or the compound synthesized two steps before the synthesis of lysine. Since we already deduced the compound synthesized immediately before lysine, we can now deduce which compound is synthesized two steps before the synthesis of lysine. Using a similar logic, we can identify the compound synthesized three, and then four, steps before the synthesis of lysine.

4.16   *Answer:*

a. In each of these diseases, the lack of an enzymatic step leads to the toxic accumulation of a precursor or its by-product. The proposed treatments are ineffective because they do not prevent the accumulation of the toxic precursor. For both diseases, the symptoms would worsen as the precursor or by-product accumulated.

b. The loss of 25-hydroxycholecalciferol 1 hydroxylase should lead to increased serum levels of 25-hydroxycholecalciferol, the precursor it acts upon. Since administration of the end product of the reaction, 1,25-dihydroxycholecalciferol (vitamin D), is an effective treatment, this disease is unlike those in part (a). It appears that this disease is caused by the loss of the reaction's end product and not the accumulation of its precursor.

4.17   *Answer:* Albinism is an autosomal recessive disorder that results from the inability to synthesize melanin from tyrosine. There are several biochemical steps involved in this biosynthetic pathway, and mutations in genes for the enzymes that carry out each of the steps can lead to albinism. Therefore, individuals can have albinism due to different autosomal recessive mutations.

The first couple, parents with albinism whose children also have albinism, have mutations affecting the same biochemical step. We can make this inference because their children have albinism, and so the mutant gene the children received from each of their parents must affect the same step of the melanin biosynthetic pathway.

The second couple, parents with albinism whose children are normally pigmented, have mutations affecting a different biochemical step. We can make this inference using the following logic. Since the children do not have albinism, we know that they are able to complete the biosynthetic pathway. However, since the children's parents have albinism, we also know that each parent gave them a mutant gene for one biosynthetic step. Since the children are able to complete the biosynthetic pathway, they must have received one normal copy of that mutant gene from the other parent. So, each parent gave their children a normal copy of a gene affecting one biosynthetic step and a mutant copy of a gene affecting a different biosynthetic step. These children are carriers of mutations affecting two different biosynthetic steps in the synthesis of melanin.

4.18   *Answer:*

a. Since normal parents have affected offspring, the disease appears to be recessive. However, since patients with 50% of GSS activity have a mild form of the disease, individuals may show mild symptoms if they are heterozygous (mutant/+) for a mutation that eliminates GSS activity. In a population, individuals having the disease may not all show identical symptoms, and some may have more severe disease than others. The severity of the disease in an individual will depend on the nature of the person's GSS mutation and, possibly, whether the person is heterozygous or homozygous for the disease allele. The alleles discussed here appear to be recessive.

b. Patient 1, with 9% of normal GSS activity, has a more severe form of the disease, whereas patient 2, with 50% of normal GSS activity, has a less severe form of the disease. Thus, increased disease severity is associated with less GSS enzyme activity.

c. The two different amino acid substitutions may disrupt different regions of the enzyme's structure (consider the effect of different amino acid substitutions on hemoglobin's function, discussed in the text). As amino acids vary in their polarity and charge, different amino acid substitutions within the same structural region could have different chemical effects on protein structure. This, too, could lead to different levels of enzymatic function. (For a discussion of the chemical differences between amino acids, see Chapter 6.)

d. By analogy with the disease PKU discussed in the text, 5-oxoproline is produced only when a precursor to glutathione accumulates in large amounts due to a block in a biosynthetic pathway. When GSS levels are 9% of normal, this occurs. When GSS levels are 50% of normal, there is sufficient GSS enzyme activity to partially complete the pathway and prevent high levels of 5-oxoproline.

e. The mutations are allelic (in the same gene), since both the severe and the mild forms of the disease are associated with alterations in the same polypeptide that is a component of the GSS enzyme. (Note that, although the data in this problem suggest that the GSS enzyme is composed of a single polypeptide, they do not exclude the possibility that GSS has multiple polypeptide subunits encoded by different genes.)

f. If GSS is normally found in fetal fibroblasts, one could, in principle, measure GSS activity in fibroblasts obtained via amniocentesis. The GSS enzyme level in cells from at-risk fetuses could be compared with that in normal control samples to predict disease due to inadequate GSS levels. Some variation in GSS level might be seen, depending on the allele(s) present. Since more than one mutation is present in the population, it is important to devise a functional test that assesses GSS activity, rather than a test that identifies a single mutant allele.

4.19   *Answer:* Proteins serve many different functions. Some examples are given in the table below.

Protein Function	Examples and Their Roles
Enzyme	DNA polymerase I—synthesizes DNA, proofreads, excises an RNA primer
	DNA ligase—seals a nick in a DNA sugar–phosphate backbone
	Phenylalanine hydroxylase—converts phenylalanine to tyrosine
	Topoisomerase—introduces/removes negative supercoils in DNA
Structural protein	Tubulin—polymerizes to form microtubules, used in chromosome segregation at anaphase
	Myosin—a muscle protein used in muscle contraction
	Actin—polymerizes to form actin filaments, which provide structural integrity to the cell
Viral protein	Proteins making up the coat of T2, TMV
Receptor	Acetylcholine receptor—binds the neurotransmitter acetylcholine, found on the surface of muscle cells
Transporter	Hemoglobin—transports oxygen
Ion channel	CFTR—transports chloride ions
Regulatory molecule	Transcription factors—determine where mRNA transcripts are produced (see Chapter 11)
Bind DNA	Single-stranded DNA-binding protein—keeps single-stranded DNA strands intact and prevents them from renaturing within a replication bubble during DNA synthesis
Antibody	Immunoglobulins—immune function
Blood type	A, B, O glycoproteins—specify blood type

4.20   *Answer:* Many examples are given in the text. Here are two:

Hb-S mutations in the β-globin gene change the sixth amino acid from the N terminus of the β-globin polypeptide. This amino acid is changed from a negatively charged, acidic amino acid (glutamic acid) to an uncharged, neutral amino acid (valine). This single amino acid change causes the β-globin polypeptide to fold in an abnormal way, which in turn causes sickling of red blood cells and sickle-cell anemia.

The most common mutation causing cystic fibrosis (CF) is a mutation in the CFTR (cystic fibrosis transmembrane regulator) gene called ΔF508. This mutation deletes three consecutive base pairs of DNA and results in the deletion of a single amino acid in the CFTR protein. This amino acid is deleted in a region of the CFTR protein important for binding ATP. Since this region contributes to the function of the protein—to transport chloride ions across cell membranes—this single amino acid deletion affects the function of the protein and causes CF.

4.21   *Answer:* Many single base-pair mutations in the β-globin gene cause amino acid substitutions at different sites in the β-polypeptide chain. They can have different effects, depending on the type of amino acid substitution and its position. Some of them, such as the Hb-S mutation described in the answer to Question 4.20, alter the charge of an amino acid and thereby affect the folding of the protein. This in turn either affects the function of the hemoglobin molecule and/or the shape of the red blood cell, causing anemia. Not all such mutations are equally severe. In the Hb-C mutation, the sixth amino acid from the N terminus of the β-polypeptide chain is changed from glutamic acid to lysine. Both of these amino acids are hydrophilic. Consequently, the conformation of the hemoglobin molecule is not as altered as in the Hb-S mutation, and the Hb-C mutation causes only mild anemia.

4.22   *Answer:*

  a. From text Figure 4.11, p. 72, Hb-Norfolk affects the α-chain whereas Hb-S affects the β-chain of hemoglobin. Since each chain is encoded by a separate gene, there remains one normal allele at the genes for each of α- and β-chains in a double heterozygote. Thus, some normal hemoglobin molecules form and double heterozygotes do not have severe anemia. However, unlike double heterozygotes for two different, completely recessive mutations that lie in one biochemical pathway, these heterozygotes exhibit an abnormal phenotype. This is because some mutations in the α- and β-chains of hemoglobin show partial dominance. In particular, Hb-S/+ heterozygotes show symptoms of anemia if there is a sharp drop in oxygen tension, so these double heterozygotes exhibit mild anemia.

  b. Both Hb-C and Hb-S affect the sixth amino acid of the β-chain. The Hb-C mutation alters the normal glutamate to lysine, while the Hb-S mutation alters it to valine. Since both mutations affect the β-chain, no normal hemoglobin molecules are present. According to the text, only one type of β-chain is found in any one hemoglobin molecule. Therefore, an Hb-C/Hb-S heterozygote has two types of hemoglobin: those with Hb-C β-chains and those with Hb-S β-chains. The individuals would exhibit anemia, perhaps intermediate in phenotype between homozygotes for Hb-C and Hb-S.

4.23   *Answer:*

  a. Individuals with Kartagener syndrome (described in Chapter 4, p. 68) are also male-sterile. Their male sterility arises because their mutations result in dynein–motor protein dysfunction that blocks microtubule movements needed for sperm motility. Based on this information, one hypothesis is that these mutants affect sperm motility. The α- and β-tubulins in these mutants might be unable either to form microtubules properly or to interact properly with other proteins, such as dynein–motor proteins, that are important for motility.

  b. First, check whether the testes of the animals have motile sperm. If they lack motile sperm, examine their sperm to assess whether microtubules are properly formed (using cell biological methods such as electron microscopy or staining with fluorescent dyes that allow microtubules to be visualized).

4.24   *Answer:* One rapid screening method would be to isolate and lyse red blood cells and then use gel electrophoresis to separate hemoglobin proteins based on their electric charge as shown in text Figure 4.8, p. 70. This screen would detect a mutation causing an amino acid substitution that also alters the electric charge of hemoglobin. It would not detect a mutation that does not alter the charge of hemoglobin and so would not detect all mutations that alter the function of hemoglobin.

4.25   *Answer:*

  a. The gel that is shown separates proteins based on their charge. The anode (the positive pole) is at the top, and the cathode (the negative pole) is at the bottom. Since the polypeptide in

Got-2^M Got-2^M homozygotes moves further toward the cathode, it is more positively charged and is therefore more basic.

b. The problem statement indicates that GOT-2 is a homodimer, a protein with two identical polypeptides bound to each other. The single bands seen in *Got-2$^+$ Got-2$^+$* and *Got-2^M Got-2^M* homozygotes indicate that each has one type of homodimer. The homodimer seen in *Got-2$^+$ Got-2$^+$* animals is more negatively charged than the homodimer seen in *Got-2^M Got-2^M* animals. The three bands seen in the *Got-2$^+$ Got-2^M* heterozygote are, in order from anode to cathode, a homodimer composed of *Got-2$^+$* polypeptides, a heterodimer composed of *Got-2^M* and *Got-2$^+$* polypeptides, and a homodimer composed of *Got-2^M* polypeptides. The different band intensities in the middle lane result from the random association of the two types of *Got-2* monomer to form dimers in the ratio of 1 *Got-2$^+$* homodimer : 2 *Got-2$^+$ Got-2^M* heterodimer : 1 *Got-2^M* homodimer.

c. The analysis in part (**b**) indicates that cells that are *Got-2$^+$ Got-2^M* heterozygotes produce two types of monomers that can combine in the ratio 1 *Got-2$^+$* homodimer : 2 *Got-2$^+$ Got-2^M* heterodimer : 1 *Got-2^M* homodimer. In contrast, the text indicates that a single cell produces only one type of β-globin polypeptide, so cells in β^{A}β^S heterozygotes produce hemoglobin with either β^A or β^S globin. When hemoglobin is analyzed by gel electrophoresis, many cells are used, so heterozygotes have two bands. The gel electrophoresis result demonstrates that in contrast to what is seen for β-globin, a *Got-2* monomer is produced from both alleles in a cell of a *Got-2$^+$ Got-2^M* heterozygote. The monomers combine at random to produce three types of dimers in the 1:2:1 ratio described in part (**b**).

4.26 *Answer:*

a. A mouse model for a human disease is a strain of mice that recapitulates some aspects of the human disease. For a human disease caused by a genetic mutation, a mouse model can be developed by using genetic engineering to produce a strain with a genetic alteration similar to that found in the human disease. For example, a mouse model for cystic fibrosis has been developed by making a mouse strain that has the same defect in their CFTR gene as do humans with cystic fibrosis. Mouse models are used to understand the genetic and cellular processes that lead to disease and to test alterative therapeutic strategies.

b. In humans, Tay–Sachs disease is caused by a mutation in the *HEXA* gene that results in the loss of *N*-acetylhexosaminidase A (Hex-A) activity. In normal individuals, Hex-A cleaves an *N*-acetylgalactosamine group from the brain ganglioside. Without Hex-A, ganglioside accumulates in brain neurons, and they degenerate. Therefore, one phenotypic feature of the human disease that a mouse model should recapitulate is the accumulation of ganglioside. How this is accomplished at the genetic level depends on whether mice have an enzyme that performs the biochemical reactions carried out by Hex-A. If mice have such an enzyme, a mouse model could be developed by deleting or otherwise mutating the gene (or genes) for that enzyme. If mice lack this biochemical function, then a mouse model could be developed by introducing a gene (or genes) that would lead to the neuronal accumulation of ganglioside. In humans, the accumulation of ganglioside leads to neurodegeneration, and this produces other disease symptoms. Therefore, one additional phenotypic requirement is that the accumulation of ganglioside leads to neurodegeneration. The phenotypic consequences of neurodegeneration caused by the accumulation of ganglioside in the mouse model may not be identical to those in humans. In humans, early symptoms include an unusually enhanced reaction to sharp sounds and a cherry-colored spot on the retina surrounded by a white halo. Later, they include rapid neurodegeneration that produces generalized paralysis, blindness, a progressive loss of hearing, and serious feeding problems. However, even if the mouse model does not display all of these features, it would still be useful since it would recapitulate some fundamental features of the human disease.

c. If neurons in the mouse model accumulate ganglioside and this leads to neurodegeneration, the model could be used to investigate the biochemical and cellular processes that lead to neurodegeneration. Understanding these processes could be instrumental in designing therapeutic strategies that could delay or prevent this neurodegeneration, and these strategies could then be tested in the mouse model to see if they prevent or diminish neurodegeneration there. The mouse model could also be used to evaluate strategies involving gene therapy, for example, strategies that introduce a functional copy of the *HEXA* gene.

4.27   *Answer:* At one level, the answer to this question is straightforward. Couples who are prospective parents can undergo genetic testing for mutations that result in enzyme deficiencies. If both members of a couple are heterozygous for mutations in the same gene, then they may elect to undergo genetic counseling to assess the risk of having an affected child and to discuss the options available to them concerning prenatal screening.

In practice, however, this question raises very complex issues. First, a decision to undergo genetic testing is associated with certain risks. While the risks associated with drawing blood for the testing procedure itself can be minimal, there are additional risks with very real, significant consequences. These include a risk of emotional discomfort upon learning that one is (or is not) a carrier, risks to personal and familial relationships, and potential risks to privacy, insurability, employment, discrimination, and stigmatization. Second, it is difficult to know which mutations to test for. Sometimes this issue can be rationally addressed if there is a clear family history of a particular inherited disease. However, this may not be the case. For example, for autosomal recessive diseases, family members may show no signs of a disease because they are heterozygous, and some individuals will not know their familial history. In addition, because the genes we have are shared within our ethnic group, the risks we have for different inherited diseases are related to our ethnicity. Given this, genetic screening and testing can raise issues related to cultural and societal values, historical (and perhaps current) levels of discrimination, and the availability and quality of health care services. Third, this question raises personal, philosophical, and religious issues. Some individuals may not be willing to undergo genetic testing out of deeply held personal beliefs. While some couples may be willing to undergo genetic testing and prenatal testing so that they can use this information in planning, they may not be willing to electively terminate a fetus who has a genetically based enzyme deficiency. With current and anticipated advances in genomics (see Chapters 8–10), these and other policy, societal, and ethical issues related to genetic screening and genetic testing are becoming more significant.

4.28   *Answer:*

a. Amniocentesis is typically done after 12 weeks of pregnancy (after the first trimester), while chorionic villus sampling can be done between 8 and 12 weeks of pregnancy. In either sampling method, there is a risk of fetal loss. While chorionic villus sampling can allow parents to learn if the fetus has a genetic defect earlier than does amniocentesis, there is more risk of fetal loss and more chance of an inaccurate diagnosis due to the contaminating presence of maternal cells.

b. These sampling methods offer parents an opportunity to learn about the genetic constitution and health of the fetus early in a pregnancy. If the fetus is diseased, early prenatal diagnosis allows parents to make an informed decision about the pregnancy. They can seek genetic counseling and consider what options might be available to them: to treat the diseased fetus *in utero*, to plan for the care of a diseased child, or to terminate the pregnancy.

c. Such a method would allow for early, *noninvasive* prenatal diagnosis. This would substantially reduce the risk to the fetus and the discomfort to the mother. Since a blood sample could be obtained by many health care professionals and shipped off-site for processing, it would also eliminate the need for a highly skilled physician and sophisticated on-site support services to perform the sampling procedure. Consequently, it would allow for more accessible prenatal testing at lower cost.

4.29   *Answer:*

a. In Caucasians, PKU occurs in about 1 in 12,000 births while CF occurs in about 1 in 2,000 births. In African-Americans and Asian-Americans, the CF frequency is 1 in 17,000 and 1 in 31,000, respectively. Given their relative frequencies in Caucasians, the decision to mandate testing for certain diseases is not based on disease frequency alone.

b. The Guthrie test is a simple clinical screen for phenylalanine in the blood. A drop of blood is placed on a filter-paper disc and the disc placed on solid culture medium containing *B. subtilis* and β-2-thienylalanine. The β-2-thienylalanine normally inhibits the growth of *B. subtilis*, but the presence of phenylalanine prevents this inhibition. Therefore, the amount of growth of *B. subtilis* is a measure of the amount of phenylalanine in the blood. The test provides an easy, relatively inexpensive means to reliably quantify blood phenylalanine levels, making it an effective preliminary screen for PKU in newborn infants.

c. Mandated diagnostic testing requires a highly accurate test—one that has very low false-positive and false-negative rates—as misdiagnosis of a genetic disease in a genetically normal individual has significant potential for emotional distress in the family of the misdiagnosed child and misdiagnosis of an affected individual as normal may delay necessary therapeutic treatment. A set of mutations with a range of different disease phenotypes may make it difficult to employ a single easy-to-use test. For example, different mutations may make it impossible to use just one DNA-based test, and non-DNA-based tests that are effective at diagnosing severe disease phenotypes may not be equally effective at diagnosing mild disease forms because they may give results that overlap with those from normal individuals.

d. Testing for PKU in newborns is essential for early intervention to prevent the toxic accumulation of phenylketones and the resulting neurological damage in early infancy. Unless it is documented that intervention in newborns is critical for CF disease management, testing for CF in newborns is less critical. Testing is warranted to confirm a diagnosis when severe CF symptoms are apparent in a newborn.

4.30   *Answer:* There are no known cures or treatments for these diseases, and individuals with these diseases do not begin to exhibit symptoms until one or more years after birth. It is difficult to justify routine testing in this situation since the information gained from testing will not affect the disease course or outcome.

4.31   *Answer:*

a. Tests can be DNA based and determine the genotype of a parent or fetus or be biochemically based and determine some aspect of the individual's physiology. For example, the Guthrie test determines the relative amount of phenylalanine in a drop of blood to assess whether an individual has PKU; enzyme assays can determine whether a person has a complete or partial enzyme deficiency; gel electrophoresis can determine whether a person has an altered α- or β-globin that might be associated with anemia. DNA-based tests assess the presence or absence of a specific mutation and are normally employed only when there is already suspicion that an individual may carry that mutation (e.g., the couple has already had an affected offspring). Biochemical tests typically focus on assessing gene function, so they are often used in screens. However, they may not provide detailed information about which gene or biochemical step is affected and require that the biochemical activity be present in the tested cell population, such as cells obtained from an amniocentesis.

b. Both PKU and Tay–Sachs disease are caused by autosomal recessive mutations through which each parent contributed one of their autosomes to the affected son, so you would use a DNA-based test to evaluate whether each parent is heterozygous for an allele present in the affected son. If any of the tested parents do not carry the mutation present in their affected son, that son has a new mutation.

c. There are multiple factors to weigh when making this decision. These include the chance that a child will be affected, the type of disease, and whether the disease can be treated effectively. Since each conception is independent, there is a one in four chance of having an affected offspring. Since there is no effective treatment for Tay–Sachs disease, having witnessed their first child suffer from this disease while knowing he could eventually die from it might strongly affect the Liebermans' decision. In contrast, in the Chávezes' case there is an effective treatment for PKU, and knowing whether a fetus is affected could help them anticipate and prepare for their child's needs.

4.32   *Answer:* Your choice!

5

Gene Expression: Transcription

Chapter Outline

Review of Key Terms, Symbols, and Concepts

In your own words, write a brief, precise definition of each term in the groups on this and the next page. Check your definitions using the text. Then develop a concept map using the terms in each list.

1	2	3
central dogma	prokaryotic RNA polymerase	RNA polymerase II
gene expression	transcription initiation	protein-coding genes
replication	promoter	mRNA, snRNA
transcription	closed, open promoter complex	regulatory elements
translation	holoenzyme	general transcription factors
primary transcript	core enzyme	regulatory factors
precursor RNA	sigma factor	core promoter
mRNA	σ^{70}, σ^{32}	promoter-proximal elements
tRNA	heat shock, stress	Goldberg-Hogness, TATA,
rRNA	consensus sequence	CAAT, GC boxes
snRNA	-10, -35 regions	enhancer element
RNA polymerase	Pribnow box	activator
RNA polymerases I, II, III	elongation	upstream activator
prokaryotic genes	proofreading activity	sequence (UAS)
eukaryotic genes	transcription bubble	TBP, TFIIB, D, E, F, H, TAF
structural gene	*rho*-dependent termination	initial committed complex
protein-coding gene	type I, II terminators	minimal transcription
nucleolus	hairpin loop	initiation complex
nucleoplasm	twofold symmetry	complete transcription
nucleus	coupled transcription	initiation complex
gene regulatory elements	and translation	preinitiation complex
5'-to-3', 3'-to-5'	transcription unit	
coding strand	leader, coding, trailer sequences	
template strand	5', 3' UTR	
nontemplate strand	monocistronic, polycistronic	
NTPs	upstream, downstream	

4	5	6
RNA polymerase II	*E. coli* RNA polymerase	spliceosome
transcription unit	RNA polymerase I	snRNPs
leader, trailer, coding sequences	RNA polymerase II	self-splicing
5′, 3′ UTR	RNA polymerase III	group I, II introns
precursor mRNA	28S, 18S, 5.8S, 5S rRNAs	protein-independent reaction
pre-, mature mRNA	bacterial rRNAs	secondary structure
posttranscriptional modification	mRNA	lariat molecule
monocistronic	tRNA	*Tetrahymena* pre-rRNA
5′ cap	snRNA	tRNA genes
5′ 7-methyl guanosine		RNA enzyme
5′–5′, 2′–5′ bonds		ribozyme
capping enzyme		RNA world hypothesis
methylation		
3′ polyadenylation		
poly(A) site, tail		
poly(A) polymerase		
CPSF, CstF, CFI, CFII, PAB II		
introns, exons		
intervening, expressed sequence		
hnRNA, gRNA		
mRNA splicing		
branch-point sequence		
3′, 5′ splice sites		
snRNA, snRNP		
spliceosome		
U1, U2, U4, U5, U6		
RNA lariat structure		
RNA editing		

Thinking Analytically

As transcription and RNA processing are central to gene expression, they have been investigated intensely. Our substantial understanding of these processes is reflected in the wealth of detailed information presented in this chapter. As was the case for understanding DNA replication, the best way to understand and retain this information is to organize the details and place them in context. As you read the chapter, continually refer to the text figures that summarize the key events of transcription and RNA processing. Try explaining the figures to yourself out loud to enhance your understanding. To clarify and solidify your understanding of the material after you have read the chapter once, go through it again and categorize its detailed information.

To start categorizing the information, develop a list of terms and identify their chemical nature. Is the term a region of DNA, of RNA, or part of a protein? After this, relate the term to its function in the overall process of gene expression. If it pertains to DNA, how does it relate to the structure of a gene or a transcription unit? If it pertains to RNA, how does it relate to the RNA being synthesized or being processed? If it pertains to a part of a protein, how is it involved in transcription or RNA processing?

To help you relate a term to its function, construct sketches of the processes of transcription and transcript processing. Diagram how the structure of a gene at the DNA level relates to the structure of its primary transcript at the RNA level. Then diagram how the structure of the primary transcript relates to the structure of the processed, mature transcript.

Next, distinguish between transcription processes and characteristics in prokaryotes and eukaryotes. While there are some similarities between prokaryotes and eukaryotes, many differences exist. It may help to list analogous sites and factors, pairing prokaryotic elements with those doing similar jobs in eukaryotes.

Questions for Practice

Multiple-Choice Questions

1. Each row of the table below lists an item composed of DNA, RNA, and/or protein. Indicate an item's chemical composition by placing an X in the appropriate column(s).

Item	DNA	RNA	Protein
sigma factor			
promoter			
terminator			
transcription factor			
regulatory factor			
Pribnow box			
transcription initiation complex			
snRNP			
spliceosome			
rho			
promoter element			
RNA polymerase core enzyme			
ribozyme			
consensus sequence			
U2			
enhancer			

2. Now indicate whether each item is found only in prokaryotes, only in eukaryotes, or in both prokaryotes and eukaryotes by placing an X in the appropriate column.

Item	Only in Prokaryotes	Only in Eukaryotes	Found in Both
sigma factor			
promoter			
terminator			
transcription factor			
regulatory factor			
Pribnow box			
transcription initiation complex			
snRNP			
spliceosome			
rho			
promoter element			
RNA polymerase core enzyme			
ribozyme			
consensus sequence			
U2			
enhancer			

3. Which of the following statements is correct?
   a. During transcription, the template strand is read in a 3′-to-5′ direction.
   b. During transcription, the template strand is read in a 5′-to-3′ direction.
   c. During transcription, the nontemplate strand is read in a 3′-to-5′ direction.
   d. During transcription, the nontemplate strand is read in a 5′-to-3′ direction.

4. Which of the following statements is correct?
   a. During transcription, an RNA strand is synthesized in the 5′-to-3′ direction.
   b. During transcription, an RNA strand is synthesized in the 3′-to-5′ direction.
   c. During transcription, DNA is synthesized in the 5′-to-3′ direction.
   d. During transcription, DNA is synthesized in the 3′-to-5′ direction.

5. Which of the following statements is *not* correct?
   a. DNA polymerases can proofread, but RNA polymerases cannot.
   b. Some RNA polymerases, but no DNA polymerases, are sensitive to α-amanitin.
   c. Only RNA polymerases can initiate the formation of a polynucleotide.
   d. RNA polymerases synthesize in a 3′-to-5′ direction, while DNA polymerases synthesize in a 5′-to-3′ direction.

6. Which one of the following is essential for RNA polymerase to bind an *E. coli* promoter?
   a. sigma factor
   b. snRNP
   c. TFIID
   d. U1

7. Which one of the following is essential for RNA polymerase II to bind a eukaryotic promoter?
   a. sigma factor
   b. *rho*
   c. TFIID
   d. U1

8. Which of the following statements is *not* correct?
   a. Prokaryotic and eukaryotic mRNAs have 5′ untranslated leader sequences.
   b. Only prokaryotic mRNAs are polyadenylated at their 3′ ends.
   c. In prokaryotes, transcription and translation are coupled.
   d. Consensus sequences can be found in both DNA and RNA.
   e. In eukaryotes, RNA splicing occurs in the nucleus.

Answers:

1. A promoter, terminator, Pribnow box, promoter element, and enhancer are composed of DNA. U2 and a ribozyme are composed of RNA. A sigma factor, transcription factor, regulatory factor, *rho,* and the RNA polymerase core enzyme are composed of protein. Consensus sequences can be found in both RNA and DNA. A transcription initiation complex contains proteins that interact with DNA. Spliceosomes and snRNPs contain both RNA and proteins.

2. Sigma factor, the Pribnow box, *rho,* and the RNA polymerase core enzyme are found only in prokaryotes (*E. coli*). A snRNP, spliceosome, ribozyme, enhancer, and U2 are found only in eukaryotes. A promoter, terminator, transcription factor, regulatory factors, transcription initiation complex, promoter element, and consensus sequence can be found in both eukaryotes and prokaryotes.

3a, 4a, 5d, 6a, 7c, 8b

Thought Questions

1. Compare and contrast each of the following groups of terms with respect to location, function, and host organism (prokaryote or eukaryote).
   a. Pribnow box and TATA element
   b. promoter elements and enhancer elements
   c. the promoters bound by RNA polymerase I, II, III
   d. rRNA genes in prokaryotes and eukaryotes

2. Do prokaryotes or eukaryotes have more RNA polymerase (per unit total protein)? Why should the two groups of organisms differ?

3. How does *rho*-dependent termination differ from *rho*-independent termination? What is the role of the hairpin loop in each of these events? Is the hairpin loop found in DNA or RNA?

4. What takes the place of sigma factor in eukaryotes?

5. Recall that there is no simple relationship between an organism's C-value and its structural and organizational complexity. Do you expect a relationship to exist between the amount of hnRNA and the structural or organizational complexity of the organism? The amount of cytoplasmic mRNA? Why or why not?

6. The promoters for RNA polymerase II have been highly conserved and thus differ little among eukaryotes. Why might this be the case? (Hint: Consider the number of genes transcribed by RNA polymerase II.)

7. Consider what will happen to an mRNA once it is processed, and then address the following questions: How precise does RNA splicing need to be? How precise does transcription initiation need to be? How precise does polyadenylation need to be?

8. What posttranscriptional modifications are routinely made to a eukaryotic mRNA? Where do they occur in the cell?

9. Some transcripts can undergo alternative splicing. What would result from including different exons in different processed mRNAs? How might pre-RNAs be spliced alternatively in different tissues?

Thought Questions for Media

After reviewing the media on the *iGenetics* website, try to answer these questions.

1. At which end of the template strand does transcription begin?

2. When transcription is complete, which strand of DNA is the final RNA molecule identical to if the thymine in DNA is replaced with uracil in RNA?

3. What purpose does the sequence AAUAAA serve in a pre-mRNA's 3' UTR?

1. Suppose a mutation in the β-globin gene introduced a new 3' splice site within its first intron.
   a. In what different ways could the mutation affect the reading frame of the mature mRNA?
   b. If the mature mutant mRNA were translated in the same reading frame after the mutant site, what would its effect be on the β-globin protein?
   c. If the mutation caused the mRNA to be translated in a different reading frame, what would be its effect on the β-globin protein? (Remember that when mRNAs are "read" out of their correct reading frames, stop codons are often introduced.)

2. Suppose a point mutation occurred in the first intron of the β-globin gene but did not change either the branch point, the 5' splice site, or the 3' splice site sequence. Could such a mutation ever affect the level of mRNA transcripts available for translation? How might your answer change if the mutation were a deletion or insertion of 100 base pairs of DNA? (Recall that the first intron is 130 base pairs long.)

3. In the iActivity, the first multiple-choice question describes two forms of beta-thalassemia: beta-plus and beta-zero. Beta-plus thalassemia occurs when a reduced amount of β-globin protein is produced, while beta-zero thalassemia occurs when no β-globin protein is produced.
   a. Do you expect the phenotypes of these forms of thalassemia to be identical in heterozygotes having a disease allele and a normal allele? Why or why not?
   b. Will they be identical in homozygotes for a disease allele? Why or why not?

Solutions to Text Questions and Problems

5.1   *Answer:* While both DNA and RNA are composed of linear polymers of nucleotides, their bases and sugars differ. DNA contains deoxyribose and thymine, while RNA contains ribose and uracil. Their structures also differ. DNA is frequently double-stranded, while RNA is usually single-stranded. Single-stranded RNAs are capable of forming stable, functional, and complex stem-loop structures, such as those seen in tRNAs. Double-stranded DNA is wound in a double helix and packaged by proteins into chromosomes, either as a nucleoid body in prokaryotes or within the eukaryotic nucleus. After being transcribed from DNA, RNA can be exported into the cytoplasm. If it is mRNA, it can be bound by ribosomes and translated. Eukaryotic RNAs are highly processed before being transported out of the nucleus. DNA functions as a storage molecule, while RNA functions variously as a messenger (mRNA carries information to the ribosome), in the processes of translation (rRNA functions as part of the ribosome, tRNA brings amino acids to the ribosome), and in eukaryotic RNA processing (snRNA functions within the spliceosome).

Both DNA polymerases and RNA polymerases catalyze the synthesis of nucleic acids in the 5'-to-3' direction. Both use a DNA template and synthesize a nucleic acid polynucleotide that is complementary to the template. However, DNA polymerases require a 3'-OH to add onto, while RNA polymerases do not. That is, RNA polymerases can initiate chains without primers, while DNA polymerases cannot. Furthermore, RNA polymerases usually require specific base-pair sequences as signals to initiate transcription.

5.2   *Answer:* The DNA sequences that are transcribed into RNA are determined using two general principles. First, signals in the DNA base sequences identify the specific region to be transcribed. Only regions bounded by transcription initiation and transcription termination signals are transcribed. In regions bounded by these signals, only one strand is ordinarily transcribed, so that transcripts are formed in a 5'-to-3' direction using a single DNA template strand. Second, transcription within a defined region occurs only if additional transcription-inducing molecules are present. Some of these molecules recognize the signals within the DNA that define the transcription unit and are used in the transcription process.

5.3   *Answer:* Both eukaryotic and *E. coli* RNA polymerases transcribe RNA in a 5'-to-3' direction using a 3'-to-5' DNA template strand. There are many differences between the enzymes, however. In *E. coli*, a single RNA polymerase core enzyme is used to transcribe genes. In eukaryotes, there are three types of RNA polymerase molecules: RNA polymerase I, II, and III. RNA polymerase I synthesizes 28S, 18S, and 5.8S rRNA and is found in the nucleolus. RNA polymerase II synthesizes hnRNA, mRNA, and some snRNAs and is nuclear. RNA polymerase III synthesizes tRNA, 5S rRNA, and some snRNAs and is also nuclear.

Each RNA polymerase uses a unique mechanism to identify those promoters at which it initiates transcription. In prokaryotes such as *E. coli*, a sigma factor provides specificity to the sites bound by the four-polypeptide core enzyme, so that it binds to promoter sequences. The holoenzyme loosely binds a sequence lying about 35 bp before transcription initiation (the −35 region), changes configuration, and then tightly binds a region lying about 10 bp before transcription initiation (the −10 region) and melts about 17 bp of DNA around this region. The two-step binding to the promoter orients the polymerase on the DNA and facilitates transcription initiation in the 5'-to-3' direction. After about eight or nine bases are formed in a new transcript, sigma factor dissociates from the holoenzyme, and the core enzyme completes the transcription process. Although the principles by which eukaryotic RNA polymerases bind their promoters are similar in that they use a set of ancillary protein factors—transcription factors—the details are quite different. In eukaryotes, each of the three types of RNA polymerases recognizes a different set of promoters by using a polymerase-specific set of transcription factors, and the mechanisms of interaction are different.

5.4   *Answer:* Prokaryotic and eukaryotic genes differ in their gene structure, in their RNA processing, and in how transcription is coupled to translation.

Structure: Prokaryotic genes are defined by an upstream promoter, an RNA-coding sequence, and a downstream terminator. While these three features also exist in eukaryotic genes, eukaryotic promoters are more complex, and nearby or distant enhancer and silencer elements can strongly affect the level of transcription of eukaryotic genes. The RNA-coding sequences of eukaryotes can be interrupted with introns. Finally, prokaryotic mRNAs are often polycistronic, containing the amino acid coding information for more than one gene. In contrast, eukaryotic mRNAs are generally monocistronic, containing the amino acid coding information from just one gene. A notable exception to this general principle is found in *C. elegans*, where polycistronic mRNAs are found at certain loci.

Processing: Prokaryotic genes lack introns, while eukaryotic genes typically have one or more introns; therefore, a transcribed region can be larger than the size of a mature mRNA. The excision of introns from primary mRNAs is only one aspect of the processing of eukaryotic RNAs. In addition, eukaryotic mRNAs are modified at both their 5′ and 3′ ends: They are capped and polyadenylated.

Coupling of transcription and translation: Since prokaryotes lack a nucleus, transcription is directly coupled to translation. In eukaryotes, mRNAs must be processed and then transported out of a nucleus before they are translated by ribosomes in the cytoplasm.

These three differences provide cell types in a multicellular eukaryote with three means to regulate gene expression. Gene expression can be regulated at each of these three levels: transcription, mRNA processing, and translation.

5.5   *Answer:* Termination of transcription in *E. coli* is signaled by controlling elements (sequences within the DNA) called terminators. Two classes of terminators exist, *rho*-independent (Type I) and *rho*-dependent (Type II). Both Type I and Type II termination events lead to the cessation of RNA synthesis and the release of both the RNA chain and the RNA polymerase from the DNA.

Type I terminators utilize sequences with twofold symmetry lying about 16–20 bp upstream of the termination point to signal the termination site (see text Figure 5.5, p. 86). The hairpin loop that forms when a twofold symmetric sequence is transcribed, plus a string of Us, lead to termination, perhaps by destabilizing the RNA–DNA hybrid in the terminator region. Type II terminators lack the structure of Type I terminators and instead use an ATP-activated *rho* protein that binds to recognition sequences in the transcribed termination region. The binding of *rho* leads to the hydrolysis of the ATP and the release of the transcript and the RNA polymerase from the DNA template.

In eukaryotes, transcription termination differs depending on the RNA polymerase under consideration. RNA polymerase I transcribes repeated 18S, 5.8S, and 28S rDNA clusters as single transcription units. Transcription of each unit is terminated at a specific site. The termination site lies in the nontranscribed spacer (NTS) between adjacent rDNA transcription units.

RNA polymerase II transcribes genes for mRNAs and some snRNAs. Transcription termination for these genes is fundamentally different from transcription termination in bacteria because these genes lack specific transcription termination sequences at their 3′ ends. mRNA transcription can continue for hundreds or thousands of nucleotides downstream of the protein-coding sequence until it is past a poly(A) site in the RNA. The poly(A) site is recognized and cleaved by a complex set of proteins. It is positioned 10 to 30 nucleotides after an AAUAAA sequence and is followed by a GU-rich or U-rich sequence. Once the RNA is cleaved, poly(A) polymerase adds A nucleotides onto the 3′-OH of the RNA to produce a poly(A) tail.

RNA polymerase III transcribes genes for 5S rRNA, tRNA and some snRNAs. Termination events for RNA polymerase III were not discussed in this chapter.

5.6   *Answer:* The Pribnow box is the −10 element of the bacterial promoter. It is located at −10 bp relative to the starting point of transcription and has the consensus sequence 5′-TATAAT-3′ (in the coding strand). A second consensus sequence is located about 35 bp before transcription initiation (the −35 region). Each of these sequences is important for the binding of RNA polymerase and initiation of RNA transcription. At the start of transcription initiation, the holoenzyme loosely binds the −35 region and then changes configuration and tightly binds the −10 region. It melts about 17 bp of DNA around this region. The two-step binding to the promoter orients the polymerase on the DNA and facilitates transcription initiation in the 5'-to-3' direction, as shown in text Figure 5.4, p. 85, and the figure below:

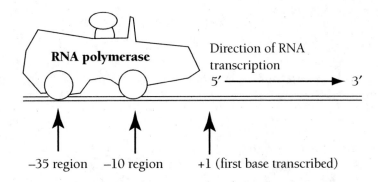

5.7 *Answer:*

a, b. There are multiple 5'-AG-3' sequences in each strand, and transcription may proceed in either direction. Determine the correct initiation site by locating the −10 and −35 consensus sequences recognized by RNA polymerase and σ⁷⁰. Good −35 (TTGACA) and −10 (TATAAT) consensus sequences are found on the top strand, starting at the 8th and 32nd bases from the 5' end, respectively, indicating that the initiation site is the 5'-AG-3' starting at the 44th base from the 5' end of that strand.

c. Transcription proceeds from left to right in this example.

d. the bottom (3'-to-5') strand

e. the top (5'-to-3') strand

5.8 *Answer:* In the figure below, possible −10 and −35 regions of each sequence are boxed and consensus sequences are in boldface type.

Gene	−35 Region	−10 Region	Initiation Region
lac	ACCCAGGCTT**TACACT**TTATGGCTTCCGGCTCG**TATGTT**GTGTGGAATTGTGAGCGG		
lacI	CCATCGAATG**GCGCAA**AACCTTTCGCGGTATGG**CATGAT**AGCGCCCGGAAGAGAGTC		
galP2	ATTTATTCCAT**GTCACA**CTTTTCGCATCTTTGT**TATGCT**ATGGTTATTTCATACCAT		
araB,A	GGATCCTAC**CTGACG**CTTTTTATCGCAACTCTC**TACTGT**TTCTCCATACCCGTTTTT		
araC	GCCGTGATTA**TAGACA**CTTTTGTTACGCGTTTT**TGTCAT**GGCTTTGGTCCCGCTTTG		
trp	AAATGAGCTG**TTGACA**ATTAATCATCGAACTAG**TTAACT**AGTACGCAAGTTCACGTA		
bioA	TTCCAAAAC**GTGTTT**TTTGTTGTTAATTCGGTG**TAGACT**TGTAAACCTAAATCTTTT		
bioB	CATAATCGAC**TTGTAA**ACCAAATTGAAAAGATT**TAGGTT**TACAAGTCTACACCGAAT		
tRNA^Tyr	CAACGTAACAC**TTTACA**GCGGCGCGTCATTTGA**TATGAT**GCGCCCCGCTTCCCGATA		
rrnD1	CAAAAAAATAC**TTGTGC**AAAAAATTGGGATCCC**TATAAT**GCGCCTCCGTTGAGACGA		
rrnE1	CAATTTTTCTA**TTGCGG**CCTGCGGAGAACTCCC**TATAAT**GCGCCTCCATCGACACGG		
RRNa2	AAAATAAATGC**TTGACT**CTGTAGCGGGAAGGCG**TATTAT**GCACACCCCGCGCCGCTG		

a. Two sequences (*rrnD1, rrnE1*) have perfect matches with the −10 consensus sequence, and one sequence (*trp*) has a perfect match with the −35 consensus sequence.

b. Examining these sequences illustrates that the identification of a consensus sequence in a promoter or another DNA sequence does not mean that the same sequence will always be present in a specific region. A consensus sequence is identified by determining the most common base at a particular position in a specified region in a large number of aligned sequences. For example, in the set of sequences shown here, the most frequently found bases in each position of the

−10 region are 5′-TATGAT-3′. The most frequent bases in all of the positions except for the fourth position match −10 region consensus sequence (5′-TATAAT-3′).

c. These are the sites that the RNA polymerase holoenzyme initially recognizes and binds to during transcription initiation.

d. It is likely to have some functional importance, perhaps because it, like these consensus sequences, is recognized by a protein.

e. Sequences closer to the consensus sequence may be more easily recognized by the RNA polymerase holoenzyme. This could result in more efficient transcription initiation so that the gene is more frequently transcribed.

5.9   Answer:

a. *E. coli* promoters vary with the type of sigma factor that is used to recognize them. More than four types of promoters exist, each having different recognition sequences. Most promoters have −35 and −10 sequences that are recognized by σ^{70}. Other promoters have consensus sequences that are recognized by different sigma factors, which are used to transcribe genes needed under altered environmental conditions such as heat shock and stress (σ^{32}), limiting nitrogen (σ^{54}), or when cells are infected by phage T4 (σ^{23}).

b. Although there is one core RNA polymerase enzyme, different RNA polymerase holoenzymes are formed from different sigma factors. Promoter recognition is determined by the sigma factor.

c. Utilizing different sigma factors allows for a quick response to altered environmental conditions (for example, heat shock, low N_2, phage infection) by the coordinated production of a set of newly required gene products.

5.10   Answer: The two cultures will have a different collection of mRNAs, as *E. coli* RNA polymerase will transcribe a different set of genes in response to a heat shock. Under heat-shock conditions, σ^{32} increases in amount and directs the core RNA polymerase to bind to the promoters of genes that encode proteins needed to cope with the heat-related stress. Hence, in response to a heat shock, genes with promoters that are recognized by σ^{70} will not be transcribed as often as are genes with promoters that are recognized by σ^{32}. This will lead to the presence of a different collection of mRNAs in the two cultures.

5.11   Answer: RNA polymerase I is located in the nucleolus and transcribes the major rRNA genes that code for 18S, 5.8S, and 28S rRNAs; RNA polymerase II is located in the nucleoplasm and transcribes the protein-coding genes to produce mRNA molecules and some snRNAs; RNA polymerase III is located in the nucleoplasm and transcribes the 5S rRNA genes, the tRNA genes, and some small nuclear RNAs. All transcription occurs in the nucleus, and only some RNAs are transported into the cytoplasm.

In the cell, the 18S, 5.8S, 28S, and 5S rRNAs are structural and functional components of the ribosome, which functions during translation in the cytoplasm. After processing, mRNAs are transported into the cytoplasm where they are translated to produce proteins. The tRNAs are also transported into the cytoplasm, where they bring amino acids to the ribosome to donate to the growing polypeptide chain during protein synthesis. Small nuclear RNAs function in nuclear processes such as RNA splicing and processing.

5.12   Answer:

a.

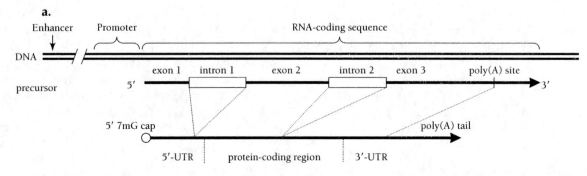

b.

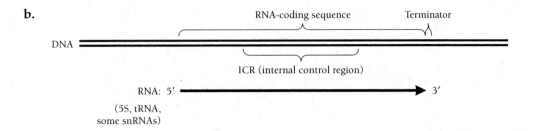

5.13   *Answer:* By convention, DNA sequence is given 5'-to-3'. This is the same polarity as the antitemplate strand, the strand that is complementary to the 3'-to-5' template strand used for transcription. By using this convention, analyzing a DNA sequence is made easier. If a region of the sequence is transcribed, the RNA will have an identical sequence, except that U will replace T.

Transcription units should be flanked at their 5' ends by promoter elements. Therefore, approach this problem by first surveying the sequence for the GC, CAAT, and TATA box consensus sequences. The figure below identifies these sequences using underlined, non-italic uppercase letters and italic notes. The approximate site of transcription initiation is noted, and the RNA-coding region of the DNA strand is italicized. An mRNA that could be produced (a conceptual mRNA) is given in lowercase letters. This mRNA has two signals (noted and underlined) that could be used by the ribosome to recognize the start and termination of translation. Initiation of a polypeptide chain is signaled by a 5'-AUG-3' codon (encoding a methionine). Chain termination is signaled by a UAA stop codon. Features of translation are described in Chapter 6.

```
              −80                    −65                   −50
           GC element              CAAT box             GC element
    5'  AGAGGGCGGT  CCGTATCGGC  CAATCTGCTC  AGAGGGCGGA


                                 −30
                               TATA box
        TTCACACGTT  GTTATATAAA  TGACTGGGCG  TACCCCAGGG


+1 (approx., conceptual)
                transcription          potential
                initiation          translation start
        TTCGAGTATT  CTATCGTATG  GTGCACCTGA  CT(...)
    mRNA    5'uauu  cuaucguaug  gugcaccuga  cu(...)


                               potential
                            translation stop
        GCTCACAAGT  ACCACTAAGC  (...)
        gcucacaagu  accacuaagc  (...)
```

5.14   *Answer:* Introns are removed from a pre-mRNA molecule by the action of a spliceosome. Consensus sequences at the intron–exon boundaries and within the intron itself are recognized by spliceosome components as the spliceosome assembles around the intronic sequence. First, U1 snRNP binds to the 5' splice site by base-pairing interactions between the U1 snRNA and the 5' splice site sequence. Then, U2 snRNP binds to a branch-point region inside of the intron. Following the association of a preassembled U4/U6/U5 particle with the bound U1 and U2 snRNPs, U4 snRNP dissociates from the complex, allowing the formation of an active spliceosome. Splicing proceeds via cleavage of the 5' exon–intron junction, attaching the 5' end of the intron sequence to a branch-point sequence via an unusual 2'-5' bond, and then cleavage at the 3' exon–intron junction. When the two exons are ligated together, a lariat structure composed of intron sequences is released. See text Figure 5.12, p. 93, and Figure 5.13, p. 94.

5.15   *Answer:*

a. The double-stranded regions represent the pairing of a processed mRNA with the DNA from which the precursor-mRNA was transcribed. Therefore, the single-stranded regions represent sequences present in DNA that are not present in the mature mRNA. Thus, the image shows that mature mRNAs are missing sequences present in DNA, and it provides evidence for the existence of introns that are spliced out of pre-mRNAs.

b. There are seven single-stranded, looped regions, so the pre-mRNA for ovalbumin has 7 introns and 8 exons.

c. The mRNA was purified from the cytoplasm. mRNAs purified from the nucleus would include pre-mRNAs that do not have all of their introns removed. As pre-mRNAs are processed, they are exported from the nucleus through nuclear pores.

5.16   *Answer:*

a. The pre-mRNA will be capped, its intron removed, and polyadenylated. So it will have 1 (5′ m⁷G cap) + 40 (exon 1) + 60 (exon 2) + 200 (poly(A) tail) = 301 bases.

b. The U1 snRNA is part of the U1 snRNP that recognizes the 5′ splice site. It recognizes this site by base pairing between the U1 snRNA and the first two bases of the intron. If the U1 snRNA has an A-to-G base substitution at the position marked by the asterisk, it will not recognize the 5′ splice site and so the intron will not be removed. The transcript would have an additional 135 intronic bases and be 436 bases long.

c. To pair with the G in the mutant U1 snRNA, the U at the asterisked site in the RNA would need to be changed to a C. The U in the RNA is encoded by an A in the DNA template strand, so an AT-to-GC DNA base-pair mutation would lead to a C at the asterisked position.

5.17   *Answer:*

a. Splicing produces two RNAs: the 100-base mature mRNA that results from the splicing of exons 1 and 2, and a lariat structure formed when the 5′ end of the intron becomes attached via a 2′–5′ phosphodiester bond to an A nucleotide within the branch-point sequence. The lariat structure will be degraded, while the spliced structure containing exons 1 and 2 will be capped and polyadenylated, with a final length of 301 bases. The following figure shows the structures produced by splicing.

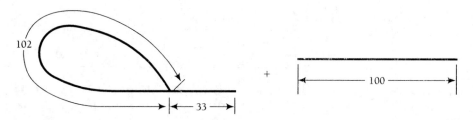

b. The mutation will prevent U1 snRNP from recognizing the 5′ splice site. Therefore, the intron will not be recognized and removed by a spliceosome and a linear, 235-base-long molecule will be found. If this molecule is capped and polyadenylated, it will be 436 bases long.

c. The mutation alters the branch-point A nucleotide as well as an adjacent A nucleotide and so will prevent U2 snRNP from binding to the branch-point sequence. The intron will not be recognized and removed by the spliceosome, and a linear 235-base-long molecule will be found.

d. This mutation alters the 3′ splice site and thus could hinder its cleavage. Since U1 snRNP will be able to identify the 5′ splice site and U2 snRNP the branch point, spliceosome formation and the splicing process can proceed until a lariat is formed. However, if the 3′ splice site cannot be cleaved by the spliceosome, exon 1 will not become spliced to exon 2, because the intron will remain in a lariat structure attached to exon 2. The following figure illustrates the structures that could be formed:

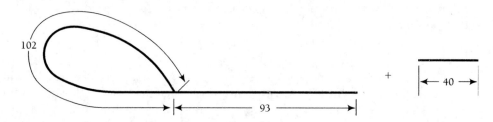

5.18   *Answer:* Group I introns are self-splicing. Unlike the removal of introns from most eukaryotic mRNAs, removal of group I introns does not require a spliceosome containing snRNAs and protein-splicing factors. In group I introns, the intron folds in a protein-independent manner to catalyze the splicing reaction.

While both splicing mechanisms result in the joining of RNA sequences flanking an intron, the more widespread use of spliceosomes to remove introns may reflect advantages associated with this mechanism. For example, it may allow greater flexibility in the sequence composition of an intron because specific secondary structures do not have to form, while still allowing for the precise removal of intronic sequences (using consensus sequences at the 5′ and 3′ splice sites and the branch point). Spliceosome processing of introns may also allow for greater diversity in intron size. The group I intron in the *Tetrahymena* pre-rRNA is 413 bp. In contrast, introns processed by spliceosomes can be from tens to thousands of base pairs. As discussed in Chapter 18, intron removal using spliceosomes can also be regulated using protein factors. This allows for an additional level of control over gene expression. Thus, splicing mechanisms using spliceosomes allow for greater diversity in intron composition and gene expression than do self-splicing mechanisms.

5.19   *Answer:* The RNA world hypothesis proposes that RNA-based life predates the present-day DNA-based life. In an RNA world, RNAs carried out catalytic reactions necessary for life in presumably primitive cells. After group I intron self-splicing was discovered in *Tetrahymena* intron RNA, RNA enzymes, or ribozymes, were developed by modifying *Tetrahymena* intron RNA and other self-cleaving RNAs so that they could function catalytically to cleave RNA molecules at specific sequences. The discovery that RNA could function as an enzyme led to the formulation of the RNA world hypothesis.

5.20   *Answer:*

a. snRNAs are found in the nucleus and are used in RNA splicing. They form snRNPs by complexing with proteins. snRNPs assemble around intronic sequences (starting with U1 snRNP binding to the 5′ splice site and U2 snRNP binding to the branch-point sequence) to form spliceosomes that remove the intronic sequences and splice together exonic sequences (see text Figure 5.13, p. 94).

gRNAs are found in the nucleus and mitochondria and are involved in RNA editing, the posttranscriptional insertion or deletion of nucleotides or the modification of one base to another. In trypanosomes where RNA editing results in the removal and insertion of U nucleotides, the gRNA pairs with the mRNA transcript and is thought to be responsible for cleaving the transcript, templating the missing U nucleotides, and ligating the transcript back together again.

b. snRNAs are highly abundant with at least 10^5 copies per cell. Their abundance reflects the large number of transcripts with introns that must be processed before the transcripts are exported from the nucleus into the cytoplasm for translation.

5.21   *Answer:*

a. The coding strand is the DNA strand that has the same sequence as the RNA except that T in DNA is replaced by U in RNA. The template strand is the DNA strand that is used as a template for RNA synthesis, and so is the strand that is complementary to the RNA. Therefore, the top (5′-to-3′) strand is the coding strand, and the bottom (3′-to-5′) strand is the template strand.

b. The RNA has been subjected to a posttranscriptional modification. In particular, the 23rd base in the RNA has been posttranscriptionally edited from a U to a G.

5.22   *Answer:* A recessive lethal is a mutation that causes death when it is homozygous—that is, when only mutant alleles are present. Heterozygotes for such mutations can be viable. Recessive lethal mutations result in death because some essential function is lacking. Neither copy of the gene functions, so the organism dies.

a. Deletion of the U1 genes will be recessive lethal, as U1 snRNA is essential for the identification of the 5′ splice site in RNA splicing. Incorrect splicing would lead to nonfunctional gene products for many genes, a nonviable situation.

b. This mutation would prevent U1 from base-pairing with 5′ splice sites and thus, by the same reasoning as in (**a**), would be recessive lethal.

c. If a deletion within intron 2 did not affect a region important for its splicing (for example, the branch point or the regions near the 5′ or 3′ splice sites), it would have no effect on the mature mRNA produced. Consequently, such a mutation would lack a phenotype if it were homozygous. However, if the splicing of intron 2 were affected and the mRNA altered, such a mutation, if homozygous, could result in the production of only nonfunctional hemoglobin, leading to severe anemia and death.

d. The deletion described would affect the 3′ splice site of intron 2, leading to, at best, aberrant splicing of that intron. If the mutation were homozygous, only a nonfunctional protein would be produced, resulting in severe anemia and death.

5.23   *Answer:* 1 (5′ m^{7}G cap) + 100 (exon 1) + 50 (exon 2) + 25 (exon 3) + 200 (poly(A) tail) = 376 bases.

5.24   *Answer:* The first two bases of an intron are typically 5′–GU–3′ and are essential for base-pairing with the U1 snRNA during spliceosome assembly. A GC-to-TA mutation at the initial base pair of the first intron impairs base pairing with the U1 snRNA, so that the 5′ splice site of the first intron is not identified. This causes the retention of the first intron in the *tub* mRNA and a longer mRNA transcript in *tub/tub* mutants. When the mutant *tub* mRNA is translated, retention of the first intron could result in the introduction of amino acids not present in the *tub*$^+$ protein or, if the intron contained a chain termination (stop) codon, premature translation termination and the production of a truncated protein. In either case, a nonfunctional gene product is produced.

The *tub* mutation is recessive because the single *tub*$^+$ allele in a *tub/tub*$^+$ heterozygote produces mRNAs that are processed normally, and when these are translated, enough normal (*tub*$^+$) product is produced to obtain a wild-type phenotype. Only the *tub* allele produces abnormal transcripts. When both copies of the gene are mutated in *tub/tub* homozygotes, no functional product is made and a mutant, obese phenotype results.

6

Gene Expression: Translation

Chapter Outline

Review of Key Terms, Symbols, and Concepts

In your own words, write a brief, precise definition of each term in the groups below and on the following page. Check your definitions using the text. Then, develop a concept map using the terms in each list.

1	2	3
protein	genetic code	translation
polypeptide	triplet code	aminoacyl-tRNA synthetase
amino acid	codon	codon recognition
α-carbon	frameshift mutation	specificity of codon recognition
R group	revertant	initiation
peptide bond	reversion	elongation
acidic, basic, neutral polar,	random copolymers	termination
neutral nonpolar amino acid	ribosome-binding assay	aminoacyl-tRNA
C, N terminus	cell-free, protein-synthesizing	charged tRNA
primary structure	system	transformylase
secondary structure	open reading frame	fMet, tRNA.fMet
tertiary structure	comma-free code	tRNA.Met
quaternary structure	nonoverlapping code	30S, 70S initiation complex
conformation	universal, degenerate,	ribosome-binding site
α-helix	redundant code	Shine--Dalgarno sequence
β-pleated sheet	start, stop codon	IF1, IF2, IF3, eIFs cap binding
heteromultimeric	sense, nonsense codon	protein
hydrogen bond	wobble hypothesis	PABP
ionic interaction		Kozak sequence
sulfur bridge		scanning model
van der Waals force		peptidyl transferase
chaperone		P, A, E sites
		EF-Tu, EF-Ts, EF-G, GTP
		translocation
		polyribosome
		polysome
		release factor
		RF1, RF2, RF3, eRF1, eRF3
		UGA, UAG, UAA codon
		ribosome recycling factor (RRF)

4	5	6
endoplasmic reticulum	tRNA	*E. coli* RNA polymerase
membrane-bound ribosome	codon	RNA polymerase I
signal hypothesis	anticodon	S-value, sedimentation rate
signal sequence	cloverleaf	30S, 50S ribosomal subunits
signal recognition particle (SRP)	stem-loop structure	70S ribosome
SRP receptor	complementary base-pairing	23S, 16S, 5S rRNA
signal peptidase	chemically modified base	40S, 60S ribosomal subunits
Golgi apparatus	pre-tRNA molecule	80S ribosome
cisternal space	*E. coli* RNA polymerase	28S, 18S, 5.8S, 5S rRNA
glycoprotein	RNA polymerase III	ribosomal protein
		rDNA, rDNA repeat unit
		rDNA transcription unit
		precursor rRNA
		ribonuclease
		spacer sequence

Thinking Analytically

Much of the material presented in this chapter is detailed and descriptive. The initiation, elongation, and termination of translation are all complex events. Each involves ribosomal subunits, RNAs, and stage-specific factors that differ in prokaryotes and eukaryotes. As in the past two chapters, placing the information in context will help you learn and retain it.

There are several levels in which to organize this chapter's information. Develop an understanding of the differences between the three types of RNAs used in translation (mRNA, rRNA, and tRNA) by contrasting what you previously learned about the formation and transcriptional organization of mRNA with new information presented in this chapter on the transcriptional organization and structure of tRNA and rRNA. Second, consider the level of spatial organization. Associate the different types of RNA (rRNA, mRNA, tRNA) and factors involved in translation with the different components of the translation machinery in the cell. Third, construct a temporal framework to follow these components through the stages of translation. For prokaryotes, and then for eukaryotes, what RNAs and factors are components of the first initiation complex? What RNAs and factors are present during elongation? What new factors are required for termination? Fourth, come back to the level of spatial organization. For eukaryotes, once proteins are synthesized, what factors are used to shuttle them to the appropriate location?

Keep in mind the polarity of DNA and RNA when analyzing DNA sequences, inferring the RNAs produced from DNA, and identifying translation reading frames in a mRNA. Transcripts are always synthesized in the 5'-to-3' direction using the 3'-to-5' DNA template strand, and polypeptides are always synthesized starting at their N terminus using codons that start relatively nearer to the 5' end of the mRNA. The rhyme "5 to 3, N to C" may help you remember the orientations of mRNA and polypeptides. Pay close attention to maintain the correct mRNA, tRNA anticodon, and DNA polarity.

One of the highlights of this chapter is the presentation of a set of elegant experiments used to decipher the genetic code. These technically demanding experiments addressed one of the fundamental questions in genetics: How is information in DNA used to code for proteins? Consider them carefully, and consider how interpreting them often uses probabilistic thinking. The product rule, which states that the frequency of two independent events occurring together is the product of their separate probabilities, allows one to deduce the appropriate codons that specify particular amino acids. Consider the following related problem:

    a. A synthetic mRNA is generated by randomly polymerizing adenine and guanine ribonucleotides. What codons would be formed, and what would be their relative frequency, if the synthesis began with a limitless mixture of 3 adenine to 1 guanine?

b. When the mRNAs generated in **(a)** are added to a cell-free translation system, polypeptides are formed that, on average, have about 55% lysine, about 19% arginine, about 19% glutamic acid, and about 7% glycine. What can you infer about codon usage from these data (without consulting a table of the genetic code)?

Answer: First, determine what possible codons (three-nucleotide combinations) could be generated. Then determine the frequency of that codon by multiplying together the probability of obtaining each base in one codon. Since there is a 3 A:1 G ratio, the chance of finding an A is $\frac{3}{4}$, and the chance of finding a G is $\frac{1}{4}$.

$$P(AAA) = (\tfrac{3}{4})^3 = 0.421875 \sim 42\%$$

$$p(AAG) = (\tfrac{3}{4})^2 (\tfrac{1}{4}) = 0.140625 \sim 14\%$$

$$p(AGA) = (\tfrac{3}{4})^2(\tfrac{1}{4}) = 0.140625 \sim 14\%$$

$$p(AGG) = (\tfrac{3}{4})(\tfrac{1}{4})^2 = 0.046875 \sim 5\%$$

$$p(GAA) = (\tfrac{1}{4})(\tfrac{3}{4})^2 = 0.140625 \sim 14\%$$

$$p(GAG) = (\tfrac{1}{4})^2(\tfrac{3}{4}) = 0.046875 \sim 5\%$$

$$p(GGA) = (\tfrac{1}{4})^2(\tfrac{3}{4}) = 0.046875 \sim 5\%$$

$$p(GGG) = (\tfrac{1}{4})^3 = 0.015625 \sim 2\%$$

Since AAA accounts for about 42% of the total codons that are translated, and only lysine constitutes at least 42% of the amino acid content of the polypeptides, AAA must encode lysine. By similar reasoning, GGG must encode glycine. Since there is only 7% glycine, and no codon alone accounts for 7% of the total codon usage, glycine must be encoded by at least two codons. GGG must be one of these, since if any other two codons encoded glycine, the amount of glycine would exceed 7%. The remaining glycine must be encoded by one of the GAG, GGA, or AGG codons, since they are represented 5% of the time. The remaining lysine must be encoded by either AAG, AGA, or GAA, as no combination of other codons would give 55% lysine. This leaves arginine to be encoded by one of the AAG, AGA, GAA codons and one of the AGG, GAG, GGA codons. Similarly, glutamic acid must be encoded by one of the AAG, AGA, GAA codons and one of the AGG, GAG, GGA codons. To make additional inferences, more experimentation (e.g., with different copolymers) must be done.

Questions for Practice

Multiple-Choice Questions

1. The term *secondary structure* refers to a polypeptide's
   a. sequence of amino acids.
   b. structure that results from local interactions between the residues of different amino acids.
   c. folding that results from local and distant interactions between the residues of different amino acids.
   d. interactions with a second polypeptide chain.

2. The eukaryotic equivalent of the Shine–Dalgarno sequence is the
   a. 60S large ribosomal subunit.
   b. 40S small ribosomal subunit.
   c. 5′ cap of the mRNA.
   d. poly(A) tail.

3. In which stage of translation is GTP *not* used?
   a. initiation
   b. elongation
   c. translocation
   d. termination

4. Which of the following are the same in both prokaryotes and eukaryotes?
   a. elongation factors
   b. stop codons
   c. the use of fMet.tRNA
   d. AUG initiation codons
   e. both b and d

5. Specificity in translation is obtained by all of the following *except*
   a. using specific tRNA synthetases for each amino acid.
   b. using an anticodon.
   c. using a degenerate triplet code having codons for each amino acid.
   d. using RNA polymerase.

6. In which of the following are coding sequences *not* found?
   a. introns
   b. exons
   c. mRNA
   d. hnRNA

7. In an unprocessed, newly synthesized eukaryotic protein,
   a. the N terminus is encoded by sequences in the 5′ region of the mRNA.
   b. the C terminus is encoded by sequences in the 5′ region of the mRNA.
   c. the first amino acid is always f-methionine.
   d. the last amino acid is always encoded by the codon AAA.

8. During translation in *E. coli*,
   a. an intact 70S ribosome binds the mRNA during initiation.
   b. Shine–Dalgarno sequences present in the mRNA align it with the 23S rRNA.
   c. both initiation and elongation require energy in the form of GTP.
   d. termination occurs when the ribosome recognizes a chain termination codon with the aid of EF-Tu.

9. The RNAs that are used in eukaryotic translation include all of the following *except*
   a. 5S rRNA.
   b. 28S rRNA.
   c. mRNA.
   d. tRNA.
   e. snRNA.

10. In eukaryotes, proteins destined to remain in the cell are distributed by all of the following *except*
    a. packaging into secretory vesicles.
    b. complexing with an SRP using an N-terminal signal sequence.
    c. using posttranslational transport.

Answers: 1b, 2c, 3d, 4e, 5d, 6a, 7a, 8c, 9e, 10a

Thought Questions

1. The following sequence of bases in *E. coli* DNA is part of a gene. Mark the region that, if transcribed, will form the first codon to be translated. Mark the region that, if transcribed, will form a Shine–Dalgarno sequence. Is the strand shown the template or nontemplate strand? (Hint: Find the initiation codon. Be careful about polarity!)

   5′-CCGCATTCCTCCGGCGGGACCTACT-3′

2. Why is the code for methionine not degenerate? (Hint: What special role does methionine play in translation?)

3. What are the components of a cell-free, protein-synthesizing system? What is the function of each?

4. Describe three complementary methods by which the genetic code was deciphered. Is any single method sufficient to completely decipher the code? What advantages and disadvantages does each method have?

5. The genetic code is nearly universal. To what extent does this indicate that the code acquired its basic form very early in the evolution of cells?

6. Consider which bases can wobble to base-pair with each other. What structural similarities exist between bases at the 3′ end of a codon that can wobble to base-pair with the base at the 5′ end of the anticodon?

7. What percentage of 70S ribosomes do you expect to be associated with mRNA in prokaryotes? What percentage of 80S ribosomes do you expect to be associated with mRNA in eukaryotes?

8. Discuss the various ways in which proteins within a cell are targeted for secretion. How can a genetic approach be used to dissect the secretory pathway?

9. How do prokaryotes and eukaryotes differ in the mechanisms they use to identify the first codon in a reading frame? In what ways are the mechanisms similar?

10. How are posttranscriptional modifications to mRNA important for translation?

Thought Questions for Media

After reviewing the media on the *iGenetics* website, try to answer these questions.

1. How does the ribosome IF–GTP complex identify where it should bind to the mRNA?
2. What are the functions of EF-Tu and EF-G in translation elongation?
3. When in translation is GTP hydrolysis required?
4. Review the A, E, and P sites on the ribosome. Which site never has a charged tRNA in it? Which site is only bound by a charged tRNA or a RF? Which site is almost always occupied by a tRNA with an attached polypeptide?
5. Peptidyl transferase provides two functions, one during translation elongation and one during translation termination. Are they the same enzymatic function?

1. Based on viewing the iActivity, what different features of a coding region mutation would cause it to be associated with a mutant phenotype?
2. What type of coding region mutations have no effect whatsoever on protein function?
3. What type of coding region mutations are likely to have little, if any, effect on protein function?

Solutions to Text Questions and Problems

6.1 *Answer:* A protein is composed of one or more polypeptides, each of which is composed of a folded, linear chain of amino acids. Proteins function in many different ways, including as enzymes to catalyze biochemical reactions, as structural molecules (e.g., actin, myosin, tubulin), as receptors (e.g., on the cell surface, for small signaling molecules such as neurotransmitters), as transporters (e.g., a protein that transports sugars across a membrane), as ion channels (e.g., the protein defective in cystic fibrosis, CFTR, transports Cl⁻ ions), and as regulatory molecules (e.g., transcription factors).

6.2 *Answer:*

a. The hemoglobin will dissociate into its four component subunits, because the heat will destabilize the ionic bonds that stabilize the quaternary structure of the protein. An individual subunit's tertiary structure may also be altered, because the thermal energy of the heat may destabilize the folding of the polypeptide.

b. The protein will denature. Its secondary and tertiary structures are destabilized by heating, so it does not retain a pattern of folding that allows it to be soluble.

c. The protein will denature when its secondary and tertiary structures are destabilized by heating. Unlike albumin, RNase will renature if cooled slowly and will reestablish its normal, functional tertiary structure.

d. It is likely that the meat proteins will be denatured when their secondary, tertiary, and quaternary structures are destabilized by the acid conditions of the stomach. Then the primary structure of the polypeptides will be destroyed as they are degraded into their amino acid components by proteolytic enzymes in the digestive tract.

e. Valine is a neutral, nonpolar amino acid, unlike the acidic glutamic acid (see text Figure 6.2, p. 104). A change in the chemical properties of the sixth amino acid may alter the function of the hemoglobin molecule by affecting multiple levels of protein structure. Since it is an amino acid substitution, it changes the primary structure of the β-polypeptide. This change could affect local interactions between amino acids lying near it, and in doing so, alter the secondary structure of the β-polypeptide. It could also affect the folding patterns of the protein and alter the tertiary structure of the β-polypeptide. Finally, the sixth amino acid residue is known to be important for interactions between the subunits of hemoglobin molecules (see text Figures 4.9–4.11, pp. 71–72) because some mutations which alter that amino acid result in sickle-cell anemia. Thus, this change could alter the quaternary structure of hemoglobin.

6.3 *Answer:*

a. The primary structure, or amino acid sequence, of the prion protein would be unchanged because the disease is caused not by a mutation, but rather by misfolding of the prion protein. One misfolded protein can convert a normally folded protein to the misfolded state, so the misfolded proteins are infectious. The secondary structure is affected because α-helical regions are misfolded into β-pleated sheets. This is likely to lead to an altered tertiary structure that results in the formation of amyloid.

b. If a genetic mutation led to an amino acid substitution, it would affect the primary structure of the prion protein. A particular amino acid substitution in the prion protein could make it more susceptible to being misfolded and lead, as in **(a)**, to changes in its secondary and tertiary structures.

6.4 *Answer:* b

6.5 *Answer:* At each position of a four-base-long codon, there will be one of four possible bases. So, there are $4 \times 4 \times 4 \times 4 = 4^4 = 256$ possible codons. This is far more than is needed to code for 20 amino acids. On the other hand, if there were only two bases in a codon, there would be only $4 \times 4 = 4^2 = 16$ possible codons, too few to uniquely specify 20 amino acids. Codons three bases long provide for $4 \times 4 \times 4 = 4^3 = 64$ possible codons.

6.6   *Answer:* The minimum word size must be able to uniquely designate 20 amino acids, so the number of combinations must be at least 20. The following table gives the number of combinations as a function of word size.

	Word Size	Number of Combinations
a.	5	$2^5 = 32$
b.	3	$3^3 = 27$
c.	2	$5^2 = 25$

6.7   *Answer:*   Stage A: $4^2 = 16$ different meaningful triplets.
Stage B: $4^2 \times 2 = 32$ different meaningful triplets.

6.8   *Answer:*

a. Proflavin causes the addition or deletion of a single DNA base pair. If this occurs within a gene's protein-coding sequence, it causes a frameshift mutation that changes the reading frame after the mutant site.

b. Wild-type r^+ phage and mutants at the *rII* locus have different growth responses in the *E. coli* B strain. An *rII* mutant produces clear plaques, while the wild-type r^+ strain produces turbid plaques. This difference allows for the selection of mutants. Therefore, to select for *rII* mutants, infect the mutagenized T4 phage into *E. coli* B and select clear plaques. Some of these will be *rII* mutants.

c. Wild-type r^+ phage, but not *rII* mutants, can grow on strain *E. coli* K-12(λ). Select for revertants by infecting the *rII* mutants into *E. coli* K-12(λ), plating the bacteria, and screening for plaques. Since only r^+ phage can grow on K-12(λ), each plaque must be formed by a revertant phage.

d. Mutation *rII*^{X} is caused by a base-pair insertion (+ mutation) that disrupts the reading frame downstream of the insertion. Not all of the revertants must affect the same base pair, because they need only to restore the reading frame. A deletion (− mutation) of the inserted base pair would precisely revert the mutation and restore the reading frame. A deletion (− mutation) of a nearby base pair, at a site just before or after the site mutated in *rII*^{X}, would restore the reading frame near the mutant site and could lead to a functional protein. The following figure illustrates how a reading frame can be restored by a second-site mutation. In the figure, nucleotides are shown in groups of three to facilitate the identification of codons, black boxes highlight the base inserted by a + mutation (the type of mutation in *rII*^{X}) and alterations to the reading frame, and a grey box highlights the base that will be deleted by a − mutation.

Wild type

DNA	5′ ATG TCT TAT TGT CTT GGG CCC... 3′
	3′ TAC AGA ATA ACA GAA CCC GGG... 5′
RNA	5′ AUG UCU UAU UGU CUU GGG CCC... 3′
Polypeptide	Met Ser Tyr Cys Leu Gly Pro...

Mutation altering the reading frame caused by the insertion of an A–T base pair (+ mutation)

DNA	5′ ATG ATC TTA TTG TCT TGG GCC C... 3′
	3′ TAC TAG AAT AAC AGA ACC CGG G... 5′
RNA	5′ AUG AUC UUA UUG UCU UGG GCC C... 3′
Polypeptide	Met Ile Leu Leu Ser Trp Ala...

Reversion restoring the reading frame caused by the deletion of a second-site − mutation.

DNA sequence prior to a 1 bp deletion:

DNA: 5' ATG ▮TC T▮A TTG TCT TGG GCC C... 3'
               3' TAC ▮AG A▮T AAC AGA ACC CGG G... 5'

Sequences following a 1-bp deletion:

DNA: 5' ATG ▮TC TAT TGT CTT GGG CCC... 3'
               3' TAC ▮AG ATA ACA GAA CCC GGG... 5'

RNA: 5' AUG ▮UC UAU UGU CUU GGG CCC... 3'

Polypeptide: Met **Ile** Tyr Cys Leu Gly Pro...

In this example, the sequence with the restored reading frame retains a missense mutation.

e. All of the revertants must result from a deletion (− mutation) of a base pair nearby the base pair inserted in the *rII*^{X} mutations, so all are double mutants. As illustrated in the figure in part **(d)**, some of the codons nearby the base pair inserted in *rII*^{X} will be altered. Consequently, the proteins produced in the revertants will have a short segment with one or more incorrect amino acids followed by the normal sequence of amino acids. Since the phage has a wild-type phenotype, the presence of the incorrect amino acids must not have eliminated the protein's function.

f. Recombination allows the mutant site introduced in the revertant to be separated from the original mutant site. Therefore, recombination would separate the two *rII* mutations and give two products: the original 1-base-pair insertion mutant (*rII*^{X}) and, since the cause of the reversion is a deletion, a 1-base-pair deletion (−) mutant. Select for revertants of the − mutant just as in part **(c)**: Infect the mutant into *E. coli* K-12(λ), plate the bacteria, and screen for plaques. Only r^+ phage can grow, so revertants will have a 1-base-pair insertion nearby or at the deleted base. Revertants of − *rII* mutants will be + *rII* mutants.

g. The *rII*^{Y} mutant is a − mutation, so combining it with another − mutant will give a double mutant having two nearby − mutations. The *rII* reading frame will not be restored, so the double mutant will be a *rII* mutant. Proflavin treatment causes a 1-base-pair insertion or deletion. Proflavin can restore the reading frame and produce r^+ phage only if it introduces a third − mutation nearly the other two. The following figure illustrates the effects of recombining two nearby − mutations onto one chromosome. A chromosome with two nearby − mutations will not have a restored reading frame, but adding a third − mutation will restore the reading frame. In the following figure, black boxes highlight the altered bases and changes to the reading frame.

Wild type (the three bases in black boxes will be deleted sequentially, from left to right)

DNA: 5' ATG ▮CT ▮A▮ TGT CTT AGG GCC... 3'
               3' TAC ▮GA ▮T▮ ACA GAA TCC CGG... 5'

RNA   5' AUG ▮CU ▮A▮ UGU CUU AGG GCC... 3'

Polypeptide   Met Ser Tyr Cys Leu Arg Ala...

Deleting one base (− mutation) alters the reading frame.

DNA sequence prior to a 1-bp deletion:

DNA   5' ATG ▮CT ▮A▮ TGT CTT AGG GCC... 3'
              3' TAC ▮GA ▮T▮ ACA GAA TCC CGG... 5'

Sequences following 1-bp deletion:

DNA   5' ATG CT▮ A▮T GTC TTA GGG CC... 3'
              3' TAC GA▮ T▮A CAG AAT CCC GG... 5'

RNA   5' AUG CU▮ A▮U GUC UUA GGG CC... 3'

Polypeptide   Met **Leu Ile Val Leu Gly**...

Deleting a second base (− mutation) further alters the reading frame.

DNA sequence prior to a second 1-bp deletion:

DNA   5′ ATG CT**T** A**TT** GTC TTA GGG CC... 3′
                  3′ TAC GA**A** T**AA** CAG AAT CCC GG... 5′

Sequences after a second 1-bp deletion:

DNA   5′ ATG CTA **T**TG TCT TAG GGC C... 3′
                  3′ TAC GAT **A**AC AGA ATC CCG G... 5′

RNA   5′ AUG CUA **U**UG UCU UAG GGC C... 3′

Polypeptide   Met **Leu Leu Ser Stop**

Deleting a third base (− mutation) restores the reading frame.

DNA sequence after two 1-bp deletions:

DNA   5′ ATG CTA **T**TG TCT TAG GGC C... 3′
                  3′ TAC GAT **A**AC AGA ATC CCG G... 5′

Sequences after a third 1-bp deletion:

DNA   5′ ATG CTA TGT CTT AGG GCC... 3′
                  3′ TAC GAT ACA GAA TCC CGG... 5′

RNA   5′ AUG CUA UGU CUU AGG GCC... 3′

Polypeptide   Met **Leu** Cys Leu Arg Ala...

In this example, one amino acid has been deleted, and one amino acid is different from that in the original reading frame when three − mutations restore the reading frame.

h. Obtaining an r^+ phage requires that the reading frame be restored. A reading frame will be restored by multiple single-base deletions only if the number of deleted bases is the same as the number of bases in a codon. Therefore, since three nearby − mutations restore the reading frame and give an r^+ phenotype, the genetic code must be triplet. Proflavin-induced revertants would not be recovered in part **(g)** unless the genetic code was triplet. The figure in part **(g)** illustrates that since amino acids are specified by three bases, three − mutations are able to restore the reading frame. Suppose that amino acids were not specified by three bases, but were instead specified by four bases. Then, as shown in the following figure, it would take four − mutations to restore the reading frame. In the following figure, nucleotides are arranged in groups of four, black boxes highlight the four bases that will be deleted and alterations to the reading frame, and aa1, aa2, aa3, . . . , aa20 represent hypothetical amino acids encoded by 4-base codons.

Wild type (the four bases in black boxes will be deleted sequentially, from left to right)

DNA   5′ AAAA **TTTT** **GGG**G CCCC AAAA TTTT GGGG CCCC... 3′
                  3′ TTTT **AAAA** **CCC**C GGGG TTTT AAAA CCCC GGGG... 5′

RNA   5′ AAAA **UUUU** **GGG**G CCCC AAAA UUUU GGGG CCCC... 3′

Polypeptide   aa1   aa2   aa3   aa4   aa1   aa2   aa3   aa4...

Deleting one base (− mutation) alters the reading frame.

DNA sequence prior to a 1-bp deletion:

DNA   5′ AAAA **TTT**T **G**GGG CCCC AAAA TTTT GGGG CCCC... 3′
                  3′ TTTT **AAA**A **C**CCC GGGG TTTT AAAA CCCC GGGG... 5′

Sequences after a 1-bp deletion:

DNA   5′ AAAA TT**TG** **G**GGC CCCA AAAT TTTG GGGC CCC... 3′
                  3′ TTTT AA**AC** **C**CCG GGGT TTTA AAAC CCCG GGG... 5′

RNA   5′ AAAA UU**UG** **G**GGC CCCA AAAU UUUG GGGC CCC... 3′

Polypeptide   aa1 **aa5 aa6 aa7 aa8 aa9 aa10**...

Deleting a second base (– mutation) further alters the reading frame.

DNA sequence prior to a second 1-bp deletion:

DNA   5′ AAAA TTTG GGGC CCCA AAAT TTTG GGGC CCC... 3′
                3′ TTTT AAAC CCCG GGGT TTTA AAAC CCCG GGG... 5′

Sequences after a second 1-bp deletion:

DNA   5′ AAAA TTGG GGCC CCAA AATT TTGG GGCC CC... 3′
                3′ TTTT AACC CCGG GGTT TTAA AACC CCGG GG... 5′

RNA   5′ AAAA UUGG GGCC CCAA AAUU UUGG GGCC CC... 3′

Polypeptide   aa1 aa11 aa12 aa13 aa14 aa11 aa12...

Deleting a third base (− mutation) further alters the reading frame.

DNA sequence prior to a third 1-bp deletion:

DNA   5′ AAAA TTGG GGCC CCAA AATT TTGG GGCC CC... 3′
                3′ TTTT AACC CCGG GGTT TTAA AACC CCGG GG... 5′

Sequences after a third 1-bp deletion:

DNA   5′ AAAA TTGG GCCC CAAA ATTT TGGG GCCC C... 3′
                3′ TTTT AACC CGGG GTTT TAAA ACCC CGGG G... 5′

RNA   5′ AAAA UUGG GCCC CAAA AUUU UGGG GCCC C... 3′

Polypeptide   aa1 aa11 aa16 aa17 aa18 aa19 aa20...

Deleting a fourth base (− mutation) restores the reading frame.

DNA sequence prior to a fourth 1-bp deletion:

DNA   5′ AAAA TTGG GGCC CCAA AATT TTGG GGCC CC... 3′
                3′ TTTT AACC CCGG GGTT TTAA AACC CCGG GG... 5′

Sequences after a fourth 1-bp deletion:

DNA   5′ AAAA TTGG CCCC AAAA TTTT GGGG CCCC... 3′
                3′ TTTT AACC GGGG TTTT AAAA CCCC GGGG... 5′

RNA   5′ AAAA UUGG CCCC AAAA UUUU GGGG CCCC... 3′

Polypeptide   aa1 aa11 aa4 aa1 aa2 aa3 aa4...

By showing that combinations of three − mutations or three + mutations were able to restore r^+ function, Crick and his colleagues were able to conclusively demonstrate that the genetic code was a triplet code.

6.9   *Answer:* Determine the expected amino acids in each case by calculating the expected frequency of each kind of triplet codon that might be formed and inferring from these what types and frequencies of amino acids would be used during translation.

    a. 4 A : 6 C gives $2^3 = 8$ codons, specifically AAA, AAC, ACC, ACA, CCC, ACA, CAC, and CAA. Since there is 40% A and 60% C,

$P(\text{AAA}) = 0.4 \times 0.4 \times 0.4 = 0.064$, or 6.4% Lys
$P(\text{AAC}) = 0.4 \times 0.4 \times 0.6 = 0.096$, or 9.6% Asn
$P(\text{ACC}) = 0.4 \times 0.6 \times 0.6 = 0.144$, or 14.4% Thr
$P(\text{ACA}) = 0.4 \times 0.6 \times 0.4 = 0.096$, or 9.6% Thr (24% Thr total)
$P(\text{CCC}) = 0.6 \times 0.6 \times 0.6 = 0.216$, or 21.6% Pro
$P(\text{CCA}) = 0.6 \times 0.6 \times 0.4 = 0.144$, or 14.4% Pro (36% Pro total)
$P(\text{CAC}) = 0.6 \times 0.4 \times 0.6 = 0.144$, or 14.4% His
$P(\text{CAA}) = 0.6 \times 0.4 \times 0.4 = 0.096$, or 9.6% Gln

b. 4 G:1 C gives $2^3 = 8$ codons, specifically GGG, GGC, GCG, GCC, CGG, CGC, CCC, and CCG. Since there is 80% G and 20% C,

$P(\text{GGG}) = 0.8 \times 0.8 \times 0.8 = 0.512$, or 51.2% Gly

$P(\text{GGC}) = 0.8 \times 0.8 \times 0.2 = 0.128$, or 12.8% Gly (64% Gly total)

$P(\text{GCG}) = 0.8 \times 0.2 \times 0.8 = 0.128$, or 12.8% Ala

$P(\text{GCC}) = 0.8 \times 0.2 \times 0.2 = 0.032$, or 3.2% Ala (16% Ala total)

$P(\text{CGG}) = 0.2 \times 0.8 \times 0.8 = 0.128$, or 12.8% Arg

$P(\text{CGC}) = 0.2 \times 0.8 \times 0.2 = 0.032$, or 3.2% Arg (16% Arg total)

$P(\text{CCC}) = 0.2 \times 0.2 \times 0.2 = 0.008$, or 0.8% Pro

$P(\text{CCG}) = 0.2 \times 0.2 \times 0.8 = 0.032$, or 3.2% Pro (4% Pro total)

c. 1 A:3 U:1 C gives $3^3 = 27$ different possible codons. Of these, one will be UAA, a chain-terminating codon. Since there is 20% A, 60% U, and 20% C, the probability of finding this codon is $0.6 \times 0.2 \times 0.2 = 0.024$, or 2.4%. All of the remaining 26 (97.6%) codons will be sense codons. Proceed in the same manner as in **(a)** and **(b)** to determine their frequency, and determine the kinds of amino acids expected. To take the frequency of nonsense codons into account, divide the frequency of obtaining a particular amino acid considering all 27 possible codons by the frequency of obtaining a sense codon. This gives

$(0.8/0.976)\% = 0.82\%$ Lys

$(3.2/0.976)\% = 3.28\%$ Asn

$(12.0/0.976)\% = 12.3\%$ Ile

$(9.6/0.976)\% = 9.84\%$ Tyr

$(19.2/0.976)\% = 19.67\%$ Leu

$(28.8/0.976)\% = 29.5\%$ Phe

$(4.0/0.976)\% = 4.1\%$ Thr

$(0.8/0.976)\% = 0.82\%$ Gln

$(3.2/0.976)\% = 3.28\%$ His

$(4.0/0.976)\% = 4.1\%$ Pro

$(12.0/0.976)\% = 12.3\%$ Ser

The chains produced likely would be relatively short due to the chain-terminating codon.

d. 1 A:1 U:1 G:1 C will produce $4^3 = 64$ different codons, all possible in the genetic code. The probability of each codon is $1/64$, so there will be a $3/64$ chance of a codon being chain terminating. With those exceptions, the relative proportion of amino acid incorporation is dependent directly on the codon degeneracy for each amino acid. Inspecting the table of the genetic code in text Figure 6.7, p. 111, and taking the frequency of nonsense codons into account yields the following table:

Amino Acid	Number of Codons	Frequency	Amino Acid	Number of Codons	Frequency
Trp	1	$1/61 = 1.64\%$	Cys	2	3.28%
Met	1	1.64%	Ile	3	$3/61 = 4.92\%$
Phe	2	$2/61 = 3.28\%$	Val	4	$4/61 = 6.56\%$
Try	2	3.28%	Pro	4	6.56%
His	2	3.28%	Thr	4	6.56%
Gln	2	3.28%	Ala	4	6.56%
Asn	2	3.28%	Gly	4	6.56%
Lys	2	3.28%	Leu	6	$6/61 = 9.84\%$
Asp	2	3.28%	Arg	6	9.84%
Glu	2	3.28%	Ser	6	9.84%

6.10   *Answer:* In population 1, the codons that can be produced encode Lys (AAA, AAG), Arg (AGG, AGA), Glu (GAG, GAA), and Gly (GGA, GGG). All of these are sense codons, so long polypeptide chains containing these amino acids will be synthesized. In population 2, the codons that can be produced are the sense codons for Lys (AAA), Asn (AAU), Ile (AUA, AUU), Tyr (UAU), Leu (UUA), Phe (UUU), and a nonsense codon (UAA). The frequency of the nonsense codon will be $(\frac{1}{4} \times \frac{3}{4} \times \frac{3}{4}) = \frac{9}{64} = 0.14$, or 14%. Thus, the polypeptides formed in population 2 will, on average, be shorter than those formed in population 1. If a nonsense codon appears about 14% of the time, there will be, on average, $1/0.14 = 7.14$ codons from one nonsense codon to the next. On average, six sense codons will lie in between a nonsense codon, so polypeptides will be synthesized that are about six amino acids long.

6.11   *Answer:*

1. Triplet: Three nucleotides specify either the insertion of an amino acid into a polypeptide chain or a chain termination event.

2. Continuous: An mRNA-coding region is read in a continuous fashion without skipping nucleotides.

3. Nonoverlapping: A coding region is read in a nonoverlapping manner. Triplets are read sequentially.

4. Nearly universal: Nearly all organisms use the same code, with exceptions found in mammalian mitochondria and the nuclear genomes of some protozoa.

5. Degenerate: More than one codon typically codes for a single amino acid.

6. Signals start and stop: The code has translation stop (chain termination) and translation start signals. AUG, which encodes methionine within a coding region, is usually used as a start codon. One of three nonsense (*not sensing* an amino acid) codons are used as chain termination codons.

7. Wobble: The 5′ base of some anticodons wobbles, so that some tRNAs can recognize multiple codons (coding for the same amino acid).

6.12   *Answer:* Though mRNA, rRNA, and tRNA are all single-stranded, each has unique features. Features unique to mRNA are a 5′ untranslated leader sequence, a protein-coding sequence, and a 3′ untranslated trailer sequence (see text Figure 5.8, p. 90). In prokaryotes, the Shine–Dalgarno sequence within the 5′ untranslated leader sequence is essential for the identification of the correct start codon by the small ribosomal subunit. In eukaryotes, the processing of mRNAs to have 5′ caps and 3′ poly(A) tails, and the removal of intronic sequences, are important for their translation (see text Figures 5.9b, 5.10, 5.11, and 5.12, pp. 90–93).

   rRNAs have three sizes in prokaryotes (5S, 16S, 23S) and four sizes in eukaryotes (5S, 5.8S, 18S, and 28S). The three prokaryotic rRNAs and three of the eukaryotic rRNAs (5.8S, 18S, and 28S) are produced by processing a single rRNA precursor transcript (the eukaryotic 5S rRNA is transcribed separately). They fold in a complex manner and have both structural and functional roles in the ribosome.

   tRNA molecules are small, about 4S, and consist of a single chain of 75 to 90 nucleotides. There is extensive base pairing between different parts of the tRNA molecule, allowing it to form a cloverleaf secondary structure having three or four loops. The tRNA molecule functions to carry amino acids to the ribosome. An amino acid is attached to its 3′ end in the cytoplasm for delivery to the ribosome. After an anticodon in loop II binds to the mRNA, the ribosome transfers the amino acid to a growing polypeptide chain. There is extensive posttranscriptional modification of tRNA bases, so that tRNAs contain modified bases such as inosine, ribothymidine, pseudouridine, dihydrouridine, methylguanosine, dimethylguanosine, and methylinosine (see text Figure 6.9).

   Therefore, mRNA, rRNA, and tRNA differ considerably in structure and have very different secondary and tertiary structures achieved by intramolecular base-pairing interactions. These interactions, in the case of rRNA and tRNA, are essential for them to fulfill their different functions. Therefore, one general hypothesis for why these molecules differ in structure is that these differences facilitate their function during translation.

6.13   *Answer:*

    a. 3

    b. 1, 2, 3, 4

    c. 3

    d. 1, 2

    e. 1 (Note that some tRNAs and rRNAs have introns.)

    f. 4

    g. 1

6.14   *Answer:*

    a. Prokaryotic and eukaryotic ribosomes each have two subunits with parallel functions and components. However, as presented in Chapter 5, the detailed constituents differ. The 70S prokaryotic ribosome has a 30S small subunit containing a 16S rRNA and 20 different proteins, and a 50S large subunit containing a 23S rRNA and 5S rRNA and 34 different proteins. The larger 80S eukaryotic ribosome has a 40S small subunit, containing an 18S rRNA and about 35 proteins, and a 60S large subunit, containing 28S, 5.8S, and 5S rRNAs and about 50 ribosomal proteins. In both eukaryotic and prokaryotic ribosomes, the proteins serve as structural units that help to organize the rRNA into key ribozyme elements.

    b. Ribosomes function in translation, which proceeds through three phases: initiation, elongation, and termination. During the initiation phase of translation, the small subunit, with the aid of initiation factors, is bound to the mRNA and the initiating aminoacyl-tRNA (tRNA.fMet in prokaryotes, an initiator Met-tRNA in eukaryotes). The large subunit binds, forming an initiation complex with the initiator tRNA in the P site of the ribosome. During elongation, a second aminoacyl-tRNA is bound to the A site in the ribosome, the peptidyl transferase activity of the ribosome catalyzes the formation of the peptide bond, a now-uncharged tRNA is released (from the E site of the large subunit), and the ribosome translocates one codon down the mRNA. Translation elongation continues, so that codons are matched to amino acids in a growing polypeptide chain, until a stop (nonsense) codon is reached. Stop codons are recognized by release factors, which initiate three processes: the release of the polypeptide from the tRNA in the P site, the release of the tRNA from the ribosome, and the dissociation of the two ribosomal subunits and the release factor from the mRNA.

6.15   *Answer:*

    a. 3'-TAC AAA ATA AAA ATA AAA ATA AAA ATA...-5' (The first fMet or Met is removed following translation of the mRNA.)

    b. 5'-ATG TTT TAT TTT TAT TTT TAT TTT TAT...-3'

    c. 3'-AAA-5' is the anticodon for Phe, and 3'-AUA-5' is the anticodon for Tyr.

6.16   *Answer:* Text Figure 6.7, p. 108, and text Table 6.1, p. 109, aid in answering this question. The answer is given in the following table:

Amino Acid	tRNAs Needed	Rationale
Ile	1	3 codons can use 1 tRNA (wobble)
Phe	1	2 codons can use 1 tRNA (wobble)
Tyr	1	"
His	1	"
Gln	1	"
Asn	1	"
Lys	1	"
Asp	1	"

Amino Acid	tRNAs Needed	Rationale
Glu	1	"
Cys	1	"
Trp	1	1 codon
Met	2	Single codon, but need one tRNA for initiation and one tRNA for elongation
Val	2	4 codons: 2 can use 1 tRNA (wobble)
Pro	2	"
Thr	2	"
Ala	2	"
Gly	2	"
Leu	3	6 codons: 2 can use 1 tRNA (wobble)
Arg	3	"
Ser	3	"
Total	32	61 codons

6.17   *Answer:* The template strand is the one read to produce the mRNA. It is complementary to the mRNA and has an opposite polarity. The nontemplate strand has the same 5'-to-3' polarity as the mRNA, and if U is replaced by T, the same sequence. Use the polypeptide segment and a table of the genetic code to determine the possibilities that exist for the first three codons of the mRNA (read 5'-to-3') and the sequence of the nontemplate DNA strand. Let N = any nucleotide, Y = a pyrimidine (C or U), and R = a purine (G or A).

amino acids: Arg — Gly — Ser

potential codons: 5'   AGR   GGN   AGY 3'
                              or   or
                            CGN   UCN

nontemplate strand sequence: 5'   AGR   GGN   AGY 3'
                                            or   or
                                          CGN   TCN

By comparing the nontemplate strand sequence to the one given, the top strand is the nontemplate strand, with the 5' end on the right side. The template strand is the bottom strand, and transcription occurs from right to left. The C terminus and the N terminus of the polypeptide segment can also be determined from this information.

```
- - - - 3'-GGCTAGCTGCTTCCTTGGGGA-5'- - - -
          |||||||||||||||||||||
- - - - 5'-CCGATCGACGAAGGAACCCCT-3'- - - -
```

Transcribed into: 3' GGC UAG CUG CUU CCU UGG GGA 5'
Translated into: C-Arg-Asp-Val-Phe-Ser-Gly-Arg-N

6.18   *Answer:* Since a dipeptide is formed, translation initiation is not affected, nor is the first step of elongation—the binding of a charged tRNA in the A site and the formation of a peptide bond. However, since *only* a dipeptide is formed, it appears that translocation is inhibited.

6.19   *Answer:*

   a. By saying that the genetic code is degenerate, we mean that more than one codon occurs for each amino acid.

   b. Two synonymous codons encode the same amino acid. Examination of the genetic code shown in text Figure 6.7, p. 108, shows that two of the four columns have amino acids that are present in more than one of the four rows. For these amino acids, a particular change in the first base of a codon will specify the same amino acid. Examine the genetic code and notice that Leu and Arg are both present in multiple rows in one column. These amino acids have codons where a mutation in the first nucleotide can result in a synonymous codon. Eight codons have this property: four of each of the six Leu and six Arg codons could have mutations in the first nucleotide that produce a synonymous codon. For Leu, synonymous codons would be produced by mutations causing a U-to-C change in the first nucleotide of codons UUA and UUG, and by mutations causing a C-to-U change in the first nucleotide of codons CUA and CUG. For Arg, synonymous codons would be produced by mutations causing a C-to-A change in the first nucleotide of codons CGA and CGG, and by mutations causing an A-to-C change in the first nucleotide of codons AGA or AGG.

   c. No amino acids have codons where a mutation in the second nucleotide can result in a synonymous codon. If such codons existed, the same amino acid would have to be present in multiple columns within one row of text Figure 6.7.

   d. Many codons have the property that mutations in the third nucleotide generate a synonymous codon. Indeed, in text Figure 6.7, any square that contains two or more codons specifying the same amino acid identifies codons with this property. To identify which codons do not have this property, examine text Figure 6.7 to identify amino acids that appear just once in 1 of the 16 squares. This will reveal that Met and Trp have codons where a mutation in the third nucleotide never generates a synonymous codon. Two codons, AUG (Met) and UGG (Trp), show this property.

   e. There are 61 sense codons and 3 nonsense codons. All of the sense codons except the two identified in part **(d)** can be changed by a single nucleotide mutation to a synonymous codon. Therefore, $(61 - 2)/61 = 59/61 = 96.7\%$ of sense codons can be changed by a single nucleotide mutation to a synonymous codon. Text Figure 6.7 indicates that the genetic code is highly degenerate. Since most of the degeneracy occurs at the third nucleotide position, mutations that affect this position often lead to synonymous codons.

   f. Though silent mutations do not alter the amino acid sequence of a protein, they can affect the rate of translation. Not all amino acyl-tRNA molecules are equally abundant, and a change from a wild-type to a synonymous codon may result in a codon being read by a rare acyl-tRNA. This will result in a slower rate of translation. A slower rate of translation may affect how chaperones interact with the newly synthesized polypeptide and alter its folding. Two polypeptides with identical amino acid sequences that are folded differently may have different functional properties. As a result, silent mutations could affect progression of disease and response to drug treatments.

6.20   *Answer:* Codon usage bias results from the more frequent use of just some of the degenerate codons for one amino acid. From the data shown here, the four codons for alanine are used frequently and at relatively similar frequencies—the largest difference between the usage of the four codons is that GCG is used about twice as much as GCU. In contrast, two of the six codons for arginine are used at much lower frequencies. For example, CGU is used about ten times more frequently than is AGG. In addition, 2 of the codons, AGA and AGG, are used much less than the other 8 codons. For example, AGG is used in only $(2,915/1,611,503) \times 100\% = 0.18\%$ of all codons and $[2,915/(32,590 + 33,547 + 6,166 + 9,955 + 4,656 + 2,915)] \times 100\% = 3.2\%$ of Arg codons.

   If one codon for an amino acid is used much more frequently than a second codon for the same amino acid, it follows that many more tRNAs are available to pair with the first codon than with the second codon. Such variation in tRNA abundance could affect the translation rate of proteins with many rarely used codons. Such proteins would be translated more slowly, since it will take longer for the less abundant tRNAs to be matched to their codons. Here, the wild-type sequence uses the more frequently used codons for arginine and alanine, as does nucleotide sequence variant 2. In contrast, nucleotide sequence variant 1 uses the less frequently utilized codons for arginine (AGA, AGG) and alanine (GCU, GCA). Thus, nucleotide sequence variant 1 should be used to try to diminish the rate of translation of the *ECs4312* mRNA since it is most likely to be translated more slowly.

6.21   *Answer:*

   a. The normal tRNA has the anticodon 5'-GGG-3', which binds to the codons 5'-CCC-3' and (because of wobble) 5'-CCU-3'. Both of these codons encode Pro (proline).

   b. The mutant tRNA has the anticodon 5'-GGA-3', which recognizes the codons 5'-UCC-3' and (because of wobble) 5'-UCU-3'. Since the amino acid that is attached to the tRNA is unaffected by a mutant anticodon, the mutant tRNA will continue to carry proline to the ribosome.

   There are two consequences of the anticodon mutation. First, since 5'-UCC-3' and 5'-UCU-3' encode Ser (serine), the mutant tRNA will compete with the normal tRNA.Ser in the cell for binding to UCC and UCU codons during the translation of an mRNA. In a percentage of UCC codons, this leads to the insertion of proline instead of serine into a polypeptide chain. Second, unless the cell normally has an additional tRNA.Pro able to bind to the codons 5'-CCC-3' and 5'-CCU-3' (e.g., a tRNA with the anticodon 5'-IGG-3'), these codons would no longer be able to be read as sense codons. Consequently, when the ribosome encounters these codons in an mRNA, it will stall and chain termination will occur. This would lead to truncated proteins.

6.22   *Answer:* The anticodon 5'-GAU-3' recognizes the codon 5'-AUC-3', which encodes Ile. The mutant tRNA anticodon 5'-CAU-3' would recognize the codon 5'-AUG-3', which normally encodes Met. The mutant tRNA would therefore compete with tRNA.Met for the recognition of the 5'-AUG-3' codon, and if successful, insert Ile into a protein where Met should be. Since a special tRNA.Met is used for initiation, only AUG codons other than the initiation AUG will be affected. Thus, this protein will have four different N terminal sequences, depending on which tRNA occupies the A site in the ribosome when the codon AUG is present there:

        Met-Val-Ser-Ser-Pro-**Ile**-Gly-Ala-Ala-**Ile**-Ser

        Met-Val-Ser-Ser-Pro-**Met**-Gly-Ala-Ala-**Ile**-Ser

        Met-Val-Ser-Ser-Pro-**Ile**-Gly-Ala-Ala-**Met**-Ser

        Met-Val-Ser-Ser-Pro-**Met**-Gly-Ala-Ala-**Met**-Ser

6.23   *Answer:* The normal tRNA recognizes the codon 5'-UAC-3', and so must have carried the amino acid tyrosine. The altered anticodon will recognize the codon 5'-UAA-3', a chain termination codon. Consequently, a tyrosine will be inserted when the nonsense codon UAA in an mRNA is positioned in the A site of the ribosome. This will result in read-through of the mRNA some of the time (when the termination factor does not compete for binding to the chain termination codon), and the addition of amino acids onto the C terminus of the protein. mRNAs having UAG and UGA chain termination codons will not be affected.

6.24   *Answer:* Aminoacylation of tRNAs occurs enzymatically using aminoacyl-tRNA synthetases. To provide for specificity in charging a tRNA, a separate aminoacyl-tRNA synthetase exists for each amino acid. This prevents an inappropriate amino acid from becoming attached to a tRNA. If an inappropriate amino acid were attached to a tRNA, the wrong amino acid would be inserted into a growing polypeptide chain, even with correct codon–anticodon base-pairing between the mRNA and tRNA.

   Aminoacyl-tRNA synthetases catalyze two sequential reactions to attach an amino acid to its appropriate tRNA. The first reaction results in the formation of an aminoacyl–AMP complex from the amino acid and ATP. The second reaction results in a covalent bond between the carboxyl group of the amino acid and the last ribose at the 3' end of the tRNA (see text Figure 6.9, p. 11).

6.25   *Answer:* In both prokaryotes and eukaryotes, the initiating codon of a transcript is AUG, recognized by a special charged tRNA (tRNA.fMet in prokaryotes, initiator Met-tRNA in eukaryotes). This first codon is recognized in part because it is in a particular context: In prokaryotes, it is near the Shine–Dalgarno sequence, while in eukaryotes, it is embedded in a Kozak sequence. It is possible that if it were mutated, the 30S (in prokaryotes) or 40S (in eukaryotes) initiation complex would not form correctly, since the initiator tRNA would not find the correct initiator codon. The consequence of this would be that the mRNA would not be translated. On the other hand, if another AUG codon was very close by (and in eukaryotic mRNAs, embedded in a Kozak-type sequence), it might be used as an initiation codon, but the mRNA might be translated at a lower efficiency.

6.26   *Answer:* In both prokaryotes and eukaryotes, protein synthesis is initiated using special initiator tRNAs. In prokaryotes, methionine is attached to tRNA.fMet by methionine-tRNA synthetase, and transformylase catalyzes the addition of a formyl group to the methionine. The resulting fMet-tRNA.fMet is used at the AUG initiation codon. In eukaryotes, the N-terminal methionine is not formylated, but a special initiator methionine-tRNA is still used.

In both prokaryotes and eukaryotes, an initiation complex containing the small ribosomal subunit, initiator factors, GTP, and the mRNA forms sequentially. In prokaryotes, after IF1, IF2, IF3, and GTP bind to the 30S ribosomal subunit, fMet-tRNA.fMet and the mRNA attach to form the 30S initiation complex. The mRNA is aligned using an internal ribosome-binding site (the Shine–Dalgarno sequence) lying near the AUG initiation codon that base-pairs with sequences at the 3′ end of the 16S rRNA. After the 50S ribosomal subunit binds, GTP is hydrolyzed and IF1 and IF2 are released, leaving a 70S initiation complex. In eukaryotes, after eIF4A binds to the 5′ cap of the mRNA, a complex of the 40S ribosomal subunit, the initiator Met-tRNA.Met, GTP, and additional eIFs bind. Only after the 40S ribosomal subunit scans and finds the initiator codon does the 60S ribosomal subunit bind. This displaces the eIFs and produces the 80S initiation complex.

In both prokaryotes and eukaryotes, chain termination is signaled by one of three stop codons (UAG, UAA, UGA). These stop codons do not code for an amino acid, but are recognized with the help of termination factors or release factors. Of the three RFs in *E. coli*, RF1 recognizes UAA and UAG, RF2 recognizes UAA and UGA, and RF3 stimulates chain termination. Eukaryotes have a single release factor, eRF, that recognizes all three stop codons. The release factors trigger release of the polypeptide from the tRNA in the P site of the ribosome, release of the tRNA from the ribosome, and dissociation of the two ribosomal subunits from the mRNA. The initiating amino acid is usually cleaved from the completed peptide.

6.27   *Answer:*

a. In bacteria, translation initiation requires three initiation factors: IF-1, IF-2, and IF-3. At the start of translation intiation, IF-1 and IF-3 are bound to the 30S subunit. IF-3 aids in the binding of the 30S subunit to mRNA and prevents binding of the 50S ribosomal subunit to the 30S subunit. IF-2 brings the initiator tRNA, fMet-tRNA.fMet, to the 30S subunit–mRNA complex with a molecule of GTP. IF-1 blocks the A site so that only the P site is available for the initiator tRNA to bind to. When the 70S initiation complex is formed when the 50S ribosomal subunit binds to the 30S subunit, GTP is hydrolyzed and the three initiation factors are released.

Elongation in bacteria requires two elongation factors: EF-Tu and EF-Ts. When an aminoacyl-tRNA binds to the codon in the A site, it is brought to the ribosome bound to EF-Tu–GTP. When the aminoacyl-tRNA binds to the codon in the A site, GTP hydrolysis releases EF-Tu–GDP. EF-Tu is recycled using EF-Ts. EF-Ts binds to EF-Tu and displaces the GDP. Next, GTP binds to the EF-Tu–EF-Ts complex to produce an EF-Tu–GTP complex simultaneously with the release of EF-Ts. An aminoacyl-tRNA binds to the EF-Tu–GTP, and that complex can bind to the A site in a ribosome when the complementary codon is exposed.

Translocation in bacteria requires the elongation factor EF-G. An EF-G–GTP complex binds to the ribosome, GTP is hydrolyzed, and translocation of the ribosome occurs along with displacement of the uncharged tRNA away from the P site. GTP hydrolysis may change the structure of EF-G to facilitate the translocation event.

In bacteria, termination requires three release factors, RF1, RF2, and RF3. These have shapes that mimic that of a tRNA and regions that read the codons. Two RFs read the stop codons: RF1 recognizes UAA and UAG, and RF2 recognizes UAA and UGA. Their binding to a stop codon triggers peptidyl transferase to cleave the polypeptide from the tRNA in the P site. After the polypeptide leaves the ribosome, RF3–GDP binds to the ribosome, stimulating the release of the RF from the stop codon and the ribosome. GTP then replaces the GDP on RF3, and RF3 hydrolyzes the GTP. This allows RF3 to be released from the ribosome.

One additional factor, the ribosome recycling factor (RRF), is required to deconstruct the remaining complex of ribosomal subunits, mRNA, and uncharged tRNA so that the ribosome and tRNA can be recycled. The shape of RRF mimics that of a tRNA. After it binds to the A site, EF-G binds and causes translocation of the ribosome, thereby moving RRF to the P site and the uncharged tRNA to the E site. The RRF releases the uncharged tRNA, and EF-G releases RRF, causing the two ribosomal subunits to dissociate from the mRNA.

b. Though eukaryotic initiation factors are used during eukaryotic translation initiation, many more are used, and some are not used in the same way as are prokaryotic initiation factors. The use of eIFs is discussed in the answer to part **(c)**. In eukaryotes, elongation is similar to that in prokaryotes: eEF-2 functions like bacterial EF-G, eEF-1A plays the role of EF-Tu, and eEF-1B has a similar role to EF-Ts. In eukaryotes, translation termination is also similar to that in bacteria. A single release factor, eRF1, recognizes all three stop codons, and eRF3 stimulates the termination events. There is no equivalent of RRF, though ribosome recycling does occur in eukaryotes.

c. During eukaryotic translation initiation, many more initiation factors (eIFs) are used. They are used during the identification of the AUG initiation codon and to stimulate subsequent translation initiation. Since Shine–Dalgarno sequences are not present in eukaryotes, eukaryotic ribosomes and eIFs use an alternative mechanism to identify the AUG initiation codon. First, eIF–4F—a multimer of several proteins, including eIF–4E and the cap binding protein—binds to the cap at the 5' end of the mRNA. Then, a complex of the 40S ribosomal subunit with the initiator Met-tRNA, several eIF proteins, and GTP binds, and together with other eIFs, scans the mRNA for an initiator AUG codon embedded in a Kozak sequence. After the 40S subunit finds and binds to this AUG, the 60S ribosomal subunit binds and displaces all eIFs except eIF–4F to produce the 80S initiation complex. The subsequent initiation of translation requires eIF–4F, as poly(A) binding protein II bound to the poly(A) tail also binds to eIF–4G, one of the proteins of eIF–4F at the cap. This loops the poly(A) tail at the 3' end of the mRNA close to its 5' end and stimulates translation initiation.

6.28   *Answer:* Multiple lines of evidence support the view that the rRNA component of the ribosome serves more than a structural role. First, the 3' end of the 16S rRNA is important for identifying where the small ribosomal subunit should bind the mRNA. It has a sequence that is complementary to the Shine–Dalgarno sequence, the ribosome-binding site (RBS) in the mRNA. Mutational analyses demonstrated that the 3' end of the 16S rRNA must base-pair with this mRNA sequence for correct initiation of translation. Second, the 23S rRNA is required for peptidyl transferase activity. Evidence that the peptidyl transferase consists entirely of RNA comes from studies of the atomic structure of the large ribosomal subunit and is supported by experiments showing that peptidyl transferase activity remains following the depletion of the 50S subunit proteins, but not after the digestion of rRNA with ribonuclease T1.

6.29   *Answer:* A eukaryotic mRNA is modified to contain a 5' 7-methyl-G cap and a 3' poly(A) tail. The 5' cap is required early in translation initiation—it binds to the eIF–4F complex just prior to the binding of a complex of the 40S ribosomal subunit, the initiator Met-tRNA, and other eIF proteins. Transcription initiation is stimulated by the looping of the poly(A) tail close to the 5' end. This occurs when the poly(A) binding protein (PAB) binds to eIF–4G, which is part of the eIF–4F complex.

6.30   *Answer:* In both prokaryotes and eukaryotes, the initiator AUG codon is present in a sequence context that helps define it as the initiator codon. In prokaryotes, the correct AUG is found downstream of a purine-rich ribosome-binding site (RBS). The RBS is complementary to a pyrimidine-rich region at the 3' end of the 16S rRNA. The formation of complementary base pairs between the mRNA and the 16S rRNA allows the ribosome to locate the correct AUG within the mRNA for the initiation of protein synthesis. In eukaryotes, the correct AUG codon is identified by scanning for an

AUG codon embedded in a Kozak sequence. After the 5' cap is bound by eIF-4F, a complex of the 40S ribosomal subunit with the initiator Met-tRNA, several eIF proteins, and GTP binds the mRNA. Together with other eIFs, the complex scans along the mRNA for an initiator AUG codon embedded in a Kozak sequence.

6.31   *Answer:* First rewrite the sequences so that the codons can be readily seen, noting the mutations (underlined):

```
Normal:    AUG UUC UCU AAU UAC (...) AUG GGG UGG GUG UAG
Mutant a:  AUG UUC UCU AAU UAG (...) AUG GGG UGG GUG UAG
Mutant b:  AGG UUC UCU AAU UAC (...) AUG GGG UGG GUG UAG
Mutant c:  AUG UUC UCG AAU UAC (...) AUG GGG UGG GUG UAG
Mutant d:  AUG UUC UCU AAA UAC (...) AUG GGG UGG GUG UAG
Mutant e:  AUG UUC UCU AAU UC.  ..)A UGG GGU GGG UGU AG.
Mutant f:  AUG UUC UCU AAU UAC (...) AUG GGG UGG GUG UGG
```

Mutants *a, b, c, d,* and *f* are point mutations in which one base has been substituted for another. Mutant *e* is a deletion of a single base that results in a shift in the reading frame of the mRNA (a frameshift mutation). Translating each sequence using the genetic code, determine the proteins that would be formed if these sequences were translated:

```
normal:  AUG UUC UCU AAU UAC ... AUG GGG UGG GUG UAG
         Met Phe Ser Asn Tyr ... Met Gly Trp Val Stop

a:       AUG UUC UCU AAU UAG ... AUG GGG UGG GUG UAG
         Met Phe Ser Asn Stop
```

Mutant *a* is a nonsense mutation and results in premature chain termination.

```
b:       AGG UUC UCU AAU UAC ... AUG GGG UGG GUG UAG
                                 Met Gly Trp Val Stop
```

Mutant *b* mutates the initiation codon, so that a polypeptide would be formed (if formed at all) using a downstream initiation codon. It results in a polypeptide missing amino acids at its N terminus.

```
c:       AUG UUC UCG AAU UAC ... AUG GGG UGG GUG UAG
         Met Phe Ser Asn Tyr ... Met Gly Trp Val Stop
```

Mutant *c* changes a base in the 3' end of the codon. This does not alter the amino acid that is inserted. It will be "silent" and have no phenotypic effect.

```
d:       AUG UUC UCU AAA UAC ... AUG GGG UGG GUG UAG
         Met Phe Ser Lys Tyr ... Met Gly Trp Val Stop
```

Mutant *d* changes a base in the 3' end of the codon. This does alter the amino acid that is inserted. It is a missense mutation, resulting in the insertion of a Lys instead of an Asn.

```
e:       AUG UUC UCU AAU UC. ..A UGG GGU GGG UGU AG.
         Met Phe Ser Asn Ser ... Trp Gly Gly Cys ?
```

Mutant *e* is a single base-pair deletion and results in a frameshift mutation that alters the reading frame of the protein. All amino acids inserted following Asn are likely to be incorrect. It is conceivable that a stop codon could be read in the region that is indicated by the . . ., leading to premature chain termination.

```
f:   AUG UUC UCU AAU UAC ... AUG GGG UGG GUG UGG
     Met Phe Ser Asn Tyr ... Met Gly Trp Val Trp..
```

Mutant *f* changes a base in the chain-terminating UAG codon so that the amino acid Trp will now be inserted. It will result in the placement of additional amino acids onto the C terminus of the protein.

6.32   *Answer:* One approach to this problem is to infer the possible coding sequence(s) that could be used for the normal protein (using N = any nucleotide, R = purine, Y = pyrimidine) and then examine this sequence to deduce what possible mutations could have resulted in the mutant proteins.

Based on the normal amino acid sequence, the mRNA sequence is:

```
amino acid sequence:    Met-Gly-Glu-Thr-Lys-Val-Val-...-Pro
  potential mRNA:  5'-AUG GGN GAR ACN AAR GUN GUN ... CCN-3'
```

In mutant 1, premature chain termination has occurred. This could have occurred if, in the DNA transcribed into the third [GAR (Glu)] codon, a G-C base pair was changed to a T-A base pair. This would lead to a UAR (stop) codon.

```
normal sequence:     Met-Gly-Glu-Thr-Lys-Val-Val-...-Pro
normal   mRNA: 5'-AUG GGN GAR ACN AAR GUN GUN ... CCN-3'
mutant   mRNA: 5'-AUG GGN UAR ACN AAR GUN GUN ... CCN-3'
mutant sequence:     Met-Gly-Stop
```

It could also have occurred if a T–A base-pair insertion mutation occurred in the DNA so that a U was transcribed in between the normal second and third codons, resulting in a UGA (stop) third codon.

```
amino acid sequence:     Met-Gly-Glu-Thr-Lys-Val-Val-...-Pro
potential mRNA:      5'-AUG GGN GAR ACN AAR GUN GUN ... CCN-3'
mutant mRNA:         5'-AUG GGN UGA RAC NAA RGU NGU N.. .CC-3'
mutant sequence:         Met-Gly-Stop
```

In mutant 2, premature chain termination has occurred after a wrong amino acid has been inserted. To explain both of these results as a consequence of a single mutational event, try either insertion or deletion mutations that would alter the reading frame. One possible explanation is that a G–C base-pair insertional mutation in the DNA resulted in a G being inserted after the third codon. If the N of the fourth codon were a U, then such a frameshifting insertion would change the Thr to Asp and also introduce a chain termination codon into the fifth codon position. If the R in the GAR coding for Glu (the third amino acid) is a G, this mutation could also be caused by a G–C or A–T base-pair insertional mutation after the first two nucleotides coding for Glu. As before, assume the N of the fourth codon is a U.

```
amino acid sequence:     Met-Gly-Glu-Thr-Lys-Val-Val-...-Pro
potential mRNA:      5'-AUG GGN GAR ACN AAR GUN GUN ... CCN-3'
mutant mRNA:         5'-AUG GGN GAR GAC UAA RGU NGU N.. .CC-3'
mutant sequence:         Met-Gly-Glu-Asp-Stop
```

In mutant 3, the situation is similar to that with mutant 2. This time, however, several wrong amino acids are inserted before chain termination. To explain all of these consequences as the result of a single mutational event, check for the consequences of deletions or insertions in the region of the second and third codons. One possible explanation is that a deletion mutation in the DNA resulted in the N of the second codon being deleted. If, as in mutant 2, the N of the fourth codon is a U, the R of the third codon is a G, the R of the fifth codon is an A, and the N of the sixth codon is an A, the mutant sequence would be obtained.

```
normal sequence:    Met-Gly-Glu-Thr-Lys-Val-Val ... Pro
normal mRNA:        5'-AUG GGN GAR ACN AAR GUN GUN ... CCN-3'
normal mRNA:        5'-AUG GGN GAG ACU AAA GUA GUN ... CCN-3'
mutant mRNA:        5'-AUG GGG AGA CUA AAG UAG UN. ..C CN-3'
mutant sequence:    Met-Gly-Arg-Leu-Lys-Stop
```

In mutant 4, the normal second amino acid (Gly) has been replaced with Arg. Arg is encoded by AGR or CGN, while Gly is encoded by GGN. If a G–C base pair were substituted for a C–G base pair in the DNA so that the first G of the second codon were replaced by a C, Arg would be inserted as the second amino acid.

```
normal sequence:    Met-Gly-Glu-Thr-Lys-Val-Val ... Pro
normal mRNA:        5'-AUG GGN GAR ACN AAR GUN GUN ... CCN-3'
mutant mRNA:        5'-AUG CGN GAR ACN AAR GUN GUN ... CCN-3'
mutant sequence:    Met-Arg-Glu-Thr-Lys-Val-Val ... Pro
```

6.33   *Answer:* Because of the redundancy in the genetic code, a number of different DNA strands could serve as coding (nontemplate) strands for this sequence. If N = any of the four nucleotides, Y = either pyrimidine nucleotide (C, T), and R = either purine nucleotide (A, G), then the amino acid sequence could be encoded by any of the following strands:

```
Met-His-    Arg   -   Arg    -Lys-Val-His-Gly-Gly
ATG CAY (AGR or CGN) (AGR or CGN) AAR GTN CAY GGN GGN
```

Calculate the number of different sequences by multiplying the possibilities (using the product and sum rules):

```
ATG CAY (AGR or CGN) (AGR or CGN) AAR GTN CAY GGN GGN
 1  × 2 ×   (2 + 4)   ×  (2 + 4)  × 2 × 4 × 2 × 4 × 4 = 18,432
```

6.34   *Answer:* Both GAA and GAG code for glutamic acid, while GUU, GUC, GUA, and GUG code for valine. The simplest explanation is that there was an AT-to-TA change in the DNA, at the 17th base pair in the coding region of the gene. In this event, the 6th codon, instead of being GAA or GAG, would be GUA or GUG and encode valine.

6.35   *Answer:*

a. If the primary mRNA for this gene is 250 kb, it must be substantially processed by RNA splicing (removing introns) and polyadenylation to a smaller mature mRNA.

b. A 1,480-amino-acid protein requires 1,480 × 3 = 4,440 bases of protein-coding sequence. This leaves 6,500 − 4,440 = 2,060 bases of 5' untranslated leader and 3' untranslated trailer sequence in the mature mRNA—about 32%.

    c. The ΔF508 mutation could be caused by a DNA deletion for the three base pairs encoding the mRNA codon for phenylalanine. This codon is UUY (Y = U or C), and the DNA sequence of the nontemplate strand is 5'-TTY-3'. The segment of DNA containing these bases would be deleted in the appropriate region of the gene.

    d. If positioned at random and solely within a gene's coding region (that is, not in 3' or 5' untranslated sequences or in intronic sequences), a deletion of three base pairs results either in an mRNA missing a single codon or an mRNA missing bases from two adjacent codons. If three of the six bases from two adjacent codons were deleted, the remaining three bases would form a single codon. In this case, an incorrect amino acid might be inserted into the polypeptide at the site of the left codon, and the amino acid encoded by the right codon would be deleted. If the 3' base of the left codon were deleted, it would be replaced by the 3' base of the right codon. Since the code is degenerate, and wobble occurs in the 3' base, this type of deletion might not alter the amino acid specified by the left codon. The adjacent amino acid would still be deleted, however.

6.36   *Answer:*

    a. The protein encoded by the *ADAM12* gene encodes a membrane-bound protein. Therefore, one initial hypothesis to explain why N-terminal amino acids are missing in the mature protein is that the protein is directed to the membrane via transport through the endoplasmic reticulum, and during this process, the N-terminal amino acids are cleaved from the growing polypeptide chain. Notice that the N-terminal sequence of the mRNA-encoded polypeptide contains many hydrophobic amino acids (see text Figure 6.3, p. 105). It is a signal sequence. As the signal sequence is synthesized by the ribosome, it becomes bound by a signal recognition particle (SRP) that blocks further translation of the mRNA until the growing polypeptide–SRP–ribosome–mRNA complex becomes bound to the ER. When the SRP binds to an SRP receptor in the ER membrane, the ribosome becomes bound to the ER, the SRP is released, and translation resumes with the growing polypeptide extending through the ER membrane into its cisternal space. Once the signal sequence is fully within the cisternal space of the ER, it is cleaved from the polypeptide by a signal peptidase (see text Figure 6.21, p. 123).

    b. The mutation would disrupt the signal sequence, so the polypeptide would no longer be directed into the ER for further processing and targeting to the cell membrane. An ADAM12 protein would be synthesized but would not be positioned correctly in the cell membrane.

6.37   *Answer:* This question asks you to conceptualize the order of the many steps that are part of gene expression. In a cell, some processes occur independently of others, while other processes are coupled together. Consequently, some of these processes cannot be placed in a precise order. It is efficient to first cluster the statements into four groups based on whether they involve transcription initiation (group 1), mRNA transcript processing and transport (group 2), translation (group 3), or protein processing (group 4), and then develop a conceptual order. Here is *one* possible order.

    1a. An activator protein binds an enhancer.

    1b. RNA pol II initiates mRNA synthesis.

    2a. An intron is removed from the Val-pre-tRNA. (This can be done anytime before the Val-tRNA is used in step 3).

    2b. The mRNA is cleaved near the poly(A) site in its 3' UTR.

    2c. Poly(A) polymerase adds 200 A's onto the 3' end of the mRNA.

    2d. Introns are removed from the mRNA by a spliceosome. (Splicing can occur before, simultaneously with, or after the polyadenylation described in steps **2b** and **2c**.)

    2e. The mRNA is transported out of the nucleus into the cytoplasm. (Note that transcription, splicing, and transport are coupled).

    3a. A specific aminoacyl tRNA synthetase charges initiator Met-tRNA. (This can be done anytime before step **3d**.)

    3b. Cap-binding protein binds the 7-^{m}G cap at the 5' end of the mRNA.

    3c. A complex of the 40S ribosomal subunit, an initiator Met-tRNA, several eIF proteins, and GTP scan for an AUG codon embedded within a Kozak sequence.

3d. Poly(A) binding protein binds the poly(A) tail and eIF-4G.

3e. A specific aminoacyl tRNA synthetase charges Val-tRNA. (This can occur anytime after **2a**.)

3f. Val-tRNA, complexed with eEF-1A and GTP, comes to the ribosome.

3g. Peptidyl transferase catalyzes the formation of a peptide bond.

3h. eEF-2–GTP binds to the ribosome.

4a. An SRP binds the N-terminal region of the growing polypeptide and blocks translation.

4b. A signal peptidase acts on the N-terminal region of the protein.

4c. Chaperones assist in a polypeptide's cotranslational folding.

3i. eRF1 recognizes a nonsense codon. (This step occurs during translation termination, so it is placed last since it will occur after a nascent polypeptide starts to be cotranslationally transported into the ER.)

6.38   *Answer:* Some genes can inhibit the activity of others. An increase in an enzyme's activity will be seen if actinomycin D blocks the transcription of a gene that codes for an inhibitor of the enzyme's activity.

7

DNA Mutation, DNA Repair, and Transposable Elements

Chapter Outline

DNA Mutation

Adaptation versus Mutation

Mutations Defined

Spontaneous and Induced Mutations

Detecting Mutations

Repair of DNA Damage

Direct Reversal Repair of DNA Damage

Excision Repair of DNA Damage

Human Genetic Diseases Resulting from DNA Replication and Repair Mutations

Transposable Elements

General Features of Transposable Elements

Transposable Elements in Bacteria

Transposable Elements in Eukaryotes

Review of Key Terms, Symbols, and Concepts

In your own words, write a brief, precise definition of each term in the groups below and on the following page. Check your definitions using the text. Then develop a concept map using the terms in each list.

1	2	3
mutation	mutagen	DNA repair
adaptation	carcinogen	mismatch repair,
fluctuation test	spontaneous mutation	proofreading
random mutation	mutation rate	direct correction, direct
base-pair mutation	mutation frequency	reversal
base-pair substitution	tautomer, tautomeric shift	mutator mutation, gene
somatic vs. germ-line	depurination, deamination	photoreactivation
mutation	mutational hot spot	light repair
gene vs. chromosomal	induced mutation	photolyase
mutation	ionizing, nonionizing	excision (dark) repair, NER
point mutation	radiation	base excision repair
transition, transversion	thymine dimer	glycosylase
mutation	SOS response	O^6-methyl-guanine
missense mutation	base analog	methyltransferase
nonsense mutation	5BU, AZT, MMS	translesion DNA synthesis
neutral mutation	base-modifying agent	SOS response, *lexA*, *recA*
silent mutation	nitrous acid, hydroxylamine	methyl-directed mismatch
frameshift mutation	intercalating agent	repair
forward mutation	acridine, proflavin	xeroderma pigmentosum
reverse mutation (reversion)	site-specific *in vitro*	ataxia-telangiectasia
true vs. partial reversion	mutagenesis	Fanconi anemia
suppressor mutation, gene	Ames test	Bloom syndrome
second-site mutation		Cockayne syndrome
intragenic, intergenic		hereditary nonpolyposis
suppressor		colon cancer
nonsense suppressor,		
suppression		

4	5	6
mutant screen	transposable element	transposable element vs.
visible mutation	transposition	retrotransposon
replica plating	transposition event	mutator gene
nutritional mutation	insertion sequence (IS)	replicative vs. conservative
auxotrophic mutation	element	transposition
conditional mutation	IS module	homologous recombination
temperature-sensitive mutant	terminal inverted repeat	deletion
resistance mutation	transposase	inversion
	target site	translocation
	target site duplication	*Ac, Ds* controlling elements
	transposon (Tn)	null mutation
	nonhomologous	autonomous element
	recombination	nonautonomous element
	composite transposon	stable allele
	noncomposite transposon	unstable (mutable) allele
	Tn*10*, Tn3	donor site
	replicative transposition	*Ty* element
	conservative (nonreplicative),	long terminal (direct) repeat
	cut-and-paste transposition	delta repeat
	simple insertion	target site duplication
	cointegrate	retrovirus
	cointegration model	reverse transcriptase
	transposase	*P* element
	resolvase	LINEs, SINEs
	β-lactamase	Alu, L1 elements

Thinking Analytically

Mutation is a fundamental process in genetics and evolution. This chapter presents the conceptual framework geneticists use to consider the origin of mutations. Then it presents a detailed discussion of the types and causes of mutation, strategies to identify mutants, the nature of mutagens and how mutagens can be identified, and the biological mechanisms used to repair mutations. The chapter closes with a discussion of transposons, ubiquitous elements in prokaryotes and eukaryotes that are capable of moving within a genome and in so doing, causing mutation. The material presented here is both highly conceptual and quite detailed. Focus first on the concepts and then, as in previous chapters, learn to use the terms and definitions to explain the concepts. To follow some of the complicated processes described in this chapter, it is essential to clearly understand the precise meaning of each term.

As you consider the molecular basis of mutation, it will help to review the chemical structure of the bases to clearly visualize the action of mutagens. Use diagrams as you consider the effects of specific mutations and repair processes on the structure of DNA. Use diagrams to follow how a mutant DNA sequence results in altered codon usage in an mRNA. Proceed methodically (and fastidiously, so as not to overlook a subtle point such as changes in polarity) through any analysis involving base-pair changes. Use terms carefully, remembering that mutations affect the bases in DNA and then, indirectly, the bases in transcribed RNA and the amino acids in proteins.

Pay especially close attention to the sections on suppressor mutations and the screening procedures used to isolate new mutations. After you organize the presented information, use diagrams and flowcharts to visualize the relationships between the terms and processes in these areas.

The material on transposons is broadly descriptive, so it will be helpful to categorize this information. Distinguish between the various categories of transposable elements by considering transposable elements from four perspectives: (1) structure, (2) mode of transposition, (3) the effect of a transposed element on the structure of a gene or chromosome, and (4) the effect of a transposed element on the function of a gene. As you read this section of the chapter, refer frequently to the text figures to visualize more clearly the different transposon structures and modes of transposition.

Questions for Practice

Multiple-Choice Questions

Match the best choice below to each of the descriptions in questions 1–8.

a. missense mutation	**e.** nonsense mutation
b. transversion mutation	**f.** transition mutation
c. neutral mutation	**g.** frameshift mutation
d. forward mutation	**h.** suppressor mutation

1. _____ A purine-pyrimidine base pair that is mutated to a different purine-pyrimidine base pair

2. _____ A point mutation in the DNA that changes a codon in the mRNA and causes an amino acid substitution that does not alter the function of the translated protein

3. _____ A DNA change in which a G–C base pair is replaced by a T–A base pair

4. _____ A mutation that results in the addition or deletion of a base pair within the coding region of a gene

5. _____ Any point mutation that is expressed as a change from the wild type to the mutant phenotype

6. _____ A base-pair change in the DNA that results in the change of an mRNA codon to either UAG, UAA, or UGA

7. _____ A mutation in the DNA that changes a codon in the mRNA and causes an amino acid substitution that may or may not produce a change in the function of a translated protein

8. _____ Any new mutation that restores some or all of the wild-type phenotype to a previously isolated mutation

9. The Ames test is used to screen for
   a. potential mutagens and carcinogens.
   b. the presence of enol forms of thymine and guanine.
   c. frameshift mutations.
   d. spontaneous mutations.

10. In the Ames test, rat liver extracts are used
    a. to chemically alter and detoxify potential mutagens.
    b. to chemically alter and toxify potential mutagens.
    c. to determine if an environmental chemical that itself is not mutagenic may become mutagenic when processed in the liver.
    d. all of the above

11. A population of cells is subjected to UV irradiation and then placed in the dark. There will be significant
    a. production of base tautomers.
    b. breakage of phosphodiester bonds.
    c. formation of pyrimidine dimers.
    d. photolyase activity.

12. Single bacterial cells sensitive to the infection of a phage are inoculated into a large number of separate culture dishes and allowed to grow in parallel. After many generations, a sample is taken from each culture, inoculated with the phage, and separately plated. Which result is expected?
    a. All plates will have similar numbers of bacterial colonies.
    b. No bacterial colonies will be seen on any of the plates.
    c. Only one plate in 10^6 will have bacterial colonies.
    d. Some plates will have no bacterial colonies, some will have a few, and some will have many.

13. How are transposition and recombination fundamentally different?
    a. Recombination requires DNA homology but transposition does not.
    b. Transposition requires DNA homology but recombination does not.
    c. Only during transposition can a piece of DNA be moved from a virus to a cell.
    d. Only during recombination can a deletion occur.

14. Which of the following can result from the insertion of a transposon in bacteria?
    a. gene inactivation
    b. an increase or decrease in transcriptional activity of a gene
    c. deletions and insertions
    d. all of the above

15. Which of the following can be consequences of transposition in eukaryotes?
    a. no effect on a nearby gene
    b. production of a mutation by insertional mutagenesis
    c. increased or decreased transcription from a nearby promoter
    d. all of the above

16. In what ways are bacterial IS and Tn elements alike?
    a. Both have inverted repeat sequences at their ends.
    b. Both integrate into target sites and cause a target site duplication.
    c. Both contain a transposase gene.
    d. Both contain antibiotic resistance genes.
    e. Both always use replicative transposition.
    f. a, b, and c
    g. all of the above

17. Reverse transcriptase is used by which two of the following transposable elements? (Mark two letters.)
    a. the *Ty* element in yeast
    b. an IS element in bacteria
    c. the Tn*10* element in bacteria
    d. an L1 element in humans

18. In a bacterial IS element, how does transposase know the boundaries of the DNA to be transposed?
    a. There are special recognition sites at the ends of the IS element.
    b. It recognizes the target site of insertion.
    c. It recognizes the IR sequences.
    d. It recognizes the delta sequences.

19. In corn, the insertion of an autonomous element within a gene results in the production of an allele that mutates at high frequency. Why?
    a. Although an autonomous element cannot excise, it is highly mutable.
    b. An autonomous element has transposase and can excise, thereby causing a mutation.
    c. Autonomous alleles are unstable if nonautonomous elements are also in the genome.
    d. Autonomous alleles generally insert into promoter regions.

20. *Ty* elements in yeast are similar to retroviruses because (choose the correct answer)
    a. both *Ty* elements and retroviruses utilize an RNA transposition intermediate.
    b. both *Ty* elements and retroviruses utilize reverse transcriptase.
    c. introns are usually found in retroviruses and *Ty* elements.
    d. both a and b

21. Which of the following is *not* true about the L1 family of LINE elements in mammals?
    a. They are retrotransposons.
    b. They comprise about 5% of the genome.
    c. All elements in one individual are full-length elements.
    d. They are capable of causing disease by insertional mutagenesis during an individual's lifetime.

Answers: 1f, 2c, 3b, 4g, 5d, 6e, 7a, 8h, 9a, 10d, 11c, 12d, 13a, 14d, 15d, 16f, 17a&d, 18c, 19b, 20d, 21c

Thought Questions

1. What is the evidence that mutations occur spontaneously and at a low frequency, regardless of selection for or against them?

2. The proofreading ability of DNA polymerases is extremely good, but not quite perfect. What error rates are associated with DNA replication, from whence do they arise, and how might this be important in evolutionary terms?

3. Distinguish between a reversion mutation, an intragenic suppressor mutation, and an intergenic suppressor mutation.

4. Distinguish between a missense and a nonsense mutation and between a missense, a silent, and a neutral mutation.

5. How would you classify the following mutations: (a) a single base change in a promoter region that affects the transcription of a gene; (b) a single base change in a promoter region that has no effect; (c) a DNA sequence difference between two strains that has no apparent phenotypic effect?

6. What is the basis for the Ames test? What are its specific merits? Are there any kinds of mutagens that it might not detect (e.g., those that specifically cause point mutations, frameshifts, small deletions, or chromosomal rearrangements)?

7. We have obtained significant insight into how DNA is repaired from studies in bacteria and yeast, as well as from the molecular genetic analyses of disease genes from humans with defective DNA repair. (a) Speculate as to the phenotype(s) of bacteria and yeast mutations that are defective in DNA repair. (b) How might comparison of these three systems be beneficial?

8. In *Drosophila*, the first mutations isolated (e.g., the first white-eyed mutant) were spontaneous. Currently, most new mutations are isolated by using mutagens. Why are mutagens currently employed, and what benefit do mutagens have for the study of genetics and development? How is site-specific *in vitro* mutagenesis used to study the function of cloned genes?

9. What spontaneous mutation rates are found in different organisms? Are these rates relatively similar or quite different? Why do you think this is so?

10. Dyes are routinely used to stain nuclei in bacteriological and histological preparations as well as to visualize DNA and RNA molecules separated by size using agarose gel electrophoresis. Some of these dyes bind to the backbone of nucleic acids (e.g., the major groove of double-stranded DNA), while others intercalate between bases. How would you specifically test whether a particular dye is mutagenic? How would you use the results of the test to design general precautions for laboratory workers using these dyes?

11. If a substance is mutagenic, is it necessarily carcinogenic? Why or why not? If a substance is carcinogenic, is it necessarily mutagenic? Why or why not?

12. Contrast conservative and replicative transposition. How can conservative transposition of the *Ac* element result in gene duplication? Can a particular IS element behave in both ways?

13. Consider how the distinction between direct and inverted repeats is central to the recognition of insertion sequences. The insertion sequence itself contains inverted terminal repeats. Thus, inverted repeats are present as part of the transposable element both before and after the insertion. On the other hand, the act of insertion results in a staggered cut in the host DNA. When the gaps are filled in after insertion, direct repeats will be generated flanking the inverted terminals of the transposable element. Indeed, insertion sequences have been identified by the presence of a pair of inverted repeats flanked by direct repeats. Using this logic, find the insertion sequence in the following single-stranded length of DNA:

CGTAGCCATTTGCGATATGCATCCGAATATCGCAAGCCATGCCA

14. In what situations can a nonautonomous element behave like an autonomous element? Give specific examples in corn and *Drosophila*.

15. Following the mobilization of *Ty* elements in yeast, two mutants were recovered that affected the activity of enzyme X. One of these mutants lacked enzyme activity and was a null mutation. The other mutant had three times as much enzyme activity. Both mutants had a *Ty* element inserted into the X gene. Generate a hypothesis to explain how this is possible.

16. What differences and similarities are there between transposable elements that utilize an RNA intermediate and those that do not?

17. What kinds of repetitive elements are SINEs and LINEs? Support for a hypothesis that a particular repetitive element is a transposon can come from analyzing its DNA sequence for open reading frames that encode transposase-like products. In humans, Alu sequences do not encode any of the enzymes that are presumably needed for retrotransposition. What aspects of their structure suggest that they might be capable of retrotransposition? What evidence is there that Alu sequences are retrotransposons capable of moving via an RNA intermediate, much like the yeast *Ty* element?

18. In humans, insertion of transposable elements has occasionally been associated with disease. An L1 element inserted into the gene for blood-clotting factor VIII resulted in hemophilia in two unrelated individuals. An Alu element insertion disrupted pre-mRNA processing at the gene for neurofibromatosis. In each case, the insertion was not in either of the affected individuals' parents and so appeared to be a result of an insertional event during the affected individuals' lifetime. Given that each of these classes of elements represents a substantial fraction of moderately repetitive DNA, how likely is it that most spontaneous mutations are due to insertional mutagenesis by L1 elements? If it is not very likely, why not?

Thought Questions for Media

After reviewing the media on the *iGenetics* website, answer these questions.

1. What are the consequences of a nonsense mutation?

2. What are the consequences if a nonsense mutation is suppressed?

3. Suppose the mutation in the *Nonsense Mutations and Nonsense Suppressor Mutations* animation was an AT-to-GC transition instead of an AT-to-TA transversion.
   a. What would be the result of this mutation on the gene's protein product?
   b. Explain how this mutation could be suppressed using a mechanism similar to that illustrated in the animation.

4. The *Mutagenic Effects of 5BU* animation shows how 5BU can introduce mutations that are either AT-to-GC transition mutations or GC-to-AT transition mutations. For each type of mutation:
   a. How many rounds of replication are involved in the formation of the mutation?
   b. In which round(s) of replication must 5BU be in its normal form?
   c. In which round(s) of replication must 5BU be in its rare form?

5. If 5BU is incorporated into DNA, but never shifts to its rare form during DNA replication, can it still cause a transition mutation?

6. Based in the information in the animation, is there a way for 5BU to cause a transversion mutation?

7. In principle, a mutagenic compound can cause either forward (new) mutations or reverse mutations.
   a. Does the Ames test assess the frequency of reverse mutations (say, *his* to *his*$^+$) or the frequency of forward mutations (say, *his*$^+$ to *his*)? How?
   b. Why is it advantageous for the Ames test to assess this type of mutation frequency?
   c. Does this strategy influence which types of mutagenic compounds can be detected using the Ames test?

8. According to the *Ames Test Protocol* animation, why is the S9 liver extract added to the bacteria during the Ames test?

9. Suppose two different transposable elements are mobilized and insert themselves into two different genes. In gene *A*, transposon IS1 inserts itself into the translated region. In gene B, transposon IS2 inserts itself at a site three base pairs downstream from the TATA box, but before the start of the transcribed region.

a. What similarities do you expect to find between the sequences of the transposable element inserted at each gene?

b. In addition to the sequence of the transposable elements, what sequence alterations do you expect to find in the region near the site of insertion?

c. What features do the sequence alterations in (b) have, and how do they arise?

d. How might the transposon insertions influence the functions of genes *A* and *B*? Are they similar or different? Why?

1. In the iActivity *A Toxic Town,* you observed that vinyl chloride causes a missense transversion mutation in the Ames test. Although the allowable EPA concentration of vinyl chloride is 2 μg/L, it is present at 140 μg/L in the groundwater of Russellville.

   a. Can you infer that it is the vinyl chloride in the drinking water that causes missense transversion mutations in the residents of Russellville? Why or why not?

   b. Suppose the concentration of vinyl chloride in a neighboring village is 2 μg/L, the EPA allowable concentration. Is the water safe to drink? What concerns, if any, would you have?

   c. Would your answers to (a) and (b) change if you knew that most of the adult residents of Russellville and the neighboring village smoked three packs of cigarettes a day?

2. In the iActivity *A Toxic Town,* 1,2-dichloroethene was not mutagenic in the Ames test, but was found in the groundwater at about six times the allowable EPA concentration. Since it is not mutagenic, why does the EPA bother to regulate how much 1,2-dichloroethene can be found in groundwater? What other factors might be used to determine the allowable groundwater concentration of a chemical?

3. Suppose that sequence analysis like that performed in the iActivity shows that a chemical causes a silent transition. Since it does not alter the amino acid sequence of a polypeptide, should you still be concerned about the chemical as a potential mutagen?

4. In the iActivity *The Genetics Shuffle,* you were able to determine that Tn*10* transposition is conservative. Does this allow you to infer whether Tn*10* transposition proceeds through a DNA or RNA intermediate?

5. Suppose you performed an experiment similar to the one illustrated in the iActivity *The Genetics Shuffle* to identify the mode of transposition of an uncharacterized transposon. You observe that none of the colonies exhibit any sectoring and that they are either blue or white. After picking several blue and several white colonies, you use PCR to amplify the region surrounding the *donor* DNA in each colony. You sequence the PCR products and compare the sequences to those of the molecules used to generate the heteroduplexes. What do you find, and how do you explain your findings?

Solutions to Text Questions and Problems

7.1   *Answer:* b

7.2   *Answer:* False. Mutations occur spontaneously at a more or less constant frequency, regardless of selective pressure. Once they occur, however, they can be selected for or against, depending on the advantage or disadvantage they confer. It is important not to confuse the frequency of mutations with selection.

7.3   *Answer:* e

7.4   *Answer:* c. The key to this answer is the word *usually*. The other choices might apply rarely, but not usually.

7.5   *Answer:* Start methodically and write out the potential codons for the normal protein. Let N represent any nucleotide, R a purine (A or G), and Y a pyrimidine (C or U). Then the codons can be written as:

	1	2	3	4	5	6	7	8	9
Normal:	Phe	Leu	Pro	Thr	Val	Thr	Thr	Arg	Trp
Codon:	UUY	UUR	CCN	ACN	GUN	ACN	ACN	CGN	UGG
		or						or	
		CUN						AGR	

Mutant 1: The alteration of all of the amino acids after codon 2 suggests that this mutation is a frameshift, either a deletion or an addition of a base pair in the DNA region that codes for the mRNA near codons 2 and 3. His is CAY, which can be generated from CCN by the insertion of a single A between the two Cs. If this is the case, one has:

	1	2	3	4	5	6	7	8	9
Mutant 1:	Phe	Leu	His	His	Gly	Asp	Asp	Thr	Val
Frameshift:	UUY	UUR	CAC	NAC	NGU	NAC	NAC	NCG	NUG
		or						or	or
		CUN						NGR	RUG

Now identify the unknown bases, given the amino acid sequence:
   To code for His, the new fourth codon must be CAC.
   To code for Gly, the new fifth codon must be GGU.
   To code for Asp, the new sixth codon must be GAC.
   To code for Asp, the new seventh codon must be GAC.
   To code for Thr, the new eighth codon must be ACG.
   To code for Val, the new ninth codon must be GUG.
Thus, one has:

	1	2	3	4	5	6	7	8	9
Mutant 1:	Phe	Leu	His	His	Gly	Asp	Asp	Thr	Val
Codon:	UUY	UUR	CAC	CAC	GGU	GAC	GAC	ACG	GUG
		or							
		CUN							

This analysis indicates that the codons used in the normal protein are:

	1	2	3	4	5	6	7	8	9
Normal:	Phe	Leu	Pro	Thr	Val	Thr	Thr	Arg	Trp
Codon:	UUY	UUR or CUN	CCC	ACG	GUG	ACG	ACA	CGG	UGG

Mutant 2: Codon 5 in mutant 2 encodes Met, instead of Val. This single change could be caused by a point mutation, where the G in codon GUG is changed to an A, leading to an AUG codon. This would occur by a CG-to-TA transition in the DNA.

Mutant 3: Mutant 3 has a normal amino acid sequence, but is prematurely terminated, indicating that a nonsense mutation occurred. The nonsense mutation occurred in the ninth codon. If an A base is substituted (for one of the Gs) or inserted (before or after the first G), one could have either UAG or UGA. Thus, either a frameshift or base substitution (CG-to-TA transition) occurred.

Mutant 4: Mutant 4 shows premature termination at codon 5 (indicating a nonsense codon there) and has missense mutations at codons 2 and 4. Compare the possible sequences of the mutant with the normal sequence to see if one mutational event can account for all of these phenomena.

	1	2	3	4	5	6	7	8	9
Normal:	Phe	Leu	Pro	Thr	Val	Thr	Thr	Arg	Trp
Normal Codon:	UUY	UUR or CUN	CCC	ACG	GUG	ACG	ACA	CGG	UGG
Mutant 4:	Phe	Pro	Pro	Arg	Stop				
Possible Mutant Codons:	UUY	CCN (CCC)	CCN (CCA)	AGR or CGN	UAA UAG UGA				

Consider codon 2 carefully. For Pro to be encoded by CCN in the mutant protein and be obtained by a single change from the second codon, Leu (in the normal protein) must be encoded by CUN. If the U were deleted (by an AT deletion in the DNA) and the N were a C, a CCC Pro codon and a frameshift would result. Codon 3 would become CCA and still code for Pro, codon 4 would become CGG and code for Arg, and codon 5 would become UGA, a nonsense codon.

Mutant 5: Mutant 5 shows an alteration of only the fourth amino acid (Thr to Ser), suggesting a point mutation. If the fourth codon were changed from ACG to UCG (by a TA-to-AT transversion in the DNA), this missense mutation would occur.

7.6   Answer:

a. If the normal codon is 5'-CUG-3', the anticodon of the normal tRNA is 5'-CAG-3'. If a mutant tRNA recognizes 5'-GUG-3', it must have an anticodon that is 5'-CAC-3'. The mutational event was a CG-to-GC transversion in the gene for the leucine tRNA. The mutant tRNA will carry leucine to a codon for valine.

b. Since a leucine-bearing (mutant) tRNA can suppress the mutation, presumably leucine is normally present at position 10.

c. The mutant tRNA recognizes the codon 5'-GUG-3', which codes for Val. In normal cells, a Val-tRNA.Valine would recognize the codon and insert valine.

d. Leu

7.7   *Answer:*

a. The temperature sensitivity of the *rpIIA^ts* mutant could be due to a single amino acid change in the protein subunit of RNA polymerase II that causes it to be nonfunctional at the restrictive temperature. If its inability to function is due to a change in its secondary or tertiary structure that prevents it from interacting with another protein during transcription, then a mutation in this second interacting protein might be compensatory. Such a mutation would effectively suppress the initial mutation, as it would allow for transcription even at the restrictive temperature.

b. A new mutation in a second protein would be an intergenic suppressor mutation. The original mutation could also be suppressed by reverting the missense mutation or by an intragenic suppressor mutation. In an intragenic suppressor mutation, a particular second site within the protein would need to be mutated so as to compensate for the initial mutation.

c. One approach is to treat *rpIIA^ts/rpIIA^ts* individuals with a mutagen and mate them to *rpIIA^ts/rpIIA^ts* individuals at the permissive temperature. A second-site suppressor could be selected for by removing the parents and shifting the progeny to the restrictive temperature. Since all of the offspring are *rpIIA^ts/rpIIA^ts*, only offspring carrying a new mutation capable of suppressing the recessive lethality of the *rpIIA^ts* mutation will survive.

d. Second-site suppressors will be quite rare and will appear at a much lower frequency than will mutations in a typical eukaryotic gene. To suppress a particular defect, a very specific new mutation must occur. Hence, the vast majority of mutations that are induced by a mutagen will lack the specific compensatory ability of a suppressor mutation.

e. Since intergenic suppressors may result from mutations in interacting proteins, this approach could be used to identify genes for proteins that interact during transcription.

7.8   *Answer:* Acridine is an intercalating agent that induces frameshift mutations. *lacZ-1* probably is a frameshift mutation that results in a completely altered amino acid sequence after some point, although it might be truncated due to the introduction of an out-of-frame nonsense codon. In either case, the protein produced by *lacZ-1* would most likely have a different molecular weight and charge. During gel electrophoresis (see text Figure 4.8, p. 70), it would migrate differently than the wild-type protein. 5BU is incorporated into DNA in place of T. During DNA replication, it can be read as C by DNA polymerase because of a keto-to-enol shift. This results in point mutations, usually TA-to-CG transitions. *lacZ-2* is likely to contain a single amino acid difference, due to a missense mutation; although it, too, could contain a nonsense codon. A missense mutation might lead to the protein's having a different charge, while a nonsense codon would lead to a truncated protein that would have a lower molecular weight. Both would migrate differently during gel electrophoresis.

7.9   *Answer:*

a. The codons read as

   5'-AUG-ACC-CAU-UGG-UCU-CGU-UAG-3'

   The last codon is a nonsense (chain termination) codon, while the others are sense codons. The chain would be six amino acids long.

b. The new sequence would be

   5'-AUG-ACC-CAU-UAG-...

   Since UAG is a nonsense (chain termination) codon, the new chain would be only three amino acids long.

7.10   *Answer:* There were eight new mutations in 94,073 normal couples. Since the phenotype is dominant, the phenotype is seen when just one of the parental genes is mutated. There were $2 \times 94,073$ copies of the gene that could have undergone mutation. Therefore, the apparent mutation rate at this locus is

$$8/(2 \times 94,073) = 8/188,146 = 4 \times 10^{-5} \text{ mutations per locus per generation}$$

7.11 *Answer:*

Nucleotide Altered	Codon					
	UAG	Code	UAA	Code	UGA	Code
First	AAG	Lys	AAA	Lys	AGA	Arg
	CAG	Gln	CAA	Gln	CGA	Arg
	GAG	Glu	GAA	Glu	GGA	Gly
Second	UUG	Leu	UUA	Leu	UUA	Leu
	UCG	Ser	UCA	Ser	UCA	Ser
	UGG	Trp	UGA	Stop	UAA	Stop
Third	UAC	Tyr	UAC	Tyr	UGC	Cys
	UAU	Tyr	UAU	Tyr	UGU	Cys
	UAA	Stop	UAG	Stop	UGG	Trp

7.12 *Answer:* In the following answer, nucleotide sequences are always given 5' to 3'.

a. Only a subset of amino acids has codons that can be changed to a nonsense codon by a single base change. The following table lists the nonsense codons, the codons produced when single nucleotide changes are made to each nonsense codon, and the amino acids these encode.

Nonsense Codon	5' Base Change	Amino Acid	Central Base Change	Amino Acid	3' Base Change	Amino Acid
UAG	CAG	Gln	UUG	Leu	UAU	Tyr
	AAG	Lys	UCG	Ser	UAC	Tyr
	GAG	Glu	UGG	Trp	UAA	Stop
UAA	CAA	Gln	UUA	Leu	UAU	Tyr
	AAA	Lys	UCA	Ser	UAC	Tyr
	GAA	Glu	UGA	Stop	UAG	Stop
UGA	CGA	Arg	UUA	Leu	UGU	Cys
	AGA	Arg	UCA	Ser	UGC	Cys
	GGA	Gly	UAA	Stop	UGG	Trp

b. A mutation affecting a tRNA's anticodon will result in a tRNA nonsense suppressor if the altered anticodon recognizes a nonsense codon. The following table lists the nonsense codons, the anticodons able to recognize them without using wobble, the anticodons produced when single nucleotide changes are made to each, the codons these recognize, and the amino acids encoded by those codons.

Nonsense Codon	Anti-codon	5' Base Change	Codon	Amino Acid	Central Base Change	Codon	Amino Acid	3' Base Change	Codon	Amino Acid
UAG	CUA	UUA	UAA	Stop	CCA	UGG	Trp	CUU	AAG	Lys
		AUA	UAU	Tyr	CAA	UUG	Leu	CUC	GAG	Glu
		GUA	UAC	Tyr	CGA	UCG	Ser	CUG	CAG	Gln
UAA	UUA	CUA	UAG	Stop	UCA	AGU	Ser	UUU	AAA	Lys
		AUA	UAU	Tyr	UAA	UUA	Leu	UUC	GAA	Glu
		GUA	UAC	Tyr	UGA	UCA	Ser	UUG	CAA	Gln
UGA	UCA	CCA	UGG	Trp	UUA	UAA	Stop	UCU	AGA	Arg
		ACA	UGU	Cys	UAA	UUA	Leu	UCC	GGA	Gly
		GCA	UGC	Cys	UGA	UCA	Ser	UCG	CGA	Arg

The table shows that the same amino acids as in part (a) have tRNAs with anticodons that can be changed by a single nucleotide mutation to a tRNA nonsense suppressor.

c. A tRNA nonsense suppressor will not always insert the correct (wild-type) amino acid into the elongating polypeptide chain. For example, consider a nonsense mutation that changes a CAG codon for Gln to UAG. One type of nonsense suppressor tRNA would insert Gln, while other types would insert Glu, Lys, Trp, Leu, Ser, or Tyr.

7.13   *Answer:*

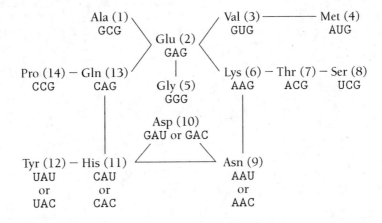

7.14   *Answer:*

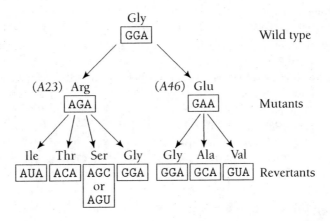

7.15   *Answer:* Using the genetic code, and letting N represent any nucleotide, R a purine, and Y a pyrimidine, the wild-type RNA can be denoted as:

```
        -Met-Phe-Ala-Asn-His-Lys-Ser-Val-Gly-
         39   40   41   42   43   44   45   46   47
                                        UCN
         AUG  UUY  GCN  AAY  CAY  AAR  or  GUN  GGN
                                        AGY
```

Since the mutants were obtained using a mutagen that causes single base-pair insertions or deletions, the mutants have frameshift mutations. Therefore, a base pair should be missing or added in codon 40. Determine which insertion or deletion gives a frameshift with the appropriate amino acid sequence by comparing the mutant amino acid sequence with that of the wild type. You will find that if the Y of codon 40 is deleted, an appropriate sequence can be obtained, providing the unknown nucleotides are as specified below:

```
        -Met-Leu-Leu-Thr-Ile-Arg-Val-Stop
         39   40   41   42   43   44   45
         AUG  UUG  CNA  AYC  AYA  ARA  GYG  UNG
              N=U  Y=C  Y=U  R=G  Y=U  N=A
```

This means that the original sequence was

-Met-Phe-Ala-Asn-His-Lys-Ser-Val-Gly-
   39   40   41   42   43   44   45   46   47
  AUG UUY GCU AAC CAU AAG AGU GUA GGN

In the revertant, the reading frame is restored at codon 46, the Val (GUG) at codon 45 is altered to a Gly (GGN), and the chain termination codon at position 46 (UAG) is altered to a Val (GUN). This would have occurred if a G was inserted before or after the first G in codon 45. One would have

-Met-Leu-Leu-Thr-Ile-Arg-Gly-Val-Gly-
   39   40   41   42   43   44   45   46   47
  AUG UUG CUA ACC AUA AGA GGU GUA GGN

7.16   Answer:

a. The Ames test measures the rate of reversion of *his* auxotrophs to wild type. It selects for *his*$^+$ revertants by spreading *his* cells on medium without histidine and with or without a mixture of rodent liver enzymes in the presence of a filter disk impregnated with a potentially mutagenic compound. The spontaneous reversion rate is measured by using a control disk. Since the spontaneous reversion rate is very low, the increase in the reversion rate due to a mutagen is readily quantifiable. This makes the Ames test highly sensitive.

b. Impregnate a set of filter disks with the herbicide, and obtain an array of *his* mutants that are caused by different types of base-pair substitution and frameshift mutations. Place impregnated filter disks on two sets of plates lacking histidine, one set with rodent liver enzymes and one set without. Then spread each type of *his* mutant on both types of plates, incubate the plates, and monitor the number of *his*$^+$ colonies that grow. Compare the number of *his*$^+$ revertants on these plates to the number of *his*$^+$ colonies seen on control plates lacking the herbicide. If the herbicide is mutagenic, there will be a significant increase in colonies on the plate without liver enzymes. If the herbicide's animal metabolites are mutagenic, there will be a significant increase in colonies on the plate with the liver enzymes.

c. A serious concern is that the herbicide might not be mutagenic in the Ames test, even though it decays in the field through the action of sunlight, flora, or environmental chemicals to a mutagenic compound. The Ames test would provide support for the herbicide being safe when it is not. This concern can be partly addressed by performing additional Ames tests on extracts of plant and soil material treated with the herbicide. It is also possible that the herbicide is mutagenic in the Ames test but that its decay products in the field are not mutagenic. In this case, the main concern would be over herbicide exposure during its application. Presumably, this would make the herbicide unsuitable for use, even if it became safer following application.

7.17   Answer:

a. Many, but not all, DNA polymerases have a proofreading capacity that causes them to stall at mismatches during DNA replication. When present, the 3'-to-5' exonuclease activity associated with the polymerase will excise mismatched bases, so that they can be replaced. See text discussion in Chapter 3, p. 40, and Chapter 7, p. 146.

b. Shortly after DNA replication, mismatches can still be repaired by using a set of enzymes that recognize and excise mismatches in the newly synthesized DNA strand. In *E. coli*, mismatch repair is initiated when single base-pair mismatches or small base-pair additions or deletions in newly replicated DNA are bound by the MutS protein. The newly replicated strand is distinguished from the parental strand by the presence of an unmethylated A nucleotide in a 5'-GATC-3' sequence close to the mismatch. The MutL and MutH proteins bring the unmethylated GATC close to the mismatch and form a complex with MutS. MutH nicks the new, unmethylated DNA strand and a section of this DNA strand, including the mismatch, is excised by an exonuclease. DNA polymerase III and ligase repair the gap, producing the correct base pair (see text Figure 7.17, p. 149).

c. In *E. coli,* the parental strand can be distinguished from the newly replicated strand by methylation of the A in the sequence 5'-GATC-3'. Because a newly replicated DNA strand is not methylated until a short time after its synthesis, hemimethylation at this frequently appearing site allows for the identification of which strand is newly synthesized. Since only the strand with the unmethylated A is nicked by the MutH protein and excised by an exonuclease during mismatch repair, only the newly synthesized strand and not the parental strand is resynthesized by DNA polymerase III.

7.18   *Answer:* Photoreactivation requires the enzyme photolyase, which, when activated by a photon of light with a wavelength between 320 and 370 nm, splits the dimers apart. Dark repair does not require light but requires several different enzymes. First, the uvrABC endonuclease makes two single-stranded nicks, on the 5' side and the 3' side of the dimer. Then an exonuclease excises the 12-nucleotide-long segment of one strand between the nicks, including the dimer. Next, DNA polymerase I fills in the single-stranded region in the 5'-to-3' direction. Finally, the gap is sealed by DNA ligase.

7.19   *Answer:*

a. Large amounts of DNA damage trigger the SOS response, in which the RecA protein becomes activated and stimulates LexA to cleave itself. Since the LexA protein functions as a repressor for about 17 genes whose products are involved in DNA damage repair, this results in the coordinate transcription of those genes. Following the repair of DNA damage and inactivation of RecA, newly synthesized LexA coordinately represses their transcription.

b. The response is mutagenic because a DNA polymerase for translesion DNA synthesis is produced during the SOS response. When this polymerase encounters a lesion, it incorporates one or more nucleotides not specified by the template strand into the new DNA across from the lesion. These nucleotides may not match the wild-type template sequence, and so this polymerase introduces mutations.

c. In mutants having loss-of-function mutations in both *recA* and *lexA*, or only in *lexA*, there would be no functional LexA protein to repress transcription of the 17 genes whose protein products are involved in the SOS response; this would result in constitutive activation of the SOS response. If the loss-of-function mutation is only in *recA*, however, heavy DNA damage would not trigger RecA protein activation, so RecA could not stimulate the LexA protein to cleave itself to induce the SOS response. Instead, the LexA protein would continue to repress the DNA repair genes in the SOS system. Such a mutant would be highly sensitive to mutagens such as UV light and X-rays.

7.20   *Answer:*

a. In its normal state, 5-bromouracil is a T analog, base-pairing with A. In its rare state, it resembles C and can base-pair with G. It will induce an AT-to-GC transition as follows:

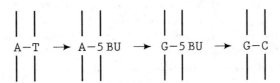

b. Nitrous acid can deaminate C to U, resulting in a CG-to-TA transition.

7.21   *Answer:* As you work on this problem, keep in mind the key findings from Luria and Delbruck's fluctuation test experiment: mutations occur spontaneously and are not the result of adaptation. This problem requires you to distinguish between spontaneous mutations, which are always occurring at a low rate, and mutations induced by mutagens, which can occur at a high rate but only following the treatment with a mutagenic agent. Mutations recovered following treatment with a mutagen are induced mutations, while mutations recovered without mutagen treatment are spontaneous. It also illustrates how a screen, if sensitive enough, can pick up rare spontaneous mutations as well as rare spontaneous revertants. Therefore, carefully examine how a screen selects for or against mutations, make inferences about how often mutations occur (from how many cell divisions occur before a selection is done or how many cells are used when a selection is performed), and under what conditions new mutations are recovered.

a. When cells were grown in the presence of 5BU, arg^+-to-arg mutations occurred because some of the cells plated on plates containing minimal medium supplemented only with arginine (both arg^+ and arg cells grow on this medium) were unable to grow on replica plates having only minimal medium (only arg^+ cells can grow on this medium). Mutations (arg-to-arg^+) also occurred during the growth of cells from an arg colony in 20 cultures containing minimal medium supplemented with arginine, since colonies were produced when the cultures were plated on minimal medium.

b. The arg^+-to-arg mutations were induced by the mutagen 5BU and are forward mutations. The arg-to-arg^+ mutations were spontaneous and are reverse mutations.

c. The induced arg^+-to-arg mutations were identified following replica plating. Colonies growing on plates supplemented with arginine can be arg^+ or arg. The arg mutant colonies were identified because they could not grow following replica plating onto medium without supplemental arginine. The spontaneous arg-to-arg^+ mutations were selected for by plating on medium without supplemental arginine.

d. The 20 cultures produced different numbers of colonies because arg-to-arg^+ mutations occurred at different points during the growth of the cultures. A culture with more colonies had a cell undergoing an earlier mutation, and this had more arg^+ descendants than did a culture with few colonies.

e. 5BU induces TA-to-CG and CG-to-TA transitions, so a second treatment with 5BU can revert 5BU-induced mutations. 5BU treatment should increase the frequency of reversion over the spontaneous frequency that was observed, so each of the cultures would produce a greater number of colonies.

f. MMS is an alkylating agent that causes GC-to-AT transitions. It would not increase the reversion rate of a 5BU-induced mutation. It might—by causing additional, second-site arg mutations—even lead to a decrease in the number of arg-to-arg^+ revertants.

7.22   *Answer:*

a, b.

```
5'-T-HX-U-A-G-BU-enol-2AP-C-BU-X-2AP-imino-3'

3'-A-C-A-T-C——— G —— T-G-A-C———C——5'
```
                                                          ◄————————————

c. If postmeiotic germ cells are treated, a single mutated site in one strand of the double helix will not be repaired until mitotic division begins during embryogenesis. Given the semiconservative replication of DNA, the normal strand will be replicated into two normal strands. If the mutated site on the other strand is not repaired, when the strand is replicated it will give rise to a double helix with two mutant strands. In this scenario, the products of DNA replication at the first mitotic division consist of one normal and one mutant helix. This will produce two different cell types, resulting in a mosaic individual.

For some mutagens, such as BU or 2AP, there is a variation in this method of mosaic production. If the BU (or 2AP) remains in the DNA strand it was incorporated into, the first mitotic division may result in a normal double helix (the new strand is copied from the old normal strand), and a double helix with the BU (or 2AP) paired to a "wrong" base (due to the rare form of BU). In this case, a mutant site will be produced on one of the daughter double helices that result after the second mitotic division (at the four-cell stage). In principle, a mutant cell could be introduced at any mitotic division when BU is incorporated in its rare form during DNA synthesis. In each case, a mosaic individual would be produced, but the later the developmental stage at which the mutation was introduced, the fewer the mutation-bearing cells.

7.23   *Answer:*

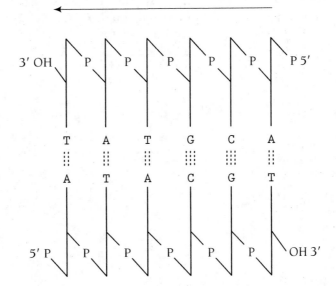

7.24   *Answer:* The absence of dG*TP* leads to a block in polymerization after the first two bases:

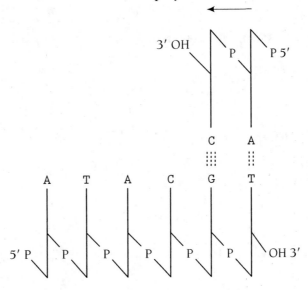

7.25   *Answer:* While the dHTP can substitute for dGTP, there is no dCTP, so polymerization cannot continue past the first base:

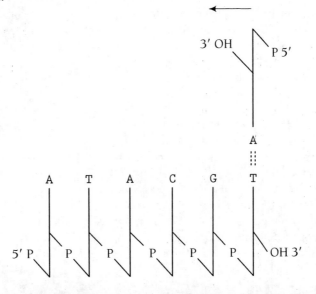

7.26 *Answer:* Pretreatment of the template with HNO_2 deaminates G to X, C to U, and A to H. X will still pair with C, but U pairs with A, and H pairs with C, causing "mutations" in the newly synthesized strand:

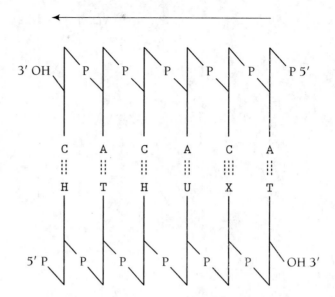

7.27 *Answer:* The dHTP will substitute for the absence of dGTP, and pair with C:

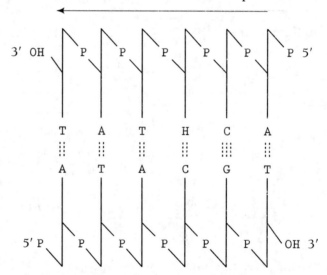

7.28 *Answer:* Answer this problem using only the data provided. First consider what is known about HA. HA causes a GC-to-AT transition and cannot revert mutations it induces. Therefore, HA cannot cause AT-to-GC transitions. HA also cannot revert the BU mutation. Consequently, BU must have caused a GC-to-AT transition.

Now consider the relationship between NA and HA. Since HA can revert NA mutations, the NA mutation was an AT-to-GC transition. This is consistent with the observation that NA can revert the HA mutation.

Now consider AP. AP cannot revert its own mutation, but it can revert the AT-to-GC transition caused by NA. Therefore the AP mutation was a GC-to-AT transition, and AP cannot induce AT-to-GC transitions. The AP mutation cannot be reverted by HA, because HA cannot induce AT-to-GC transitions. AP also could not revert the GC-to-AT transitions caused by BU or HA.

Because BU can revert its own GC-to-AT mutation, it can induce AT-to-GC transitions. Therefore, BU can revert the GC-to-AT mutations caused by AP and HA.

Because NA can cause AT-to-GC transitions, NA could revert the GC-to-AT transition caused by BU. It cannot be determined from these data whether NA can induce GC-to-AT transitions. If it can induce GC-to-AT transitions, it could revert its own mutations; if it cannot, it would not be able to revert its own mutations.

Mutation Induced by	Proportion of Mutations Reverted by				Base-Pair Substitution Inferred
	BU	AP	NA	HA	
BU	+	−	+	−	GC-to-AT
AP	+	−	+	−	GC-to-AT
NA	+	+	?	+	AT-to-GC
HA	+	−	+	−	GC-to-AT

7.29   *Answer:*

   a. The codon for Met is 5'-AUG-3'. This would be encoded by 3'-TAC-5' in the template DNA strand, which pairs with 5'-ATG-3' in the nontemplate DNA strand. In this case, the A in the nontemplate strand was deaminated to form hypoxanthine and paired with C in the template strand. The new template was 3'-CAC-5', and the new codon was 5'-GUG-3', coding for Val.

   b. In the mutant in **(a)**, the template strand was 3'-CAC-5', and the nontemplate strand was 5'-GTG-3'. Since hydroxylamine acts on cytosine bases, it would act on the template strand. If it acted at the 3'-C, DNA replication would result in the nontemplate strand becoming 5'-ATG-3'. After an additional round of replication, one of the daughter cells would have a template strand that is 3'-TAC-5'. Thus, hydroxylamine could be used to obtain revertants.

7.30   *Answer:* Nitrous acid deaminates C to make it U. U pairs with A, so treatment with nitrous acid leads to CG-to-TA transitions. Analyze how this treatment would affect the codons of this protein. Use N to represent any nucleotide and Y to represent a pyrimidine (U or C). Then the codons for Pro are CCN, the (relevant) codons for Ser are UCN, the codons for Leu are CUN, and the codons for Phe are UUY. (Nucleotides are written in the 5'-to-3' direction, unless specifically noted otherwise.)

   The codon CCN for Pro would be represented by CCN in the nontemplate DNA strand. Deamination of the 5'-C would lead to a nontemplate strand of UCN and a template strand of 3'-AGN-5'. This would produce a UCN codon encoding Ser. Deamination of the middle C would lead to a nontemplate strand of CUN and a template strand of 3'-GAN-5', producing a CUN codon encoding Leu.

   Further treatment of either mutant would result in deamination of the remaining C and a template strand of 3'-AAN-5'. This would result in a UUN codon. Since we are told that Phe is obtained, N must be C or U, and the template strand must be 3'-AAA-5' or 3'-AAG-5'.

   To explain why further treatment with nitrous acid has no effect, observe that nitrous acid acts via deamination and that T has no amine group. If the template strand were 3'-AAA-5', the nontemplate strand would have been TTT. Since T cannot be deaminated, nitrous acid will have no effect on the nontemplate strand.

7.31   *Answer:* Use the revertant frequencies under the heading "None" to estimate the spontaneous reversion frequency.

   ara-1: BU and AP, but not HA or a frameshift, can revert *ara-1*. Both BU and AP cause CG-to-TA and TA-to-CG transitions, while HA causes only CG-to-TA transitions. If HA cannot revert *ara-1*, it must require a TA-to-CG transition to be reverted and must be caused by a CG-to-TA transition.

   ara-2: BU, AP, and HA, but not a frameshift, can revert *ara-2*. Since HA causes only CG-to-TA transitions, *ara-2* must have been caused by a TA-to-CG transition.

   ara-3: By the same logic as that for *ara-2*, *ara-3* must have been caused by a TA-to-CG transition.
   Provided that this is a representative sample, mutagen X appears to cause both TA-to-CG and CG-to-TA transitions. It does not appear to cause frameshift mutations.

7.32   *Answer:* One of the most striking parallels between human and bacterial DNA repair systems has come from the analysis of mutations that affect mismatch repair (see Question 7.17 and its answer above). Mutations in any of the four human genes *hMSH2*, *hMLH1*, *hPMS1*, and *hPMS2* result in an increased accumulation of mutations in the genome and a hereditary predisposition to hereditary nonpolyposis colon cancer (HNPCC). Mutations in the *E. coli* genes *mutS* and *mutL* also result in an increased accumulation of mutations, and the normal alleles of these genes are essential for the initial stages of mismatch repair. The human gene *hMSH2* is homologous to *E. coli mutS*, and the other three human genes are homologous to *E. coli mutL*, indicating that aspects of mismatch repair are shared in these two organisms.

Examples of additional human genetic defects that lack functions required for DNA repair include xeroderma pigmentosum, ataxia telangiectasia, Fanconi anemia, Bloom syndrome, and Cockayne syndrome (see text Table 7.1, p. 150). While the specific DNA repair process affected by these mutations may not yet be sufficiently characterized for a direct comparison with a homologous process in *E. coli*, it has become clear that there are parallels in the types of repair processes that exist in the two organisms. For example, xeroderma pigmentosum and Fanconi anemia both affect repair of DNA damage induced by UV irradiation, whose mechanism of repair is well understood in *E. coli*.

7.33   *Answer:*

a. As the descendants of a bacterial cell form a colony on a solid surface, they divide and gradually spread radially in a gradually expanding ring. Suppose that at one point during the growth of a *lac* colony, a cell on the periphery spontaneously mutates to *lac*⁺. As the colony grows outward, the descendants of the *lac*⁺ cell will form a wedge-shaped sector. Since *lac*⁺ cells turn red on MacConkey-lactose medium, this will appear as a red (*lac*⁺) sector in an otherwise white (*lac*) colony.

b. Mutator mutations lead to an increased frequency of spontaneous mutations. Here, a mutator mutation would lead to an increased frequency of *lac*-to-*lac*⁺ reversions, and *lac*⁺-to-*lac* mutations would occur in the descendants of the revertants. The colonies would be white with multiple red, wedge-shaped sectors. In some of the red sectors, there would be white sectors.

c. Mutator mutations affect functions involved in DNA repair. For example, the *mutD* mutator gene mutation of *E. coli* encodes the ε subunit of DNA polymerase III, the primary replication enzyme in *E. coli*. The *mutD* mutants are defective in 3′-to-5′ proofreading activity, so that many incorrectly inserted nucleotides are left unrepaired. A *lac* mutation caused by a transition or transversion could be corrected during DNA replication by a mismatch that goes unrepaired due to the mutator mutation, producing a *lac*⁺ cell. Its descendants would produce a red sector within the white colony. In a subsequent cycle of DNA replication, a second unrepaired mismatch could introduce a new *lac* mutation, producing a white sector within the red sector.

7.34   *Answer:* Insertion elements (IS elements) are simpler in structure than transposons and have a transposase gene flanked by perfect or nearly perfect inverted repeat sequences (IR sequences). The more complex transposable elements (Tn elements) exist in two forms, composite transposons and noncomposite transposons. Composite transposons have a central gene-bearing region flanked by IS elements. Transposition of these elements, and the genes they contain (e.g., genes for antibiotic resistance), occurs because of the function of the IS elements. Noncomposite transposons also contain genes but do not terminate with IS elements. However, they do have inverted terminal repeated sequences that are required for transposition.

Both types of elements can integrate into target sites with which they have no homology, where they cause target site duplications. The transposition of IS elements and composite transposons requires use of the host cell's replicative enzymes and the transposase encoded in the element. Noncomposite transposons can transpose by two different mechanisms. Tn3-like noncomposite transposons utilize a replicative transposition mechanism employing a cointegrate—a fusion between a transposable element and the recipient DNA. Genes within Tn3 code for the enzymes transposase and resolvase that are needed for its transposition. Tn10-like composite transposons can move by a conservative (nonreplicative) transposition.

Upon insertion, all of the elements can cause mutations by a number of different mechanisms, including disruption of a gene's coding sequence or regulatory region.

7.35   *Answer:* The structure and, at a general level, the function of eukaryotic and prokaryotic transposable elements are very similar. For example, both Tn and *Ac* elements have genes within them and have inverted repeats at their ends. Both prokaryotic and eukaryotic elements may affect gene function in a variety of ways, depending on the element involved and how it integrates into or nearby a gene. The integration events of eukaryotic elements, like those of most prokaryotic transposable elements, involve nonhomologous recombination. Some eukaryotic elements, such as *Ty* elements in yeast and retrotransposons, move via an RNA intermediate, unlike the IS and Tn prokaryotic elements.

7.36   *Answer:* The left inverted repeat of the IS element has been removed, so that the two ends of this IS element are no longer homologous. The element will not be able to move out of this location and insert into another site.

7.37   *Answer:*
  a. i.   The transposon Tn*3* is a transposable element whose transposition requires its DNA replication. Its transposition is illustrated in the cointegration model shown in text Figure 7.22, p. 154. When the donor DNA containing the transposable element fuses with the recipient DNA, the transposable element becomes duplicated with one copy located at each junction between the donor and recipient DNA. After this cointegrate is resolved into two products, each has one copy of the transposable element.
   ii.   The bacterial Tn*10* element and the corn *Ac* element transpose without DNA replication using conservative transposition. After transposition, the element is lost from its original site of insertion.
   iii.   *Ty* elements in yeast and *copia* elements in *Drosophila* transpose by an RNA intermediate. After synthesis of an RNA copy of the integrated DNA sequence, reverse transcription results in a new element that integrates at a new chromosomal location.
  b.   Evidence that the inverted or direct terminal repeats found in transposable elements are essential for their transposition comes from the observation that mutations altering these sequences eliminate the ability of an element to transpose. These sequences are recognized by transposase during a transposition event.
  c.   yes

7.38   *Answer:* Deletions, inversions, and translocations can occur when homologous recombination occurs between two identical transposons inserted in different locations in the genome. To see how this occurs, draw out the chromosomes produced when a crossover occurs between two transposons inserted in different locations and orientations in the genome. If two transposons are inserted in the same orientation in one chromosome, pairing and homologous recombination between them results in a deletion of the segment lying between them. If two transposons are inserted in an opposite orientation in one chromosome, pairing and homologous recombination between them results in an inversion of the segment lying between them. If two transposons are inserted in different chromosomes, pairing and homologous recombination between them will result in a reciprocal translocation. Whether the translocation results in two single-centromere chromosomes or in a dicentric and acentric chromosome will depend on the orientation and position of the elements relative to their respective centromeres.

7.39   *Answer:* The extra 111 amino acids plus the one base-pair shift indicates that 334 base pairs were inserted into the G6Pase structural gene. Insertion of sequences is consistent with an initial *Ty* transposition into the G6Pase gene that was followed by recombination between its two deltas. Recombination between the two deltas would excise the *Ty* element but leave delta sequences behind in the G6Pase gene. Delta elements are 334 base pairs long and 70% AT, and therefore have the characteristics of the inserted sequence. If the delta element were positioned so that it world be translated and not generate a stop codon, it would yield the 111 new amino acids and one extra base pair, which would cause the frameshift. The two extra amino acids at the C-terminal end of G6Pase were added presumably because the frameshift did not allow the normal termination codon to be read.

7.40   *Answer:* Since introns are spliced out only at the RNA level, a transposition event that results in the loss of an intron (such as that used by *Ty* elements) indicates that the transposition occurred via an RNA intermediate. Thus, A is likely to move via an RNA intermediate. The lack of intron removal during B transposition suggests that it uses a DNA-to-DNA transposition mechanism (either conservative or replicative, or some other mechanism).

7.41   *Answer:*

   a. The ability to modify a pest species genetically may provide a means to develop better strategies for pest control. For insects harboring parasites that affect human and animal populations (e.g., mosquitoes that are hosts to malaria), the ability to modify the insect host genetically may provide a means to influence the reproduction of a human or animal pathogen.

   b. By analogy with the information used to develop *P* element–mediated transformation in *Drosophila*, it is essential to understand the mode of transposition of the element and to have identified the essential features of the element that allow it to transpose (the nature of the transposase and its regulation, the sequences the transposase recognizes to mediate transposition, etc.).

8

Genomics: The Mapping and Sequencing of Genomes

Chapter Outline

Review of Key Terms, Symbols, and Concepts

In your own words, write a brief, precise definition of each term in the groups below and on the following page. Check your definitions using the text. Then develop a concept map using the terms in each list.

1	2	3
genomics	molecular cloning	physical map
structural genomics	DNA clone	virtual chromosome
functional genomics	recombinant DNA	genomic library
comparative genomics	cloning vector	chromosome library
Human Genome Project (HGP)	restriction enzyme	cDNA, complementary DNA
Human Genome Organization (HUGO)	restriction site	cDNA library
descriptive science	restriction endonuclease	partial digestion
hypothesis-driven science	restriction digest	insert size
	twofold rotational symmetry	agarose gel electrophoresis
	sticky, staggered, blunt ends	DNA ladder, DNA size markers
	5', 3' overhang	ethidium bromide, SYBR green
	anneal	cosmid, phage vector
	ligate, DNA ligase	artificial chromosome
	plasmid vector	BAC, YAC vector
	polylinker, multiple cloning site	*ori*, F-factor origin
	origin, *ori*	*TEL, CEN, ARS* sequences
	selectable marker, *amp*R	*TRP1, URA3* markers
	unique restriction site	flow cytometry
	blue/white colony screening	oligo(dT) chains
	β-galactosidase	reverse transcriptase
	transformation	RNase H
	electroporation	DNA polymerase I, ligase
	vector recircularization	restriction site linker, linker
	alkaline phosphatase	adapter
	pBluescript II	subcloning

4	5
DNA sequencing	annotation
dideoxy sequencing	single nucleotide polymorphism (SNP)
pyrosequencing	DNA marker
template DNA	haplotype
oligonucleotide primer, primer	genetic recombination
universal sequencing primer	recombination hot, cold spot
T7, SP6 primer	tag SNP
pBluescript II	DNA microarray, chip
deoxynucleotide	SNP chip
dideoxynucleotide	hybridization
DNA polymerase	haplotype map, hapmap
3'-to-5' DNA exonuclease	open reading frame (ORF)
sequencing ladder	cDNA, microRNA
complementary sequence	NCBI, TIGR, NHGRI, GOLD
pyrophosphate	gene density
pyrogram	gene-rich region
whole-genome shotgun (WGS) sequencing approach	gene desert
	C-value paradox
sequencing, assembly, finishing	repetitive DNA
computer algorithm	Bacteria, Archaea, Eukarya
fold coverage	*Arabidopsis* 2010 project
draft sequence	data mining
Celera	homology, homologous gene

Thinking Analytically

The material in each section of this chapter builds on that of the previous section. Consequently, mastering the material in this chapter requires you to develop an integrated understanding of related topics. After reading through the chapter, check your general understanding of each section by outlining an answer to each of the key questions posed at the beginning of the chapter. Review the chapter material until you have a secure understanding of the general answers to the key questions. This will help you to contextually organize and retain the details in each section of this chapter, which in turn will help you develop an integrated understanding of this material.

This chapter presents the core set of techniques and ideas used to clone, sequence, and annotate genomes. Many of these have been developed by coupling fundamental genetic principles with technological advances. For example, the development of the ability to clone DNA required the synthesis of information from bacterial genetics (e.g., how to transform cells, how to design and use selectable markers, how to perform bacterial crosses, how to design plasmids); DNA replication (the discovery, characterization, and purification of DNA polymerases and ligases); and the discovery, characterization, and purification of restriction enzymes. As you learn about the methods used to clone and sequence genomes, reflect on how they rely on a synthesis of information from different areas of genetics and biochemistry.

Learning the material in this and the next two chapters requires you to understand the logic and fundamental genetic principles behind multiple laboratory and analytical techniques. While it would be helpful to have firsthand experience with all of them, this is unlikely to be an option. Indeed, the current repertoire of techniques used for cloning, sequencing, and analyzing genomes is so great and so rapidly advancing that no one scientist has firsthand experience in all of them. Still, scientists learn to think effectively about them and apply them to their research questions. You too can do this. Start by thinking through the steps of a new method and considering the rationale for each step. This will give you an understanding of how the method works. Then carefully examine how it is used in a specific application.

Ask yourself, "What is the objective of using this method in the application?" Once you have explored several different methods, consider how they can be used together to achieve an experimental goal and which methods can be used interchangeably.

One challenge associated with understanding the material of this chapter is to visualize manipulations of DNA that cannot be directly sensed (with the eyes, ears, nose, or touch). Like material from the physical sciences—chemistry and physics—that considers molecular interactions, the material in this chapter requires visualization and abstract conceptualization. While the results of techniques presented in this chapter cannot be directly sensed, they are based on understanding and developing a mental image of the molecular structure, function, and activity of nucleic acids and proteins in test tubes, cells, and viruses under defined environmental conditions. When the techniques produce reasonable, expected results, they validate and sometimes expand our understanding of the structure and function of these molecules. For example, we have never *seen* the actual base sequences of a fragment of DNA, but we have developed a model of DNA structure from experimentation. *If* that model is correct, then techniques such as dideoxy sequencing and pyrosequencing of DNA should work. As you learn about an experimental method, identify the models being used. Consider how the results obtained with the method would be altered if the model were incorrect.

Once a genome has been sequenced and the sequence assembled, its sequence is analyzed and annotated. Many of the strategies used to analyze and annotate a genome draw on information you have learned about in prior chapters. For example, genes are identified within a newly sequenced segment of DNA by scanning the DNA for sequence features associated with promoters, open reading frames, and intron–exon boundaries. These features were presented in earlier chapters on transcription and translation. Therefore, if you have trouble understanding the strategies used to annotate a genome, return to earlier chapters and review their material to clarify unclear concepts. Once you have a solid understanding of earlier material, you can strengthen your understanding of how a genome is annotated by reflecting on how the logic that underlies the analysis of sequence data is derived from understanding fundamental aspects of gene structure and organization.

The analysis of different genomes has provided insight into the similarities and differences between the genomes of different organisms. As was the case for similarly detailed material in earlier chapters, it will be easier to retain this material if you organize it into a contextual framework.

Finally, step back and consider that modern genetics increasingly interfaces with many different aspects of human health, agriculture, and human society. Reflect on the future directions for genomic studies and on the ethical, legal, and social issues that have arisen with the advent of sequencing the human genome. Ask yourself which of the outcomes need to be carefully monitored and regulated. Step back and think outside the box wherein scientists only pursue information and research for its own sake, justified by the potential for positive benefit to society. What dangers are associated with genomics? How, as a society, can we ensure that the "good" of genomics is utilized while minimizing its dangerous aspects?

Questions for Practice

Multiple-Choice Questions

1. In addition to the human genome, which of the following genomes were sequenced as part of the Human Genome Project?
   a. budding yeast
   b. nematode
   c. *E. coli*
   d. fruit fly
   e. all of the above

2. Which of the following is the best description of the goals of *functional* genomics?
   a. identifying a large set of SNPs within an annotated genome sequence
   b. understanding how and when each gene of the genome is used
   c. understanding the evolution of and biological differences between several species through a comparison of their genomes
   d. identifying the location of gene and nongene sequences within a sequenced genome

3. Which of the following statements about restriction enzymes is *not* true?
   a. All restriction enzymes cut DNA between the 3′ carbon and the phosphate moiety of the phosphodiester bond.
   b. Restriction enzymes are only found in bacterial cells.
   c. A restriction enzyme produced by a bacterium does not cleave that bacterium's DNA, because the bacterium methylates the site recognized by the restriction enzyme.
   d. All restriction enzymes recognize sites in DNA that have twofold rotational symmetry.

4. Which of the following is a feature that is useful, but not required, in a plasmid-cloning vector?
   a. An origin of DNA replication (*ori*).
   b. A dominant selectable marker such as *amp*^{R}.
   c. One or more unique restriction cleavage sites.
   d. A sequence that can facilitate sequencing of inserts using a universal sequencing primer.

5. A researcher wants to construct a genomic library in a plasmid vector with 4-kb inserts. He identifies a restriction enzyme that recognizes a 6-bp site that cleaves DNA, on average, every 4 kb and leaves sticky ends. He plans to completely digest the genomic DNA with this enzyme and then ligate the fragments into a similarly cleaved, alkaline-phosphatase treated plasmid vector. When he shares his plans with a colleague, the colleague advises him to prepare genomic DNA fragments in a different manner, specifically by partially digesting the genomic DNA with an enzyme that recognizes a more frequently appearing site and then selecting 4-kb fragments using gel electrophoresis. Whose approach is best, and why?
   a. The researcher's approach is best. All of the DNA fragments can be cloned, and none of the genome's information will be lost.
   b. The approach suggested by the colleague is best. If the DNA were completely digested, some fragments would be too large and some too small to clone. Partial digestion and size selection ensures that all of the fragments can be cloned and that none of the genomes information will be excluded when the library is formed. It also ensures that any particular sequence can be found in multiple clones in the library, so that an analysis of overlapping clones can be used to reconstruct the sequence of a particular genomic region.

6. On what basis does agarose gel electrophoresis separate DNA molecules?
   a. By charge: DNA molecules with more negatively charged phosphates move through the gel at a greater rate than do DNA molecules with fewer negatively charged phosphates.
   b. By size: Smaller DNA molecules move through the gel at a greater rate than do larger DNA molecules.
   c. By size and charge: Larger DNA molecules have more negatively charged phosphates than do smaller DNA molecules, so they move through the gel at different rates.
   d. By shape: Larger DNA molecules form different three-dimensional structures than do smaller DNA molecules, and the gel distinguishes between these structures.

7. What is meant by an SNP haplotype?
   a. a set of specific SNP alleles at particular SNP loci that is close together in one small region of a chromosome
   b. a small group of genetically linked SNPs
   c. a description of all of the SNPs present on one chromosome of one individual
   d. the SNP alleles that are possible at one chromosomal site in different chromosomes present in a population
   e. both a and b

8. A cDNA and a cloned fragment of genomic DNA share sequences from one ORF of a mouse. What differences do you expect to see between the cDNA and genomic DNA sequences?
   a. None; they should be identical.
   b. The cDNA might have intronic sequences.
   c. The genomic DNA might have promoter sequences.
   d. The genomic DNA might have a poly(A) tail.
   e. both b and c

9. DNA microarrays are
   a. aligned sets of printed DNA sequences, ordered according to their chromosomal positions.
   b. ordered grids of DNA molecules of known sequence fixed at known positions on a solid substrate.
   c. aligned sets of printed SNPs in a database.
   d. ordered grids of homologous genes from different organisms.

10. Which of the following statements is *not* true of archaean genomes?
    a. Some have large main circular chromosomes as well as multiple circular extrachromosomal elements.
    b. The genes involved in energy production, cell division, and metabolism are similar to their counterparts in bacteria.
    c. The genes involved in DNA replication, transcription, and translation are similar to their counterparts in eukaryotes.
    d. They have a higher GC content compared to either bacteria or eukaryotes.

11. Why could Celera Genomics obtain only the sequence of about 97% of the genomes of *Drosophila* and humans?
    a. In both organisms, simple telomeric sequences are very difficult to sequence, and these make up about 3% of the genome.
    b. In both organisms, long ribosomal DNA repeats make up about 3% of the genome. Since these are identical, it is impossible to sequence each individual repeat.
    c. In both organisms, approximately 3% of the sequences were in error.
    d. In both organisms, heterochromatic regions mostly near the centromeres are unclonable, making sequences in these regions impossible to obtain.

12. Why are antibiotic resistance markers important components of plasmid cloning vectors?
    a. The plasmid must have resistance to accept DNA inserts.
    b. They allow identification of bacteria that have taken up a plasmid.
    c. They ensure the presence of the *ori* site.
    d. They ensure that the plasmid can be cut by a restriction enzyme.

13. The restriction enzyme *Bam*HI cleaves a phosphodiester bond between two G–C base pairs at a six-base-pair site. The 5'-to-3' sequence of one of the sites is GGATCC. Which statement is true?
    a. *Bam*HI leaves a 5' overhang.
    b. *Bam*HI leaves a 3' overhang.
    c. *Bam*HI leaves a blunt end.
    d. DNA cleaved by *Bam*HI cannot be religated.

Answers: 1e, 2b, 3b, d, 4d, 5b, 6a, 7e, 8e, 9b, 10d, 11d, 12b, 13a

Thought Questions

1. What is the difference between hypothesis-driven science and descriptive science? In what types of circumstances is descriptive science necessary? How does descriptive science enhance hypothesis-driven science? Are there any circumstances where descriptive science is unwarranted?

2. What kinds of organisms naturally make restriction enzymes? Of what use are they to the organism where they are naturally made?

3. What properties does a tag SNP have? Why are tag SNPs useful? Discuss whether a tag SNP developed for use in one population works equally well in another population.

4. Three neighboring haplotypes are present in one region of a chromosome in the order A-B-C. A recombination hot spot lies between B and C. Which haplotypes will be inherited together more often, A and B, A and C, or B and C? Explain why.

5. Why is it important to use linkers when cloning cDNAs?

6. Two approaches to genome annotation are to: (a) compare cDNA and genomic DNA sequence; and (b) use computer algorithms to search the sequence of both DNA strands for protein-coding genes. What are the differences between these approaches, what are the disadvantages of each approach, and why are both approaches needed?

7. What are the ranges of sizes of bacterial genomes? Does the size of a bacterial genome positively correlate with the number of genes it has? Consider where bacteria with small genomes live. Hypothesize what factors allow some bacteria to have much smaller genomes than other bacteria.

8. For each of the organisms whose genomes are described in the text, tabulate the percentage of the protein-coding genes with unknown functions. What different hypotheses can you offer as to why so many protein-coding genes have unknown functions? How might you test your hypotheses?

9. What is meant when two genes in different species are referred to as homologs? What properties do you expect two homologous genes to have? Consider two homologous protein-coding genes. Which do you expect to be more similar: their DNA sequences or the amino acid sequences of their proteins? Explain why.

10. What are the arguments for and against the ability of states or the federal government to collect genetic data on their populace?

Thought Questions for Media

After reviewing the media on the *iGenetics* student website, try to answer these questions.

1. After shearing the DNA to fragments that are approximately 2 kb in size, why are the DNA fragments treated with SI nuclease?

2. What features must a plasmid cloning vector have in order to identify clones with inserts, and to obtain the end-sequences of inserts, in an efficient manner?

3. After the 2-kb DNA fragments are cloned into plasmid vectors, they are transformed into bacteria, the plasmids isolated, and their inserts sequenced. Since only about 500 bp of insert DNA can be obtained from each end of an insert, how is the remaining 1 kb of DNA obtained?

4. How are overlapping clones identified to construct a clone contig?

5. Why might there be gaps in an assembled sequence?

1. What is the rationale behind deleting the *STA1*, *STA2*, and *STA2K* genes?

2. Why is it important to *entirely* delete each of the *STA1*, *STA2*, and *STA2K* genes?

3. Why are there differences between the beers made with the three recombinant yeast strains, since each has a deletion of a gene responsible for glucoamylase production?

4. Why is the *CUP1* gene needed in these experiments? How would you demonstrate that it had no effect on fermentation characteristics or beer quality?

5. Refer to the frame that asks you to insert the *STA1* gene into the YEpD vector. Suppose there were two *Sna*BI sites flanking the *STA1* gene. Even though there is a unique *Sna*BI site in the YEpD vector, why wouldn't you use it instead of the *Bgl*II site?

Solutions To Text Questions and Problems

8.1   *Answer:* A DNA clone is a section of a DNA molecule that has been inserted into a vector molecule, such as a plasmid, phage, BAC, or YAC, and then replicated to form many identical copies when the vector is transformed into cells and the cells are propagated. Cloning genomic DNA involves several steps. After genomic DNA is isolated, it is manipulated so that it can be inserted into the cloning vector. This involves partially cleaving the DNA using a restriction enzyme to produce molecules with sticky ends and then selecting molecules of the desired size by agarose gel electrophoresis. The sticky ends of the insert DNAs are then annealed to complementary sticky ends in a similarly cleaved cloning vector, the nicks in the phosphodiester backbone are sealed using DNA ligase, and the recombinant molecule is transformed into a host cell. The host cell is propagated, and the DNA clone can be purified from the cells.

8.2   *Answer:* Examples of methods that utilize the hydrogen bonding in complementary base pairing include: (1) the binding of complementary sticky ends present in a cloning vector and a DNA fragment prior to their ligation by DNA ligase; (2) the annealing of a labeled nucleic acid to a complementary single-stranded DNA fragment on a microarray; (3) the annealing of an oligo(dT) primer to a poly(A) tail during the synthesis of cDNA from mRNA; and (4) the annealing of a primer to a template during a DNA sequencing reaction. In each case, base pairing allows for nucleotides to interact in a sequence-specific manner essential for the procedure's success. The binding of complementary sticky ends present in a cloning vector and DNA fragment position the fragment and the vector so that DNA ligase, which requires that base-pair matches flanking a gap in the phosphodiester backbone are correct before it can seal the nick in the phosphodiester backbone, can covalently attach the insert and vector molecules. Since the annealing of a labeled nucleic acid to a complementary single-stranded DNA fragment on a microarray is based on complementary base pairing, it allows the microarray be used for the detection of specific sequences. The annealing of an oligo(dT) primer to a poly(A) tail during the synthesis of cDNA from mRNA requires complementary base pairing between the primer and mRNA, which in turn defines where reverse transcriptase will initiate RNA-directed DNA synthesis. In a similar way, the binding of a primer to a template at the start of a DNA sequencing reaction requires complementary base pairing between the sequences in the primer and the template, which in turn defines where the DNA sequencing reaction will start.

8.3   *Answer:* Restriction enzymes serve to protect their hosts from infection by invading viruses and degrade any potentially infectious foreign DNA taken up by the cell (for example, by transformation). Since restriction enzymes digest DNA (restrict it) at specific sites, any foreign DNA will be cut up. To protect its own DNA from digestion by its restriction enzyme(s), a bacterium modifies (methylates) the sites recognized by its own restriction enzymes. This prevents cleavage at these sites.

8.4   *Answer:* The average length of the fragments produced indicates how often, on average, the restriction site appears. If the DNA is composed of equal amounts of A, T, C, and G, the chance of finding one specific base pair (A–T, T–A, G–C, or C–G) at a particular site is $\frac{1}{4}$. The chance of finding two specific base pairs at a site is $(\frac{1}{4})^2$. In general, the chance of finding n specific base pairs at a site is $(\frac{1}{4})^n$. Here, $1/4{,}096 = (\frac{1}{4})^6$, so the enzyme recognizes a six-base-pair site.

8.5   *Answer:*

a. The enzyme recognizes a sequence that has two G–C base pairs, two C–G base pairs, one A–T base pair, and one T–A base pair in a particular order. Since 40% of the genome is composed of G–C base pairs, the chance of finding a G–C or C–G base pair is 0.20, and the chance of finding an A–T or a T–A base pair is 0.30. The chance of finding these six base pairs with this sequence is $(0.20)^4 \times (0.3)^2 = 0.000144$. A genome with 3×10^9 base pairs will have about 3×10^9 different groups of 6-bp sequences. Thus, the number of sites in the human genome is $(0.000144) \times (3 \times 10^9) = 432{,}000$.

b. 3×10^9 bp$/432{,}000$ sites $= 1/0.000144 = 6{,}944$ bp between sites.

c. The chance of finding these six base pairs in a sequence having 80% A-T base pairs is $(0.10)^4 \times (0.4)^2 = 0.000016$, so two *Avr*II sites will be $1/0.000016 = 62,500$ bp apart.

8.6 *Answer:* Since 40% of the base pairs in human DNA are G-C, the probability of finding a G-C or C-G base pair is 0.20 and the probability of finding a T-A or A-T base pair is 0.30. (This assumes that in any region of the genome, there will be an average of 40% G-C or C-G base pairs.) The probability of finding a particular restriction enzyme recognition sequence is given in the following table.

Enzyme	Recognition Sequence	Probability of Finding the Sequence	Average Distance Between Sites
*Bam*HI	5'-GGATCC-3' 3'-CCTAGG-5'	$(0.2)^4(0.3)^2 = 0.000144$	$1/0.000144 = 6,944$ bp
*Eco*RI	5'-GAATTC-3' 3'-CTTAAG-5'	$(0.2)^2(0.3)^4 = 0.000324$	$1/0.000324 = 3,086$ bp
*Not*I	5'-GCGGCCGC-3' 3'-CGCCGGCG-5'	$(0.2)^8 = 0.00000256$	$1/0.00000256 = 390,625$ bp
*Hae*III	5'-GGCC-3' 3'-CCGG-5'	$(0.2)^4 = 0.0016$	$1/0.0016 = 625$ bp

8.7 *Answer:*

a. In a random sequence that is 25% each A, G, C, and T, the chance of finding a 6-bp site is $(\frac{1}{4})^6 = 1/4,096$, and the chance of finding an 8-bp site is $(\frac{1}{4})^8 = 1/65,536$. In such a sequence, *Apa*I, *Hind*III, *Sac*I, and *Ssp*I should produce fragments that average 4,096 bp in size, and *Srf*I and *Not*I should produce fragments that average 65,536 bp in size.

b. i. The large variation in average fragment sizes when one restriction enzyme is used to cleave different genomes could reflect: (1) the nonrandom arrangements of base pairs in the different genomes (e.g., there is variation in the frequencies of certain sequences that are part of the restriction site in the different genomes); and/or (2) the different base compositions of the genomes (e.g., genomes that are rich in A-T base pairs should have fewer sites for enzymes recognizing sites containing only G-C base pairs).

ii. The large variation in fragment sizes when the same genome is cut with different enzymes that recognize sites having the same length could reflect: (1) the nonrandom arrangement of base pairs *in that genome*; and/or (2) the base composition *of that genome*.

iii. If the sequence of *Mycobacterium tuberculosis* was random and contained 25% each of A, G, T, and C, enzymes recognizing a 6-bp site should produce fragments that are about 16-fold smaller than enzymes recognizing an 8-bp site. That this is not the case here suggests that at least one of these assumptions is incorrect. Two possibilities are that the genome of *Mycobacterium tuberculosis* is very rich in G-C base pairs and poor in A-T base pairs, and/or that there is a nonrandom arrangement of base pairs so that 5'-AA-3', 5'-TT-3', 5'-AT-3', and/or 5'-TA-3' sequences are rare. (The data given for *Sac*I suggest that the sites 5'-AG-3' and 5'-CT-3', which are part of the *Hind*III site, are not rare.)

8.8 *Answer:* All cloning vectors have three cardinal features: the ability to replicate within a host cell conferred by an origin of replication (e.g., an *ori* in bacterial plasmids, an *ARS* in YACs), a dominant marker that allows for their selection in a host cell (e.g., antibiotic resistance in bacterial vectors, an auxotrophic marker in YACs), and one or more unique restriction sites for DNA insertion. Many different types of vectors have been developed. Three types are bacterial plasmids, bacterial artificial chromosomes (BACs), and yeast artificial chromosomes (YACs). In addition to the three required features mentioned previously, YACs also have *CEN* sequences to ensure their proper segregation during cell division. These vectors differ in the amount of DNA they hold and how they are used. Plasmids typically hold less than 10 kb of DNA, can replicate at a high copy number within bacterial cells, and are used for many different purposes (in addition to those described in this chapter, more are discussed in text Chapters 9 and 10). When a genome is sequenced, they are used during the shotgun cloning of 2-kb and 10-kb inserts. BACs hold up to 300 kb of DNA and are present in a single copy in bacterial cells. They are the preferred vector for large clones in physical mapping studies of genomes because they do not undergo rearrangements, as do YACs. Two disadvantages to using *E. coli* cloning vectors are that very AT-rich sequences are difficult to clone in *E. coli*, and some sequences are poisonous to *E. coli* when cloned. YACs can hold between 0.2 and 2 Mb of DNA and are present in one copy per cell. Since they can hold large inserts, they have been useful for the construction of physical maps of the genome. However, their usefulness is limited because that they can undergo rearrangements and are often chimeric (holding DNA from more than one site in the genome).

8.9   *Answer:* In addition to the three cardinal features described in the answer to Question 8.8, the pBluescript II plasmid has several features that make it useful for constructing and cloning recombinant DNA. It has an origin of replication that results in it being present in a high copy number that facilitates purification of plasmid DNA. It contains many unique restriction sites in a polylinker or multiple cloning site that facilitates cloning fragments of DNA obtained after cleavage with a variety of restriction enzymes. Its polylinker is inserted near the 5′ end of the *lacZ* gene, which encodes β-galactosidase. Cells harboring a plasmid with an intact *lacZ* gene form blue colonies when grown on media with the β-galactosidase substrate X-gal. Cells harboring a plasmid whose *lacZ* gene has been interrupted by a cloned segment of DNA will not express functional β-galactosidase and will be white. Thus, blue/white screening can be performed to determine if a bacterial colony harbors a plasmid with DNA insertion. The pBluescript II plasmid also contains phage promoters flanking each side of the polylinker. These promoters are used to make *in vitro* RNA copies of the cloned DNA. Finally, the pBluescript II plasmid contains sequences flanking the polylinker that are complementary to universal sequencing primers. This allows an insert to be sequenced without prior information about its sequence. During the sequencing of a genome, it is particularly useful to work with a plasmid present in a high copy number so that plasmid DNA can be more easily purified, perform blue/white screening to detect colonies harboring plasmids with inserts, and use a set of universal sequencing primers to easily obtain the sequence inserted into different clones.

8.10   *Answer:*

a. To clone the DNA fragment, you must prepare the pBluescript II vector so that it has the same sticky ends as those of the DNA fragment, and so that it does not recircularize when you mix the vector with DNA ligase. Therefore, linearize the circular pBluescript II vector by digesting it with the enzyme *Pst*I. Then, treat the digested vector with alkaline phosphatase to remove its 5′ phosphates. This leaves only 5′-OH groups at its two ends, and so prevents its recircularization when mixed with DNA ligase. If the plasmid is not prevented from recircularizing, most of the colonies that are produced following transformation will not have inserts. After treating the vector with phosphatase, mix it with the 2-kb DNA fragment, and add DNA ligase. Since the insert DNA has not been treated with phosphatase, it retains 5′ phosphate groups and its 5′ ends can be ligated to the sticky ends of the digested vector. Then, transform *E. coli* with the ligation reaction, and plate the cells on medium containing ampicillin and X-gal. The presence of ampicillin in the medium ensures that only bacteria containing the pBluescript II plasmid will grow. The presence of X-gal allows colonies with inserts to be identified. If the fragment was not inserted into the *Pst*I site, the *lacZ* gene will function, β-galactosidase will be made, X-gal will be cleaved, and the colony will be blue. If the fragment was inserted into the *Pst*I site, it will have disrupted the *lacZ* gene, no β-galactosidase will be made, and the colony will be white.

b. To verify that you have cloned the fragment, independently confirm the results obtained using the blue/white screening. Select white colonies and prepare plasmid DNA from each colony. Digest the prepared DNAs with *Pst*I, and separate the digestion products by size using agarose gel electrophoresis. A colony with the correct insert should produce two bands: a 2-kb band corresponding to the insert and a 3-kb band corresponding to the pBluescript II vector.

8.11 *Answer:* If the enzyme is not inactivated, the restriction enzyme produced by the *hsdR* gene will cleave any DNA transformed into *E. coli* with the appropriate recognition sequence. This will make it impossible to clone DNA with the recognition sequence that is not methylated at the A in this sequence.

8.12 *Answer:* The *recA* mutation assists in preventing recombination between the host chromosome and the plasmid vector. This restricts propagation of the plasmid to the cytoplasm and maintains the integrity of cloned sequences. It also makes the host cell less viable if it is accidentally released into the environment, because it is less efficient at DNA repair and sensitive to UV light.

8.13 *Answer:* A genomic library made in a plasmid vector is a collection of plasmids that have different yeast genomic DNA sequences in them. Like two volumes of a book series, two plasmids in the library will have identical vector sequences but different yeast DNA inserts. Such a library is made as follows:

1. Isolate high-molecular-weight yeast genomic DNA by isolating nuclei, lysing them, and gently purifying their DNA.

2. Cleave the DNA into fragments that are 5–10 kb, an appropriate size for insertion into a plasmid vector. This can be done by cleaving the DNA with *Sau*3A for a limited time (i.e., performing a *partial* digest) and then selecting fragments of an appropriate size by either sucrose density centrifugation or agarose gel electrophoresis.

3. Digest a plasmid vector such as pBluescript II with *Bam*HI. This will leave sticky ends that can pair with those left by *Sau*3A. Treat the digested plasmid with alkaline phosphatase to prevent it from recircularizing when mixed with DNA ligase.

4. Mix the purified, *Sau*3A-digested yeast genomic DNA with the prepared plasmid vector and DNA ligase.

5. Transform the recombinant DNA molecules into *E. coli*.

6. Recover colonies with plasmids by plating on media with ampicillin (pBluescript II has a gene for resistance to this antibiotic) and with X-gal (to allow for blue/white colony screening to identify plasmids with inserts). Each colony will have a different yeast DNA insert, and all of the colonies comprise the yeast genomic library.

In a BAC vector, much larger DNA fragments—200 to 300 kb in size—would be used.

8.14 *Answer:* Marisol's strategy will ensure that the inserts are representative of all of the genomic sequences. Partial digestion of genomic DNA will generate a population of overlapping fragments representative of the entire genome. When the library is screened, multiple overlapping clones from a region will be identified. Mike's strategy works in principle, but in practice has drawbacks. Analyzing a region requires each adjacent restriction fragment from that region to be cloned and recovered in a screen of a genomic library. Given the small size of the restriction fragments, the library will need to contain a very large number of clones, and screening the library to find all of the adjacent clones in a region will be very laborious. In addition, large genes will be split into multiple pieces. Hesham's strategy is the least desirable. While using ionizing radiation to introduce double-strand breaks will result in the random fragmentation of DNA and produce a population of overlapping genomic DNA fragments, it will also introduce other types of DNA damage (see text Chapter 7). Damage to the DNA may prevent its successful cloning, and sequences that can be cloned are unlikely to be identical to the genomic DNA, because bacterial DNA repair processes will lead to alterations in the DNA sequence.

8.15 *Answer:* Use a restriction site linker, a short segment of double-stranded DNA that contains a restriction site. The linker can be efficiently ligated onto blunt-ended DNA fragments. Digestion of the resulting DNA fragments with the restriction enzyme will then produce fragments with sticky ends. Their sticky ends allow for efficient ligation into plasmids digested with the same restriction enzyme. See text Figure 8.16, p. 197. To clone DNA fragments that have the restriction site found in the linker, use an adapter—a short, double-stranded piece of DNA with one sticky end and one blunt end.

8.16   *Answer:* From the text, $N = \ln(1 - p)/\ln(1 - f)$, where N is the necessary number of recombinant DNA molecules, p is the probability of including one particular sequence, and f is the fractional proportion of the genome in a single recombinant DNA molecule. Here, $p = 0.90$ and $f = (2 \times 10^5)/(3 \times 10^9)$, so $N = 34,538$.

8.17   *Answer:*

a. The chance the biochemist will find the antifreeze gene if he sequences the insert of just one clone from a library is f, where f is the fractional proportion of the genome in a single DNA clone. For the plasmid library, $f = (7 \times 10^3)/(2 \times 10^9) = 3.5 \times 10^{-6}$. For the BAC library, $f = (2 \times 10^5)/(2 \times 10^9) = 1 \times 10^{-4}$. For the YAC library, $f = (1 \times 10^6)/(2 \times 10^9) = 5 \times 10^{-4}$.

b. If N is the necessary number of recombinant DNA molecules, p is the probability of including one particular sequence, and f is the fractional proportion of the genome in a single recombinant DNA molecule, $N = \ln(1 - p)/\ln(1 - f)$. Here, $p = 0.95$. Use the values for f determined in part (a). For a plasmid vector, $N = \ln(1 - 0.95)/\ln[1 - 3.5 \times 10^{-6}] = 8.6 \times 10^5$. For a BAC vector, $N = \ln(1 - 0.95)/\ln[1 - (1 \times 10^{-4})] = 3.0 \times 10^4$. For a YAC vector, $N = \ln(1 - 0.95)/\ln[1 - (5 \times 10^{-4})] = 6.0 \times 10^3$.

c. Plasmid clones are easier to manipulate than BAC or YAC clones. Their high copy number in bacterial cells facilitates their purification. This, and the ease of constructing plasmid libraries with inserts that are less than 10 kb, makes them useful for sequencing genomes using a whole-genome shotgun approach. The sequence of the ends of the inserts in many different clones can be obtained and then used to assemble the sequence of the genome. However, plasmid vectors they hold less DNA than BAC or YAC vectors. Therefore, for situations such as that described in this problem, where a particular clone must be identified in a library, many more clones need to be analyzed when a plasmid library is used.

  BACs are artificial bacterial chromosomes and are present in cells in just one copy. BACs accept inserts up to 300 kb and have the advantage that they can be manipulated just like bacterial plasmids (though their purification is not as simple as plasmids). Sequences cloned into BACs are stable and do not undergo rearrangements in the host. This property has made BAC vectors the preferred vector for making large clones in physical mapping studies of genomes. Two disadvantages of BACs (and other cloning vectors for *E. coli*) are that AT-rich DNA fragments do not clone well, and some DNA sequences are toxic to *E. coli*.

  YACs are artificial chromosomes grown in yeast cells. They have been used to clone very large DNA fragments (between 0.2 and 2.0 MB) and so are useful for creating physical maps of large genomes such as the human genome. They have two disadvantages. First, during the cloning process, a fraction of YAC vectors accept two or more inserts, forming a chimeric YAC. A second problem is that portions of the insert DNA are frequently deleted or otherwise modified in the yeast host cell, or undergo recombination with other DNA in the host cell. This confounds and slows down the sequence assembly process, since these modified clones contain rearranged DNA inserts that are not identical to DNA in the genome, and the overlap between different YAC clones can sometimes be misleading.

d. Recombinant molecules containing AT-rich sequences do not clone well in *E. coli*, so if the Antarctic fish has a very AT-rich genome and a genomic library were propagated in *E. coli*, some of the sequences in the genome would not be present in the library. Therefore, the library would not be representative of all the sequences in the genome of the fish.

8.18   *Answer:*

a. If 500 nucleotides of sequence are recovered from each dideoxy sequencing reaction, approximately, $500 \times (13,543,099 + 10,894,467) = 1.22 \times 10^{10}$ nucleotides were sequenced, corresponding to $(1.22 \times 10^{10}$ nucleotides$/(3 \times 10^9$ bp/haploid genome$) \approx$ fourfold coverage.

b. Clones must be sequenced from libraries with different sized inserts so that sequences can be assembled in locations where repetitive DNA elements are inserted. If a plasmid with a 2-kb insert has a unique sequence at one end but a repetitive sequence at the other end, it will not be possible to continue to assemble the sequence past this plasmid because many clones in the library have the same repetitive sequence, and they come from all over the genome. Since many repetitive sequences are about 5 kb in length, sequencing plasmids with 10-kb inserts circumvents this problem. Some of the 10-kb inserts will have a sequence at one end that overlaps the unique sequence in the plasmid with the 2-kb insert as well as a unique sequence at their other end that lies past the repetitive element and can be assembled with unique sequence from other plasmids.

c. The sequence of the central region is obtained from the sequence of overlapping clones during sequence assembly.

8.19 *Answer:*

a. In a DNA sequencing reaction, the annealing of a sequencing primer to one strand of a double-stranded DNA fragment defines the point from which DNA sequence can be obtained. If the sequence of an insert in pBluescript II is unknown, it is not possible to design and synthesize a sequencing primer targeted directly to it. To circumvent this issue, the pBluescript II vector has universal sequencing primer sites that flank the multiple cloning site. As shown in text Figure 8.9, p. 184, in pBluescript II, the T7 universal sequencing primer anneals near the *Kpn*I site, and the SP6 universal sequencing primer anneals on the other side of the multiple cloning site. These sequencing primers are positioned so that DNA polymerase can extend from the primer to obtain the sequence of the ends of the insert.

b. If dideoxy sequencing is used, only several hundred bases of sequence are obtained from one sequencing reaction. Let us consider the case where a sequencing reaction produces 500 bases of sequence. To obtain the sequence of the entire 7-kb insert, first obtain the sequence of the ends of the insert using the universal primers present in the pBluescript II vector. In a second step, use that sequence to design new primers that are about 450 bases from the ends of the insert, and use these to obtain an additional 500 bases of DNA sequence. Assemble this sequence with that obtained previously based on the overlap between the sequences—you will have about 950 bases of sequence at each end. Take a third step: design primers that are about 900 bases from the ends of the insert, use them in a third set of sequencing reactions to obtain an additional 500 bases of DNA sequence, and assemble this sequence onto the one you already have. Continue to design primers based on the newly obtained sequence, and use them to "walk" through the sequence in this manner until you have obtained the sequence of the entire insert. The sequence obtained from one end of the insert will be reversed and complementary to the sequence obtained from the other end of the insert.

c. While you could in principle use the "primer walking" method described in part (b) to obtain the sequence of a 200-kb insert in pBeloBAC11, it would be tedious and time-consuming. In addition, if there were repetitive sequences within the insert, you might run into problems—if you inadvertently designed a primer within a repetitive sequence, you would not obtain unambiguous sequence information from that primer. It is more efficient to obtain the insert's sequence by using a whole-genome shotgun cloning approach. Make a plasmid library with 2-kb and 10-kb inserts from the pBeloBAC11 clone, sequence the ends of the inserts from enough clones to obtain sevenfold coverage, and then assemble that sequence using computerized algorithms.

8.20 *Answer:* The whole-genome shotgun approach to sequencing a genome obtains many 500-nucleotide sequences at once and then assembles them into a continuous sequence for each chromosome. It relies on technology that generates a great many sequence reads very quickly and then computerized algorithms to identify overlaps and build long stretches of continuous sequence. In contrast, the biochemist's approach proceeds stepwise. Even if technology were used so that each sequence read were obtained quickly, the process of obtaining the entire genome's sequence would be slow since each clone would be analyzed before the next clone would be sequenced. In addition, the biochemist's approach cannot be used to assemble the entire sequence of a genome. The biochemist's approach obtains DNA sequence from clones of just one size. Since repetitive elements are dispersed throughout the genome, if a repetitive element is present at one end of a clone, it is not possible to know how to align the sequence from that clone with the sequence from other clones containing the same repetitive element. The whole-genome shotgun approach circumvents this problem by sequencing clones with different sized inserts.

Coverage refers to the number of nucleotides that are sequenced compared to the number of nucleotides in the genome. If a genome is sequenced with sevenfold coverage, sevenfold more nucleotides were sequenced than are present in the genome. Since clones are sequenced at random, so some regions will be sequenced twice just by chance. Therefore, if just the number of nucleotides in a genome were sequenced (onefold coverage), some regions would not be sequenced and there would be gaps in the assembled sequence. A genome sequenced with greater coverage has a decreased probability of having gaps in its sequence. In addition, greater coverage will result in more regions of the genome having been sequenced multiple times. This facilitates a comparison of overlapping sequences from different clones and allows errors in the assembled and finished sequence to be minimized.

8.21   *Answer:* After the primer anneals to the fragment, DNA polymerase will extend the primer at its 3' end by adding nucleotides that are complementary to the template. As the primer is extended, some chains will be prematurely terminated when a labeled dideoxynucleotide is incorporated. Since the four dideoxynucleotides are labeled with different fluorescent dyes, the extension products that terminate with the same base will have the same fluorescent label and be detected as distinct, labeled bands after separation using capillary gel electrophoresis. Therefore, the order of fluorescent peaks can be used to determine the sequence.

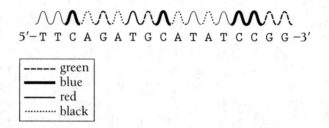

5'–T T C A G A T G C A T A T C C G G –3'

------ green
■■■■ blue
——— red
········· black

8.22   *Answer:* Both dideoxy chain-termination sequencing and pryosequencing start with a DNA template, DNA polymerase, and a sequencing primer. However, dideoxy chain-termination sequencing detects the sequence of a nucleotide chain using a chain-termination mechanism, while pyrosequencing does not. In dideoxy chain-termination sequencing, four different fluorescently labeled dideoxynucleotides are present in a DNA synthesis reaction where the sequencing primer is extended by DNA polymerase. When a fluorescently labeled dideoxynucleotide is incorporated into a growing polynucleotide chain, chain termination occurs. When the extension products are separated by size using capillary gel electrophoresis, the order of fluorescent peaks can be used to determine the sequence.

In contrast, pyrosequencing determines a sequence by enzymatic detection of the pyrophosphate released when a nucleotide is incorporated by DNA polymerase as it extends a new DNA strand. In pyrosequencing, a single-stranded DNA molecule is attached to a solid, microscopic bead and placed in the microscopic well of a pyrosequencer. A sequencing reaction mixture is added that contains a primer, DNA polymerase, and three other enzymes. The four dNTPs are added sequentially to and removed from the pyrosequencing reaction so that only one dNTP is present in the reaction at any one time. If, when a dNTP is added to the reaction, it is complementary to the first unpaired base in the template strand, DNA polymerase will add it to the primer and a molecule of pyrophosphate will be released. A second enzyme in the reaction uses the pyrophosphate to produce ATP, and a third enzyme uses the energy stored in the newly produced ATP to generate light. The pyrosequencer detects and quantifies the amount of light released and correlates it to which dNTP was present in the reaction. In this way, the base added to the growing DNA strand is determined. The process is continued cyclically so that over many cycles, the sequence complementary to the template strand sequence is obtained.

Pyrosequencing is advantageous for large-scale sequencing projects because it allows for the gathering of massive amounts of sequence data. A pyrosequencer has about 200,000 microscopic wells. In each, a different pyrosequencing reaction can be carried out. If each well contains a bead with a single-stranded template DNA prepared from a different clone in the same plasmid vector, a reaction mixture with a universal sequencing primer can be used to obtain about 20 million nucleotides of genome sequence in about 6 hours.

8.23   *Answer:* Not all SNPs lead to an alteration in phenotype. Some are silent. For example, if a SNP does not lie in a DNA sequence that is transcribed, or does lie in a transcribed sequence but after mRNA processing does not alter the amino acid inserted into a polypeptide chain, it will not cause a missense or nonsense mutation and could be silent. If a SNP does also not lie in a gene regulatory region, it will not affect a gene's function and could also be silent.

8.24 *Answer:*

a. A SNP marker is a single nucleotide polymorphism—a simple, single base-pair alteration present in some individuals at one particular chromosomal site.

b. A haplotype is a set of specific SNP alleles at particular SNP loci that lie close together in one small region of a chromosome. Differences in SNP alleles in different members of a population will lead to a population having a set of haplotypes. Because recombination is uncommon in a small region of the genome, SNPs in one small region of a chromosome tend to be inherited together. Genetic recombination happens in recombination hot spots and is far rarer in recombination cold spots. SNPs at a set of loci lying within a recombination cold spot will tend to be inherited together in a population and result in a haplotype that is shared in different members of the population.

c. A hapmap is a haplotype map—a complete description of all of the haplotypes known in a set of tested human populations, including information on their chromosomal location.

d. A tag SNP is a SNP within a haplotype whose genotype can be used to identify the other SNP alleles in the haplotype. SNPs within a haplotype are inherited together because they lie in a recombination cold spot. This makes it possible to infer what SNP alleles are present in a haplotype using a single measurement, that of the tag SNP.

e. By using hybrid cell lines containing a single copy of chromosome 21, the researchers could infer exactly what alleles were present on a single chromosome. Suppose they had instead analyzed samples obtained from the blood of different individuals that contained two copies of chromosome 21. Then, they would not be able to determine the arrangement of SNP alleles on one copy of chromosome 21. For example, consider two SNP loci, *A* and *B*, in one region of chromosome 21 and an individual who has the genotype *A1 A2 B1 B2*. The individual could have alleles *A1* and *B1* on one copy of chromosome 21 and *A2* and *B2* on the other copy, or *A1* and *B2* on one copy of chromosome 21 and *A2* and *B1* on the other copy. By using hybrid cell lines with just one copy of chromosome 21, the researchers were able to determine which SNP alleles were present in one haplotype.

f. i. Though a population may have many different SNP alleles and haplotypes, not all of these will be seen in members of just one family. Since individuals within a family share more of their genome, they will share more haplotypes than unrelated individuals will. Consequently, if the cell lines were established from blood samples drawn at a large family reunion, there would be fewer haplotypes than if the lines were established from unrelated individuals. If there are fewer haplotypes, there should also be fewer tag SNPs. Indeed, since recombination is generally infrequent in any one chromosomal region (see text Chapter 14), related individuals are expected to share haplotypes over larger segments of their genome. Therefore, fewer tag SNPs can be used to identify their haplotypes.

   ii. Some SNPs may only have arisen in certain populations, and so some haplotypes may be seen only in certain populations. In addition, some haplotypes may be more frequent in a particular population. Therefore, individuals whose ancestors originate from the same geographical region, though unrelated as family members, are likely to share more haplotypes than do individuals whose ancestors originate from distinct geographical origins. Therefore, the number of haplotypes and the number of tag SNPs is likely to be fewer in individuals with ancestors from the same geographical region than in individuals with ancestors from different geographical regions.

8.25 *Answer:* A tag SNP is a SNP having alleles that can identify the alleles at other SNPs in a haplotype. To identify a tag SNP, identify the haplotypes present in a set of samples and then determine whether a SNP within that haplotype can uniquely specify the haplotype.

In this dataset, start to identify haplotypes by comparing pairs of samples. Focusing initially on two columns of the table, proceed down the columns row by row to identify pairs of cell lines that share neighboring SNP alleles in one chromosomal region. At some point as you proceed down the columns, two cell lines that shared neighboring SNP alleles in earlier rows will no longer share the same SNP allele. This likely marks the end of a shared haplotype. Draw a line underneath the last row where SNP alleles are shared, and scan the rows above the line to see if any other samples share the haplotype you have identified. Shade or color-code the squares within the table to keep track of the haplotype. Once you have identified a haplotype in one set of adjacent rows, examine the remaining columns in a similar manner to identify the other haplotypes in that region. Shade or color-code these and then proceed further down the table, analyzing additional rows in the same manner as before, to identify the next set of haplotypes. After you have completed an analysis of all rows of the table, go back and see if any neighboring haplotypes can be combined and extended. Finally, examine the haplotype regions to identify tag SNPs—SNPs with alleles that uniquely specify the haplotype. One approach to this is to exclude SNPs with alleles that are seen in more than one haplotype, since these cannot serve as tag SNPs.

In the following table, SNP alleles belonging to a haplotype are similarly shaded, horizontal lines separate regions with different haplotypes, and tag SNPs are in bold.

Cell Line

1	2	3	4	5	6	7	8	9	10
A1	A1	A2	A3	A1	A3	A2	A3	A1	A2
B1	B1	B2	B3	B2	B3	B2	B3	B1	B2
C3	C3	C1	C2	C1	C2	C1	C2	C3	C1
D4	**D4**	**D3**	**D2**	**D1**	**D2**	**D3**	**D2**	**D4**	**D3**
E1	E1	E2	E2	E3	E2	E2	E2	E1	E2
F2	F1	F2	F2	F2	F1	F2	F2	F2	F2
G3	**G2**	**G3**	**G3**	**G1**	**G2**	**G1**	**G3**	**G1**	**G3**
H1	H1	H1	H1	H2	H1	H2	H1	H2	H1
I3	**I1**	**I3**	**I3**	**I2**	**I1**	**I2**	**I3**	**I2**	**I3**
J2	J1	J2	J2	J2	J1	J2	J2	J2	J2
K1	K1	K1	K1	K2	K1	K2	K1	K1	K1
L2	L1	L2	L2	L1	L1	L1	L2	L2	L2
M1	**M1**	**M2**	**M1**	**M1**	**M2**	**M2**	**M1**	**M2**	**M1**
N2	**N2**	**N1**	**N2**	**N2**	**N1**	**N1**	**N2**	**N1**	**N2**
O1	O1	O1	O1	O1	O2	O1	O1	O1	O2
P2	P1	P2	P1	P2	P1	P1	P1	P2	P1
Q2	Q2	Q2	Q2	Q2	Q1	Q2	Q2	Q2	Q1
R3	**R1**	**R3**	**R1**	**R3**	**R2**	**R1**	**R1**	**R3**	**R2**
S1	S2	S1	S2	S1	S1	S2	S2	S1	S1
T1	T1	T1	T1	T1	T1	T1	T1	T1	T1
U2	U1	U2	U1	U2	U2	U1	U1	U2	U2
V2	V2	V2	V2	V2	V2	V2	V2	V2	V2
W2	W3	W1	W2	W1	W3	W1	W1	W3	W1
X1	X2	X1	X1	X3	X2	X3	X1	X2	X3
Y2	**Y1**	**Y4**	**Y2**	**Y3**	**Y1**	**Y3**	**Y4**	**Y1**	**Y3**
Z1	Z1	Z2	Z1	Z2	Z1	Z2	Z2	Z1	Z2

SNPs D, G, I, M, N, R, and Y can serve as TagSNPs because these have alleles that are unique to each haplotype. The following table summarizes the haplotypes identified by alleles at these TagSNPs (the TagSNP allele is in bold):

TagSNP(s)	Haplotype
D	A1 B2 C1 **D1** E3
	A3 B3 C2 **D2** E2
	A2 B2 C1 **D3** D2
	A1 B1 C3 **D4** E1
G, I	F2 **G1** H2 **I2** J2 K2 L1
	F1 **G2** H1 **I1** J1 K1 L1
	F2 **G3** H1 **I3** J2 K1 L2
M, N	**M1 N2**
	M2 N1
R	O1 P1 Q2 **R1** S2 T1 U1 V2
	O2 P1 Q1 **R2** S1 T1 U2 V2
	O1 P2 Q2 **R3** S1 T1 U2 V2
Y	W3 X2 **Y1** Z1
	W2 X1 **Y2** Z1
	W1 X3 **Y3** Z2
	W1 X1 **Y4** Z2

The 26 SNPs define 5 sets of haplotypes, so a minimum of 5 TagSNPs are needed to differentiate between them.

8.26 *Answer:* Compare the SNPs present in individuals assigned to different racial groups using DNA chips (probe arrays) containing thousands of SNPs that are representative of SNPs throughout the entire genome. That is, use a probe array that has, for each of several thousand representative SNPs, a set of oligonucleotides that match the common allele and all possible variant alleles. Each hybridization will assess the SNP alleles present in one individual, performed by labeling fragments of genomic DNA from one individual as target DNA and hybridizing the labeled DNA to a SNP probe array. An individual's SNP alleles (and whether they are homozygous or heterozygous) will be determined by observing the pattern of fluorescence on the probe array and comparing this to the locations of the oligonucleotides for each SNP allele. The percentage of SNPs that are shared between individuals assigned to different racial groups can be determined by comparing the results of hybridizations with target DNA from individuals from different racial groups. If tag SNPs were detected using this approach, one could quantify the percentage of haplotypes that are shared in different racial groups.

8.27 *Answer:* Prepare a DNA microarray consisting of oligonucleotides that collectively represent the entirety of the normal dystrophin gene, including SNPs known to be present in normal individuals as well as known point mutations. It is important to consider that some sites in the gene will be polymorphic in normal individuals; multiple probes able to detect the various SNPs found in a particular region of the gene will need to be placed on the microarray. Isolate DNA from the blood of an individual affected with muscular dystrophy, label it with a fluorescent dye, and hybridize the chip with the labeled DNA under conditions that require a precise match between the labeled DNA and the oligonucleotide probes on the DNA microarray. The site of the mutation can be located by identifying the region of the gene where no hybridization signal is seen in any of the oligonucleotide probes that detect normal sequences. If the mutation corresponds to a previously known point mutation, the probe(s) able to detect that mutation should show a hybridization signal.

8.28 *Answer:* During *assembly*, the raw sequence obtained from genome sequencing projects are pieced together in the order they are found in the genome. This is done by aligning overlapping sequences and, when a sequencing read containing unique sequence at one end terminates with repetitive sequence, identifying other clones containing unique sequences that span the length of the repetitive element. The assembly process produces a working draft of a genomic sequence. A working draft of a genome sequence contains many gaps that must be filled in, as well as sequencing errors. The *finishing* process fills in these gaps and addresses the errors. It results in a highly accurate sequence with less than one error per 10,000 bases and as many gaps as possible filled in. After the complete sequence of a genome is obtained, it is annotated. During *annotation*, genes and other important sequence features (e.g., repetitive elements, SNPs) are identified. Genes can be identified by comparing genomic sequence to cDNA sequences obtained from sequencing clones in cDNA libraries. Genes and other important sequence features can also be predicted through the analysis of sequences using computerized algorithms. SNPs can be identified by comparing the sequences of different individuals in a population. Annotation begins the process of assigning functions to all of the genes of an organism.

8.29   *Answer:* A cDNA library is a large collection of cloned DNA sequences that are complementary to and derived from mRNAs. cDNAs are synthesized from mRNA using the enzyme reverse transcriptase, which uses an RNA template to synthesize a DNA strand.

The first step in the preparation of a cDNA library is the isolation of cellular mRNAs. Cellular RNA is passed over a column to which oligo(dT) chains are attached. These bind the A nucleotides in the poly(A)+ mRNA. The captured mRNAs are released from the column and then used as a template in a reverse transcription reaction primed with oligo(dT). This generates double-stranded DNA–mRNA molecules. To convert these to double-stranded cDNAs, RNase H is used to partially degrade the RNA strand in the hybrid DNA–mRNA, DNA polymerase I is used to synthesize new DNA fragments using the partially degraded RNA fragments on the single-stranded DNA as primers, and DNA ligase is used to ligate the new DNA fragments. There are two ways to generate sticky ends on a cDNA so that it can be efficiently cloned. In one, a restriction site linker is ligated onto the ends of the cDNA. For this method to work, methylated nucleotides must be used during the synthesis of the cDNA. Then, after an unmethylated linker is added to the cDNA's ends, the linker, but not the cDNA, will be cleaved by a restriction enzyme. The second method to add sticky ends onto the ends of the cDNA is to ligate it to an adapter—a molecule with one blunt and one sticky end.

The annotation of a genome can be aided by sequencing clones from cDNA libraries. Libraries that contain cDNA sequences contain neither introns nor non-transcribed sequences. Therefore, sequence analysis of cDNAs provides a reliable way to define the exact boundaries of exons. It also provides evidence that a genomic sequence is transcribed. One caveat is that not all of the cDNAs produced in a cDNA library will be full length. However, even if the cDNA is an incomplete copy of an mRNA, it can identify a region that contains a gene during the annotation process. Computer algorithms can take advantage of this and predict the rest of the coding region.

8.30   *Answer:* Repetitive sequences pose at least two problems for sequencing eukaryotic genomes. Highly repetitive sequences associated with centromeric heterochromatin consist of short, simple repeated sequences. These are unclonable, making it impossible to obtain the complete genome sequence of organisms with them. More complex repetitive sequences, such as those found within euchromatic regions, can be cloned and sequenced. However, since they can originate from different genomic locations and a whole-genome shotgun sequencing approach provides only short sequences, the assembly of overlapping sequences can be ambiguous. Repetitive sequences are especially problematic for assembling sequences from clones with small inserts (~2 kb). Here, one end of a clone can be unique sequence while the other may be repetitive sequence. It is therefore not possible to identify an overlapping clone from the same region of the genome, since many clones from different genomic regions have the same repetitive sequence. Some of the ambiguities can be resolved by comparing these sequences to overlapping sequences generated from sequencing clones with larger inserts, say, of about 10 kb. Since many repetitive sequences are only about 5 kb in length, a larger insert is likely to contain the repetitive sequence flanked by unique sequence.

8.31   *Answer:* At a molecular level, a gene is a sequence that encodes an RNA or polypeptide product. Not all genes encode polypeptides. For example, ribosomal RNA, transfer RNA, and microRNA genes do not encode polypeptides. Genes that are transcribed into mRNA encode polypeptides, and the mRNAs have an open reading frame, or ORF. An ORF is a sequence in the processed mRNA that encodes a polypeptide. It begins with a start codon (typically AUG, see text Chapter 6) and ends at a stop codon.

Not all sequences that are identified as ORFs function as genes. For example, some sequences that appear to be an ORF based on computerized genomic sequence analysis may not be transcribed if their genomic region lacks appropriate regulatory sequences. When computerized algorithms are used to identify ORFs in prokaryotes, they are quite accurate. However, the genomes of eukaryotes are more complex, and the presence of introns confounds computerized analyses. Hence, some ORFs are missed and some ORFs are identified that do not function as part of a gene.

8.32 *Answer:*

a. Since prokaryotic ORFs should reside in transcribed regions, they should follow a bacterial promoter containing consensus sequences recognized by a sigma factor. For example, promoters recognized by σ^{70} would contain -35 (**TTGACA**) and -10 (**TATAAT**) consensus sequences. A Shine–Dalgarno sequence (**UAAGGAGG**) used for ribosome binding should be found within the transcribed region, but before the ORF. Nearby should be an **AUG** (or **GUG**, in some systems) start codon. This should be followed by a set of in-frame sense codons. The ORF should terminate with a stop (**UAG**, **UAA**, and **UGA**) codon.

b. Eukaryotic introns are sequences in the RNA-coding region that are transcribed but not translated. They will be spliced out of the primary mRNA transcript before it is translated. If not accounted for, they could introduce additional amino acids, frameshifts, and chain-termination signals.

c. The small average size of exons relative to the range of sizes for introns makes it challenging to predict whether a region with only a short set of in-frame codons is used as an exon. Such regions could have arisen by chance or be the remnants of exons that are no longer used due to mutation in splice site signals.

d. Eukaryotic introns typically contain a **GU** at their 5′ ends, an **AG** at their 3′ ends, and a **YNCURAY** branch-point sequence 18 to 38 nucleotides upstream of their 3′ ends. To identify eukaryotic ORFs in DNA sequences, scan sequences following a eukaryotic promoter for the presence of possible introns by searching for sets of these three consensus sequences. Then try to translate sequences obtained if potential introns are removed, testing whether a long ORF with good codon usage can be generated. Since alternative mRNA splicing exists at many ~~ge~~nes, more than one possible ORF may be found in a given DNA sequence.

~~Answ~~er: An annotation can vary in its level of completeness depending on what can be inferred ~~based~~ on homology and what experimental data are available. An annotation could include:

~~1. T~~he location of a transcribed region depicted graphically with links embedded within the symb~~ols~~ used to depict transcripts
   Physical map coordinates
     i. Links to cDNA clones, SNPs, and other DNA markers in the region
   Genetic map coordinates
     i. Links to genes, mapping data in the region
  c. Location of introns, exons, alternative splice sites, alternative promoters, poly(A) addition sites, etc.
     i. Physical map coordinates
     ii. Graphical depictions of transcript structures

2. The types of evidence for a transcribed region
  a. Prediction based on computer algorithms that assess possible sequences of a promoter, conceptual ORF(s), appropriate splicing sites, homology with other genes, etc.
  b. Analysis of cDNAs
  c. Documentation of splice sites, alternative transcript forms by comparison of cDNA and genomic sequences, etc.

3. The inferred function of the gene product
  a. Links to reports, database entries, publications

    b. Evidence supporting the inferred function
      i. Inferences based on homology
      ii. Experimental evidence
    c. Information on pathways and processes involving the gene

4. Information on gene expression levels
    a. Information on where the gene is expressed
    b. Information on levels of expression in different tissues

5. Information about gene regulation
    a. Genes regulated in a similar manner
    b. Unique features of the gene and its regulation

8.34   *Answer:*

a. Comparison of cDNA and genomic DNA sequences can define the structure of transcription units by elucidating the location of the intron–exon boundaries, poly(A) sites, and the approximate locations of promoter regions. Comparison of different full-length cDNAs representing the same gene can identify the use of alternative splice sites, alternative poly(A) sites, and alternative promoters.

b. The analysis of full-length cDNAs provides information about an entire open reading frame, information about the site at which transcription starts and where the promoter lies, and the location of the poly(A) site. Partial-length cDNAs might provide some but not all of this information. While multiple cDNA sequences could be compared and assembled to obtain more information, assembling cDNAs is challenging because of the use of alternative splice sites, alternative promoters, and/or alternative poly(A) sites.

c. Genes are not uniformly distributed among different chromosomes, and some chromosomes have more genes than others do. While consistent with the finding that chromosomes have gene-rich regions and gene deserts, more data is needed to infer the relationship between the density of genes on a chromosome and how gene-rich it is. For example, a chromosome with many small genes could still have regions classified as gene deserts.

d. Two possible explanations are that: (1) some regions of the genome sequence are incorrectly assembled (e.g., due to the large numbers of repetitive sequences they contain), so the cDNAs are unable to be mapped to just one region; and (2) some of the genes are in regions that have not yet been assembled (e.g., because they are difficult to clone or sequence using current technologies). As the genome sequence is revised, these issues should be resolved.

8.35   *Answer:* Sequencing of genomes of the Archaea genomes has shown that their genes are not uniformly similar to those of Bacteria or Eukarya. While most of the archaean genes involved in energy production, cell division, and metabolism are similar to their counterparts in Bacteria, the genes involved in DNA replication, transcription, and translation are similar to their counterparts in Eukarya.

8.36   *Answer:* This answer considers sequencing efforts in three organisms, the bacterium *Haemophilus influenzae*, the archaean *Methanococcus jannaschii*, and the eukaryotic insect *Drosophila melanogaster*. The text describes the rationale for and the results of sequencing the genomes of many other organisms.

    The genome of *H. influenzae* was chosen as the first cellular organism to have its genome sequenced because its genome size is typical among bacteria, and its GC content is close to that of human. These features suggested that methods developed to sequence its genome could be applied to other bacteria and be instructive for sequencing the human genome. Since it can cause ear and respiratory tract infections, sequencing its genome could provide insights into aspects of disease pathogenesis. *Methanococcus jannaschii* is a hyperthermophilic methanogen, and the rationale for sequencing its genome was in part to provide insights into its evolutionary origins and its relationship to the Bacteria and the Eukarya. Other motivations could have been to understand the genes that allow it to survive and flourish under extreme conditions. The genome of *Drosophila melanogaster* was sequenced because this organism has been the subject of much genetics research and has contributed to our understanding of the molecular genetics of development. Insights from sequencing its genome would further expand our understanding of the genetic regulation of development.

Annotation of the *H. influenzae* genome revealed that it has 1,737 predicted protein-coding genes comprising 87% of its genome. Of these, 469 (27%) did not match any protein in the database or matched only proteins designated hypothetical. This was an early indication that when a genome is sequenced, there will be many predicted genes with unknown functions, and that these functions must be discovered using hypothesis-driven science. Annotation of the *M. jannaschii* genome revealed a similar number of ORFs (1,682 on the main chromosome, 56 on 2 plasmids). It showed that most of the genes involved in energy production, cell division, and metabolism are similar to their counterparts in the Bacteria, whereas most of the genes involved in DNA replication, transcription, and translation are similar to their counterparts in the Eukarya. This affirmed the existence of the Archaea as a third major branch of life on Earth. Annotation of the *D. melanogaster* genome revealed a euchromatic genome 118.4 Mb in size (~60 Mb is unclonable due to its highly repetitive nature) that contained just 14,015 genes. These genes have a similar diversity of functions to those identified in the worm, *C. elegans*, even though they are fewer in number. Strikingly, this number is only twice that in yeast, a less organizationally complex organism. One conclusion is that higher complexity in animals does not require a correspondingly larger repertoire of gene products, or that alternative splicing allows for additional complexity without adding new genes to the genome. A second insight gained from sequencing the *Drosophila* genome was that the fly has homologs for well over half of the genes currently known to be involved in human disease, including cancer. This has allowed the development of fly models for some human diseases.

8.37 *Answer:* In general, genes make up most of the genome of Bacteria and Archaea. Since gene density in these branches of life is very high, there will be a general relationship between the number of genes and genome size. In contrast, there is a wide range of gene densities in Eukarya, and they show a trend of decreasing gene density with increasing complexity. Consider some of the data for eukaryotes presented in the text: the yeast *S. cerevisiae* has a genome about 12 Mb in size with about 5,700 protein-coding genes; the nematode *C. elegans* has a genome about 100 Mb in size with 20,443 genes; and the fruit fly *D. melanogaster* has a genome about 178 Mb in size with 14,015 genes. Worms and flies have genomes that are about 12.5 and 14.8 times that of yeast, respectively, but have gene numbers that are only 3.6 and 2.5 times that of yeast, respectively. In addition, worms have about 45% more genes than do flies, even though worms have about 43% less DNA than flies. Therefore, the number of genes in Eukarya is not always related to genome size.

8.38 *Answer:* Some of the data from the text on gene numbers and genome sizes is tabulated in the following table.

Organism	Approximate Genome Size (in Mb)	Estimated Gene Number
H. influenzae	1.83	>1,737*
E. coli	4.64	>4,288*
M. jannaschii	1.7	>1,738*
S. cerevisiae	12.07	>6,607*
C. elegans	100.3	20,443
D. melanogaster	178.4	14,015
A. thaliana	120	25,900
O. sativa	389	56,000
H. sapiens	3,000	24,867
M. musculus	2,700	25,200
C. familiaris	2,500	17,500

*The number shown does not include non-protein coding genes.

The data in the table indicate that there is no straightforward relationship between gene number and organizational complexity. For example, two plants, *O. sativa* (rice) and *A. thaliana* have more genes than do humans, and humans have fewer genes than do mice or worms. Therefore, there appears to be a gene-number paradox. In this dataset, if gene density is crudely estimated as the number of genes divided by the size of the genome (ignoring the amount of repetitive DNA sequence), lower gene density does appear to be related to organizational complexity. Humans, mice, and dogs, the most organizationally complex organisms that are listed here, have the highest gene density. However, we also know from an analysis of the human genome that there are gene-rich regions and gene deserts. Therefore, gene density is not constant in eukaryotic organisms. This, and the limited numbers of species for which this information exists, make it difficult to make the case that organizational complexity is related to gene density.

8.39 *Answer:*

a. The main ethical, legal, social, and policy issues associated with the human genome project are:
   i. The fair use of genetic information
   ii. Maintaining privacy and confidentiality
   iii. Whether an individual's genetic differences have a psychological impact and lead to stigmatization
   iv. How genetic information is used in reproductive decision making, and reproductive rights
   v. Clinical issues relevant to the education of health-service providers, patients, and the general public in genetic capabilities, scientific limitations, and social risks; and relevant to the implementation of standards and quality-control measures in testing procedures
   vi. Uncertainties associated with gene tests for susceptibilities and complex conditions linked to multiple genes and gene–environment interactions
   vii. Conceptual and philosophical implications regarding human responsibility, free will versus genetic determinism, and concepts of health and disease
   viii. Health and environmental issues concerning genetically modified foods and microbes
   ix. Commercialization of products including property rights and accessibility of data and materials

b. Legislation is needed to protect individuals from discrimination based on information derived from genetic tests. For example, it is necessary to prevent insurers and employers from discriminating against individuals based on their genetic makeup. In the United States, the Genetic Information Nondiscrimination Act (GINA) became law on May 21, 2008. It forbids insurance companies from discriminating through reduced coverage or pricing based on a person's genetic code. It prohibits employers from making adverse employment decisions based on a person's genetic code. Neither insurers nor employers are allowed to request or demand a genetic test.

c. Pros of gene testing are that it can clarify a diagnosis, direct a physician toward appropriate treatments, allow families to avoid having children with devastating diseases, and identify people at high risk for conditions that may be preventable. Cons of gene testing are that gene tests do not always give clear results, because some tests only indicate whether a person is at increased risk for a disease; some gene tests are done for one disease but have the potential to indicate risk for several diseases; like any laboratory test, they are subject to laboratory error; they can provoke anxiety since they are not always straightforward to interpret, and there are not currently medical treatments for all diseases that can be diagnosed with a gene test; and they subject individuals to discrimination and stigmatization that can outweigh the benefits of testing.

d. Gene tests performed in presymptomatic individuals can identify whether a person is at risk for developing a disease, while gene tests performed in symptomatic individuals can be used to clarify the diagnosis of a particular disease. For example, if a gene test is used to assess the presence of a mutation that causes Huntington's disease in an individual with symptoms like those of Huntington's disease, it can confirm or disaffirm the diagnosis of Huntington's disease. The same test could be performed in someone whose parent died from Huntington's disease to inform them whether they carry the mutant allele. Testing in these two cases will have different psychological impacts on the person being tested. If the test reveals that the symptomatic individual has the Huntington's disease mutation, it may assist the physician in developing a therapeutic strategy. If the test reveals that the asymptomatic individual also has the Huntington's disease mutation, being aware of having a mutation that leads to an early death may lead to anxiety that requires psychiatric intervention.

e. At the present time in the United States, there are no federal regulations and only a few state regulations to evaluate the accuracy and reliability of genetic testing. Most genetic tests developed by laboratories are categorized as services. The Food and Drug Administration (FDA) does not regulate these.

9

Functional and Comparative Genomics

Chapter Outline

Functional Genomics

Comparative Genomics

Review of Key Terms, Symbols, and Concepts

In your own words, write a brief, precise definition of each term in the groups below. Check your definitions using the text. Then develop a concept map using the terms in each list.

1	2	3
functional genomics	gene knockout, knockdown	comparative genomics
bioinformatics	loss-of-function, null allele	linkage disequilibrium
reverse genetics	polymerase chain reaction (PCR)	haplotype block
annotation	target DNA sequence	copy number change
sequence similarity search	template, primer	representational oligonucleotide
query, subject sequence	*Taq* DNA polymerase	microarray analysis (ROMA)
homology, homologous gene	denaturation, annealing,	Virochip
BLAST	extension	SARS
open reading frame (ORF)	linear DNA deletion module	coronavirus
domain	target vector	metagenomics
FUN gene	homologous recombination	environmental genomics
orphan family	nonhomologous recombination	microbiome
single orphan	embryonic stem (ES) cells	
transcriptome, transcriptomics	RNA interference (RNAi)	
DNA microarray; gene,	Slicer	
DNA chip	antiviral system	
Cy5, Cy3	transgene	
pharmacogenomics	shRNA	
proteome, proteomics		
HUPO		
protein array, microarray, chip		
capture array		

Thinking Analytically

The goal of functional genomics is to understand the function of all of a genome's genes and nongene sequences. Achieving this goal requires both experimentation and computer modeling. As you study this material, consider how experimental and computer modeling approaches complement each other. Identify the limitations of each type of analysis. Then consider how one type of analysis can lead to questions that can be addressed by the other, and how both types of analysis are necessary to achieve the broad goal of functional genomics.

The analysis of the sequence of entire genomes has led to new insights into the structure and function of genomes and has paved the way for new types of functional and comparative genomic analyses. For example, sequence information was necessary to identify SNPs systematically, and the analysis of SNPs in haplotypes allowed the construction of haplotype blocks and haplotype maps. The availability of haplotype maps in turn paved the way for comparative genomic analyses to identify regions of the genome that have undergone recent positive selection against disease. Analyze the material in this chapter to identify other types of analyses that became possible only after genome sequence information was available. Then consider how these analyses have led to new areas of research with practical applications. This should help you better understand the types of biological questions and human problems that comparative genomics can address.

Questions for Practice

Multiple-Choice Questions

1. Which of the following statements is *not* true?
   a. A domain is part of a polypeptide sequence that tends to fold and function independent of the rest of the polypeptide.
   b. Proteins can have multiple domains.
   c. Domains are encoded by single exons.
   d. Two proteins that perform dissimilar functions can share a domain.

2. In a PCR, what determines the segment of DNA that will be targeted for amplification?
   a. the use of a thermostable DNA polymerase
   b. extending annealed primers at 72°C
   c. using primers that flank the segment and identifying specific annealing conditions
   d. the number of cycles used for amplification

3. A linear DNA deletion module is used to knock out a target gene in yeast. What leads to the production of a null allele?
   a. nonhomologous recombination
   b. the insertion of a *kan*^{R} module into the gene
   c. the use of PCR primers
   d. denaturation of the target gene

4. What is the best way to select for mouse ES cells that have had a deletion module incorporated at a target site?
   a. Select against nonhomologous transformants by growth on media with neomycin only.
   b. Select against nonhomologous transformants by growth on media with ganciclovir only.
   c. Select against nonhomologous transformants by growth on media with both neomycin and ganciclovir.
   d. Start individual cultures from each transformed ES cell without neomycin or ganciclovir in the media. Evaluate the location of the deletion module in each culture using PCR.

5. Which of the following best describes a gene that is a single orphan?
   a. It lacks even a single ORF.
   b. It has an ORF with an unknown function similar to just one gene in a different species.
   c. It has an ORF with an unknown function and is found only in one species.
   d. It has an ORF with an unknown function similar to multiple genes found in other species.

6. DNA microarrays are
   a. aligned sets of printed DNA sequences, ordered according to their chromosomal positions.
   b. ordered grids of DNA molecules of known sequence fixed at known positions on a solid substrate.
   c. aligned sets of printed SNP-containing oligonucleotides in a database.
   d. ordered grids of homologous genes from different organisms.

7. Which of the following laboratory investigations is most likely to benefit from using a capture array?
   a. identifying the proteins bound by a drug
   b. comparing liver proteins in normal rats to those in rats fed large doses of ethanol
   c. diagnosing the presence of an infectious agent
   d. determining the mRNA expression profile of yeast cells at different stages of sporulation
   e. both b and c

8. A genome of a new bacterial species has just been sequenced. What should you do first if you want to identify all of the organism's genes and assign each a function?
   a. Perform a sequence similarity search.
   b. Use a probe array to identify the gene expression profile in a bacterial culture.
   c. Use a PCR-based deletion strategy to create a collection of mutant strains that have 500 base-pair segments deleted at 1-kilobase intervals throughout the genome.
   d. Search for ORFs using a computerized algorithm.

9. In a hybridization used to detect SNPs using a DNA microarray, what is considered the probe and what is considered the target?
   a. The probe consists of fluorescently labeled genomic DNA; the target is a set of oligonucleotides on the DNA microarray.
   b. The target consists of fluorescently labeled genomic DNA; the probe is a set of oligonucleotides on the DNA microarray.
   c. The probe consists of Cy3-labeled cDNA and Cy5-labeled cDNA; the target is a set of oligonucleotides on the DNA microarray.
   d. The target consists of Cy3-labeled cDNA and Cy5-labeled cDNA; the probe is a set of oligonucleotides on the DNA microarray.

10. When a DNA microarray is used to evaluate differences in gene expression, what is considered the probe and what is considered the target?
    a. The probe is fluorescently labeled genomic DNA; the target is a set of oligonucleotides on the DNA microarray.
    b. The target is fluorescently labeled genomic DNA; the probe is a set of oligonucleotides on the DNA microarray.
    c. The probe consists of Cy3-labeled cDNA and Cy5-labeled cDNA; the target is a set of oligonucleotides on the DNA microarray.
    d. The target consists of Cy3-labeled cDNA and Cy5-labeled cDNA; the probe is a set of oligonucleotides on the DNA microarray.

11. Which of the following objectives can be achieved with certainty by applying computerized algorithms to analyze prokaryotic, but not eukaryotic, genome sequences?
    a. Identifying the locations of all protein-coding regions.
    b. Identifying the locations of known repeated sequences.
    c. Identifying the locations of known transposable elements.
    d. Identifying the locations of all rRNA genes.

12. Which one of the following methods could be used to knock down the expression of a specific gene?
    a. Introducing a transgene that produces a shRNA targeted to that gene.
    b. Introducing a deletion module for that gene into the genome using homologous recombination.
    c. Introducing a deletion module for that gene into the genome using nonhomologous recombination.
    d. Introducing a transposon into the coding region of that gene.

13. What is metagenomics?
    a. a comparative analysis of genomes from geographically distinct regions
    b. a comparative analysis of the genomes in members of one species
    c. a comparative analysis of the sequence of one genome obtained using different sequencing methods
    d. the analysis of genomes in entire communities of microbes

14. What is BLAST?
    a. the Basic Local Alignment Search Tool, used for homology searches when a DNA or amino acid sequence is compared to other sequences in a database
    b. the Big Linear Accelerator Sequencing Tool, a device funded by the Department of Energy that is able to read 10,000 bp of DNA from one sequencing reaction
    c. the Best Legal Analysis of Sequence Technology, a document from the American Bar Association that legally analyzes situations faced by biotechnology companies that introduce genetically modified organisms into the environment
    d. the Beer Legal Age Screening Tool, a DNA chip used to detect the length of simple telomeric repeats (Since these shorten with each cell division in somatic cells, this can be used to quickly determine whether an individual is over the legal drinking age.)

Answers: 1c, 2c, 3b, 4c, 5c, 6b, 7e, 8d, 9b, 10d, 11a, 12a, 13d, 14a

Thought Questions

1. What is the difference between a haplotype and a haplotype block? How do haplotype blocks arise? Do they change over many generations, or are they stable through many generations?

2. What information was required to construct the Virochip? How does using the Virochip facilitate the identification of a new virus whose sequence is not identical to those used to construct the Virochip?

3. Will two homologous genes always have a high degree of sequence similarity? Explain why or why not.

4. How are the challenges faced by proteomics different from the challenges faced by genomics?

5. What is pharmacogenomics? How can it, when combined with the use of DNA chips, be useful to develop drugs that are tailored to the needs of individuals?

6. DNA microarrays can be used to distinguish between two similar cancers affecting the same tissue. How is this done, and why might this be therapeutically helpful?

7. Some human diseases, such as some ulcers, are associated with particular bacterial flora. How might a metagenomic approach be helpful to determine if a particular disease is associated with an altered bacterial flora?

8. What method could you employ to determine whether a particular disease is associated with variation in the number of copies of different segments of the genome? What controls would you perform?

9. What is meant when two genes are referred to as homologs? For a gene encoding a protein product, explain whether it is better to search for homologs based on DNA sequence or amino acid sequence.

10. Explore the NCBI website for BLAST at http://www.ncbi.nlm.nih.gov/BLAST/. What different forms of BLAST have been developed, and for what are they used? Why is it important statistically to evaluate matches between an obtained sequence and sequences in a database as similar sequences are identified?

11. After the human genome sequence was completed, searches were performed to identify possible genes. What different criteria might be applied quickly to provide evidence that a DNA sequence is part of a functional gene? (Hint: Think about the value of homology searches.)

12. Within different ethnic groups, some haplotype blocks are more common than others are. Consequently, for diseases influenced by genetic factors, different ethnic groups vary in their frequency of disease alleles. What challenges does this present for genetic testing and for preventative medicine based on the identification of genetically at-risk populations?

Thought Questions for Media

After reviewing the media on the *iGenetics* website, try to answer these questions.

1. Why is it important to expose the microarray to two differently labeled probes simultaneously, instead of using two microarrays with a single probe on each?

2. What are the sources of the tissues for the mRNA samples used to develop the probes for the microarrays? How important is it for the tumor tissue sample to be composed only of tumor cells and not to be a mixture of tumor and normal cells?

3. Is the selection of drugs for Maeve's therapy based on a genotype? Tumor cells usually harbor multiple somatic mutations and often contain chromosomal rearrangements. If the drug selection is based on a genotype, is it based on her genotype or the genotype of the tumor? If not, what is it based on?

4. Specific genes are placed on microarrays. What information was needed to design the microarray used in this investigation?

5. How can microarrays help in identifying more effective breast cancer therapies?

1. The animation illustrated how microarrays can be designed to identify mutations in a gene as well as to analyze differences in patterns of gene expression.
   a. What differences are there in the design of these two types of microarrays?
   b. What differences are there in labeling the target DNA samples for these two types of analyses?

2. Based on the animation illustrating how gene expression is analyzed using DNA microarrays, discuss how characterization of the transcriptome allows us to gain a more complete understanding of normal cellular events.

3. How are cDNAs labeled in a microarray experiment?

4. Suppose that in a microarray experiment, 97% of the spots are yellow. Does this indicate that the experiment is unlikely to yield valuable information? Explain why or why not.

Solutions to Text Questions and Problems

9.1   *Answer:* Bioinformatics is the use of computers and information science to study genetic information and biological structures. It results from the fusion of biology, mathematics, computer science, and information science. It has become an important field with the widespread use of databases holding sequence, genetic, functional, structural (e.g., protein structure), and bibliographic information. It is used when a genome is sequenced to assemble genome (and other) sequences, find genes within databases containing sequence and genetic information, align sequences to determine their degree of matching, predict gene structure, and identify the locations of putative genes. In functional genomics, it is used to predict the function of genes based on homology to DNA or amino acid sequences and to analyze information on gene function (e.g., databases containing information on how the function of a gene can alter the transcriptome or proteome). In comparative genomics, it is used to compare homologous gene sequences and compare genomes in terms of similarities and differences between gene and nongene sequences.

9.2   *Answer:* Physically, a gene is a sequence of DNA that includes a transcribed DNA sequence and the regulatory sequences that direct its transcription (e.g., the promoter). Genes produce RNA (mRNA, rRNA, snRNA, tRNA, siRNA, and miRNA) and protein products. Functionally, genes can be identified by the phenotypes of mutations that alter or eliminate the functions of their products. In contrast, an ORF is a potential open reading frame, the segment of an mRNA (mature mRNA in eukaryotes) that directs the synthesis of a polypeptide by the ribosome. Therefore, genes have features that ORFs do not, including transcribed and untranscribed sequences and introns. We have experimental evidence for some ORFs (cDNA sequence, detected protein products), but the existence of other ORFs is predicted only from genomic sequence information.

Two general approaches can be used to determine the function of ORFs having unknown functions. First, computerized sequence similarity searches using programs such as BLAST can be performed to compare the ORF sequence and all sequences (DNA or protein) in a database. The extent of sequence similarity is used to infer whether the ORF encodes a protein with the same or similar function to that of a gene in a database. Since proteins can have multiple functional domains (e.g., a catalytic domain and a DNA-binding domain), sometimes this approach gives only partial insight into the function of the ORF's protein product. Second, an experimental approach can be used to investigate the function of the gene identified by the ORF. This may involve analyzing knockout mutations and analyzing the resulting mutant phenotype. In organisms such as humans where this experimental approach would be unethical, a gene in a model organism that encodes its homolog can be investigated instead. This approach may include demonstrating that the ORF encodes a protein and characterizing its protein product.

9.3   *Answer:*

a. Regions of similarity in a dot plot can be identified by scanning the plot for diagonal stretches of dots. If both DNA sequences are given 5′-to-3′, then diagonals that proceed continuously down and to the right identify regions with identical sequence. A mostly continuous diagonal proceeding down and to the right identifies a region with sequence similarity. In the dot plots shown here, regions with sequence similarity are shaded in grey. Two different shades of grey are used. A darker shade of grey is used to indicate regions that show the highest degree of sequence similarity. A lighter shade of grey is used to identify regions that show sequence identity over at least three nucleotides.

     i.

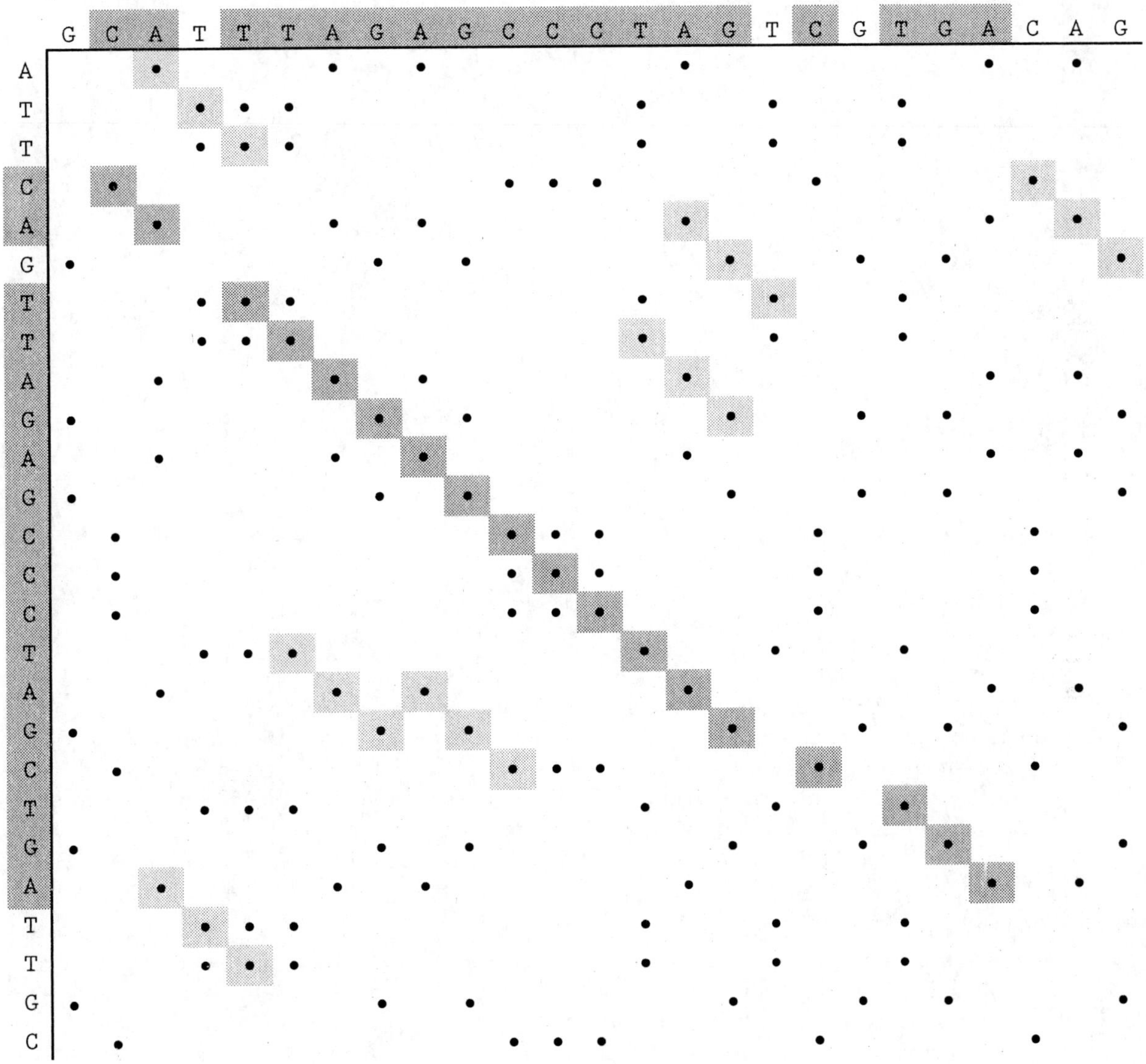

ii.

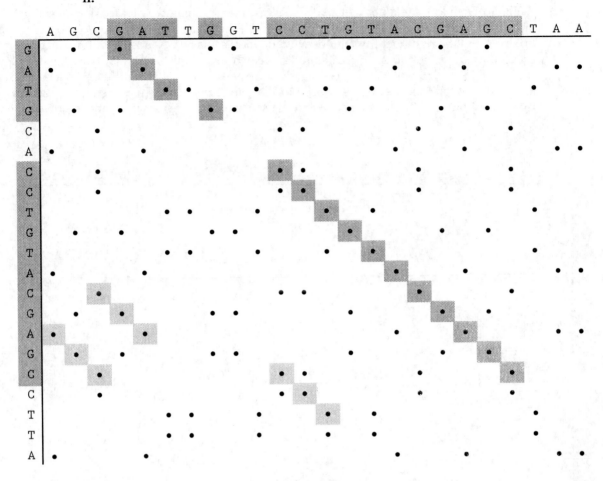

b. Inspection of the dot plots reveals regions with different amounts of sequence similarity. Therefore, the BLAST program needs a strategy to identify which alignment provides the greatest amount of sequence similarity. Within a region of sequence similarity, there are different ways to evaluate gaps. In each of the dot plots shown above, there are gaps that could reflect nucleotide substitutions, insertions, or deletions. Therefore, the BLAST program must also address when a gap should be introduced into an alignment, whether it should be extended, and whether it is preferable to introduce a mismatched base or a gap in an alignment.

9.4   *Answer:*

a, b.   In this case, use BLAST to compare the cDNA sequence to human genomic DNA sequence. This will allow you to align regions of the cDNA with sequences in the human genome from which it is derived. A cDNA is prepared from a mature, processed mRNA, so genomic regions lying between exons are introns that were transcribed but removed from a pre-mRNA. Therefore, comparing cDNA and genomic DNA sequences will allow you to determine not only the chromosomal location of the gene but also the sequence coordinates of the different exons and the approximate intron and exon boundaries. Once you have the chromosomal location and sequence coordinates of the gene, you can search databases to see if any disease mutations are known in that region.

c.   The protein domains present in the polypeptide encoded by the cDNA can offer clues as to the function of the protein. For example, a protein might have a DNA-binding domain indicating that it might be involved in the regulation of chromosome structure or transcription. Protein domains with similar functions tend to have conserved amino acid sequences. Therefore, use BLAST to compare the amino acid sequence of the ORF to amino acid sequences of known polypeptides. This will let you identify conserved protein domains that can provide insight into the potential function of the protein. If you compared the cDNA sequence to other cDNA sequences, you might find some matches. However, these matches might not reflect conserved amino acid sequences.

9.5   *Answer:* A protein domain is a part of a polypeptide sequence that tends to fold and function independently of the rest of the polypeptide. Therefore, a conserved domain is a sequence of amino acids in a polypeptide sequence that tends to fold and function independently of the rest of the polypeptide and in which some or all of the amino acids are conserved in similarly functioning domains found in other polypeptides. Domains serve to provide different functional properties to polypeptides, and polypeptides often have several distinct domains. Therefore, finding one or several different conserved domains in a polypeptide can lead to testable hypotheses about its function. For example, identifying a DNA-binding domain in a polypeptide suggests that the polypeptide has the potential to interact with DNA. If the polypeptide also has a domain that interacts with a known class of transcription factors, one testable hypothesis is that the polypeptide functions in the regulation of transcription when it is bound to DNA.

9.6   *Answer:* None of the inferences can be made without additional information and analyses. The question statement only indicates that the best match is to the *HprK* gene. The question statement does not describe the quality of the match or the region(s) that have significant sequence similarity to *HprK*. It also leaves us without a critical piece of information we need to make inferences about the potential function of this DNA fragment—we do not know whether the DNA fragment contains a gene that encodes a protein product. To address this issue, the DNA fragment should be examined for the presence of an open reading frame (ORF), and the amino acid sequence of this ORF should be compared to that of *HprK* and other known kinases. To conclude that the DNA fragment encodes a gene encoding a kinase, a kinase domain should be found within the ORF. To infer that the DNA fragment encodes a gene homologous to *HprK*, it should have an ORF, and the ORF's amino acid sequence should have significant sequence similarity to the protein produced by *HprK* in regions that are important for its biological function. However, even if the DNA fragment contains a gene that appears to be homologous to *HprK*, that gene may not function to regulate carbohydrate metabolism. We cannot exclude that it has evolved to function in or regulate a different, though perhaps related, biochemical process. When a sequence alignment provides information about functional domains present in a new protein and its homology to known proteins, it suggests hypotheses about the functions of the new protein that still must be tested experimentally.

9.7   *Answer:*
   a. A single orphan gene is a gene whose open reading frame (ORF) has an unknown function and for which homologs have not been identified in another organism. An orphan family is a set of homologous genes whose function is unknown.
   b. It is likely that the gene was initially referred to as an orphan because initial sequence analysis did not show enough evidence to identify it unequivocally as a homolog of a known gene. The question statement indicates that the polypeptide produced by the *RORC* gene has both DNA- and ligand-binding domains. It could be that when it was initially identified, it was one of many genes with these domains and so it could be identified as a receptor, but additional information was unavailable to assign it a specific function or identify its homologs. Since the gene is similar to a gene in mice essential for the formation of lymphoid tissue, one testable hypothesis is that it functions as a hormone receptor that interacts with DNA during the formation of lymphoid tissue in humans. However, this remains a hypothesis that requires testing. If it is the homolog of that mouse gene, one might also expect that the two genes function in similar biochemical pathways during the formation of lymphoid tissue. This problem raises the general issue that sequence information alone is sometimes insufficient to identify homologous genes and predict gene function.

9.8   *Answer:* To amplify a specific region, one needs to know the sequences flanking the target region so that primers able to amplify the target region can be designed. Once primers are synthesized, the polymerase chain reaction can be assembled. It contains a DNA template (genomic DNA, cDNA, or cloned DNA), the pair of primers that flank the DNA segment targeted for amplification, a heat-resistant DNA polymerase (*Taq*), the four dNTPs (dATP, dTTP, dGTP, and dCTP), and an appropriate buffer (see text Figure 9.3, p. 222).

9.9   *Answer:* The polymerase chain reaction uses repeated cycles of denaturation, annealing, and extension. In the denaturation step, the reaction mixture is heated to 94°C to denature the DNA template. The annealing and extension steps are carried out at lower temperatures. By using a DNA polymerase able to withstand short periods at very high temperatures, the same reaction mixture can be subjected to multiple cycles of denaturation—there is no need to add additional DNA polymerase as the reaction proceeds through additional cycles. Usually, DNA polymerases purified from a thermophilic bacterium are used. For example, *Taq* DNA polymerase is purified from *Thermus aquaticus*, a bacterium that normally lives in hot springs. Since the bacterium normally lives in very hot environments, it has evolved to produce enzymes that are heat stable.

9.10   *Answer:* PCR is a much more sensitive and rapid technique than cloning. Many millions of copies of a DNA segment can be produced from one DNA molecule in only a few hours using PCR. In contrast, cloning requires more DNA (ng to μg quantities) for restriction digestion and at least several days to proceed through all of the cloning steps.

9.11   *Answer:* As shown in text Figure 9.3, p. 222, two unit-length, double-stranded DNA amplimers are produced after the third cycle of PCR from one double-stranded DNA template molecule. If each step of the PCR process is 100% efficient, the number of amplimers geometrically increases in each subsequent cycle: In the fourth cycle, there will be four amplimers, in the fifth cycle there will be eight amplimers, and more generally, in the nth cycle there will be 2^{n-2} amplimers. In the 30th cycle, there will be $2^{28} = 2.68 \times 10^8$ molecules. A larger number of initial template molecules will lead to a proportional increase in amplimer production.

a. $10 \times 2^{28} = 2.68 \times 10^9$ molecules

b. $1{,}000 \times 2^{28} = 2.68 \times 10^{11}$ molecules

c. $10{,}000 \times 2^{28} = 2.68 \times 10^{12}$ molecules

Consider these answers with respect to the experimental observation that about 5 ng of DNA (about 2.3×10^9 copies of a 200-bp DNA fragment) is detected readily on an ethidium-bromide-stained agarose gel.

9.12   *Answer:* Use homologous recombination with a target vector to obtain a null allele. Design a target vector that, when a portion of it is integrated into the yeast chromosome by homologous recombination, inactivates the normal gene by the insertion of a *kan*^{R} gene. Use the two plasmids that are diagrammed in the question statement to construct the linear DNA deletion module.

First, cleave the plasmid containing the *kan*^{R} gene with *Eco*RI and *Hae*III, and isolate the 3-kb insert containing the *kan*^{R} gene using agarose gel electrophoresis. Since the fragment is cloned into the pBluescript II vector, and that vector is about 3 kb in size, it may be difficult to separate the insert from the vector by agarose gel electrophoresis. One approach to solve this problem is to identify an additional restriction enzyme that cleaves the vector sequence but does not cleave the insert sequence (see text Figure 8.4, p. 176). If that restriction enzyme is also added to the digest, the vector will be cleaved into two fragments that each are smaller than 3 kb. This will allow the insert sequence to be more easily separated from the vector fragments.

Second, cleave the *YFG* plasmid with *Eco*RI and *Hae*III. This will produce two fragments that are 1.6 kb and 5.2 kb in size (the 5.2-kb fragment has the vector sequence (~3.0 kb) plus the 5′ (1.0 kb) and 3′ (1.2 kb) regions of *YFG*. Isolate the 5.2-kb fragment using agarose gel electrophoresis, and mix it and DNA ligase with the 3.0-kb fragment from the first digest that contains the *kan*^{R} gene. This will produce a target vector in pBluescript II. The insert is diagrammed in the following figure, where B and E are PCR primers that can be used to confirm the presence of the 3.0-kb fragment containing the *kan*^{R} gene.

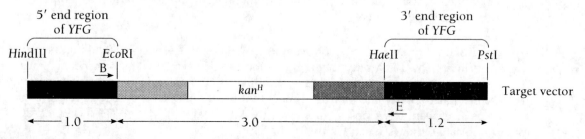

Third, transform the ligated plasmid into *E. coli*, and select for plasmids with the desired inserts using two antibiotics. Adding ampicillin to the medium will select for bacterial colonies that harbor pBluescript II plasmids, while adding kanamycin will select for pBluescript II plasmids with the *kan*^R gene. Note that blue/white screening is not effective here, since both of the starting plasmids, if transformed, will produce white colonies. PCR with the primers B and E can be used to confirm that colonies that grow have a 3.0-kb fragment inserted between the *Eco*RI and *Hae*III sites. If the 1.6-kb fragment has not been replaced with the 3.0-kb fragment containing the *kan*^R gene, PCR with primers B and E should produce a fragment a bit more than 1.6 kb in size, while if the *kan*^R gene has been inserted, this PCR should produce a fragment a bit more than 3.0 kb in size.

Fourth, transform the targeting vector into yeast, and grow the yeast on media containing kanamycin to select for colonies with the *kan*^R gene. Since the pBluescript II plasmid does not have a yeast ARS sequence to allow it to replicate, colonies will exhibit kanamycin resistance only if the *kan*^R gene has been inserted into the yeast genome. If this occurs by homologous recombination and the *kan*^R gene has been inserted into the chromosome at the *YFG* gene, then the *YFG* gene will be knocked out. In the following figure illustrating this situation, the white regions at the right and left ends of the figure represent genomic sequences flanking (or part of) the *YFG* gene, and A–F are PCR primers that can be used to confirm that the *YFG* gene has been successfully knocked out.

Successful insertion of *kan*^R module into *YFG*

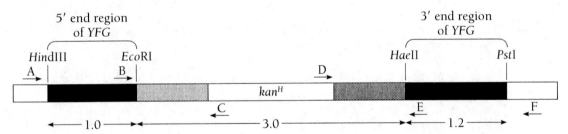

A *YFG* gene knockout can be confirmed by performing three separate PCR reactions. In the figure above, primers A and F are designed against regions that flank the 5′ and 3′ *YFG* sequences present in the targeting vector. These primers can be used in a PCR amplification to evaluate whether the *kan*^R module in the targeting vector has been inserted into the *YFG* gene. Such a PCR amplification will produce a product that is a bit over 5.2 kb in size if the *kan*^R module has been inserted into the *YFG* gene and a product that is a bit over 3.8 kb in size if the *kan*^R module has not been inserted into the *YFG* gene. Two additional PCR amplifications, one with primers A and C, and one with primers D and F, will confirm that the *kan*^R module has been inserted into the *YFG* gene. These PCR amplifications will only give a product if the *kan*^R module has been inserted into the *YFG* gene. Since PCR amplification can fail for a variety of reasons, a negative result (no PCR product) with these primers does not necessarily indicate that the *kan*^R module has been inserted elsewhere in the genome via nonhomologous recombination.

9.13   *Answer:*

a. ES cells are embryonic stem cells—cells derived from a very early embryo that retain the ability to differentiate into cell types characteristic of any part of the organism. They can be grown in culture and transformed with a gene-targeting vector. Then, cells that do not have a gene knockout are excluded by adding neomycin, which selects for cells with the gene-targeting vector, and ganciclovir, which selects for cells where the gene-targeting vector was incorporated via homologous recombination (see text Figure 9.5, p. 226). The surviving cells are tested (using PCR) for the presence of the knockout mutation and then placed in a blastocyst mouse embryo that is implanted into a female for development. During development, the transformed ES cells provide progenitor cells for the germ line so that when the mouse is mated, the knockout mutation is passed on to the next generation.

b. A chimera is a genetic mosaic, an animal with two distinct tissue types. Chimeras arise because the ES cells containing the knockout mutation are genetically different from the embryos they are placed in for development—the ES cells are from a homozygous agouti mouse, while the blastocyst embryos they will be placed in have been harvested from a homozygous black mouse. This difference in coat color genes allows chimeric pups to be readily identified.

c. When the chimeric pups mature and are mated with nontransgenic black mice, they will pass the gene knockout to some of their progeny if some of their germ line consists of the transformed cells. Since the transformed cell had two copies of the agouti gene, these progeny will have one copy of the agouti gene (from the transformed cell) and one copy of the black gene (from the mate). The progeny will be agouti because agouti is dominant to black. To determine if an agouti offspring also is heterozygous for the knockout gene, isolate its DNA using a cheek scraping, a drop of blood, or a tail snip, and perform a PCR-based test to determine whether the neo^R gene is present. Since the neo^R gene was in the gene-targeting vector, animals with it are heterozygous for the gene knockout.

9.14   *Answer:* A knockout mouse is a mouse in which the gene has been made nonfunctional, for example, by deleting part of it. Under the first hypothesis, heterozygotes develop the disease because they have only half the normal dose of the gene's function. If this hypothesis is correct, then heterozygous mice having a knockout allele and a normal allele will also have only half of the normal dose of the gene's function, and so these mice should develop symptoms of the disease. If they do not develop symptoms of the disease, this hypothesis would not be supported. The second hypothesis, that the missense mutation alters the protein to interfere with a normal process, should then be investigated further.

9.15   *Answer:*

a. The kan^R gene present in the yeast target vector described in the text provides a means to select yeast colonies that have taken up the kan^R gene. Homologous recombination in yeast is quite common, so colonies that have taken up the kan^R gene are likely to have integrated the kan^R module at the desired gene. This is because that gene is targeted for homologous recombination by the yeast sequences that flank the kan^R gene in the target vector. PCR can then be used to confirm that the gene has been knocked out by the insertion of the kan^R module. In most other organisms, homologous recombination is rare. Most often, nonhomologous recombination results in the target vector becoming integrated at a site different from the gene being targeted. Therefore, two markers are used in mice. The neo^R gene marker is used in much the same way as the kan^R gene marker in the yeast system—as a selectable insertion module to knock out a gene. Growing transformed ES cells in medium containing neomycin selects for cells that have the neo^R gene from the target vector integrated into their genome. The second marker is the *tk* gene. The target vector (see text Figure 9.5, p. 226) is designed so that the *tk* gene is not inserted when the target vector is integrated into the genome via homologous recombination, but is often inserted when the target vector is integrated into the genome via nonhomologous recombination. The drug ganciclovir inhibits the growth of cells with an active *tk* gene, so ganciclovir is used to select cells lacking the *tk* gene and cells in which homologous recombination is likely to have occurred.

b. The figure on the facing page shows a mouse target vector with the features of the one in text Figure 9.5a, p. 226, the result of its integration into the genome via homologous and nonhomologous recombination, and primers that could be used to confirm that an ES cell able to grow in the presence of neomycin and ganciclovir is a transformant resulting from homologous recombination.

   Primers A and D are designed using chromosomal sequences just outside the region of the gene present in the target vector, while primers B and C are designed against sequences within the neo^R gene. If homologous recombination has occurred, two PCR amplifications, one with primers A and C, and one with primers B and D, should each give products whose size can be predicted from the location of the primers within the targeted gene and the neo^R module of the targeting vector. These PCR amplifications will only give a product if homologous recombination has occurred. If nonhomologous recombination has occurred, the primer pairs will bind to sequences that are either distant from each other on the same chromosome or on different chromosomes, and so no amplification product will be detected. If a positive result is not obtained with PCR, it may not be due to nonhomologous recombination. Another possible explanation is that the PCR reaction failed (for example, due to nonoptimal experimental conditions) even though homologous recombination occurred. In such circumstances, an alternate method, such as Southern blotting (see text Chapter 10, pp. 261–262), can be employed.

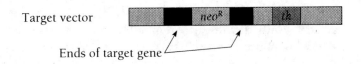

Target vector

Ends of target gene

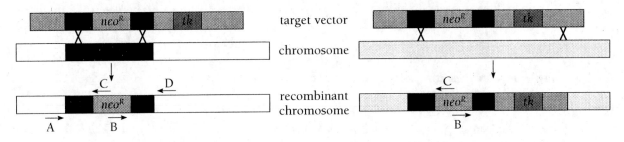

Integration via Homologous Recombination   **Integration via Nonhomologous Recombination**

target vector

chromosome

recombinant
chromosome

9.16 *Answer:* Two approaches to knocking out or knocking down gene function without a gene-targeting vector are to generate mutants by transposon insertion and to use RNA interference methods to knock down gene function. A transposon inserted into the coding region of a gene should disrupt its function. However, since transposon insertion cannot be targeted to a specific gene, a collection of mutants with different transposon insertions must be screened to identify a mutation in a specific gene. In *Mycoplasma genitalium*, about 2,000 transposon insertions were characterized to identify how many protein-coding genes are required for the organism to survive. In a diploid organism, most gene knockouts due to a transposon insertion are likely to be viable as heterozygotes, so a collection of mutants generated by transposon insertion could be obtained and screened to identify transposon inserts in or near particular genes. This method requires detailed knowledge of the transposons in an organism, including information about how they can be mobilized to insert at different locations in the genome. Therefore, it is restricted to organisms where that information is available.

The RNA interference (RNAi) method introduces dsRNA molecules complementary to a specific mRNA into cells. Once in the cell, the dsRNAs trigger the cell's RNAi pathway to render the mRNA nonfunctional (see text Figure 9.6, p. 228). This method requires information about an mRNA sequence so that a gene-specific dsRNA can be designed, and a means to introduce the dsRNA into cells. If these are available, RNAi can be used in a number of organisms without extensive modification. Indeed, it has been used in *Caenorhabditis elegans*, *Drosophila*, mice, and plants.

9.17 *Answer:* The text presents information on the results of screens that assess the consequences of individually knocking out or knocking down all of the genes in the bacterium *M. genitalium*, the yeast *S. cerevisae*, the nematode *C. elegans*, and the fly *D. melanogaster*. In *M. genitalium*, transposon insertion was used to knock out the function of genes. Since the loss of a vital gene would result in organismal lethality, this screen evaluated how many of the genes of this bacterium are required for the organism to survive. Insertions in at least 100 genes were viable, suggesting that most of the estimated 265 to 340 genes are required for the organism to survive in the lab. In the yeast, a gene deletion approach revealed that about 4,200 of the 6,600 ORFs are nonessential. Of these, about half show no significant change in phenotype when many areas of cell function—including cell cycle events, meiosis, DNA synthesis, RNA synthesis and processing, protein synthesis, DNA repair, energy metabolism, and molecular transport mechanisms—are assessed. In the worm and the fly, RNAi screens typically find that between 10 and 25% of the RNAi gene knockouts or knockdowns result in detectable phenotypes. In these organisms, additional screens that assess very specific phenotypes have been successful at suggesting functions for some of the genes that did not seem to have a clear defect in initial genome-wide screens.

We have gained considerable insights into functional genomics from these screens. In each of the screens, a substantial number of genes were not required for viability, and the loss of many of those genes did not lead to readily apparent phenotypes in a laboratory environment. These genes may be important for the organism to survive outside of the laboratory environment or function in processes that can only be identified in screens for more specific phenotypes. Indeed, since additional

RNAi screens that assessed specific phenotypes have provided insight into the function of some of these nonessential genes, it is important to keep in mind that what we learn from such genome-wide screens depends in part on how we assess phenotypes.

9.18   *Answer:*

a. On chromosome V and the X chromosome, genes are distributed uniformly. However, especially on chromosome V, conserved genes are found more frequently in the central regions. In contrast, inverted and tandem-repeat sequences are found more frequently on the arms. It appears that at least on chromosome V, there is an inverse relationship between the frequency of inverted and tandem repeats and the frequency of conserved genes.

b. Since there are fewer conserved genes on the arms, there appears to be a greater rate of change on chromosome arms than in the central regions.

c. Yes, since increased meiotic recombination provides for greater rates of exchange of genetic material on chromosomal arms.

9.19   *Answer:* The transcriptome is the set of RNAs present in a cell at a particular stage and time, while the proteome is the set of proteins present in the cell at that stage and time.

a. It is likely that the proteome has more total as well as more unique members. It is likely that it has more total members since multiple copies of a protein can be translated from a single mRNA transcript. It is also likely that it has more unique members since a given transcript, in principle, can give rise to different protein isoforms. Proteins can be modified posttranslationally or cotranslationally in different ways, including phosphorylation, glycosylation, methylation, and proteolytic processing. If proteins translated from a single transcript are modified in different ways, multiple protein isoforms are produced.

b. This analysis could be performed using DNA chips. RNA could be isolated from the nervous system of different developmental stages, and the transcriptional profile in each stage could be assessed using DNA chips. To do this type of analysis, RNA from one developmental stage would be labeled with one fluorochrome—say, a fluorescent green dye. RNA from a second developmental stage would be labeled with another fluorochrome—say, a fluorescent red dye. The labeled probes would be hybridized to the DNA chip, and the relative red : green fluorescence bound to a single site on the chip would be used to infer the relative amounts of gene expression of the gene located at that site on the chip. This could be done for many different developmental stages.

c. For the proteome, one would need to assess changes in the proteins produced over time. Thus, one would isolate proteins from the nervous system of different developmental stages and assess the relative abundance of individual proteins using an analytical method such as quantitative two-dimensional gel electrophoresis.

9.20   *Answer:*

a. Use an approach similar to that taken by Pat Brown and Ira Herskowitz to follow changes in gene expression during yeast sporulation (see text discussion on pp. 230–232 and Figure 9.7, p. 231. Inoculate two yeast cultures—one will be a reference sample and grown at the normal temperature, while the other will be an experimental sample and subjected to a heat shock. Remove aliquots of the yeast cells from each culture at time points just before and after exposure of the experimental culture to a short heat shock. Isolate mRNA from each aliquot of yeast cells, label the mRNA with Cy3 (reference samples) and Cy5 (experimental samples), and allow these targets to hybridize to a probe array (a DNA chip) onto which has been spotted an entire set of yeast ORF probes generated by PCR. Scan the chip and extract the data to determine which genes show altered patterns of expression following the heat shock.

b. This question raises an important issue. Just because a gene's transcription is altered in response to heat shock does not mean that the gene's function (or absence of function) is necessary to survive the heat shock. For example, a gene could be downregulated in response to heat shock as part of a more general cellular response to limit the synthesis of new proteins that are not required to survive the heat shock. You can evaluate whether a particular gene is required to survive a heat shock by determining if a mutant lacking the gene's function can survive a heat shock.

You are fortunate to be working with yeast, because knockout mutations exist for each of the approximately 6,600 ORFs (see text Figure 9.4, p. 224, for a description of how these mutations were induced). About 4,200 of these are viable and can be used in this approach. For each gene you identify in **(a)**, obtain a knockout mutant strain, subject it to heat shock, and determine whether the mutant remains viable. If the mutant cannot survive a heat shock, the normal gene is required for a protective response following heat shock. If the mutant can survive a heat shock, the normal gene may not be needed for the protective response. Alternatively, it may play only a modest role in the protective response. This approach will not work for genes where knockout mutations are inviable (because they eliminate essential gene functions). An alternate approach is to isolate a conditional or a partial loss-of-function mutation that can be cultured and then assess whether heat shock alters the viability of these cells.

9.21   *Answer:* Use microarray analysis to determine if patients who respond to therapy have a different pattern of gene expression in their blood cells than do patients who fail to respond to therapy. Prepare cDNA from the mRNA isolated from the blood cells of individual leukemia patients, label the cDNAs with fluorescent dyes, and use them in a microarray analysis. For example, label cDNA from a patient who responds to the therapy with Cy3, and label cDNA from a patient who fails to respond to the therapy with Cy5. Mix the labeled cDNAs together and allow them to hybridize to a probe array containing oligonucleotides from many different genes, as shown in text Figure 9.7, p. 231. Then identify the set of genes whose pattern of expression differs in the two patients. Repeat the experiment using different pairs of patients to identify the set of genes that shows consistently greater (or lesser) expression in patients who respond to therapy. The hypothesis that two (or more) different types of leukemia are present in this patient population would be supported if there are consistent differences in the gene expression patterns between patients who respond to therapy and patients who fail to respond to therapy. The pattern of gene expression could be further evaluated as a clinical marker.

9.22   *Answer:* One approach is to use model organisms (e.g., transgenic mice) that have been developed as models to study a specific human disease. Expose them and a control population to specific environmental conditions and then simultaneously assess disease progression and alterations in patterns of gene expression using microarrays. This would provide a means to establish a link between environmental factors and patterns of gene expression that are associated with disease onset or progression.

9.23   *Answer:* A DNA microarray has DNA probes (oligonucleotides, PCR-amplified cDNA products) bound to a solid substrate (a glass slide, membrane, microtiter well, or silicon chip), while a protein chip has proteins immobilized on solid substrates. Protein arrays are probed by labeling target proteins with fluorescent dyes, incubating the labeled target with the probe array, and measuring the bound fluorescence using automated laser detection. One type of protein chip is a capture array, where a set of antibodies is bound to a solid substrate and used to evaluate the level and presence of target molecules in cell or tissue extracts. A capture array can be used in disease diagnosis (to evaluate whether a specific protein associated with a disease state is present) and in protein expression profiling (evaluation of the proteome qualitatively and quantitatively).

9.24   *Answer:*

a. When a new mutation occurs on a chromosome, it is associated with a specific set of haplotypes because the new allele is flanked by the specific SNP alleles that are present on that chromosome. This set of neighboring haplotypes is called a haplotype block. As the chromosome with the mutation is passed on—and over generations, spreads through the population—the mutation will segregate with the haplotype block on which it originated. During meiosis, recombination events will occur between the chromosome bearing the mutation and a homologous chromosome that may have a different set of haplotypes. If recombination occurs near the mutation, new haplotypes will be introduced onto the chromosome bearing the mutation. This will lead to a gradual reduction in size of the haplotype block that segregates with the mutation. This leads to the expectation that more recently introduced mutations will be associated with larger haplotype blocks than are older mutations. Therefore, large haplotype blocks are thought to have origins that are more recent.

b. For a haplotype containing *HBB* to have undergone positive selection, that haplotype must confer some selective advantage. Therefore, it is reasonable to hypothesize that one or more mutations occurred in a haplotype that provided some selective advantage. Since Hb-A/Hb-S heterozygotes are more resistant to malarial infection, it is also reasonable to hypothesize that these mutations might affect Hb-A, either at the level of its expression or at the level of an amino acid substitution. However, from just this information, we cannot be certain that the haplotype that underwent positive selection had an Hb-A mutation. It could be that a mutation in a nearby gene could also confer a selective advantage.

9.25   *Answer:*

a, b, and **c.** Use representational oligonucleotide microarray analysis (ROMA) to identify which genes differ in copy number between a reference individual and sets of ASD and normal individuals. For each individual to be evaluated, isolate genomic DNA and digest it with a restriction enzyme that leaves a single-stranded overhang. Design and synthesize a single-stranded DNA adapter molecule so one of its ends is complementary to the overhang and its other end is complementary to a PCR primer. Anneal the adapter to the overhang of the restriction fragments, and ligate it to the fragments using DNA ligase. Then use PCR to amplify all of the restriction fragments in the presence of nucleotides labeled with Cy3 (green) or Cy5 (red). To determine which genes are deleted or duplicated in ASD individuals, prepare a reference target DNA by labeling DNA from a reference individual with Cy5 (red), and prepare experimental target DNAs by labeling DNA from different ASD individuals with Cy3 (green). Mix the reference target DNA with one experimental target DNA, and allow these to hybridize to a DNA microarray containing oligonucleotide probes representing genes in the 16p11.2 region [for part **(a)**] or, alternatively, probes representing genes throughout the genome [for part **(c)**]. Red spots identify probes from genes that have a decreased copy number (deletion) in an ASD individual, green spots identify probes from genes that are present in increased copy number (duplication) in an ASD individual, and yellow spots identify probes from genes present in the same copy number in the reference and ASD individuals. To investigate if the same regions have altered copy number in normal individuals [for part **(b)**], compare the reference target DNA to target DNA samples prepared from normal individuals.

9.26   *Answer:*

a. The data shown in the table suggest that mutations in an ancestor of *M. leprae* have led to the inactivation of many genes into pseudogenes. The genes of *M. leprae* and *M. tuberculosis* are about the same size, but only about 50% of *M. leprae*'s genome encodes genes, while about 91% of *M. tuberculosis*'s genome encodes genes. This appears to result from mutations in ancestors of *M. leprae* introducing 1,116 pseudogenes, compared to the six in *M. tuberculosis*. To understand why *M. leprae* might have so many pseudogenes, it is helpful to consider the results of experiments that analyze the effects of individually knocking out all of the genes in an organism. As discussed in the text and the solution to Question 9.17, a significant number of genes in some genomes can be knocked out without leading to lethality or an obviously abnormal phenotype. This result suggests the hypothesis that such genes are not used for vital processes, even though they might be needed for the organism to survive in non-laboratory environments. This suggests the following hypothesis to explain why *M. leprae* has so many more pseudogenes than *M. tuberculosis*: *M. leprae* has accumulated a large number of pseudogenes because the functions provided by those genes to an ancestor of *M. leprae* are no longer required for growth when the organism has infected skin cells, nerves, or mucous membrane cells. Those cell types may be able to provide *M. leprae* with functions that were lost when pseudogenes were formed. A corollary to this hypothesis is that this situation generally does not hold for *M. tuberculosis*.

b. To assess what enzymatic functions the two bacteria can carry out, characterize the types of enzymes that are encoded by ORFs present in the two genomes. For each ORF, perform a BLAST search to determine what domains are present in the polypeptide encoded by the ORF, identify potential homologs from other species, and examine the enzymatic functions associated with the homologs. Characterizing the spectrum of enzymatic functions represented in the set of homologs will let you estimate what different enzymatic functions are present in each organism.

c. One possibility to explain why *M. leprae* cannot be cultured is that the skin, nerve, and mucous membrane cells that it grows in provide it with nutrients that are required for its growth. Identifying the enzymatic functions present in *M. tuberculosis* that are missing in *M. leprae* could provide some clues as to what these nutrients are, because the enzymatic functions *M. leprae* is missing could be important in the synthesis of such nutrients. A culture medium with those nutrients could be tested for its ability to support growth of *M. leprae*.

9.27   *Answer:*

a. From the website http://nihroadmap.nih.gov/hmp/index.asp, the goals of the human microbiome project (HMP) are to: (1) determine whether individuals share a core human microbiome; (2) understand whether changes in the human microbiome can be correlated with changes in human health; (3) develop the technological and bioinformatic tools needed to support these goals; and (4) address the ethical, legal, and social implications raised by human microbiome research.

b. From the website http://hmp.nih.gov, there are three projects being pursued by the HMP. The first project is to collect the genomic sequences of about 600 microbes from cultured and uncultured bacteria. These data will be combined with other data to provide a reference collection of about 1,000 genomes that can serve as a benchmark against which further sequence data can be compared. The second project is to use sequencing of the 16S rRNA to characterize the complexity of microbial communities at individual body sites, and to determine whether there is a core microbiome at each site. The body sites that will be studied include the gastrointestinal, female urogenital, nasal, and pharyngeal tracts, the oral cavity, and the skin. The third project is an expansion of the second project. It involves metagenomic whole-genome shotgun sequencing of samples taken from human subjects. Together, these three projects will provide insights into the genes and pathways present in the human microbiome, which will help meet the first goal of the HMP described in the answer to part **(a)**. Presumably, the third goal of developing technological and bioinformatic tools will be a component of these projects.

9.28   *Answer:*

a. The Virochip is a DNA microarray with oligonucleotide probes for about 20,000 genes representing the very large number of viruses with sequenced genomes. When labeled target DNA is prepared from an unknown virus and mixed with the probes on the chip, it will hybridize to similar sequences. The pattern of sequence similarities that is observed can be used to identify the type of virus that the target DNA was derived from. In this way, it was determined that SARS patients all had a novel coronavirus.

b. Target DNA prepared from a new virus will hybridize to sequences on the Virochip that are similar to it. Thus, if the new virus is related to a known virus, the Virochip should be useful to detect and classify it.

9.29   *Answer:*

S, A, F, C	Aligning DNA sequences within databases to determine the degree of matching
A, F, C	Identification and description of putative genes and other important sequences within a sequenced genome
F	Characterizing the transcriptome and proteome present in a cell at a specific developmental stage or in a particular disease state
S	Preparing a genomic library containing 2-kb and 10-kb inserts
C	Comparing the overall arrangements of genes and nongene sequences in different organisms to understand how genomes evolve
F	Describing the function of all genes in a genome
F, C	Determining the functions of human genes by studying their homologs in nonhuman organisms

F _____   Developing a capture array

S _____   Developing a physical map of a genome

A, F, C _____   Developing DNA microarrays (DNA chips)

S _____   Obtaining a working draft of a genome sequence by assembling overlapping DNA sequences

S, C _____   Whole-genome shotgun sequencing of a DNA sample isolated from a bacterial community growing in a hot spring in Yellowstone National Park

F, C _____   Identifying homologs to human disease genes in organisms suitable for experimentation

S, A _____   Identifying a large collection of SNP DNA markers within one organism

A _____   Cloning and sequencing cDNAs from one organism

C _____   Using a Virochip to characterize a new infection

F _____   Making gene knockouts and observing the phenotypic changes associated with them

C _____   Using microarray analysis to type SNPs in a population of individuals

10

Recombinant DNA Technology

Chapter Outline

Review of Key Terms, Symbols, and Concepts

In your own words, write a brief, precise definition of each term in the groups below and on the following page. Check your definitions using the text. Then develop a concept map using the terms in each list.

1	2	3
genetic engineering	library screening	restriction map
recombinant DNA	cDNA, complementary DNA	Southern blot analysis, Southern blotting
cloning vector	cDNA library	northern blot analysis, northern blotting
plasmid vector	expression vector	polymerase chain reaction (PCR)
lambda vector	genomic library	subcloning
bacterial lawn	autoradiogram	reverse-transcriptase PCR (RT-PCR)
plaque	autoradiography	real-time quantitative PCR, real-time PCR
shuttle vector	replica plating	SYBR green
forced, directional cloning	random-primer labeling	site-specific mutagenesis
transcribable vector	hexanucleotide random primers	humanization
T7, T3, SP6 promoter	Klenow fragment	alternative pre-mRNA splicing
probe	radioactive labeling	hybrid dysgenesis
riboprobe	nonradioactive labeling	P-element
PCR cloning vector	digoxigenin-dUTP	yeast two-hybrid system
	alkaline phosphatase	interaction trap assay
	chemiluminescent substrate	reporter gene
	colorimetric substrate	Gal4p, AD, BD
	complementation	
	epitope	
	heterologous probe	
	oligonucleotide probe	
	consensus sequence	
	guessmer	
	GenBank	

4	5
DNA polymorphism	gene therapy
gene	somatic cell therapy
allele	germ-line cell therapy
indel	transgene
DNA typing, fingerprinting, profiling	transgenic cell
DNA marker	transformation
SNP	transfection
STR, microsatellite, SSR	biotechnology
VNTR, minisatellite	plant genetic engineering
monolocus, single-locus probe	*Agrobacterium tumefaciens*
multilocus probe	crown gall disease
RFLP	Ti plasmid
multiplex PCR	T-DNA
PCR-RFLP analysis method	virulence (vir) region
ASO hybridization analysis	electroporation
reverse ASO hybridization	gene gun
genetic testing	antisense mRNA
DNA molecular testing	edible vaccine
prenatal diagnosis	pharming
newborn screening	
carrier (heterozygote) detection	
exclusion, inclusion result	

Thinking Analytically

Genetic engineering uses the techniques of cloning, DNA manipulation, and transformation to alter the structure and characteristics of genes to address biological questions and to develop solutions for problems that can be addressed by biotechnology. Advances in genetic engineering come from two sources: developing new technology and applying previously developed techniques in new combinations or in different ways. Consider PCR as an example. PCR was developed using the key insight that DNA segments can be amplified using multiple rounds of DNA synthesis. Since then, many applications have been developed by combining PCR with other molecular methods: PCR-amplified DNA can be cloned by using specially designed PCR cloning vectors; PCR is used for DNA typing by combining it with restriction digestion in PCR-RFLP; and it is used to quantify DNA copy number and gene expression in real-time PCR. Therefore, as you consider the material in this chapter, reflect on how different experimental objectives have been achieved by combining different modular, molecular genetic techniques. As you approach a new method, identify how it works by breaking it down into its component parts. Identify the component techniques that you have seen before, such as restriction digestion, plasmid cloning, or PCR, and then consider how the method integrates these techniques with new or additional ones to achieve an experimental objective.

Questions for Practice

Multiple-Choice Questions

For Questions 1–10, match each experimental goal with the techniques useful to attain it. Multiple or alternative techniques may be used to achieve one goal. Some techniques will be used more than once.

Techniques	Experimental Goal
_____	**1.** Amplify a specific genomic DNA sequence.
_____	**2.** Rapidly assess whether a restriction site is present at one site in the genome.
_____	**3.** Try to exonerate a convicted rapist with DNA evidence.
_____	**4.** Identify cDNA clones that express a certain epitope.
_____	**5.** Evaluate which of two alternatively spliced exons is expressed in a tissue.
_____	**6.** Test whether an animal has been poached from a game reserve.
_____	**7.** Identify plasmids having a particular DNA sequence insert.
_____	**8.** Test whether a package of hamburger contains a pathogenic strain of *E. coli*.
_____	**9.** Determine the levels of expression of a particular mRNA at different developmental stages.
_____	**10.** Determine the size of a fragment of DNA inserted into a plasmid vector.

Techniques:

- **a.** restriction mapping
- **b.** restriction digestion
- **c.** PCR
- **d.** RT-PCR
- **e.** real-time PCR
- **f.** express a protein using an expression vector
- **g.** northern blot analysis
- **h.** Southern blot analysis
- **i.** lifts of bacterial colonies or plaques
- **j.** agarose gel electrophoresis
- **k.** DNA sequencing
- **l.** analyses using a multilocus probe
- **m.** analyses of microsatellites

11. Which of the following could be done as part of a humanization process?
    - **a.** Use site-directed mutagenesis to make a mouse protein more like the human protein.
    - **b.** Replace a genomic copy of a gene with the human homolog.
    - **c.** In a model organism, knock out the homolog of a human gene and then transform a transgene with the human homolog.
    - **d.** all of the above

12. When a PCR reaction is performed using genomic DNA as a template, a 1.5-kb product is amplified. When the same reaction is set up using cDNA as a template, a 0.8-kb product is amplified. A likely explanation for the different-sized products is that
    - **a.** primers always bind to different sequences in different templates.
    - **b.** there is a mutation in the genomic DNA.
    - **c.** there is an intron in the gene.
    - **d.** the cDNA is degraded.

13. Which of the following techniques would be the best to use to determine whether a segment of the genome is duplicated or deleted?
    - **a.** PCR followed by gel electrophoresis
    - **b.** RT-PCR followed by gel electrophoresis
    - **c.** real-time PCR

14. A researcher wants to obtain a clone of a gene using information about the gene's sequence obtained using whole-genome shotgun sequencing so that she can experimentally analyze its promoter. What should she do?
    - **a.** Use a labeled oligonucleotide probe to screen a genomic library.
    - **b.** Use a labeled oligonucleotide probe to screen a cDNA library.
    - **c.** Use a labeled antibody to screen an expression library.
    - **d.** Use the sequence information to design primers for PCR, use PCR to amplify the genomic segment of interest, and then clone the segment into a PCR-cloning vector.

15. What can you ascertain by performing a northern blot analysis?
  a. information about the restriction sites present in a particular region of the genome
  b. information about the levels of mRNA present in a tissue
  c. whether a multilocus probe is present
  d. whether one or both of two alternatively spliced mRNAs are expressed in a tissue

Answers: 1c; 2b, c; 3c, j, k, l, m; 4f, i; 5d, j, k; 6c, j, k, l, m; 7i; 8c, e, k, j; 9d, e, g, j; 10a, b, j; 11d; 12c; 13c; 14a, d; 15b, d

Thought Questions

1. Contrast PCR, RT-PCR, and real-time RT-PCR in terms of their templates, products, and applications.

2. For what different purposes would you choose to analyze a SNP, a STR, or a VNTR?

3. What is involved in introducing a transgene into a plant? How is this process fundamentally different from that used for introducing a transgene in animals?

4. Address the following questions to explore the kinds of results that could be obtained on a Southern blot made with genomic DNA.
  a. DNA is digested with a restriction enzyme that cuts at a defined 6-bp sequence having 2 G–C base pairs and 4 A–T base pairs. The genome has 40% G–C base pairs. What is the *average* fragment size?
  b. The cleaved DNA is separated by size using agarose gel electrophoresis. When the gel is stained, a smear of DNA is seen. Why is a smear and not one or a few bands of DNA seen?
  c. The DNA is transferred in a Southern blot to a membrane. When sequences transferred to the membrane are hybridized to a unique-sequence probe made from a fragment that is 4.0 kb in length, bands that are 0.5, 3.0, and 9.0 kb are seen. How do you interpret this result?
  d. The same blot is hybridized with a probe that has homology to moderately repetitive DNA. The probe has been made from a fragment that is 1.2 kb in size. The blot has about 40 bands, ranging in size from 3 to 17 kb. How do you interpret this result?

5. Construct a restriction map of a 10-kb DNA fragment using the following data:

Enzymes Used	Sizes of Fragments (in kb)
*Eco*RI	1, 4, 5
*Bam*HI	4, 6
*Hind*III	0.8, 1.5, 7.7
*Eco*RI and *Bam*HI	1, 2, 3, 4
*Eco*RI and *Hind*III	0.5, 0.8, 1, 3.2, 4.5
*Bam*HI and *Hind*III	0.8, 1.5, 2.5, 5.2
*Bam*HI, *Eco*RI, and *Hind*III	0.5, 0.8, 1, 2, 2.5, 3.2

6. Suppose you have cloned 11 kb of eukaryotic genomic DNA that includes a single gene. After analyzing the sequence of about 500 bp at each end of the clone, you believe you have evidence that these sequences contain the 5′ UTR and 3′ UTR sequences of the gene. What might this evidence be? How can you use the information you have in hand, together with Southern and northern blot analyses and PCR, to: (a) identify the length of the primary transcript of the gene; (b) identify the length of the mature mRNA of the gene; and (c) obtain a cDNA copy of the mature mRNA of the gene?

Thought Questions for Media

After reviewing the media on the *iGenetics* website, try to answer these questions.

1. In the animation depicting restriction mapping, how is agarose gel electrophoresis able to separate fragments of cleaved DNA?

2. The rotating disk method is effective for orienting restriction fragment sites in a circular molecule relative to each other. Explain how it works.

3. Sometimes, when the rotating disk method is being used to locate restriction enzyme sites relative to each other, overlaying maps does not allow sites to be positioned. In some cases, an alternative mirror image map must be used. Why?

4. How could you modify the rotating disk method to map linear DNA fragments?

5. Automated DNA sequencers have made sequencing DNA both cheaper and easier. Why is it still important to know how to construct a restriction map?

6. The calibration curve shown in the animation is not linear over the entire length of the gel. However, it is approximately linear between about 1,000 and 10,000 base pairs. Why might it be linear over only part of the length of the gel?

7. Each of two enzymes, enzyme I and enzyme II, cuts a plasmid giving fragments of 2,506 and 5,160 bp. What is the best means to determine quickly and unambiguously how many different sites these enzymes recognize and their positions relative to each other?

8. From the animation on the yeast two-hybrid system, what is meant by a "bait gene"? How does the "bait" allow you to "fish" for interacting proteins?

9. When a yeast two-hybrid screen is done, what is the genotype of the transformed yeast strain? Why are both uracil *and* tryptophan left out of the medium on which the transformed yeast are grown?

10. Suppose a cDNA for the Y gene is fused to the Gal4 AD. This cDNA is expressed in a yeast cell that also expresses a cDNA for the X gene that is fused to the Gal4 BD, and which has a UAS_G promoter upstream of the *lacZ* gene. A blue colony is seen when the yeast is plated on a medium with X-gal. What control could you do to ensure that the Y-Gal4 AD fusion protein activates *lacZ* expression specifically through its interaction with the X-Gal4 BD fusion protein, and not through some other mechanism?

11. How is a yeast two-hybrid screen done?

12. In the animation on plant genetic engineering, what features in the T plasmid define the DNA sequences that will be transferred to the plant nucleus? Why are the *vir* genes not transferred?

13. What different types of *vir* genes are there, and how does each function in transferring T DNA into the plant genome? What is the purpose of placing an antibiotic resistance gene in the *vir* region of T vectors?

14. What is the basis for Roundup™ resistance in crop plants?

15. What different types of DNA sequences need to be engineered into T DNA to confer Roundup resistance? How should these be arranged?

16. Normally, *Agrobacterium tumefaciens* infections are harmful to plants. Why are infections by strains carrying T-vector plasmids not harmful?

17. Outline the steps you would take to obtain a stock of seeds for Roundup-resistant plants from a plant whose leaf has been infected with an appropriate strain of recombinant *A. tumefaciens*.

18. In the animation on DNA molecular testing, what properties of SNPs distinguish them from other types of DNA polymorphisms?

19. In the example shown in the animation, an SNP led to a single amino acid change that led to disease. Are all, or even most, SNPs likely to be associated with a phenotype?

20. Are all SNPs also RFLPs?

21. How can SNPs be detected if they affect a restriction site? If they do not affect a restriction site?

1. In the iActivity where you created a genetically modified brewing yeast for beer, what is the rationale behind deleting the *STA1*, *STA2*, and *STA2K* genes?

2. Why is it important to delete *entirely* each of the *STA1*, *STA2*, and *STA2K* genes?

3. Why are there differences between the beers made with the three recombinant yeast strains, since each has a deletion of a gene responsible for glucoamylase production?

4. Why is the *CUP1* gene needed in these experiments? How would you demonstrate that it had no effect on fermentation characteristics or beer quality?

5. Refer to the frame that asks you to insert the *STA1* gene into the YEpD vector. Suppose there were two *Sna*BI sites flanking the *STA1* gene. Even though there is a unique *Sna*BI site in the YEpD vector, why would you not use it instead of the *Bgl*II site?

6. Reflect on the iActivity where you combed through "fur"ensic evidence. For one primer pair, how many different PCR products can be obtained in one individual? How many different alleles can be detected with one primer pair?

7. For five primer pairs, how many different PCR products can be obtained in one individual? How many different alleles can be detected with five primer pairs?

8. Are alleles detected as STRs dominant, recessive, or neither? Why?

9. For one primer pair, how many different patterns of PCR products can be obtained in two individuals? For five primer pairs, how many different patterns of PCR products can be obtained in two individuals?

10. Why is it important in forensics to perform DNA typing on loci that are highly polymorphic?

11. How is the profile probability used to determine the likelihood that two matching samples come from the same individual?

12. What is the advantage of using fluorescent primers and multiplex PCR? If you want to test multiple loci using PCR, what information would you need to know about each pair of primers before labeling them and using them in a multiplex PCR?

Solutions to Text Questions and Problems

10.1   *Answer:*

    a. Vectors have been developed for transforming yeast as well as plant and animal cells. These are useful for studying cloned eukaryotic genes in a eukaryotic environment, commercial production of eukaryotic gene products (for example, drugs and antibodies), developing gene therapy, engineering crop plants, and developing transgenic animals.

    b. Shuttle vectors are cloning vectors that can replicate in two or more host organisms. They are used to introduce DNA into organisms other than *E. coli*. A typical shuttle vector has the ability to replicate in *E. coli*, where it is usually easier and faster to perform initial cloning and engineering steps. Once the appropriate recombinant DNA molecule is constructed in *E. coli*, it can be transferred into another organism without further subcloning.

    c. A yeast shuttle vector should contain dominant selectable markers for both yeast (for example, *URA3*, which provides for uracil-independent growth when the vector is transformed into a *ura3* yeast) and *E. coli* (for example, ampicillin resistance); several unique restriction enzyme sites suitable for cloning foreign DNA; and, if it is not integrated into the yeast chromosome, sequences that allow it to replicate autonomously, as a plasmid, in both yeast cells and bacteria.

10.2   *Answer:* The λ-phage vectors described in the text grow using a lytic cycle and cannot undergo a lysogenic cycle. After these phage infect a bacterial cell, they reproduce within the cell and then lyse the cell to release their progeny. When a single phage infects a cell growing within a layer of agar containing many growing bacterial cells, the phage progeny released when that cell is lysed infect neighboring bacterial cells. After multiple cycles of bacterial infection and lysis, a plaque—a clearing in the agar where all of the cells in one region have been killed by phage lysis—is produced. The killing of the host bacterial cell by the phage is advantageous for working with DNA clones because each plaque contains a large number of identical phage. Therefore, each plaque on a lawn of bacterial cells provides a source of phage that can be collected to continue work with the cloned DNA they contain. Phage libraries can be screened in similar ways to those used for screening plasmid libraries in bacteria, but they have two advantages: phage vectors accept larger inserts than do plasmids; and many more plaques can "fit" on a plate than can bacterial colonies. Therefore, using a phage vector allows a much larger set of clones and a greater amount of "insert" DNA to be screened on one bacterial plate than would be the case if a plasmid vector were used.

10.3   *Answer:* As discussed in text Chapter 8, a complementary DNA, or cDNA, is a DNA copy of an mRNA. A cDNA library is a collection of clones containing the different cDNAs synthesized from the entire population of mRNA of a particular (usually eukaryotic) tissue or cell. It is constructed as follows: Initially, the mRNAs are isolated from the tissue or cell where they are expressed. The mRNA molecules are purified from the other RNAs present in cells by passing the total cellular RNA over an oligo-dT column, which binds the poly(A) tails of the mRNAs. After the other RNAs are washed through the column, the poly(A)$^+$ mRNAs are eluted from the column. Then, cDNAs are synthesized by annealing an oligo(dT) primer to the poly(A) tail of each mRNA and using the enzyme reverse transcriptase to synthesize a single-stranded DNA copy of each mRNA strand. This results in a collection of DNA–mRNA hybrids. RNase H is added to degrade the mRNA strands partially, leaving single-stranded complementary DNAs with short mRNA fragments attached. DNA polymerase I is added to synthesize a second DNA strand using the short mRNAs as primers. DNA ligase is used to ligate the DNA fragments of the second strand together. Finally, linkers or adapters are ligated onto the ends of the cDNAs (if linkers are used, the linkers are cleaved to generate sticky ends), and each member of the resulting collection of double-stranded DNAs is ligated into a restriction site in a cloning vector and propagated. Since there is a population of mRNA molecules in a particular tissue or cell, this procedure produces a population of clones, or a library, containing different cDNA inserts, that reflects the population of mRNA present in a particular tissue or cell (see text Figures 8.15, p. 196, and 8.16, p. 197).

    If a cDNA library is constructed using mRNA isolated from a particular tissue, the cDNA inserts represent partial copies of genes transcribed in that tissue. Thus, each clone can be used to identify a gene expressed in that tissue. A cDNA library can be screened for cloned copies of particular mRNA transcripts either by using the same methods that are used to screen genomic libraries or by performing an expression screen. For example, just as for genomic libraries, a cDNA library could be screened by using a DNA probe containing part of the gene of interest, by using a heterologous probe, or by using an oligonucleotide probe. However, since a cDNA is a mature mRNA copy of a gene, if the cDNA library has been made in an expression vector, the cDNA can be expressed (that is, transcribed and the transcript translated). In this case, the protein encoded by a cDNA can be produced in a bacterial cell. If an antibody is available that binds to a protein expressed in a particular tissue, the antibody can be radioactively or nonradioactively labeled and used as a probe to identify clones expressing the protein. Such clones have cDNAs that encode the protein. Cloning in an expression vector is shown in text Figure 10.1, p. 250, and this method of screening an expression vector library is demonstrated in detail in text Figure 10.5, p. 257.

10.4   *Answer:* Use an expression vector. Expression vectors have the signals necessary for DNA inserts to be transcribed and for these transcripts to be translated. In prokaryotes, the vector should have a prokaryotic promoter sequence upstream from the site where the cDNA is inserted, and possibly, a terminator sequence downstream of this site. In eukaryotes, a eukaryotic promoter would be needed, and a poly(A) site should be provided downstream from the site where the cDNA is inserted. If the cDNA lacked a start codon, a start AUG codon embedded in a Kozak consensus sequence would be needed upstream from the site where the cDNA is inserted so that the transcript can be efficiently translated. In the event that the cDNA lacked a start codon, care must be taken during the design of the cloning steps to ensure that the open reading frame (ORF) of the cDNA is in the same reading frame with the start codon provided by the vector.

10.5   *Answer:* It would be preferable to use cDNA. Human genomic DNA contains introns, while cDNA synthesized from cytoplasmic poly(A)+ mRNA does not. Prokaryotes do not process eukaryotic precursor mRNAs having intron sequences, so genomic clones will not give appropriate translation products. Since cDNA is a complementary copy of a functional mRNA molecule, the mRNA transcript will be functional, and when translated human (pro-)insulin will be synthesized.

10.6   *Answer:* If genomic DNA had been used, there could be concerns that an intron in the genomic DNA was not removed, since *E. coli* does not process RNAs like eukaryotic cells do. However, the cDNA is a copy of a mature mRNA, so this should not be a concern. Some other potential concerns are as follows.

First, in order for insulin to be expressed, it must be inserted in the correct reading frame, so that premature termination of translation does not occur and the correct polypeptide is produced. Therefore, check whether the insulin sequence is inserted in the correct reading frame.

Second, depending on the nature of the sequence inserted, a fusion protein with β-galactosidase, and not just human insulin, may have been produced. The polylinker in pBluescript II is within the β-galactosidase gene. Sequences inserted into the polylinker, if inserted in the correct reading frame (the same one as used for β-galactosidase), will be translated into a β-galactosidase–fusion protein. This protein would be greater in size than human insulin. This may not be acceptable, depending on the intended use of the recombinant protein. If a fusion protein were acceptable, it would be important to ensure that only the ORF (the open reading frame) of the insulin gene is properly inserted into the polylinker of the pBluescript II vector.

Third, a complete copy of the human mRNA transcript for insulin may have been used, and not just the open reading frame. If transcribed, it would have features of eukaryotic transcripts but not features required for prokaryotic translation. Indeed, some of its 5'-UTR and 3'-UTR sequences may interfere with prokaryotic transcription and translation. For example, it will lack a Shine–Dalgarno sequence to specify where translation should initiate and identify the first AUG codon. In the pBluescript II vector, a Shine–Dalgarno sequence is supplied after the promoter for the *lacZ* gene, since without an insert in the polylinker, β-galactosidase is produced. However, the cDNA may have 5'-UTR sequences that interfere with translation initiation in prokaryotes, or that contain stop codons, terminating translation of the β-galactosidase–fusion protein.

Fourth, the cDNA may encode a protein that is posttranslationally processed in eukaryotic cells to become human insulin. The protein produced in *E. coli* may not be processed by *E. coli*. Depending on the type of posttranslational modification, it may be possible to modify (engineer) the cDNA to produce a protein similar to human insulin without requiring it to be posttranslationally modified by *E. coli*.

10.7   *Answer:*

a. Use restriction digestion to cleave the cloned cDNA so that most of the cDNA's ORF is released by restriction digestion. Choose restriction enzymes so that the fragment containing most of the cDNA's ORF can be cloned directionally into the expression vector and allow the expression of a fusion protein containing the ORF and the six-histidine tag. Since the ORF includes *Xho*I and *Eco*RI sites close to its beginning and a *Pst*I site close to its end, most of the ORF can be released from the vector in which the cDNA is cloned by digesting the clone with either *Xho*I or *Eco*RI and *Pst*I. However, to clone this fragment into the expression vector in the correct orientation, the beginning of the ORF must be inserted near the translation start site, and the end of the ORF must be inserted near the six-histidine tag. The *Xho*I, *Eco*RI, and *Pst*I sites in the expression vector shown in text Figure 10.B, p. 289, are located such that directional cloning can be done only if both the vector and cDNA clone are cleaved with *Xho*I and *Pst*I. Then, the *Xho*I-*Pst*I fragment from the cDNA clone can be inserted into the expression vector in an orientation that will produce the desired fusion protein. Cleavage with *Eco*RI and *Pst*I would invert the orientation of the cDNA fragment in the expression vector and not produce the desired fusion protein. Even if the ORF is inserted in the correct orientation, a fusion protein might not be produced. The insert might lead to a frameshift, so that the open reading frame is not maintained within the inserted sequence, and the desired fusion protein cannot be produced.

b. If the cDNA had no *Xho*I, *Pst*I, or *Eco*RI sites, one approach would be to clone the ORF from the cDNA using a PCR-based strategy. Design one PCR primer targeted to sequence near the beginning of the ORF and incorporate into its 5' end either an *Xho*I or *Pst*I site. Design a second PCR primer targeted to sequence near the end of the ORF and incorporate into its 5' end an *Eco*RI site. Perform PCR amplification with these primers using the cDNA as a template, and digest the product of the PCR amplification with either *Xho*I or *Pst*I (depending on the site incorporated into the primer) and *Eco*RI. Ligate the product of the restriction digestion into a similarly cleaved expression vector, and transform this into *E. coli*. To ensure that a fusion protein is produced, carefully design the PCR primers so that the open reading frame is maintained after the digested fragment is ligated into the expression vector.

10.8   *Answer:* If a cloning vector containing an unpaired T is prepared, the unpaired A nucleotide left at the end of a fragment amplified by a PCR can be advantageously used to clone the amplification product efficiently. The cloning of blunt-ended DNA fragments is not very efficient, and the A–T base pairing between the amplification product and the vector provides a sticky end that makes cloning more efficient.

10.9   *Answer:* In gel electrophoresis, DNA fragments are separated by size. Since DNA is negatively charged due to its phosphates, it will migrate toward the positive pole in an electric field. Since, in an agarose gel, smaller DNA fragments will move more readily through the pores in the gel, smaller DNA fragments move through the gel more rapidly than larger DNA fragments. (Although larger DNA fragments have more phosphate groups and hence more *total* negative charge, they have the same amount of charge density (negative charge per unit mass) as smaller DNA fragments. Hence, the DNA is separated by size in this gel, not by charge.) To determine the sizes of the fragments produced by a restriction digest or the size of a PCR product, the DNA sample should be loaded into one well of an agarose gel and a size standard, or marker, DNA sample should be loaded into another well of the gel. A current should be applied to induce the DNA samples to migrate through the gel. After electrophoresis, the gel should be stained with a dye that binds DNA, such as ethidium bromide. Ethidium bromide will complex with DNA and fluoresce under ultraviolet light. The fluorescent image should be photographed, and the distance each DNA band has migrated from the loading should be measured. Since the molecular sizes of the DNA fragments in the marker lane are known, a calibration curve can be drawn to relate the DNA size (in log kb) to the migration distance (in mm). Then the migration distance for the DNA band of the PCR product can be measured. By comparing it to the calibration curve, its size can be determined (see text Figures 8.8, p.181, and 10.2, p. 252).

10.10   *Answer:* Sort out the results for the first enzyme by tabulating the results:

Complete Digestion		Partial Digestion	
Fragment	Size (bp)	Fragment	Size (bp)
a	2,000	d-a-c	3,600
b	1,400	a-d-b	3,100
c	900	c-b-d	3,000
d	700	a-c	2,900
Total plasmid	5,000	d-a	2,700
		b-c	2,300
		d-b	2,100

Consider the following: If an enzyme cuts a circular molecule once, it will produce one fragment. If an enzyme cuts a circular molecule twice, it will produce two fragments. (Diagram these situations to convince yourself of this.) Since four fragments are produced when enzyme I completely cleaves the plasmid, enzyme I must cut the plasmid at four sites. A partial digestion occurs when not all four sites are cut. For the partial digestion fragments that contain three fragments, two cuts were made in neighboring sites. Thus, the *d-a-c* fragment was released when two cuts were made at sites flanking fragment *b*, the *a-d-b* fragment was released when two cuts were made at sites flanking fragment *c*, and the *c-b-d* fragment was released when two cuts were made at sites flanking fragment *a*. For the partial digestion fragments containing only two fragments, cuts were made that flank both fragments. Thus, *a* is next to *c*, *d* is next to *a*, *b* is next to *c*, and *d* is next to *b*. This information can be used to order the fragments in the plasmid. Since *a* is next to *c* and *d*, the order must be *c-a-d*. Since *b* is next to *c* and *d*, the order must be *d-b-c*. Since *d* is next to *a* and *b*, the order must be *a-d-b*. Thus, the order of fragments in the plasmid is *c-a-d-b*.

When the plasmid is cleaved with both enzyme I and enzyme II, six fragments are produced. This indicates that the two enzymes together recognize six sites. Since enzyme I cleaves at four sites, enzyme II must cleave at two sites. Since the 1,400- and 900-bp fragments produced when enzyme I cleaves the plasmid remain intact in the double digestion, and the 2,000- and 700-bp fragments do not remain intact in the double digestion, enzyme II must cleave at sites within the 2,000- and 700-bp fragments (*a* and *d*). Given the 1,200- and 800-bp fragments produced with the double digestion, enzyme II must cleave *a* 800 bp from an enzyme I site. Given the 400- and 300-bp fragments produced with the double digestion, enzyme II must cleave *d* 300 bp from an enzyme I site. This gives the following map:

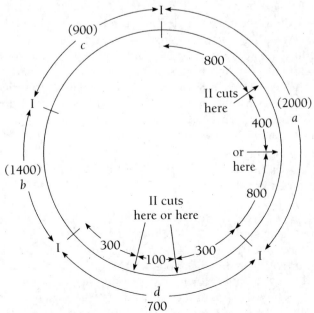

The ambiguities in enzyme II site positions could be resolved if one knew what size fragments were produced when the plasmid was digested to completion with enzyme II alone.

10.11   *Answer:* Construct a map stepwise, considering the relationship between the fragments produced by double digestion and the fragments produced by single-enzyme digestion. Start with the larger fragments. The 1,900-bp fragment produced by digestion with both A and B is a part of the 2,100-bp fragment produced by digestion with A, and the 2,500-bp fragment produced by digestion with B. Thus, the 2,500-bp and 2,100-bp fragments overlap by 1,900 bp, leaving a 200-bp A-B fragment on one side and a 600-bp A-B fragment on the other. One has:

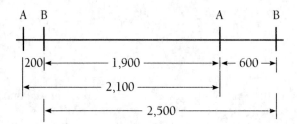

The map is extended in a stepwise fashion, until all fragments are incorporated into the map. The restriction map is:

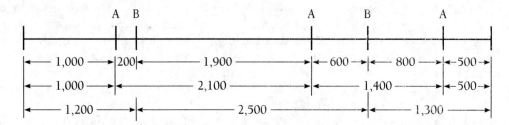

10.12   *Answer:*

   a. Text Table 8.1, p. 174, indicates that the *Bgl*II enzyme leaves a 5'-GATC overhang and that the *Pst*I enzyme leaves a 3'-ACGT overhang. If the multiple cloning site (MCS) of the pBluescript II vector could be cleaved to leave these overhangs, the 4.5-kb fragment could be cloned directionally into the vector. Examination of the restriction enzyme sites available in the MCS of pBluescript II reveals a *Pst*I site, but no *Bgl*II sites. There are multiple approaches to obtain the required 5'-GATC overhang. One approach is to examine the MCS further to determine whether cleaving any of its sites leaves the same kind of overhang as *Bgl*II. A comparison of the sites in the MCS to the enzymes described in text Table 8.1 identifies a *Bam*HI site that, if cut, would leave a 5'-GATC overhang, just like that of *Bgl*II. Thus, cleaving the vector with *Bam*HI would produce the appropriate sticky end. To directionally clone the insert, cleave the pBluescript II vector with *Pst*I and *Bam*HI, allow the fragment to anneal to the sticky ends in the vector, and use DNA ligase to seal the gap in the phosphodiester backbones.

   Another approach to obtain appropriate sticky ends for directional cloning is to cut the polylinker with the enzyme *Sma*I (which leaves blunt ends), ligate a linker containing a *Bgl*II site onto the blunt end, and cleave the modified vector with *Bgl*II and *Pst*I.

   b. Transform the ligated DNA into a host bacterial cell, and plate the cells on bacterial medium containing ampicillin and a substrate (X-gal) for β-galactosidase that turns blue when cleaved. This selects for bacterial colonies that harbor pBluescript II plasmids and allows for blue/white screening to identify colonies that have plasmids with inserts. Pick white colonies (which have an interrupted *lacZ* gene, and so β-galactosidase is not produced and the substrate is not cleaved) and isolate plasmid DNA from them. Cleave the DNA with restriction enzymes, and analyze the products using agarose gel electrophoresis to verify that the appropriate-sized fragments are recovered. Digestion with *Eco*RI should give two fragments, one that is 2,691 + 490 = 3,451 bp (vector plus the 490-bp *Eco*RI fragment of the insert) and one that is 4,500 − 490 = 4,010 bp (the insert minus the 490-bp fragment of the insert). A set of double digests (*Eco*RI + *Pst*I; *Eco*RI + *Bam*HI) will also be informative.

10.13   *Answer:*

    a. Assuming the cDNA is cloned, she should isolate a fragment of the cDNA inserted into the vector, label it as described in text Box 10.1, p. 259, and use the probe to screen a genomic DNA library, as shown in text Figure 10.6, p. 258.

    b. Genomic clones provide for the analysis of gene structure: intron–exon boundaries, transcriptional control regions, and polyadenylation sites. This analysis is important for evaluating how a gene's expression is controlled. Since mutations in regulatory regions can affect the expression of the gene, analysis of these regions is important for understanding the molecular basis of a mutation.

10.14   *Answer:* Screen the BAC library in a manner similar to that used for screening other libraries (shown in text Figures 10.5, p. 257 and 10.6, p. 258) as follows:

    1. Determine how many BACs you need to screen. Based on the answer to Question 8.16 and assuming mice and humans have similarly sized genomes, you would need to screen about 35,000 BACs to be 90% sure of obtaining a BAC clone with the gene.

    2. Plate *E. coli* cells harboring the BACs onto bacterial plates with growth medium that selects for the presence of the BACs.

    3. Either pick individual BAC-containing colonies, grow them up in microtiter plates, and then array them into grids on membranes (as is done for the cDNA clones in text Figure 10.5), or use a velveteen surface and replica plating to inoculate the bacterial colonies onto the surface of membranes.

    4. After the BAC-containing bacterial colonies have grown, remove the membrane filters with the colonies from their culture dishes, lyse the bacteria that are growing on them, and allow the denatured DNA to bind the filter.

    5. Make a probe by using the cDNA template and random-primer labeling as described in Box 10.1, p. 259, in the text.

    6. Incubate the probe with the DNA filters in a heat-sealable plastic bag and allow the probe to hybridize to complementary BAC sequences that are bound to the filters.

    7. Wash the filters free of unbound probe and then detect the location of the hybridized probe using autoradiography for a radioactively labeled probe or chemiluminescent detection for a nonradioactively labeled probe.

    8. Pick the BAC colonies that have sequences complementary to the probe based on the locations of the hybridization signal.

10.15   *Answer:* The antibodies that recognize the purified enzyme should be used to screen a cDNA expression library as shown in text Figure 10.5, p. 257.

    1. Prepare cDNAs using mRNA isolated from a mouse tissue where phosphofructokinase is abundant. See text Figure 8.15, p. 196.

    2. Clone the cDNAs into a plasmid expression vector using linkers. See text Figures 8.16, p. 197, and 10.1, p. 250.

    3. Transform *E. coli* with the cDNA clones, and plate the bacteria on a medium that selects for the presence of plasmids.

    4. Transfer individual colonies to microtiter dishes and then grow and store the bacteria.

    5. Print colonies to a membrane filter, and grow them on the medium to express the protein products of the cloned cDNAs.

    6. Remove the filters from their medium, lyse the cells *in situ*, and allow the protein products to be bound to the filters.

    7. Label the antibodies with radioactivity, and incubate the labeled antibodies with the membrane filters.

    8. Wash off unbound antibody, and use autoradiography to detect the location of bound antibody.

    9. Pick the bacterial colonies that align with the radioactive signal, grow them up, and purify the cDNA-bearing plasmids from these colonies.

10.16   *Answer:* She should clone the genes by complementation. Transform each mutant with a library containing wild-type sequences and then plate the transformants at an elevated, restrictive temperature. Colonies that grow have a plasmid that complements the cell division mutation—they are able to overcome the functional deficit of the mutation because the plasmid has provided a copy of the wild-type gene. Purify the plasmid from these colonies, and characterize the cloned gene. The shuttle vector would also contain a selectable maker, such as URA3, for selection of transformants in yeast. If the cell division mutants were also made into *ura3* mutants, then transformants could be selected for using URA3. However, in this case, the temperature-sensitive phenotype of the cell division mutants enables the direct selection for transformants receiving the wild-type gene.

10.17   *Answer:* Since the actin amino acid sequence is conserved, the DNA sequence will be somewhat conserved as well. Therefore, use the cloned cDNA for human actin as a heterologous probe to screen the yeast genomic library for the yeast actin gene. Proceed essentially as described in text Figure 10.6, p. 258. Since the genomic library of yeast has been prepared in a bacterial plasmid vector, bacterial colonies and not phage will be transferred to filters. After cell lysis, the plasmid DNA will bind to the filters so that colonies with inserts can be identified using the heterologous probe.

10.18   *Answer:* Compare the amino acid sequence to the genetic code, and design a "guessmer"—a set of oligonucleotides that could code for this sequence. Here, the guessmer would have the sequence 5'-ATG TT(T or C) TA(T or C) TGG ATG AT(T, C or A) GG(A, G, T, or C) TA(T or C)-3', and be composed of 96 different oligonucleotides. Synthesize and then label these oligonucleotides, and use them as a probe to screen a cDNA library as described in text Figure 10.5, p. 257.

10.19   *Answer:*

    a.   The lane with genomic DNA will have a smear, for there are many *Eco*RI sites in a genome and the distances between these sites will vary. The smear reflects the large number and many different sizes of *Eco*RI fragments. Since *Eco*RI recognizes a 6-bp site, the average size will be about 4,096 bp (assume the genome is 25% A, G, C, and T), and more intense staining will be seen around this size. The pBluescript II plasmid has a single *Eco*RI restriction site into which the 10-kb insert has been cloned, so the lane with plasmid DNA will have two bands: the genomic DNA insert at 10 kb and the plasmid DNA at 3 kb.

    b.   The probe will detect the 10-kb *Eco*RI fragment specifically, so a signal will be seen in each lane at 10 kb.

10.20   *Answer:* The gel is soaked in an alkaline solution to denature the DNA to single-stranded form. It must be bound to the membrane in single-stranded form so that the probe can bind in a sequence-specific manner using complementary base pairing.

10.21   *Answer:*

    a.   She should see a 2.0-kb band because the 2.0-kb probe is a single-copy genomic DNA sequence.

    b.   LINEs are moderately repetitive DNA sequences, which may be distributed throughout the genome. Since the LINE has an internal *Eco*RI site, each LINE in the genomic DNA will be cut into two fragments by *Eco*RI during preparation of the Southern blot. When the blot is incubated with the probe, both fragments will hybridize to the probe. The size of the fragments produced from each LINE element will vary according to where the element is inserted in the genome and where the adjacent *Eco*RI sites are. Hence, there will be many different-sized bands seen on the genomic Southern blot.

    c.   As in **(b)**, there will be many different-sized bands on the genomic Southern blot. The sizes of the bands seen reflect the distances between *Eco*RI sites that flank a LINE. All of the bands will be larger than the element because the element is not cleaved by *Eco*RI. Counting the number of bands can give an estimate of the number of copies of the element in the genome.

    d.   Since the heterozygote has one normal chromosome 14, the probe will bind to the 3.0-kb *Eco*RI fragment derived from the normal chromosome 14. If the translocation is a reciprocal translocation, the remaining chromosome 14 is broken in two, and attached to different segments of chromosome 21. Since chromosome 14 has a break point in the 3.0-kb *Eco*RI fragment, the 3.0-kb fragment is now split into two parts, each attached to a different segment of chromosome 21. Consequently, the 3.0-kb probe spans the translocation break point and will bind to two different fragments, one from each of the translocation chromosomes. The sizes of the fragments are determined by where the adjacent *Eco*RI sites are on the translocated chromosomes. Thus, the blot will have three bands, one of which is 3.0 kb.

e. Since the *TDF* gene is on the Y chromosome, no signal should be seen in a Southern blot prepared with DNA from a female having only X chromosomes.

10.22   *Answer:*

   a. *Not*I recognizes an 8-bp site, while *Bam*HI recognizes a 6-bp site. Eight-bp sites appear about one-sixteenth as frequently than do 6-bp sites; hence, the *Not*I fragments are larger, relatively speaking, than the *Bam*HI fragments.

   b. There are many *Bam*HI fragments in the BAC DNA insert, while there are fewer fragments in each *Not*I fragment. Digesting first with *Not*I allows regions of the BAC to be evaluated in an orderly, systematic manner and allows for the *Bam*HI fragments containing the gene to be identified more precisely and then purified.

   c. Since the 47-kb fragment is the only *Not*I fragment that has sequences hybridizing to the cDNA, it contains the gene.

   d. The 10.5-, 8.2-, 6.1-, and 4.1-kb *Bam*HI fragments contain the gene, since they hybridize to the cDNA probe.

   e. The RNA-coding region is about 28.9 kb. It is larger than the cDNA because genomic DNA contains intronic sequences.

10.23   *Answer:*

   a. If Sara has no information about the sequence of the 47-kb *Not*I fragment, she should digest the pBluescript II and 47-kb *Not*I fragment DNAs with *Bam*HI. Then she should separate the digestion products of the 47-kb *Not*I fragment by size using gel electrophoresis and purify the 6.1-, 10.5-, 4.1-, and 8.2-kb genomic DNA fragments. Then she should set up four ligation reactions, one with each of the purified genomic DNA fragments and some of the *Bam*HI-digested pBluescript II DNAs. Then she should separately transform each of the ligations into *E. coli* and select for bacterial colonies with pBluescript II having genomic DNA inserts. That is, she should plate the bacteria on media with ampicillin (to select for the presence of pBluescript II) and X-gal. Colonies with inserts will be white, while colonies without inserts will be blue. (X-gal will be metabolized to a blue compound by β-galactosidase if the *lacZ* gene in pBluescript II has not been disrupted by a genomic DNA insert.) Finally, she should verify that the white colonies from each transformation have the desired genomic DNA inserts. She should grow up representative white colonies, purify plasmid DNA from them, digest the plasmid DNA with *Bam*HI, and separate it by size using gel electrophoresis. Colonies with the correct insert should show a 3-kb band (corresponding to the size of the pBluescript II vector) and a band corresponding to the size of the appropriate genomic *Bam*HI fragment.

   An alternative approach is to set up just a single ligation and transformation, mixing together all of the fragments produced by the *Bam*HI digestion of the *Not*I fragment with the *Bam*HI digestion of pBluescript II, and then sort out later which colonies have which genomic DNA inserts by plasmid purification and *Bam*HI restriction digestion.

   b. Sara should use the sequence information to design four sets of primers that can be used in PCR amplifications to amplify each of the four desired fragments. She should design primers that will amplify a template that spans just beyond an adjacent pair of *Bam*HI sites so that the amplification products can be cleaved with *Bam*HI and then cloned into pBluescript II as described in the answer to part **(a)**.

10.24   *Answer:* If the same gene functions in the brain, the gene should be transcribed into a precursor mRNA, processed to a mature mRNA, and then translated to produce the functional enzyme. Thus, transcripts for the gene should be found in the brain. To address this issue, label the cloned DNA and use it to probe a northern blot having either total RNA or purified poly(A)+ mRNA isolated from brain tissue. If the mRNA is not abundant, preparing a northern blot with purified poly(A)+ mRNA should provide additional sensitivity. If the mRNA is particularly rare, it may be prudent to use mRNA isolated from a specific region of the brain.

An alternate, quite sensitive approach would be to sequence the cloned DNA, analyze the sequence to identify the coding region, and then design PCR primers that could be used to amplify cDNA made from mRNA isolated from various brain regions. To perform this RT-PCR (reverse transcriptase PCR), isolate mRNA, reverse-transcribe it into cDNA, and then perform PCR. Obtaining an RT-PCR product in such an investigation would provide evidence that the gene is transcribed in the brain. In this alternative method, it would be important to be sure that no genomic DNA was present in the PCR amplification mixture because the gene for the enzyme would be found in genomic DNA in both tissues.

10.25   *Answer:*

   a. Since both cDNAs hybridize to the same bands on a genomic Southern blot, they are copies of mRNAs transcribed from the same sequences. Therefore, it is likely that they are from the same gene.

   b. Different-sized bands on the northern blot indicate that the primary mRNA for this gene may be processed differently in brain and liver tissue. For example, it is possible that the 0.8-kb size difference between the two bands reflects a 0.8-kb intron that is spliced out in brain tissue but is not spliced out in liver tissue.

   c. A riboprobe is prepared by transcribing a template strand in the presence of a labeled nucleotide. Consequently, it is a single-stranded probe. A Southern blot is made with double-stranded DNA, so hybridization signal can be detected on a Southern blot because a single-stranded probe will be able to bind to a complementary DNA strand immobilized on the blot. In contrast, a northern blot is made with single-stranded RNA. Signal will be seen on a northern blot only if the probe is complementary to the sense-stranded RNA on the blot. That is, signal will be seen only if an antisense-strand probe is prepared. Since signal is seen on a Southern blot with a riboprobe, we know that the probe is able to hybridize to a complementary sequence. Therefore, no signal is seen on a northern blot because the riboprobe has the same sequence and polarity as the sense-stranded RNA on that blot.

   d. The two cDNAs are copies of mRNAs found in two different tissues. The northern blot indicates that there are some differences between the mRNAs in the different tissues. Thus, it is not surprising that the restriction maps are not identical. Note that the ends of the restriction maps are identical (the same *Eco*RI-*Hin*dIII and *Bam*HI fragments), while the internal regions are not (the brain cDNA lacks the 0.5-kb *Eco*RI-*Hin*dIII fragment and some of each adjoining fragment).

   e. The genomic Southern blot gives an indication of the gene organization at the DNA level, while the cDNA maps give an indication of the structure of the mRNA transcript(s). When the cDNA is used to probe genomic DNA sequences, it will hybridize to any sequences that are transcribed. Since restriction sites in the genome do not delineate where the transcribed regions are, the probe will hybridize to genomic DNA fragments that are only partly transcribed. That is, the probe will hybridize to transcribed sequences that are "connected to" nontranscribed sequences. Thus, the large (7.8-, 7.4-, 6.1-, and 3.6-kb) bands reflect the hybridization of parts of the cDNA to genomic DNA fragments that are only partly transcribed. Since they are the same fragment sizes that appear in the liver cDNA, the smaller fragments (2.0, 1.4, and 1.3 kb) represent fragments that are entirely transcribed. Based on these data, a possible gene organization is illustrated below:

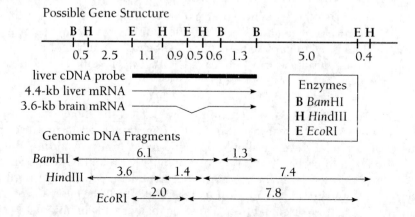

10.26   *Answer:* Isolate RNA from the livers of the alcohol-fed and control rats. Measure the levels of mRNA for alcohol dehydrogenase by either: (1) separating the RNA by size using gel electrophoresis, preparing a northern blot, and hybridizing it with a probe made by labeling a cDNA for the alcohol dehydrogenase gene; or (2) using RT-PCR or real-time quantitative PCR.

10.27   *Answer:*

a. Since *Taq* DNA polymerase lacks proofreading activity, base-pair mismatches that occur during replication go uncorrected. This means that some of the molecules produced in the PCR process will contain errors relative to the starting template. Enzymes with proofreading activity significantly reduce the introduction of errors.

b. If an error is introduced in the first few cycles of PCR amplification, most of the derivative DNA molecules produced during subsequent cycles of PCR amplification will also contain the error. This happens since molecules produced in earlier cycles of PCR serve as templates for molecules synthesized in later cycles of PCR. Consequently, if an error is introduced in a later cycle in the PCR amplification process, fewer molecules will have the error.

10.28   *Answer:* The insert Katrina sequenced was obtained from genomic DNA, while the inserts Marina sequenced were obtained from PCR. *Taq* DNA polymerase introduces errors during PCR, so that individual double-stranded molecules that are amplified during PCR may have small amounts of sequence variation. If PCR products are sequenced directly, a population of molecules is sequenced and the amount of variation is small enough that it may not be noticed—at a particular position in the sequence, only a very small number of molecules have an error. However, when PCR products are cloned, each independently isolated plasmid has an insert derived from a different double-stranded DNA PCR product, so that errors will be apparent.

10.29   *Answer:* Site-specific mutagenesis uses primers that have been modified to incorporate a mutation at a particular site. As shown in text Figure 10.10, p. 266, two separate PCR amplifications are performed to amplify two overlapping DNA segments that together span one region. The products of each PCR reaction overlap by the length of a primer in the center of the region. In the area where the two DNA segments overlap, the PCR primers do not exactly match the template sequence, but they incorporate a mutation at one site. The resulting two PCR products are mixed, denatured, and allowed to reanneal. In some cases, the overlapping ends of the different PCR products will anneal. DNA polymerase can then extend the 3′ ends to generate a double-stranded DNA molecule that spans the entire region. The entire region, now containing an alteration in DNA sequence at one central site, can then be amplified by using PCR and primers that flank the region. The product with the altered site can then be cloned and used to replace the wild-type sequence in a cell.

10.30   *Answer:* Design primers so that you can use PCR to amplify a segment of each orphan gene. Then prepare RNA from yeast at sequential stages of sporulation and use reverse transcriptase to reverse transcribe each RNA sample into cDNA. To measure the expression of each of the orphan genes in the different stages of sporulation, quantify the amount of each gene's cDNA in the different cDNA preparations using real-time PCR with SYBR® Green (see text Figure 10.9, p. 265).

10.31   *Answer:* First, use site-specific mutagenesis to introduce a single-base change into the cDNA to alter the primary structure of the metalloprotease gene product. For example, change the codon for the second amino acid in the consensus sequence, glutamate (GAA or GAG; see text Figure 6.7, p. 108), to the codon for alanine (GCA or GCG). While glutamate is an acidic amino acid, alanine is a neutral, nonpolar amino acid (see text Figure 6.2, p. 104). If glutamate is essential for proteolytic activity, the altered protein should not have proteolytic activity. After completing the site-specific mutagenesis (described in text Figure 10.10, p. 266), replace a segment of the wild-type cDNA sequence with the altered sequence. Then express the protein product of the wild-type cDNA (as a positive control) and that of the mutant cDNA, and purify the proteins that are produced. Measure the metalloprotease activity of each protein in the biochemical assay to determine whether the second amino acid must be glutamate for the protein to have proteolytic activity.

10.32 *Answer:* Humanization is the process by which a gene from a model experimental organism such as a mouse is modified to be more like its human homolog. In humanization, the mouse gene is modified using site-directed mutagenesis to change a cloned copy into something more similar to the human gene. Humanized genes have been used in several ways. One use has been to humanize antibodies that have been developed in mice that are useful in treating disease (such as cancer), so that the antibody does not generate an antigenic response when used in a human. Another use is to provide organisms for additional research on the human gene. The modified gene can be evaluated in a mouse by using knockout techniques to replace the mouse's genomic copy with the mutated version, or by knocking out the mouse gene and then adding a transgene expressing the human gene. A mouse with a humanized version of the gene can then be tested for its reaction to a candidate drug.

10.33 *Answer:*

a. The probe hybridizes to the same genomic region in each of the 10 individuals. Different patterns of hybridizing fragments are seen because of polymorphism of the *EcoRI* sites in the region. If a site is present in one individual but absent in another, different patterns of hybridizing fragments are seen. This provides evidence of restriction fragment length polymorphism. To distinguish between sites that are invariant and those that are polymorphic, analyze the pattern of bands that appear. Notice that the sizes of the hybridizing bands in individual 1 add up to 5 kb. This is also the size of the band in individual 2 and the largest hybridizing band. This suggests that there is a polymorphic site within a 5.0-kb region. This is indicated in the diagram below, where the asterisk over site *b* depicts a polymorphic *EcoRI* site:

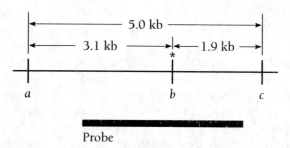

Notice also that the size of the band in individual 3 equals the sum of the sizes of the bands in individual 4. Thus, there is an additional polymorphic site in this 5.0-kb region. Since the 1.9-kb band is retained in individual 4, the additional site must lie within the 3.1-kb fragment. This site, denoted *x*, is incorporated into the diagram below. Notice that, because the 1.0-kb fragment flanked by sites *a* and *x* is not seen on the Southern blot, the probe does not extend into this region.

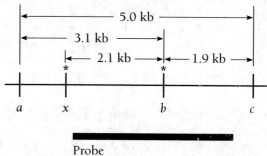

Depending on whether *x* and/or *b* are present, one will see either 5.0-, 3.1-, and 1.9-kb; 2.1- and 1.9-kb; or 4.0-kb bands. In addition, if an individual has chromosomes with different polymorphisms, one can see combinations of these bands. Thus, individual 5 has one chromosome that lacks sites *x* and *b* and one chromosome that has site *b*. The chromosomes in each individual can be tabulated as follows:

Individual	Sites on Each Homolog	Homozygote or Heterozygote?
1	*a, b, c*	homozygote
2	*a, c*	homozygote
3	*x, c*	homozygote
4	*x, b, c*	homozygote
5	*a, c/a, b, c*	heterozygote
6	*x, c/a, b, c*	heterozygote
7	*a, b, c/x, b, c*	heterozygote
8	*a, c/x, c*	heterozygote
9	*a, c/x, b, c*	heterozygote
10	*x, c/x, b, c*	heterozygote

b. Since individual 1 is homozygous, chromosomes with sites at *a*, *b*, and *c* will be present in all of the offspring, giving bands at 3.1 and 1.9 kb. Individual 6 will contribute chromosomes of two kinds, one with sites at *x* and *c* and one with sites at *a*, *b*, and *c*. Thus, if this analysis is performed on their offspring, two equally frequent patterns will be observed: a pattern of bands at 3.1 and 1.9 kb and a pattern of bands at 4.0, 3.1, and 1.9 kb. This is just like the patterns seen in the parents.

10.34 *Answer:* Chromosomes bearing CF mutations have a shorter restriction fragment than chromosomes bearing wild-type alleles. Both parent lanes (M and P) have two bands, indicating that each parent has a normal and a mutant chromosome. The parents are therefore heterozygous for the CF trait. The fetus lane (F) shows only one (lower molecular weight) band. The size of the band indicates that the fetus has only mutant chromosomes. The intensity of the band is about twice that of the same-sized band in the parent lanes. This is because the diploid genome of the fetus has two copies of the fragment, while the diploid genome of each parent only has one. Since the fetus is homozygous for the CF trait, it will have CF.

10.35 *Answer:*

a. Use the PCR-RFLP method: Isolate genomic DNA from the individual with Parkinson disease, and use PCR to amplify the 200-bp segment of exon 4; purify the PCR product, digest it with *Tsp*45I, and resolve the digestion products by size using gel electrophoresis. The normal allele will contain the *Tsp*45I site, and so produce 120- and 80-bp fragments. The mutant allele will not contain the *Tsp*45I site, and so produces only a 200-bp fragment.

b. Homozygotes for the normal allele will have 120- and 80-bp fragments; homozygotes for the mutant allele will have a 200-bp fragment; heterozygotes will have 200-, 120-, and 80-bp fragments.

c. Use RT-PCR to amplify a DNA copy of the mRNA, and digest the RT-PCR product with *Tsp*45I. First, isolate RNA from the tissue. Then make a single-stranded cDNA copy using reverse transcriptase and an oligo(dT) primer. Then amplify exon 4 of the cDNA using PCR, digest the product with *Tsp*45I, and separate the digestion products by size using gel electrophoresis. If a 200-bp fragment is identified in a heterozygote, then the mutant allele is transcribed. If only 120- and 80-bp fragments are identified, then the mutant allele is not transcribed. Note that to assess expression of either allele accurately, it is essential that the RT-PCR reaction be performed on a purified RNA template without contaminating genomic DNA.

10.36 *Answer:* One approach to evaluating the presence of a defined set of alleles is to use reverse ASO hybridization and multiplex PCR. In this approach, several different regions of the gene are amplified in one test tube using PCR and radioactive dNTPs. The radioactively labeled PCR product is used as a probe for hybridization with many different ASOs (allele-specific oligonucleotides) bound to a membrane filter. Each ASO bound to the filter contains a different sequence variant (wild-type or mutant). On the autoradiograms, the dot to which the PCR product binds indicates the allele that the individual has. Inspection of the signal on the autoradiogram allows us to infer whether the individual has any of the mutant alleles used in the test.

If the region being evaluated is very large, an alternate approach is to design a DNA microarray that has oligonucleotides that match the wild-type sequences and known sequence variants (polymorphisms and mutations) throughout the gene that is being evaluated, fluorescently label target DNA from an individual, and hybridize the DNA to the probe array. Since the oligonucleotide locations of the probes for different segments and mutant variants of the gene are known on the probe array, the observed pattern of fluorescence indicates which DNA sequences are present in the individual. This information can be used to determine whether the individual has a mutation in the gene, and if so, where it is and whether it is the same as a known mutation.

10.37   *Answer:* There are three major classes of DNA polymorphisms: single-nucleotide polymorphisms (SNPs), short tandem repeats (STRs, also known as simple sequence repeats or SSRs and microsatellites), and a variable number of tandem repeats (VNTRs, also known as minisatellites).

SNPs are single base changes. If they alter a restriction site, they can be detected as restriction fragment length polymorphisms (RFLPs). RFLPs can be assessed in a Southern blot made using genomic DNA and a probe that spans the SNP (see text Figure 10.14, p. 270, and Questions 10.33 and 10.34) or using the PCR-RFLP method (see text Figure 10.15, p. 271). Chromosomal aberrations can also result in an RFLP (for example, a deletion that removes the site, a chromosomal rearrangement that repositions the site). Not all SNPs will affect a restriction site. Independent of whether they affect a restriction site, SNPs can be detected using allele-specific oligonucleotide (ASO) hybridization analysis (see text Figure 10.16, p. 271) or using DNA microarrays (see text Figure 8.14, p. 194).

VNTRs and STRs are tandemly repeated sequences. STRs have 2- to 6-bp DNA sequences tandemly repeated from a few times to about 100 times. Because the overall length of an STR is relatively short, PCR is the preferred method for analyzing STR polymorphic loci. This is illustrated in text Figure 10.17, p. 272. VNTRs are similar to STRs, but have repeats from seven to a few tens of base pairs long. The length of VNTRs precludes the use of PCR as a convenient way to analyze them. More often, they are detected by restriction enzyme digestion (using enzymes that flank the repeat), Southern blotting, and probing with a labeled DNA fragment containing several copies of the repeating sequence. There are two types of VNTR loci, unique loci and multicopy loci. Probes that detect only one VNTR locus are monolocus probes, while probes that detect VNTRs at multiple sites in the genome are multilocus probes.

10.38   *Answer:* A SNP is a single nucleotide polymorphism. Since a single base change can alter the site recognized by a restriction endonuclease, a SNP can also be a RFLP, or restriction fragment length polymorphism. Since simple tandem repeats (STRs) and variable number tandem repeats (VNTRs) are based on tandemly repeated sequences (repeats that are 2 to 6 bp long for STRs, and from seven to tens of bp long for VNTRs), they will not usually be SNPs.

10.39   *Answer:* If the hypothesis proposed by these researchers is correct, the selective breeding strategy has resulted in two rat populations that differ in DNA sequence at a gene for the synthesis of a catecholamine. Consider, as the simplest case, that there is one SNP—it may be considered either a mutation or a polymorphism—at this gene that is responsible for the behavioral and biochemical differences. Since SNPs are common, occurring at a frequency of about one per 350 bp, the SNP that causes the phenotype is tightly linked to other nearby SNPs. Since crossing-over will not separate the tightly linked SNPs very often, the selective breeding strategy will have selected for the causal SNP as well as the SNPs that are tightly linked to it, including some of the SNPs that we can assay. Under the researchers' hypothesis, then, some of the SNPs that we can assay should be more frequent in one of the two rat populations. Identifying such SNPs will localize a region of the gene for further study to identify the causal DNA sequence change.

Therefore, we should detect which SNPs are present in the genomic DNA (isolated from a drop of blood or a tail snipping) of representative individuals of the two rat populations using PCR-RFLP (see text Figure 10.15, p. 271) or the ASO hybridization method (see text Figures 10.16, p. 271, and

10.20, p. 275) and then determine whether any of the SNPs are present at a different frequency in the two rat populations. If we find a region of the gene where SNPs consistently differ between the two rat populations, our data will support the researchers' hypothesis.

The hypothesis might also be evaluated by sequencing the gene in representative individuals from each rat population. Depending on the size of the gene and the method used for sequencing, it might be cumbersome to sequence the potentially large region containing the gene and its promoter, coding region, enhancers, and silencers from multiple individuals. Sequencing would almost certainly reveal differences since SNPs are frequent, but we would be unable to evaluate their significance without data from many individuals in each population. The method presented here is much more efficient because it allows us to screen the entire region in multiple individuals drawn from each population.

10.40 *Answer:* Mapping studies localize a gene associated with a trait by following the presence or absence of the trait in offspring of crosses where recombination has occurred to produce individuals with different genetic constitutions. Mapping studies relate the presence or absence of the trait to the specific alleles found in the offspring. If an individual is homozygous for an allele at an STR, all of their gametes have the same STR allele whether or not recombination occurs. Such an STR cannot be used as a marker to distinguish between recombinant and nonrecombinant offspring classes, and it will be found equally in offspring with and without a specific trait. Therefore, it will not be useful for mapping studies. In a population, individuals will be more often heterozygous for STRs with more alleles and higher levels of heterozygosity. The recombinant and nonrecombinant offspring classes may be distinguished in individuals heterozygous for an STR, making crosses informative for mapping studies.

If an STR has few alleles and a low heterozygosity, many individuals in a population will share the same STR genotypes. Therefore, there will be many individuals in the population who, by chance alone, will share the same genotype as a test subject, and the STR will not be very useful for DNA fingerprinting studies.

10.41 *Answer:* DNA fingerprinting is the characterization of an individual in terms of the set of DNA markers the person has. For DNA fingerprinting, DNA markers are usually chosen so that they are highly polymorphic in a population, and they may include RFLPs, simple tandem repeat polymorphisms that are 2 to 6 bp long (STRs, microsatellites), and variable numbers of tandem repeat polymorphisms that are from seven to tens of bp long (VNTRs, minisatellites). VNTRs can be derived either from just one locus or from more than one locus (monolocus or multilocus probes). Since all individuals except for identical (monozygotic) twins have different genomes, individuals of a species differ in terms of their DNA fingerprints.

Each parent donates one allele at a DNA marker to his or her offspring. Therefore, the set of DNA markers a child has come from his or her parents. If two parents and a child are tested, all of the DNA markers present in the child must also be present in the set of markers in the two parents. However, the parents can have additional markers, since they donate only one of their two alleles at each marker. If a child has no alleles in common with a suspected parent, the suspected individual can be excluded from consideration as the child's parent. If alleles are shared, the likelihood that the set of alleles came from the suspected parent must be calculated and compared with the likelihood that the set of alleles came from another person. If the alleles present in the child and one known parent are known, then one can infer at least some of the alleles that were contributed by the other parent. Usually, multiple DNA markers are used to minimize possible inaccuracy and provide for a better statistical evaluation of the results, showing that the results obtained are not based on sampling variation. The calculation of the relative odds that a set of alleles derives from a suspected parent or from another person depends on knowing the frequencies of the marker alleles in the child's ethnic population. These types of data should be used together with other non-DNA-based evidence to support a claim of parentage.

In forensic science laboratories, DNA fingerprinting is used to match or exclude the DNA fingerprint of a suspected individual with the DNA fingerprint provided by physical evidence (blood, skin, hair, semen, saliva, etc.) gathered at the scene of a crime. As in the analysis for parentage, DNA fingerprinting is very useful for excluding suspects who do not share alleles with that found in the physical evidence. Inclusion results, results where an individual is positively identified as being responsible for a crime, are more difficult to obtain. As for parentage, a calculation of the relative odds that a set of alleles derive from a suspect or from another person must be made, and this requires good population statistics. In addition, there must be evidence that there were no errors in collecting or processing samples. Thus, DNA evidence is often more useful for excluding suspects than for proving their guilt, and when used to support guilt, must usually be supported by additional, non-DNA-based evidence.

10.42 *Answer:* James and Susan Scott are not the parents of "Ronald Scott." There are several bands in the fingerprint of the boy that are not present in either James or Susan and thus could not have been inherited from either of them (e.g., bands a and b in the figure below). In contrast, whenever the boy's DNA exhibits a band that is missing from one member of the Larson couple, the other member of the Larson couple has that band (e.g., bands c and d). Thus, each band in the boy's DNA could not have been inherited from one or the other of the Larsons. These data thus support an argument that the boy is, in fact, Bobby Larson. These data should be used together with other non-DNA-based evidence to support the claim that the boy is Bobby Larson.

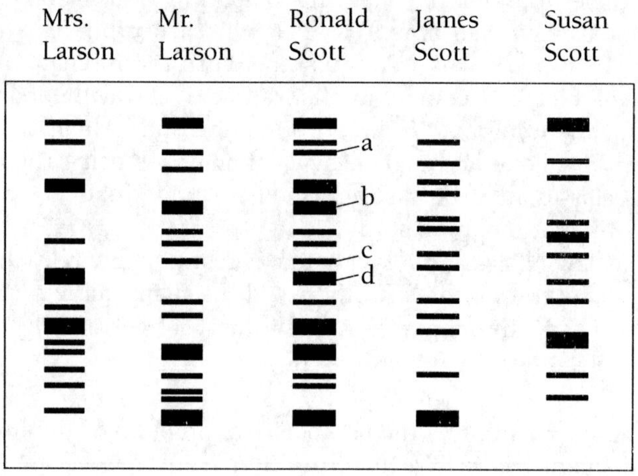

10.43 *Answer:*

a. The PCR method requires very small (nanograms) amounts of template DNA, and if the primers are designed to amplify only small regions, even DNA that is degraded partially can be used. In contrast, VNTR methods require larger amounts (micrograms) of intact DNA because restriction digests are used to produce relatively large (kb-size) fragments that are then detected by Southern blotting. Some of the DNA samples used in forensic analysis are found in crime scenes and may be stored for years, so that they may often be degraded and not be present in large amounts. STR methods can still be used on such samples, while VNTR methods cannot.

b. Multiplexing PCR reactions ensures that (1) the different STR results obtained in the reaction are all derived from a single DNA sample (laboratory labeling and pipetting errors are minimized), and (2) limited amounts of DNA samples are used efficiently.

c. P(random match) = $(0.112 \times 0.036 \times 0.081 \times 0.195)$ = 6.4×10^{-5}. About one person in 15,702 would be misidentified by chance alone using just these four markers.

d. P(random match) = $(0.112 \times 0.036 \times 0.081 \times 0.195 \times 0.062 \times 0.075 \times 0.158 \times 0.065 \times 0.067 \times 0.085 \times 0.089 \times 0.028 \times 0.039)$ = 1.7×10^{-15}. About one person in 5.94×10^{14} would be misidentified by chance alone using all 13 markers.

10.44 *Answer:*

a. This relatively small sample possesses many of the known alleles at these three loci: it has 5 of the 7 known THO1 alleles, 9 of the 20 known D21S11 alleles, and 10 of the 15 known D18S51 alleles. Individuals that have only one marker allele are homozygous for that allele. For example, Patron B is homozygous for the 162-bp allele of THO1. Since one individual can have at most two alleles at one locus, the presence of three and four marker alleles in the DNA sample obtained from the victim's fingernails indicates the presence of two different DNA samples—that of the victim and a person she had scratched.

b. The victim has the 221- and 239-bp alleles at the D21S11 locus. The DNA sample from her fingernail scraping has these alleles and the 225- and 233-bp alleles. Assuming that she scratched her assailant and not her mud-wrestling opponent, the police should investigate further individuals with the 225- and 233-bp alleles at D21S11, patrons C, E, and R.

c. The victim has the 162- and 170-bp alleles at the THO1 locus. The DNA sample from her fingernail scraping has these alleles and the 174-bp allele. This means that the assailant has the 174-bp allele. The assailant could be homozygous for the 174-bp allele or also have the 162- or the 170-bp allele. Patrons C, E, and R all have the 174-bp allele and either the 162- or 170-bp allele. Thus, the information from the THO1 locus does not allow us to distinguish between patrons C, E, and R.

   The victim has the 292- and 304-bp alleles at the D18S51 locus. The DNA sample from her fingernail scraping has these alleles and the 280- and 300-bp alleles. Only patron C has the 280- and 300-bp alleles. Therefore, the police should investigate patron C further.

10.45 *Answer:* Use an interaction trap assay (the yeast two-hybrid system). Fuse the coding region of a protein produced by *fruitless* (obtained from an open reading frame within a cDNA) to the sequence of the Gal4p BD, and cotransform this plasmid into yeast with a plasmid library containing the GAL4p AD sequence, which is fused to protein sequences encoded by different cDNAs from the *Drosophila* brain. Purify colonies that express the reporter gene (see text Figure 10.13, p. 269). In these colonies, the transcription of the reporter gene was activated when the AD and BD domains were brought together by the interactions of the *fruitless* protein with an unknown protein encoded by one of the brain cDNAs. Isolate and characterize the brain cDNA found in these yeast colonies.

10.46 *Answer:*

a. This strategy is problematic for two reasons. First, this strategy is likely to push the species further toward extinction because it eliminates several hundred individuals. Second, it is labor intensive and costly.

b. This is the best strategy: It is essentially noninvasive and does not harm the organisms, and it is efficient and cost effective.

c. This strategy would not accomplish the experimental objective. The yeast two-hybrid system is used to identify proteins that interact with a cloned protein, which is not the objective here.

d. This strategy may not work for several reasons. First, the SNP may not be able to be assessed using the RFLP method, because not all SNPs alter restriction sites. Second, Southern blot analysis usually requires DNA from more than just a few cells. If a restriction enzyme were identified that cleaved the sequence containing the SNP, PCR-RFLP would be a more reasonable choice. See text Figure 10.15, p. 271.

10.47 *Answer:* The STR loci of interest here contain from 2 to 6 CAG repeats, and lie in different regions of the genome of the endangered species. One approach to identify the different loci containing these types of repeats is to isolate DNA from a small amount of blood or tissue from the endangered species, prepare a genomic library with relatively small (several kb) inserts in a plasmid or λ vector, and screen the library with a labeled oligonucleotide probe that is composed of a short stretch of CAG repeats as described in text Figure 10.6 (p. 258). Clones that hybridize to the probe will contain CAG repeats. You can determine whether any of the loci containing CAG repeats have polymorphic lengths of CAG repeats in the population by sequencing the inserts in the clones; using the sequences flanking the repeat to design primers for PCR amplification; isolating DNA from tissue samples taken from multiple members of the population (use a tissue such as blood or saliva in an animal, or a leaf cutting in a plant, so that entire organisms do not need to be sacrificed for DNA collection); amplifying the different loci containing CAG repeats using PCR and template DNA from the different individuals; and separating the amplification products by size using gel electrophoresis. If the endangered species is related to an organism with a sequenced genome or for which STRs have been characterized, it could be more efficient to start with a bioinformatic approach. The genome of the related species could be searched for loci containing CAG repeats. If those loci are known to be polymorphic in the related species, primer sets that can be used in PCR to amplify the repeats in that species could be evaluated in for use in the endangered species.

10.48   *Answer:* In this gene therapy experiment, T cells were isolated from the patient and a viral vector was used to introduce the normal adenosine deaminase gene. The cells were then reintroduced into the patient.

10.49   *Answer:* DNA can be introduced into animal cells by using transfection methods, virus-related vectors, and electroporation. DNA can also be injected into embryos. A variety of vectors with eukaryotic origins of replication, selectable markers, and regulatory elements can be used to direct foreign gene expression in animal cells.

In contrast, the transformation of dicotyledonous plant cells is mediated by the Ti plasmid of *Agrobacterium tumefaciens*. The Ti plasmid has a 30-kb T-DNA region flanked by two repeated 25-bp sequences that are involved in T-DNA excision. When *A. tumefaciens* interacts with the host plant cell, it excises the T-DNA and transfers it to the nucleus of the plant cell. There, the T-DNA integrates into the nuclear genome. To transform plant cells, genes are placed in transformation vectors derived from Ti plasmids and between the 25-bp border sequences of the T-DNA, transformed into *A. tumefaciens*, and the plant cells are infected with *A. tumefaciens*.

To transform monocotyledonous plants, electroporation and gene gun methods are used to introduce DNA into plant cells. Transformed cells are selected (using co-transformed markers) and used to regenerate whole plants.

10.50   *Answer:* There is clearly a huge potential for success in crop modification. In addition to the examples presented in the text, visit the web pages listed below, two of many that describe the potential value of modified, vitamin-A-enhanced rice (golden rice) or mustard (golden mustard). Such products, in principle, could help millions of people suffering from vitamin A deficiency, which is associated with blindness and increased disease susceptibility.

http://www.goldenrice.org/

http://www.rff.org/Publications/Pages/PublicationDetails.aspx?PublicationID=18891

A quick Internet search using "golden rice" or "GMO" identifies mostly organizations opposing the use of GMOs. There are multiple reasons consumers have concerns about GMOs. First, some individuals find that this type of genetic alteration is in conflict with their culturally held views of the spiritual integrity of living organisms. Second, some individuals feel that the dangers associated with genetically modified organisms are unknown or not well enough understood. For example, a gene placed in a particular crop species might be transferred laterally, perhaps via some infectious agent, to another species, where it is undesirable; the gene may confer properties that are deleterious to the environment, which only appear years after introduction and which would not be apparent in controlled testing environments; the altered strain may deleteriously alter existing ecological balances; the altered gene may negatively impact human health in unknown ways; there may be significant concerns about food safety. Third, there are concerns about the maintenance of genetic diversity in crops. What will be the effect on seed stocks if only a few highly desirable strains of some crops are grown? Will this lead to crops having increased susceptibility to pathogens? Fourth, there are economic concerns: How ethically sound are the business practices of companies involved in these efforts? Should science be financed by corporations? Are these developments in the best interests of underdeveloped nations? Finally, it is a new and largely unknown area. Much is unknown. At a time regulatory agencies are entering a new territory, they are being offered conflicting "expert" opinions.

11

Mendelian Genetics

Chapter Outline

Review of Key Terms, Symbols, and Concepts

In your own words, write a brief, precise definition of each term in the groups below. Check your definitions using the text. Then develop a concept map using the terms in each list.

1	2
heritable trait, character	probability
gene, particulate factor	product rule
locus, loci	sum rule
allele, allelomorph	principle of segregation
genotype	principle of independent assortment
phenotype	branch diagram, Punnett square
dominant, dominance	chi-square (χ^2) test
recessive	goodness-of-fit test
wild-type allele	null hypothesis
loss-of-function, gain-of-function mutation	expected values
null mutation	P
heterozygote, heterozygous	significance
homozygote, homozygous	degrees of freedom
self-fertilization, selfing	pedigree analysis
cross-fertilization, cross	proband, propositus, proposita
true-breeding, pure-breeding	$1:1, 3:1$, all : none ratios
principle of uniformity	wild-type allele
P, F_1, F_2, F_3 generation, cross	rare homozygote
monohybrid, dihybrid, reciprocal cross	AA, $A-$, Aa, aa
gamete, zygote	loss-of-function, gain-of-function mutation
hybrid, dihybrid, trihybrid individual, cross	recessive, dominant trait
testcross	recessive, dominant pedigree
haploid, diploid	
gene segregation	
principle of segregation	
principle of independent assortment	

Thinking Analytically

There are different levels of understanding of Mendelian genetics. You can certainly obtain some understanding of this material from a careful reading and outlining of the chapter, especially if you pay attention to detail and the logic of Mendel's experiments. Indeed, understanding why Mendel's approach gave insights into the principles of inheritance when those for thousands of years before him failed is a substantial accomplishment. However, it is through solving problems that you will develop a practical, useful understanding of this material. As in earlier chapters, solving the problems in this chapter will not only reinforce what you have read, but will help you develop an understanding of the relationships between terms, ideas, and facts.

With some effort, you can discover one of the multiple "right" approaches to solving a Mendelian genetics problem. Pursuing any number of "right" approaches will reinforce your understanding of Mendelian genetic principles and help you gain a deeper understanding of relationships you read about in the chapter. Be warned, however, that there is also a "wrong" approach, previously described in Chapter 2 of this guide. The approach you take will influence the quality of your understanding of Mendelian genetics, so adopting a productive problem-solving stategy is discussed here once more. In the wrong approach, you read through the problem and then see if you can understand an answer presented in this guide. When you read a solution to a problem, you have not yourself devised the solution, so you have not developed the skills to analyze the situation, apply your knowledge of Mendelian principles, and identify a path that leads to a solution. You may understand the answer, but you won't have developed any of the skills to solve a similar problem. On an exam you will be stuck, and the purpose of doing the problems—to gain a deeper understanding of Mendelian principles— will have been thwarted.

Taking a "right" approach helps you develop a deeper understanding. This is not the same thing as finding *the* correct answer, usually because there is more than one approach to solving the problem. Here are some pointers:

1. Read the problem straight through without pausing. Get the sense of what it is about.
2. Then read it again, slowly and critically. This time,
   a. Jot down pertinent information.
   b. Assign descriptive gene symbols. Use a dash (e.g., $--$ or $A\ -$) when unsure of a genotype.
   c. Scan the problem from start to finish and then from the end to the beginning, and carefully analyze the *terms* used in the problem. Often, clues to the answer can be found in the way the problem is stated. (Geneticists use very precise language!)
3. If you are unsure how to continue, ask yourself, "What are the options here?"
   a. Write down all the options you perceive.
   b. Carefully analyze whether a particular option will provide a solution.
4. When you think you have a solution, read through the problem once more and make sure that your analysis is consistent with *all* the data in the problem. Try to see if there is a more general principle behind the solution or, for that matter, a clearer or more straightforward solution.
5. If you do get stuck (and everyone does!), DO NOT GO IMMEDIATELY TO THE ANSWER KEY. This will only give you the *illusion* of having solved the problem. On an exam, or in real life, there won't be an answer key available. Learn to control the temptation "to just know the answer" and go on to another problem. Come back to this one another time, perhaps the next day. Your mind may be able to use the time to sort through loose ends.
6. If you cannot solve the problem after coming back to it a second time, read through the answer key. Then close the answer key and try the problem once more. The next day, try it a third time without the answer key.

Applying Rules of Probability

Some problems on Mendelian genetics make extensive use of two rules of probability:

Product rule: The probability of two independent events occurring simultaneously is the product of their individual probabilities.

Sum rule: The probability of either one of two independent, mutually exclusive events occurring is the sum of their individual probabilities.

To apply these rules in the context of solving problems, first consider the possible outcomes of a situation. Then identify the mutually exclusive independent events leading to these outcomes. Apply the rules after rephrasing the question. Suppose there are two mutually exclusive independent events, A and B. If you can rephrase the question to ask for the chance that *both A and B* occur (together), multiply the individual probabilities: $P(\text{A and B}) = P(\text{A}) \times P(\text{B})$. If you can rephrase the question or statement to ask for the chance that *either A or B* occurs (separately), add the individual probabilities: $P(\text{A or B}) = P(\text{A}) + P(\text{B})$.

Questions for Practice

Multiple-Choice Questions

1. A dominant gene is one that
   a. suppresses the expression of genes at all loci.
   b. masks the expression of neighboring gene loci.
   c. masks the expression of a recessive allele.
   d. masks the expression of all of the above.

2. A dihybrid is an individual that
   a. is heterozygous for every gene.
   b. is heterozygous for two genes under study.
   c. is the result of a testcross.
   d. is used for a testcross.

3. The cross of an uncertain genotype with a homozygous recessive genotype at the same locus is a
   a. pure-breeding cross.
   b. monohybrid cross.
   c. testcross.
   d. dihybrid cross.

4. The genotypic ratio of the progeny of a monohybrid cross is typically
   a. 1:2:1.
   b. 9:3:3:1.
   c. 27:9:9:9:3:3:3:1.
   d. 3:1.

5. A typical phenotypic ratio of a dihybrid cross with dominant and recessive alleles is
   a. 9:1.
   b. 1:2:1.
   c. 3:1.
   d. 9:3:3:1.

6. Pedigrees showing rare recessive traits
   a. have about half of the progeny affected when one parent is affected.
   b. have heterozygotes that are phenotypically affected.
   c. have about $3/4$ of the progeny affected when both parents are affected.
   d. often skip a generation.

7. In a chi-square test, a P value equal to 0.04 tells one that
   a. there is a 4% chance the hypothesis is correct.
   b. there is a 4% chance the hypothesis is incorrect.
   c. if the experiment were repeated, chance deviations from the expected values as large as those observed would be seen only 4% of the time.
   d. if the experiment were repeated, chance deviations from the expected values as large as those observed would be seen at least 96% of the time.

8. In a chi-square test, a P value equal to 0.04 indicates that
   a. the hypothesis is unlikely to be true.
   b. the hypothesis is false and must be rejected.
   c. the hypothesis is true.
   d. the hypothesis is likely to be true.

9. Gain-of-function mutations are associated with all of the following except
   a. dominant traits.
   b. new properties in a gene.
   c. phenotypes in heterozygous individuals.
   d. a decrease in the normal activity of a gene.

10. Two parents affected with a genetic disease have five children, all of whom are affected. With regards to the family, which one of the following statements *must* be true?
    a. Both parents must have at least one mutant allele; the trait might be dominant or recessive.
    b. Both parents must be homozygous for a recessive trait.

    c. At least one parent must be homozygous.

    d. At least one parent must be homozygous for a dominant trait.

11. How many different genotypes are obtainable from the cross *Aa Bb* × *Aa Bb*?

    a. 3

    b. 4

    c. 9

    d. 16

12. What is the chance of obtaining a heterozygous individual from a testcross?

    a. 0%

    b. 50%

    c. at least 50%

    d. 100%

Answers: 1c, 2b, 3c, 4a, 5d, 6d, 7c, 8a, 9d, 10a, 11c, 12c

Thought Questions

1. Over a period of many years, numerous attempts were made to understand how physical traits are passed from one generation to the next. Gregor Mendel was first to make a breakthrough. How do you account for his success, in light of years of failure before him?

2. What led to the rediscovery of Mendel's work?

3. **a.** Clearly distinguish between an allele, a gene, and a locus.

    b. Can you see an analogy between a gene and an allele and
   - a digit and an index finger?
   - a canine and a German shepherd?
   - a dime and a mint 1954 dime?

    Where do these analogies break down?

4. Why might the term *degrees of freedom* be so named, and why (for the problems in this chapter) is it equal to $n-1$?

5. Why are the frequencies of harmful recessive mutant alleles usually higher than the frequencies of harmful dominant mutations, even though individuals with the recessive trait are rare?

6. Construct a decision-making tree (a flowchart) that can be used to decide if a pedigree shows a dominant or recessive trait.

7. Why is it important to know if a trait is common or rare when analyzing a pedigree?

8. Must wild-type alleles always be dominant?

9. Why are loss-of-function mutations usually recessive and gain-of-function mutations usually dominant?

Thought Questions for Media

After reviewing the media on the *iGenetics* website, try to answer these questions.

1. What is the difference between a locus, a gene, and an allele? Can these terms be used interchangeably?

2. What is the difference between a phenotypic ratio and a genotypic ratio? Can these ever be the same in the offspring of a cross?

3. When a true-breeding plant is self-fertilized, why aren't plants with different traits ever produced? If two true-breeding plants are crossed, why do all of the offspring have just one phenotype?

4. In a cross between two true-breeding plants differing in two characteristics, will the F$_1$ offspring always exhibit both traits of just one parent? Will they always be dihybrids?

5. What does it mean for "genes on different chromosomes to behave independently in the production of gametes"?

6. How many types of gametes are produced by a monohybrid? By a dihybrid?

7. How many different zygote genotypes can be produced in a monohybrid cross? In a dihybrid cross?

8. How many different zygote phenotypes can be produced in a monohybrid cross? In a dihybrid cross?

9. Why doesn't a recessive trait ever appear in a heterozygote? How do we know that the recessive allele is still present in a heterozygote?

1. Two tagged tribbles wander out of the iActivity tribble laboratory and show up in your bed. One is tagged "male *bb ss* (solid yellow)," and one is tagged "female *Bb Ss* (spotted brown)." You recall that spotted (*S*) is dominant to solid (*s*) and brown (*B*) is dominant to yellow (*b*) and that tribbles reproduce quickly. You seize this opportunity to make a (small) fortune selling spotted yellow tribbles. What crosses would you do to develop a true-breeding, spotted yellow strain? Since it is important to keep the population of non-spotted yellow tribbles to a minimum, you want to be sure that the animals chosen for the strain are true breeding. How can you do this, since they cannot be selfed?

2. As you read the morning paper at breakfast, you notice that a (tiny) reward has been posted by the iActivity tribble laboratory for three missing tribbles. All the ad says in describing them is that one is a heterozygote and two are homozygotes. Midway through breakfast, three untagged tribbles waddle across your plate. One is a solid brown male, one is a solid brown female, and the third is a spotted brown male. Assuming that these animals were not just stained with coffee, could they be the missing tribbles? If so, how would you determine, using crosses with just these animals, which animal is heterozygous, which animals are homozygous, and if the homozygotes are both homozygous dominant, both homozygous recessive, or one is homozygous dominant and one is homozygous recessive?

Solutions to Text Questions and Problems

11.1   *Answer:* Consider two ways to solve this problem.

   1. First, notice that this is a situation akin to Mendel's crosses. In such crosses, dominant traits mask the appearance of recessive traits, and when a true-breeding dominant plant is crossed to a true-breeding recessive plant, all the F_1 progeny show the dominant trait. Here the dominant trait is red, the recessive trait is yellow, and the parents are true breeding, since they are homozygous.

   a. Just as in Mendel's crosses, the F_1 plants will be heterozygous and all show the dominant red trait.

   b. The F_2 plants that result from the cross of two F_1 heterozygotes will also show the same ratios seen by Mendel, that is, 3 dominant : 1 recessive, or 3 red : 1 yellow.

   c. When an F_1 plant is crossed back to the red parent, a heterozygous plant is crossed to a true-breeding dominant plant. Here, each offspring receives a dominant allele from the red parent, and so all the progeny must show the dominant red phenotype.

   d. When an F_1 plant is crossed back to the yellow parent, a heterozygous plant is crossed back to a true-breeding recessive plant. This is akin to one of Mendel's testcrosses, and so the progeny should show a 1:1 ratio of red : yellow plants.

   2. Assign R as the allele symbol for dominant red color, and r as the allele symbol for recessive yellow color.

   a. Then the initial cross between two homozygous plants can be depicted as $RR \times rr$, and the F_1 progeny obtain an R allele from the red parent and an r allele from the yellow parent. Therefore, they are all heterozygotes and are Rr. Because the R (red) allele is dominant to the r (yellow) allele, the Rr progeny are red.

   b. The F_2 are obtained from $Rr \times Rr$ and so will be composed of 1 RR : 2 Rr : 1 rr types of progeny. There will be 3 red (RR or Rr) : 1 yellow (rr).

   c. The F_1 crossed back to the red parent can be depicted as $Rr \times RR$. All the progeny will obtain an R allele from the red parent; the progeny can be written as $R-$ (either RR or Rr), and all will be red.

   d. The F_1 crossed back to the yellow parent can be depicted as $Rr \times rr$. There will be two equally frequent types of progeny, Rr and rr. Thus, half the progeny will be red and half yellow.

11.2   *Answer:* A plant that is genotypically $Aa\ WxWx$ has two types of gametes: $A\ Wx$ and $a\ Wx$ (notice that Wx is a symbol for one allele, not two). In a testcross, this plant is crossed to one homozygous for recessive alleles at both the color gene and the waxy gene, $aa\ wxwx$. The gametes of this plant are all $a\ wx$. This cross can be illustrated in the following Punnett square:

		Gametes of $Aa\ WxWx$	
		$A\ Wx$	$a\ Wx$
Gametes of $aa\ wxwx$	$a\ wx$	$Aa\ Wxwx$	$aa\ Wxwx$

Progeny will be of two equally frequent genotypes: $Aa\ Wxwx$ and $aa\ Wxwx$. Thus, half will be colored (Aa), half will be colorless (aa), and all will have normal starch ($Wxwx$).

11.3   *Answer:* In the F_2, there is a 3:1 colored : colorless phenotypic ratio. This reflects a 1 CC : 2 Cc : 1 cc genotypic ratio, where colored (C) is dominant to colorless (c). Thus, there are two types of colored plants (CC, Cc) that are present in a 1 CC : 2 Cc ratio. If one is picked at random, there is a $\frac{1}{3}$ chance of picking a homozygous CC plant, and a $\frac{2}{3}$ chance of picking a heterozygous Cc plant. If selfed, the CC plant will produce only CC (colored) plants, while the Cc plant will produce both colored and colorless plants (in a 3:1 ratio). Thus, to see more than one type of plant in the progeny, a Cc plant must be chosen initially. The chance of this is $\frac{2}{3}$. (Notice that the question asks for the chance that a particular colored plant will have two types of progeny, and *not* for the ratio of progeny types when two types are seen.)

11.4 *Answer:*

 a. Since rough (*R*) is dominant over smooth (*r*), a rough parent is *RR* or *Rr* (i.e., *R*–). A cross between a rough and smooth guinea pig is *R*– × *rr*. If the cross is *RR* × *rr*, then all the progeny will be *Rr* and be rough. If the cross is *Rr* × *rr*, then half the progeny will be *Rr* (rough) and half will be *rr* (smooth). The 8 rough : 7 smooth progeny ratio approximates a 1:1 *Rr* : *rr* ratio, and so the initial cross must have been *Rr* × *rr*. The rough progeny must be *Rr*, while the smooth progeny must be *rr*.

 b. If one of the rough F$_1$ animals is mated back to its rough parent, the cross is *Rr* × *Rr*. This cross would produce both rough (*R*–) and smooth (*rr*) progeny in a 3:1 ratio.

11.5 *Answer:* First, depict the phenotypes as genotypes: A polled animal exhibiting the dominant, hornless condition can be depicted as *P*–, while a horned animal exhibits the recessive condition and must be *pp*. Therefore, the three crosses and their progeny can be depicted as

Cow		×	Polled Bull	Progeny	
Phenotype	Genotype		Genotype	Phenotype	Genotype
A: horned	*pp*	×	*P*–	horned	*pp*
B: polled	*P*–	×	*P*–	horned	*pp*
C: horned	*pp*	×	*P*–	polled	*P*–

Now follow how each set of parents contributed alleles to their progeny. In the crosses with cows A and B, a horned, *pp* offspring can be obtained only if each parent contributes a recessive *p* allele to the progeny. Therefore both the polled bull and cow B must be heterozygous: Each is *Pp*. With this information, both the crosses with cows A and C appear to be testcrosses (*Pp* × *pp*) and will produce 1:1 phenotypic ratios of polled (*Pp*) and horned (*pp*) progeny. The cross with cow B is a cross between two heterozygotes (*Pp* × *Pp*) and will produce a 3:1 phenotypic ratio of polled to horned progeny.

11.6 *Answer:* The ratio of 28 purple to 10 white plants is close to 3:1. A 3:1 ratio means that the purple plant that was initially selfed must have been heterozygous, or *Pp*. A cross of *Pp* × *Pp* would yield progeny with a genotypic ratio of 1 *PP* : 2 *Pp* : 1 *pp*. Thus, among the purple progeny, there would be ⅓ *PP* homozygotes and ⅔ *Pp* heterozygotes. Since the homozygous *PP* plants are the only purple plants that will breed true, only ⅓ of the purple-flowered progeny will breed true.

11.7 *Answer:* Notice that the two crosses give very different results. Use both sets of results to answer the question. In the cross of black female X with the brown male, the 9 black and 7 brown progeny approximate a 1:1 phenotypic ratio. This suggests that this cross is similar to a testcross and might be depicted *Bb* × *bb*. However, it is not clear from this cross alone which color trait is dominant. This question can be answered by considering the cross of black female Y with the brown male, where only black progeny are seen. This is like a cross between two true-breeding individuals where black is dominant to brown, *BB* × *bb*. Thus, the brown male is homozygous recessive (*bb*), female X is heterozygous (*Bb*), and female Y is homozygous dominant (*BB*).

11.8 *Answer:* In this question, note that the trait that is being examined is the *response* of plants to a virus. One envisions that crosses are performed between plants, and then, instead of looking at flower color or seed shape to score a trait, plants are individually tested for their response to viral infection. A cross of a plant showing only local lesions to one showing systemic lesions gives only plants that show local lesions, suggesting the hypothesis that a local lesion response is dominant to a systemic lesion response. If the allele for the local lesion response is depicted as *L*, and the allele for the systemic lesion response as *l*, the parental generation can be written as *LL* × *ll*. Then, the F$_1$ would be all *Ll* and the F$_2$ would be 1 *LL* : 2 *Ll* : 1 *ll*, or 3*L*– : 1*ll*.

   Use a chi-square test to assess how well this hypothesis fits with the observed numbers of 785 local lesion and 269 systemic lesion plants.

Class	Observed	Expected	d	d^2	d^2/e
plants with local lesions	785	790	-5	25	0.031
plants with systemic lesions	269	264	5	25	0.093
Total	1,054	1,054	0	—	$\chi^2 = 0.124$

$\chi^2 = 0.124$; df $= 1$; $0.70 < P < 0.90$

The chi-square test indicates that, in experiments similar to this one, a deviation at least as great as that observed here would be seen about 80% of the time. Therefore, the hypothesis is accepted as possible.

To further evaluate the hypothesis that the local lesion response is dominant to the systemic lesion response, testcross the F_2 plants to true-breeding plants that show a systemic lesion response (i.e., are *ll*). The progeny of this testcross can then be assayed for their response to viral infection so that the genotype of the F_2 can be determined. One would expect $^2/_3$ of those F_2 plants showing a local lesion response to be heterozygotes (i.e., *Ll*). When they are test-crossed, half of their progeny should show local responses and half systemic responses. The remaining $^1/_3$ will be *LL* and give only progeny with local responses.

11.9   *Answer:* Here, two independently assorting genes affecting eye pigment are being followed. The symbols suggested in the problem follow the convention that symbols are based on the pheno-types of mutants. Here, *bw* is used to represent the recessive, mutant allele causing brown eyes. *Bw* represents the dominant, normal allele at this locus. We infer that this gene controls the production of scarlet granules since they are lacking in the brown-eyed mutant. By the same reasoning, *st* is used to represent the recessive, mutant allele causing scarlet eyes, and *St* is the dominant, normal allele at this locus. We infer that the locus controls the production of brown granules. When writing the genotypes of the flies being crossed, be certain to write the alleles present at both genes.

a.   Our first task is to assign genotypes to the P and F_1 generations. Brown-eyed flies lack scarlet granules, so they must be *bwbw* (no scarlet) and *St–*; these flies do make brown granules. Note that they can be either *bwbw StSt* or *bwbw Stst*, and that we cannot tell their exact genotype yet. Using similar reasoning, scarlet-eyed flies must be *Bw– stst*. We can determine the exact geno-type of these P generation flies by considering what progeny they produce. Since each parent can be either of two genotypes, four different crosses are possible. These are illustrated in the following branch diagrams:

i.   brown eyes × scarlet eyes
bwbw StSt × BwBw stst

bwbw × BwBw   *StSt × stst*

         Bwbw ——————— *Stst* ⟶ *Bwbw Stst*
(scarlet granules)   (brown granules)   (all red eyes)

ii.   brown eyes × scarlet eyes
bwbw Stst × BwBw stst

bwbw × BwBw   *Stst × stst*

                              $^1/_2$ *Stst* ⟶ $^1/_2$ *Bwbw Stst*
                              (brown granules)   (red eyes)
         Bwbw
(scarlet granules)
                              $^1/_2$ *stst* ⟶ $^1/_2$ *Bwbw stst*
                              (no brown granules)   (scarlet eyes)

iii. brown eyes × scarlet eyes
   bwbw StSt × Bwbw stst

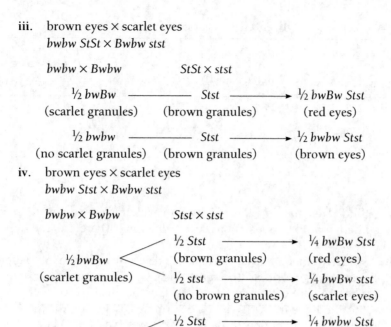

   bwbw × Bwbw   *StSt × stst*

   ½ *bwBw* —————— *Stst* ————→ ½ *bwBw Stst*
   (scarlet granules)   (brown granules)   (red eyes)

   ½ *bwbw* —————— *Stst* ————→ ½ *bwbw Stst*
   (no scarlet granules) (brown granules)   (brown eyes)

iv. brown eyes × scarlet eyes
   bwbw Stst × Bwbw stst

   bwbw × Bwbw   *Stst × stst*

   ½ *bwBw*
   (scarlet granules)
       ½ *Stst* ————————→ ¼ *bwBw Stst*
       (brown granules)   (red eyes)
       ½ *stst* ————————→ ¼ *bwBw stst*
       (no brown granules)   (scarlet eyes)

   ½ *bwbw*
   (no scarlet granules)
       ½ *Stst* ————————→ ¼ *bwbw Stst*
       (brown granules)   (brown eyes)
       ½ *stst* ————————→ ¼ *bwbw stst*
       (no brown granules)   (white eyes)

Notice that even though the parents in each of the above crosses look the same, their progeny are not. The only way all red-eyed progeny can be obtained is if the cross is that shown in **(i)**. To see if the observed F$_2$ is consistent with this view, use a branch diagram:

red eyes × red eyes
Bwbw Stst × Bwbw Stst

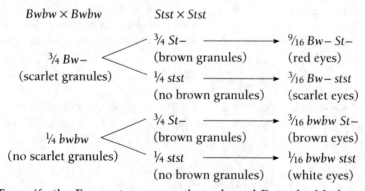

   Bwbw × Bwbw   *Stst × Stst*

   ¾ *Bw–*
   (scarlet granules)
       ¾ *St–* ————————→ ⁹⁄₁₆ *Bw– St–*
       (brown granules)   (red eyes)
       ¼ *stst* ————————→ ³⁄₁₆ *Bw– stst*
       (no brown granules)   (scarlet eyes)

   ¼ *bwbw*
   (no scarlet granules)
       ¾ *St–* ————————→ ³⁄₁₆ *bwbw St–*
       (brown granules)   (brown eyes)
       ¼ *stst* ————————→ ¹⁄₁₆ *bwbw stst*
       (no brown granules)   (white eyes)

b. To verify the F$_1$ genotype, cross the red-eyed F$_1$ to doubly homozygous recessive white-eyed flies of the genotype *bwbw stst*. One expects to see a 1:1:1:1 ratio of red : brown : scarlet : white flies, as shown in the following branch diagram.

red eyes × white eyes
Bwbw Stst × bwbw stst

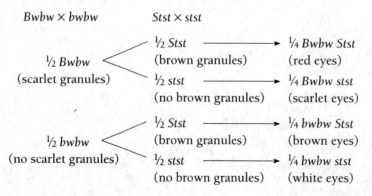

   Bwbw × bwbw   *Stst × stst*

   ½ *Bwbw*
   (scarlet granules)
       ½ *Stst* ————————→ ¼ *Bwbw Stst*
       (brown granules)   (red eyes)
       ½ *stst* ————————→ ¼ *Bwbw stst*
       (no brown granules)   (scarlet eyes)

   ½ *bwbw*
   (no scarlet granules)
       ½ *Stst* ————————→ ¼ *bwbw Stst*
       (brown granules)   (brown eyes)
       ½ *stst* ————————→ ¼ *bwbw stst*
       (no brown granules)   (white eyes)

11.10   *Answer:* First notice that white seeds are always *gg* while grey seeds are either *GG* or *Gg*. Thus, one can assign partial genotypes (either *G–* or *gg*) based on the phenotypes of the parents. The problem is to determine whether a grey parent is *GG* or *Gg*. In monohybrid crosses, there are three kinds of phenotypic ratios that can be generated. The cross *Gg* × *Gg* gives a 3 grey (*G–*):1 white (*gg*) ratio, the cross *Gg* × *gg* gives a 1 grey (*Gg*):1 white (*gg*) ratio, and the crosses *GG* × *gg* and *GG* × *G–* give all grey (*G–*) progeny. As the first cross of grey × white gives a 1:1 ratio, it must be *Gg* × *gg*. As the second cross of grey × grey gives a 3:1 ratio, it must be *Gg* × *Gg*. As the third cross of grey × white gives all grey, it must be *GG* × *gg*. In the fourth cross, only grey progeny are produced. The genotype of one of the parents must be *GG*, but the genotype of the other can only be specified as *G–*. One has:

| Parents | Progeny | | Female Parent |
Female × Male	Grey	White	Genotype
grey × white	81	82	*Gg*
grey × grey	1,183	9	*Gg*
grey × white	74	0	*GG*
grey × grey	90	0	*GG* or *G–*

11.11   *Answer:* As the farmer starts with a pair of black babbits, he must be starting with animals that are either *BB* or *Bb*. Since his pair is not true breeding, and indeed gives a 3:1 ratio of black to white progeny, he must have two heterozygotes, or *Bb* babbits. Therefore, one expects to find a 1 *BB*:2 *Bb* genotypic ratio among the black F_1 progeny that were not sold.

a. Consider that for a white babbit to be obtained in a cross between a pair of F_1 babbits, both babbits must be *Bb* in genotype, and a *bb* offspring must be produced by these parents. Now ascertain the chance of these events occurring. If one picks randomly among the black F_1 progeny, there will be a ⅓ chance of picking a *BB* individual and a ⅔ chance of picking a *Bb* individual. The chance of two *Bb* parents giving a *bb* offspring is ¼. Using the product rule, one has

P(white offspring) = P(both F_1 babbits are *Bb* and a *bb* offspring is produced)
= P(both F_1 babbits are *Bb*) × P(*bb* offspring)
= (⅔ × ⅔) × (¼)
= ⅑

b. If he crosses an F_1 male (*Bb* or *BB*) to the parental female (*Bb*), two types of crosses are possible. The crosses and probabilities are
  i. *Bb* (F_1 male) × *Bb* (parental female) P = ⅔ × 1 = ⅔.
  ii. *BB* (F_1 male) × *Bb* (parental female) P = ⅓ × 1 = ⅓.
Here, only the first cross can produce white progeny, ¼ of the time. Using the product rule, the chance that this strategy will yield white progeny is
p = ⅔ (chance of *Bb* × *Bb* cross) × ¼ (chance of *bb* offspring) = ⅙.

c. As neither of the strategies in **(b)** work very well, evaluate other potential strategies (use trial and error). One that works better in the long run, but is more work initially, is as follows. Re-mate the initial two black babbits (which we have determined to be *Bb*) to obtain a white male offspring [P = ¼ (white *bb*) × ½ (male) = ⅛]. Retain this male (note that the fertility of white males is not affected) and breed it back to its mother. This cross would be *Bb* × *bb* and give ½ white (*bb*) and ½ black (*Bb*) offspring. The progeny of this cross could be used to develop a "breeding colony" consisting of black (*Bb*) females and white (*bb*) males. These would consistently produce half white and half black offspring.

11.12   *Answer:* Wild-type alleles typically encode a product for a particular biological function. Mutations that cause the gene's product (e.g., its protein product) to be absent, partially functional, or nonfunctional are likely to result in a decrease or loss of that biological function. Such mutations are called loss-of-function mutations. They are usually recessive because the function of a single copy of a wild-type allele in a heterozygote is usually sufficient to produce enough gene product to provide for a normal phenotype. A mutation that produces no functional gene product (e.g., a mutation that leads to the production of a protein having no function) are complete loss-of-function, or null mutations.

An example of a loss-of-function mutation is Mendel's wrinkled pea mutation. The dominant, round-pea allele (*S*) encodes a starch-branching enzyme (SBEI). The recessive, wrinkled-pea allele (*s*) has an 800-bp-long transposon inserted within the *S* gene, so that it does not produce SBEI. The absence of SBEI results in developing *ss* seeds having a higher water content and larger size. As they mature, they lose a larger proportion of their volume, leading to the wrinkled seed phenotype.

Gain-of-function mutations result in gene products with new functions and properties. These types of mutations produce gene products with different enzymatic or functional properties, or different temporal or spatial patterns of expression. One example is the dominant mutation in the *FGFR3* (fibroblast growth factor receptor 3) gene that causes achondroplasia, dwarfism resulting from defects in long-bone growth. The normal FGFR3 protein is a membrane-embedded receptor. When a growth factor binds to the receptor and activates it, the receptor triggers a cascade of molecular reactions in the cell that lead to specific cellular responses affecting growth and development. The normal form of the FGFR3 protein is thought to regulate bone growth by acting in a negative pathway to limit ossification, the formation of bone from cartilage. Its regulatory effects are the strongest on the long bones, where FGFR3 function is carefully controlled. The dominant, gain-of-function mutation produces a continuously active receptor that causes heterozygotes to have significantly shortened long bones—achondroplasia.

11.13 *Answer:*

a. To determine whether a mutation is a loss-of-function mutation, determine whether it will result in a decrease or loss of the biological function of the gene. Since many loss-of-function mutations cause the gene's product to be absent, partially functional, or nonfunctional, changes at the DNA level that result in a decreased gene transcription or translation, or fail to produce a functional protein product, are typically associated with loss-of-function mutations. Using these criteria, mutations 1, 3, 5, and 7 are loss-of-function mutations.

To determine whether a mutation is a gain-of-function mutation, determine if it results in gene products with new functions and properties. Gain-of-function mutations are often associated with changes at the DNA level that lead to gene products with different enzymatic or functional properties, or different temporal or spatial patterns of expression. By these criteria, mutations 2, 4, 6, and 8 are gain-of-function mutations.

b. Mutations that cause sickness in heterozygotes will show dominant inheritance, while mutations that cause sickness only in homozygotes will show recessive inheritance. Mutation 1 will be recessive since homozygotes will have no enzyme activity and be sick, while heterozygotes will have 50% of reference activity and be normal. Mutation 2 will be dominant, since heterozygotes (and homozygotes) will have enzyme expression in the heart and be sick. Mutations that affect transcription initiation will affect the amount of mRNA available for translation and thus affect how much enzyme is produced. Whether mutations 3 and 4 lead to sickness and show an inheritance pattern depends on how much these mutations affect transcription initiation. Mutation 3 will not be dominant, since heterozygotes will have one normal allele and so have at least 50% of the reference activity. It will be recessive only if the decrease in transcription initiation at the two mutant alleles in homozygotes leads to less than 50% of reference activity. Mutation 4 will be dominant only if the increase in transcription initiation of the one mutant allele in a heterozygote, together with normal levels of transcription at the normal allele, leads to more than 150% of reference activity. If this is not the case, it will be recessive only if the increase in transcription initiation of the two mutant alleles in homozygotes leads to more than 150% of reference activity. Mutation 5 results in a truncated, nonfunctional protein, so it will be recessive just like mutation 1. Mutation 6 will be dominant since heterozygotes will be sick: they will have 250% of reference activity (200% from the mutant allele plus 50% from the normal allele). Mutation 7 will be recessive since homozygotes will be sick: they will have 20% of reference activity. Heterozygotes will be normal since they will have 60% of reference activity (10% from the mutant allele plus 50% from the normal allele). We cannot predict whether mutation 8 will have a phenotype, since there may or may not be a phenotypic consequence when the enzyme acts on additional substrates.

11.14   *Answer:* This question makes use of two concepts about gene function in diploids. The first is that each allele of a gene in a diploid contributes to the observed phenotype. The second is that a deletion mutation is a null mutation (a complete loss-of-function mutation) since a deletion of a gene prevents the production of any gene product.

   a. We are told that the *v* allele results in the loss of an enzyme activity, so it is a loss-of-function mutation. This conclusion is supported by the phenotypes of *del(v) v* and *vv* animals. Both of these genotypes have identical, bright red, mutant eyes. Thus, the *v* mutation behaves like a deletion that produces no gene product, so it is a loss-of-function mutation. Animals that are *Vv* and *del(v) V* have normal, brick red colored eyes just like *VV* animals because the wild-type *V* allele produces enough enzyme to provide a normal phenotype.

   b. Since *del(L) l* animals have a normal phenotype, we can infer that a heterozygote with a null mutation and a normal allele (*l*) shows a normal phenotype and that one copy of the normal allele is sufficient to provide a normal phenotype. The *Ll* animals do not show this normal phenotype, so the *L* allele is not a loss-of-function mutation like a deletion. It must be a gain-of-function mutation.

   c. Since *del(N) n* animals have a mutant phenotype, we can infer that the gene function provided by one copy of the normal allele (*n*) is insufficient to provide a normal phenotype. Since *Nn* and *del(N) n* animals have identical mutant phenotypes, *N* appears to be a complete loss-of-function (null) allele, just like *del(N)*.

11.15   *Answer:* Since you are told that each parent is homozygous, the parental genotypes can be determined from their phenotypes. One has a white (*pp*) spiny (*SS*) plant crossed to a purple (*PP*) smooth (*ss*) plant. This initial information can be used with branch diagrams to solve each part of the problem as follows:

   a.   P: white, spiny × purple, smooth
          $pp\,SS$ × $PP\,ss$
   Gametes: *p S*   *P s*
   F_1: *Pp Ss* (purple, spiny)

   b. $F_1 \times F_1$: *Pp Ss × Pp Ss*

   $Pp \times Pp$ $Ss \times Ss$

   $\frac{3}{4}\,P-$ ⟨ $\frac{3}{4}\,S-$ ⟶ $\frac{9}{16}\,P-\,S-$ (purple, spiny)

   $\frac{1}{4}\,ss$ ⟶ $\frac{3}{16}\,P-\,ss$ (purple, smooth)

   $\frac{1}{4}\,pp$ ⟨ $\frac{3}{4}\,S-$ ⟶ $\frac{3}{16}\,pp\,S-$ (white, spiny)

   $\frac{1}{4}\,ss$ ⟶ $\frac{1}{16}\,pp\,ss$ (white, smooth)

   c. $F_1 \times$ white, spiny: *Pp Ss × pp SS*

   $Pp \times pp$ $Ss \times SS$

   $\frac{1}{2}\,Pp$ —— $S-$ ⟶ $\frac{1}{2}\,Pp\,S-$ (purple, spiny)

   $\frac{1}{2}\,pp$ —— $S-$ ⟶ $\frac{1}{2}\,pp\,S-$ (white, spiny)

   d. $F_1 \times$ purple, smooth: *Pp Ss × PP ss*

   $Pp \times PP$ $Ss \times ss$

   $P-$ ⟨ $\frac{1}{2}\,Ss$ ⟶ $\frac{1}{2}\,P-\,Ss$ (purple, spiny)

   $\frac{1}{2}\,ss$ ⟶ $\frac{1}{2}\,P-\,ss$ (purple, smooth)

11.16   *Answer:* Using branch diagrams, one has:

a. *PP ss × pp SS*

$$PP × pp \qquad ss × SS$$
$$Pp \text{———} Ss \longrightarrow \text{all } Pp\ Ss \text{ (purple, spiny)}$$

b. *Pp SS × pp ss*

$$Pp × pp \qquad SS × ss$$
$$½ Pp \text{———} Ss \longrightarrow ½ Pp\ Ss \text{ (purple, spiny)}$$
$$½ pp \text{———} Ss \longrightarrow ½ pp\ Ss \text{ (white, spiny)}$$

c. *Pp Ss × Pp SS*

$$Pp × Pp \qquad Ss × SS$$
$$¾ P\text{–} \text{———} S\text{–} \longrightarrow ¾ P\text{–} S\text{–} \text{ (purple, spiny)}$$
$$¼ pp \text{———} S\text{–} \longrightarrow ¼ pp\ S\text{–} \text{ (white, spiny)}$$

d. *Pp Ss × Pp Ss*

$$Pp × Pp \qquad Ss × Ss$$

¾ P–
- ¾ S– ⟶ 9/16 P– S– (purple, spiny)
- ¼ ss ⟶ 3/16 P– ss (purple, smooth)

¼ pp
- ¾ S– ⟶ 3/16 pp S– (white, spiny)
- ¼ ss ⟶ 1/16 pp ss (white, smooth)

e. *Pp Ss × Pp ss*

$$Pp × Pp \qquad Ss × ss$$

¾ P–
- ½ Ss ⟶ 3/8 P– Ss (purple, spiny)
- ½ ss ⟶ 3/8 P– ss (purple, smooth)

¼ pp
- ½ Ss ⟶ 1/8 pp Ss (white, spiny)
- ½ ss ⟶ 1/8 pp ss (white, smooth)

f. *Pp Ss × pp ss*

$$Pp × pp \qquad Ss × ss$$

½ Pp
- ½ Ss ⟶ ¼ Pp Ss (purple, spiny)
- ½ ss ⟶ ¼ Pp ss (purple, smooth)

½ pp
- ½ Ss ⟶ ¼ pp Ss (white, spiny)
- ½ ss ⟶ ¼ pp ss (white, smooth)

11.17   *Answer:* Try fitting the data to a model in which catnip sensitivity/insensitivity is controlled by a pair of alleles at one gene. Hypothesize that since sensitivity is seen in all of the progeny of the initial mating between catnip-sensitive Cleopatra and catnip-insensitive Antony, sensitivity is dominant. Let *S* represent the sensitive allele, and *s* the insensitive allele. Then the initial cross would have been *S*− × *ss*, and the progeny are *Ss*. If two of the *Ss* kittens mate, one would expect 3 *Ss* (sensitive) : 1 *ss* (insensitive) kittens. In the mating with Augustus, the cross would be *Ss* × *ss*, and should give a 1 *Ss* (sensitive) : 1 *ss* (insensitive) progeny ratio. The observed progeny ratios are not far off from these expectations.

An alternative hypothesis is that sensitivity (*s*) is recessive, and insensitivity (*S*) is dominant. For Antony and Cleopatra to have sensitive (*ss*) offspring, they would need to be *Ss* and *ss*, respectively. When two of their *ss* progeny mate, only sensitive, *ss* offspring should be produced. Since this is not observed, this hypothesis does not explain the data.

11.18 *Answer:* First use the symbols for the alleles specifying each trait and the information about which allele is dominant or recessive to make initial assignments of possible genotypes. For example, if a plant is white, it must have a dominant *W* allele, but as it may be either *WW* or *Ww*, it would be initially noted as *W*−. If a plant is yellow, it has to be *ww*. Then, by considering just one pair of allelic traits at a time, and recalling the Mendelian progeny ratios you have seen [a 1:1 ratio follows from a testcross (*Aa* × *aa*), an all-to-none ratio follows if at least one parent is homozygous dominant (*AA* × *A*− or *aa*), and a 3:1 ratio follows from a monohybrid cross (*Aa* × *Aa*)], you can ascertain whether a parental *W*− plant is *Ww* or *WW*.

Cross	Parents	Progeny
a.	white, disk × yellow, sphere *WW Dd* *ww dd*	½ white, disk; ½ white, sphere
b.	white, sphere × white, sphere *Ww dd* *Ww dd*	¾ white, sphere; ¼ yellow, sphere
c.	yellow, disk × white, sphere *ww DD* *WW dd*	all white, disk
d.	white, disk × yellow, sphere *Ww Dd* *ww dd*	¼ white, disk; ¼ white, sphere; ¼ yellow, disk; ¼ yellow, sphere
e.	white, disk × white, sphere *Ww Dd* *Ww dd*	⅜ white, disk; ⅜ white, sphere; ⅛ yellow, disk; ⅛ yellow, sphere

11.19 *Answer:* First consider just one pair of alleles, say *A* and *a*. Since the cross is *Aa* × *Aa*, the progeny will be 1 *AA* : 2 *Aa* : 1 *aa*, or 3 *A*− : 1 *aa*.

a. Since the three genes assort independently, one can use the product rule to determine the chance of obtaining an *A*− *B*− *C*− offspring.

P = (chance of *A*−)(chance of *B*−)(chance of *C*−)
P = (¾)(¾)(¾)
P = (²⁷⁄₆₄)

b. Since the chance of obtaining an *AA* offspring will be ¼, and the three genes assort independently, use the product rule to determine the chance of obtaining an *AA BB CC* offspring.

P = (chance of *AA*)(chance of *BB*)(chance of *CC*)
P = (¼)(¼)(¼)
P = (¹⁄₆₄)

You can also solve this problem by setting up a branch diagram, or much more laboriously, by setting up a Punnett square.

11.20 *Answer:* First note that the problem asks only for the *appearance* of the offspring of the various crosses, and not the genotypes. Then write out the genotype of the parental cross: *tt GG ss* × *TT gg SS*.

a. For each pair of traits, a homozygous dominant plant is crossed to a homozygous recessive plant. Thus, all the F₁ progeny will show the dominant trait, and be tall, green, and smooth (*Tt Gg Ss*).

b. The F₂ results from selfing the F₁ (i.e., *Tt Gg Ss × Tt Gg Ss*). The appearance of the F₂ is most readily determined by employing a branch diagram.

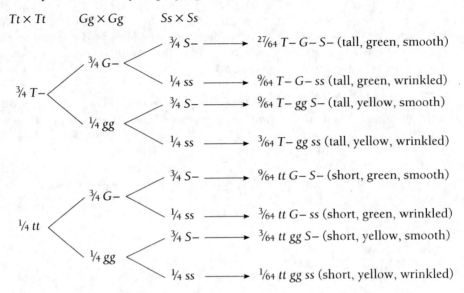

$Tt × Tt$ $Gg × Gg$ $Ss × Ss$

¾ T–
 ¾ G–
  ¾ S– ⟶ ²⁷/₆₄ T– G– S– (tall, green, smooth)
  ¼ ss ⟶ ⁹/₆₄ T– G– ss (tall, green, wrinkled)
 ¼ gg
  ¾ S– ⟶ ⁹/₆₄ T– gg S– (tall, yellow, smooth)
  ¼ ss ⟶ ³/₆₄ T– gg ss (tall, yellow, wrinkled)

¼ tt
 ¾ G–
  ¾ S– ⟶ ⁹/₆₄ tt G– S– (short, green, smooth)
  ¼ ss ⟶ ³/₆₄ tt G– ss (short, green, wrinkled)
 ¼ gg
  ¾ S– ⟶ ³/₆₄ tt gg S– (short, yellow, smooth)
  ¼ ss ⟶ ¹/₆₄ tt gg ss (short, yellow, wrinkled)

c. The branch diagram of the cross *Tt Gg Ss × tt GG ss* is:

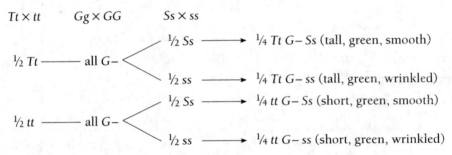

$Tt × tt$ $Gg × GG$ $Ss × ss$

½ Tt ——— all G–
  ½ Ss ⟶ ¼ Tt G– Ss (tall, green, smooth)
  ½ ss ⟶ ¼ Tt G– ss (tall, green, wrinkled)

½ tt ——— all G–
  ½ Ss ⟶ ¼ tt G– Ss (short, green, smooth)
  ½ ss ⟶ ¼ tt G– ss (short, green, wrinkled)

d. The branch diagram of the cross *Tt Gg Ss × TT gg SS* is:

$Tt × TT$ $Gg × gg$ $Ss × SS$

all T–
  ½ Gg ——— all S– ⟶ ½ T– Gg S– (tall, green, smooth)
  ½ gg ——— all S– ⟶ ½ T– gg S– (tall, yellow, smooth)

11.21   *Answer:* In order for an individual to be pigmented, they must have one of each of the dominant *C* and *O* alleles and not have any of the dominant *I* alleles. That is, they must be *C– O– ii*.

a. White Silkie (*CC oo ii*) × White Wyandotte (*cc OO ii*). These are two true-breeding strains at each of three genes and differ from each other at two loci, the *C/c* and *O/o* loci. The progeny will be dihybrids, are all *Cc Oo ii*, and are all pigmented.

b. White Leghorn (*CC OO II*) × White Wyandotte (*cc OO ii*). These two are also true breeding at each of three genes, and differ from each other at two loci, the *C/c* and *I/i* loci. Their progeny will be dihybrids, are all *Cc OO Ii*, and are all white (because of *Ii*).

c. Wyandotte-Silkie F₁ (*Cc Oo ii*) × White Silkie (*CC oo ii*). As both parents are *ii*, all the progeny will be as well, and so if they are *C– O–*, they will be pigmented. The proportions of white and pigmented progeny can be determined by using a branch diagram or considering each locus separately as follows: At the *C/c* locus, the cross is *Cc × CC*, so all the progeny will be *C–*. At the *O* locus, the cross is *Oo × oo*, a testcross, so half the progeny will be *Oo* and half will be *oo*. Thus, half of the progeny will be *C– Oo ii* and be pigmented, and half will be *C– oo ii* and be white.

11.22   *Answer:*

  a. First assign gene symbols for each of the traits. Let Y represent yellow and y green seeds, P represent purple and p white flowers, A represent axially positioned and a terminally positioned flowers, and I represent inflated and i pinched pods. Then determine as much information as you can about genotypes from the phenotypes that are given. The initial yellow seed produced a parent plant with purple, axially positioned flowers and inflated pods, so it had all four dominant alleles and was $Y{-}\ P{-}\ A{-}\ I{-}$. Determine whether the parent plant is homozygous or heterozygous at each gene by considering the types of offspring it produces when selfed. Selfing a homozygote never produces recessive offspring, while selfing a heterozygote produces 25% recessive offspring. Since selfing of the parent produces only yellow seeds, and since recessive traits for the flower color, flower position, and pod shape genes are seen when two F_1 seeds are sown, the parent is $YY\ Pp\ Aa\ Ii$. The F_1 plant with terminally positioned purple flowers, pinched pods, and yellow seeds is $YY\ P{-}\ aa\ ii$, and the F_1 plant with axially positioned white flowers, pinched pods, and yellow seeds is $YY\ pp\ A{-}\ ii$.

  b. The seeds were produced by the cross $YY\ Pp\ Aa\ Ii \times YY\ Pp\ Aa\ Ii$. Recognizing that this is a cross of two trihybrid individuals will let you predict that the phenotypic ratio in the offspring will be 27:9:9:9:3:3:3:1. You can also use a branch diagram such as that in text Figure 11.14, p. 311, to show that if the seeds are sown, they will produce yellow-seeded plants that are $^{27}/_{64}$ purple, axially positioned flowers with inflated pods; $^{9}/_{64}$ purple, axially positioned flowers with pinched pods; $^{9}/_{64}$ purple, terminally positioned flowers with inflated pods; $^{9}/_{64}$ white, axially positioned flowers with inflated pods; $^{3}/_{64}$ purple, terminally positioned flowers with pinched pods; $^{3}/_{64}$ white, terminally positioned flowers with inflated pods; $^{3}/_{64}$ white, axially positioned flowers with pinched pods; and $^{1}/_{64}$ white, terminally positioned flowers with pinched pods.

11.23   *Answer:* Although this problem can be solved using a branch diagram, the branch diagram analysis of six genes is tedious. Therefore, approach it by considering the general relationship that exists between the number of possible genotypes and phenotypes. At any one locus having alleles that act in a dominant recessive fashion, there are two possible phenotypes ($A{-}$ and aa) and three possible genotypes (AA, Aa, and aa). When several independently assorting loci are considered, the number of possibilities grows according to the number of combinations of alleles possible. For two loci, independent assortment of the alleles at each locus allows for $2 \times 2 = 4$ phenotypes (two possible phenotypes at each locus assorted with either of two possible phenotypes at a second locus) and 3×3 genotypes (three possible genotypes at one locus assorted with any of three possible genotypes at a second locus). For three loci, independent assortment of the alleles at each locus allows for $2 \times 2 \times 2 = 8$ phenotypes and $3 \times 3 \times 3 = 27$ genotypes. For n loci, the relationship becomes 2^n possible phenotypes and 3^n possible genotypes.

   To determine the frequency of a particular phenotypic or genotypic class, consider that at one locus, an F_1 hybrid cross gives $^3/_4$ phenotypically dominant and $^1/_4$ phenotypically recessive progeny and $^1/_4$ homozygous dominant, $^1/_2$ heterozygous, and $^1/_4$ homozygous recessive progeny. The fraction of progeny of a particular genotypic or phenotypic class can be determined by considering the combinations that are possible. For example, for two independently assorting loci A/a and B/b, $^3/_4$ of the progeny of a cross of $Aa\ Bb \times Aa\ Bb$ will show the $A{-}$ phenotype and $^3/_4$ of the progeny will show the $B{-}$ phenotype. When independent assortment of these two loci is considered, $^3/_4 \times ^3/_4 = ^9/_{16}$ of the progeny will show both the $A{-}$ and the $B{-}$ phenotypes. (Multiply the individual probabilities using the product rule.) Thus, when n loci are involved, $(^3/_4)^n$ of the progeny will show all dominant phenotypes, $(^1/_4)^n$ of the progeny will show all recessive phenotypes, $(^1/_4)^n$ of the progeny will be homozygous dominant at all loci, $(^1/_4)^n$ of the progeny will be homozygous recessive at all loci, and $(^1/_2)^n$ of the progeny will be heterozygous at all loci.

  a. For six loci, $3^6 = 729$ possible genotypes will be seen.

  b. Notice that the question asks for how many of the *genotypes* will be homozygous. For just one locus, two (AA, aa) of three possible (AA, Aa, aa) genotypes are homozygous. Thus, for six loci, $2^6 = 64$ genotypes will be homozygous for all loci. Note that included in these genotypes are those that are homozygous dominant at each locus, those that are homozygous recessive at each locus, and those that are homozygous dominant at one or more loci and homozygous recessive at the other loci.

c. In a monohybrid cross, $\frac{1}{4}$ of the progeny will be homozygous dominant. For the F_2 in this cross, $(\frac{1}{4})^6 = 1/4,096$ of the progeny will be homozygous dominant. Notice that this fraction of the progeny derives from a single genotype.

d. In a monohybrid cross, $\frac{3}{4}$ of the progeny show a dominant phenotype. For the F_2 in this cross, $(\frac{3}{4})^6 = 729/4,096 = 17\%$ of the progeny will show all six dominant phenotypes.

11.24 *Answer:*

a. The cross is *aa BB CC* × *AA bb $c^h c^h$*. Since the parents are true breeding at each of three different loci, the F_1 must be a trihybrid, or *Aa Bb Cc^h*. The F_1 will be agouti with black hairs and pigmented over the entire body. In the F_2, a branch diagram will identify eight possible phenotypic classes: agouti, black, full pigmentation (*A– B– C–*); nonagouti, black, full (*aa B– C–*); agouti, brown, full (*A– bb C–*); nonagouti, brown, full (*aa bb C–*); agouti, black, Himalayan (*A– B– $c^h c^h$*); nonagouti, black, Himalayan (*aa B– $c^h c^h$*); agouti, brown, Himalayan (*A– bb $c^h c^h$*); and nonagouti, brown, Himalayan (*aa bb $c^h c^h$*).

b. F_2 animals that are non-Himalayan, black, and agouti have the genotype *A– B– C–*. Among the *A–* animals, $\frac{2}{3}$ are *Aa*. Among the *B–* animals, $\frac{1}{3}$ are *BB*. Among the *C–* animals, $\frac{2}{3}$ are *Cc^h*. Thus, among all of the non-Himalayan black agouti F_2, $\frac{2}{3} \times \frac{1}{3} \times \frac{2}{3} = \frac{4}{27}$ are *Aa BB Cc^h*.

c. From the cross *Aa Bb Cc^h* × *Aa Bb Cc^h*, $\frac{1}{4}$ of the progeny will be *bb* and show brown pigment. This will be the case regardless of whether the animals are pigmented over their entire body or are Himalayan. Thus, $\frac{1}{4}$ of the Himalayan mice will show brown pigment. (Be careful not to misread this question: It does *not* ask what proportion of the progeny are both brown *and* Himalayan.)

d. From the cross *Aa Bb Cc^h* × *Aa Bb Cc^h*, $\frac{3}{4}$ of the progeny will be *B–* and show black pigment. This will be the case regardless of whether the animals are agouti or nonagouti. Thus, $\frac{3}{4}$ of the agouti mice will show black pigment. (Be careful not to misread this question: It does *not* ask what proportion of the progeny are both black *and* agouti.)

11.25 *Answer:* First, assign symbols to the alleles, and write down the cross. Let solid color be *S* and spotted be *s*. Then, if a true-breeding, solid-colored dog is bred to a spotted dog, the cross is *SS* × *ss*, the F_1 all *Ss*, and interbreeding the F_1 will give $\frac{3}{4}$ *S–* (solid) and $\frac{1}{4}$ *ss* (spotted) progeny.

a. The chance that the first puppy born is spotted is just the chance of getting an *ss* offspring from an *Ss* × *Ss* cross, or $\frac{1}{4}$.

b. The chance of getting four puppies all having solid coats is the chance of getting an *S–* offspring the first time, *and* the second time, *and* the third time, *and* the fourth time. Apply the product rule to get $p = \frac{3}{4} \times \frac{3}{4} \times \frac{3}{4} \times \frac{3}{4} = \frac{81}{256}$.

11.26 *Answer:* First, infer partial genotypes of the mother and her four kittens from their phenotypes.

Cat	Phenotype	Inferred Partial Genotype
mother	long hair, white hair with blue eyes	*ll W–*
kitten 1	long hair, white hair with blue eyes	*ll W–*
kitten 2	short hair, grey hair with dark eyes	*L– ww*
kitten 3	long hair, grey hair with dark eyes	*ll ww*
kitten 4	short hair, white hair with blue eyes	*L– W–*

Since kitten 3 is homozygous for the recessive alleles at each gene, we know that this kitten received a recessive allele for each gene from its mother. Therefore, the mother is *ll Ww* and has two types of gametes, *l W* and *l w*. If there is single paternity, the father must have contributed an *l –* gamete to kitten 1, an *L w* gamete to kitten 2, an *l w* gamete to kitten 3, and an *L –* gamete to kitten 4. This is possible if he is *Ll –w* (short hair, unknown hair or eye color). Therefore, the phenotypes seen in this litter can be explained by a single paternity. This litter does not show evidence for multiple paternities solely based on these phenotypes.

11.27 *Answer:*

a. It is important to *think through* this problem, and not just plug numbers into a chi-square formula. Here, we want to test the hypothesis of factor segregation. The hypothesis states that each allele in a monohybrid will segregate into gametes independently, so that zygotes have a half-chance of obtaining either allele from a heterozygous parent. Drawing a Punnett square shows that a 3:1 ratio of progeny phenotypes would be expected from an $F_1 \times F_1$ cross. Mendel observed 705 red and 224 white plants in the F_2, a ratio of 3.14:1. Thus, this ratio seems consistent with his hypothesis.

b. To test *how* significant this result is, use the χ^2 test to determine how frequently these types of numbers would be obtained in similar experiments.

Class	Observed	Expected	d	d^2	d^2/e
red	705	697	8	64	0.09
white	224	232	−8	64	0.28
Total	929	929	0	—	$\chi^2 = 0.37$

$$\chi^2 = 0.37;\ df = 1;\ 0.50 < P < 0.70$$

According to the χ^2 test, then, Mendel's result is consistent with this hypothesis. More specifically, in approximately 60% of similar experiments, one would expect a deviation (i.e., a value of χ^2) as great as or greater than this one. One therefore fails to reject the hypothesis.

11.28 *Answer:* First, use the symbols defined in the problem to write the genotypes of the parents and expected offspring if the two loci assort independently. One has

P: *CC pp* × *cc PP*

$F_1 \times F_1$:   *Cc Pp* × *Cc Pp*

F_2:   9 *C–P–* : 3 *C–pp* : 3 *cc P–* : 1 *cc pp*

    (9 cut, purple : 3 cut, green : 3 potato, purple : 1 potato, green)

If the two loci assort independently then, one expects to see a 9:3:3:1 phenotypic ratio in the F_2. Therefore, test the hypothesis of independent assortment using the χ^2 test.

Class	Observed	Expected	d	d^2	d^2/e
cut, purple	189	180	9	81	0.45
cut, green	67	60	7	49	0.81
potato, purple	50	60	−10	100	1.66
potato, green	14	20	−6	36	1.80
Total	320	320	0	—	$\chi^2 = 4.72$

$$\chi^2 = 4.72;\ df = 3;\ 0.10 < P < 0.20$$

Therefore, in experiments similar to this one, a deviation at least as great as that observed here would be seen about 20% of the time. Thus, the hypothesis of two independently assorting genes is accepted as being possible.

11.29 *Answer:* The F_1 is produced from a cross between two true-breeding plants, so you can infer which traits are dominant from the phenotypes of the F_1. You can then use this information to assign gene symbols. Tall is dominant to short, so let T represent tall and t represent short. Purple is dominant to white, so let P represent purple and p represent white. Axially positioned flowers are dominant to terminally positioned flowers, so let A represent axially positioned flowers and a represent terminally positioned flowers. Then rewrite the crosses and their offspring so that you can follow the inheritance of the alleles:

P: *TT AA PP* (tall, axial, purple) × *tt aa pp* (short, terminal, white)

F₁: *Tt Aa Pp* (tall, axial, purple)

Tt Aa Pp (tall, axial, purple F1) × *tt aa pp* (short, terminal, white) gives

> 164 *Tt aa ww* (tall, terminal, white)
> 144 *Tt Aa ww* (tall, axial, white)
> 156 *Tt aa Pp* (tall, terminal, purple)
> 176 *Tt Aa Pp* (tall, axial, purple)
> 138 *tt aa pp* (short, terminal, white)
> 149 *tt Aa ww* (short, axial, white)
> 182 *tt aa Pp* (short, terminal, purple)
> 166 *tt Aa Pp* (short, axial, purple)

Examining the rewritten data suggests the hypothesis that the cross between the tall, axial, and purple F₁ to short, terminal, and white is a trihybrid testcross with three independently assorting genes. A trihybrid testcross with three independently assorting genes is expected to produce eight equally frequent progeny classes. Test this hypothesis using a chi-square test.

Class	Observed (o)	Expected (e)	d (= o − e)	d²	d²/e
tall, terminal, white	164	159.375	4.625	21.39	0.134
tall, axial, white	144	159.375	−15.375	236.39	1.483
tall, terminal, purple	156	159.375	−3.375	11.39	0.071
tall, axial, purple	176	159.375	16.625	276.39	1.734
short, terminal, white	138	159.375	−21.375	456.89	2.867
short, axial, white	149	159.375	−10.375	107.64	0.675
short, terminal, purple	182	159.375	22.625	511.89	3.212
short, axial, purple	166	159.375	6.625	43.89	0.275
Total	1,275	1,275	0	—	$\chi^2 = 10.451$

$\chi^2 = 10.451$; df = 7; $0.10 < P < 0.20$

Based on the χ^2 test, we would observe a deviation at least as great as that observed here between 10 and 20% of the time if the crosses were repeated. Therefore, we should accept as possible the hypothesis that the cross has three independently assorting genes.

11.30   *Answer:* First summarize what you know about the mating types:

"*A*" = *A– B–*, "*B*" = *aa B–*, "*C*" = *aa bb*, "*D*" = *A– bb*

Then rewrite the table in terms of what is known.

	Mating Type of Progeny			
Cross	A A– B–	B aa B–	C aa bb	D A– bb
"A" × "B" A– B– × aa B–	24	21	14	18
"A" × "C" A– B– × aa bb	56	76	55	41
"A" × "D" A– B– × A– bb	44	11	19	33
"B" × "C" aa B– × aa bb	0	40	38	0
"B" × "D" aa B– × A– bb	6	8	14	10
"C" × "D" aa bb × A– bb	0	0	45	45

Notice that a cross involving mating type *C* is similar to a testcross, because *C* is *aa bb*. The progeny ratios in crosses involving "*C*" will therefore reflect the gametes from the non-"*C*" parent. In the cross of "*B*" × "*C*," both the parents are *aa*, and the 1 *B* : 1 *C* (1 *aa B*– : 1 *aa bb*) ratio in the progeny reflects the fact that "*B*" is *Bb*. Therefore, "*B*" is *aa Bb*. In the cross "*C*" × "*D*," both parents are *bb*, and the 1 *C* : 1 *D* progeny ratio indicates that "*D*" is *Aa*. "*D*" is therefore *Aa bb*. To determine the genotype of "*A*," consider that the cross of "*A*" × "*C*" produces progeny of all four mating types. This would be expected only if "*A*" were *Aa Bb*.

11.31 *Answer:* The initial cross is *Ww Rr* × *W r*. Note that since males are haploid, they have only one set of chromosomes. As a consequence, their gametes are only of one kind (e.g., the *W r* male will have only *W r* gametes) and their phenotype can be used to directly infer their genotype.

   a. The progeny females will be ½ *W*– *Rr* (black-eyed, wax sealers) and ½ *W*– *rr* (black-eyed, resin sealers).

   b. As males arise from unfertilized eggs, they receive chromosomes only from their mother. The progeny males will be ¼ *W R* (black-eyed, wax sealers), ¼ *W r* (black-eyed, resin sealers), ¼ *w r* (white-eyed, resin sealers), and ¼ *w R* (white-eyed, wax sealers).

   c. The egg fertilized by the mutation-bearing sperm results in a *Cc* female. Since fertilization occurs in flight, only males that are *C* contribute genes to the next generation. Hence the first generation arises from the cross *Cc* × *C*. There is a ½ chance of obtaining daughters that are *Cc*. Such a daughter can be fertilized only by a *C* male, so that the chance of her having a *Cc* daughter is also ½. The chance of having a *Cc* granddaughter is thus ½ × ½ = ¼. Such granddaughters will have wingless males if they are prolific. Thus, the probability that wingless males will be found in a hive founded two generations later by one of Madonna's granddaughters is the probability that the granddaughter is *Cc*, or ¼.

   d. $(½)^4 = \frac{1}{16}$.

11.32 *Answer:* For pedigree A, parents not showing the trait in generation I have a daughter that exhibits the trait. This is typical of a cross of two heterozygotes giving a homozygous recessive, affected individual: *Aa* × *Aa* (two normal parents) give 3 *A*– (normal) : 1 *aa* (affected). If this were the case, individuals II-2 and II-3 could be carriers (i.e., be *Aa*). If individual II-3 is a carrier and his spouse is homozygous recessive (*aa*), generation III would arise from the cross *Aa* × *aa*, and the 1:1 ratio of affected to unaffected individuals seen would be expected. Thus, pedigree A is consistent with the trait being recessive.

   In pedigree B, the trait is present in half of the individuals in generations I and II, but in none of those of generation III. However, the parents of generation III do not themselves exhibit the trait. This is consistent with the trait being dominant. With this view, individual I-1 would be *aa* and individual I-2 would be *Aa*. Half of their progeny would be expected to show the trait, as is observed. Furthermore, unaffected parents should have unaffected offspring, as is seen in generation III. Notice, however, that the pedigree is also consistent with a recessive trait that is not rare. In this case, individual I-1 would be heterozygous, and the cross in generation I would be *Aa* × *aa*, giving the 50% affected progeny seen in generation II. Although individual II-6 would have to be *Aa*, if her spouse was *AA*, all the children would be normal.

11.33 *Answer:*

   a. If the allele responsible for the trait is recessive to the normal allele, then to have affected offspring in generation II, the mother (individual I-1) must be heterozygous (i.e., be *Aa*). If she were homozygous for the normal allele (i.e., *AA*), all the offspring would be *A*– and be normal. If she were heterozygous, the cross in the first generation would be *Aa* × *aa*, and one would expect about 50% affected and 50% normal offspring. This is close to what is observed, and so the mother is *Aa*.

   b. Because the father is affected with a recessive trait, he must be *aa*.

   c. Since the father is homozygous for the recessive allele, all the children must have inherited an abnormal allele from their father. If they inherited a normal, dominant allele from their mother, they will not be affected (*Aa*: II-1, II-3, II-4), whereas if they inherited the abnormal, recessive allele from their mother, they will be affected (*aa*: II-2, II-5).

d. Given that the parents are *Aa* × *aa*, one expects a 1:1 ratio of affected to unaffected children. For the five offspring shown, one sees a ratio of 2:3, which, given the number of offspring, approximates a 1:1 ratio. Remember that each birth is independent of the others, and while, if many progeny are seen, one should see about a 1:1 ratio, for small numbers of progeny, the ratios may be significantly off from what is expected. Indeed, even if the couple were to have more unaffected children, the pedigree would still be consistent with the inheritance of a recessive trait. (Can you show that if the pedigree is taken on its own, *without any information about whether the trait is dominant or recessive*, the pedigree is also consistent with the inheritance of a dominant trait?)

11.34   *Answer:*

a. In each of the pedigrees, every affected individual has an affected parent. This is consistent with the trait in each pedigree being inherited as a dominant allele. Suppose this is so, and let *A* be the dominant allele for the trait. Unaffected individuals in each pedigree are *aa*. In pedigree A, I-2, II-2, II-4, II-7, II-8, III-2, IV-2, and IV-4 must be *Aa*, and II-1, III-3, III-4, III-5, III-6, III-8, III-9, IV-6, IV-7, IV-8, IV-9, and IV-10 are either *AA* or *Aa*. In pedigree B, all affected individuals are *Aa*.

In pedigree A, the trait appears relatively often and there are two instances where two affected parents (II-1 and II-2, III-5, and III-6) have all affected children. While these instances suggest that the trait in pedigree A could be modeled as a recessive condition, there are also two affected parents (II-7 and II-8) who do not have all affected offspring. This is inconsistent with the inheritance of a recessive condition, so the trait in pedigree A must be caused by a dominant allele.

b. As we inferred in part **(a)**, the trait is inherited as a dominant allele in both pedigrees. With the additional information, we can infer that all affected individuals must be *Aa*. In pedigree A, individuals II-1, III-3, III-4, III-5, III-6, III-8, III-9, IV-6, IV-7, IV-8, IV-9, and IV-10 cannot be homozygous. They must have inherited a dominant *A* allele from one parent and a recessive *a* allele from the other parent.

c. The cross is *Aa* × *Aa*. Since *AA* individuals do not survive, the expected genotypic ratio in offspring is *2 Aa : 1 aa*. Therefore, there is a $^2/_3$ chance the child will be affected.

11.35   *Answer:* First draw the pedigree. Then try to fit the "unreasonableness" trait to a dominant (*A*– = affected, *aa* = unaffected) or recessive character (*A*– = unaffected, *aa* = affected), as shown below:

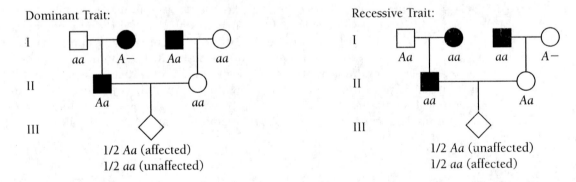

In the diagrams above, the woman is II-2, her husband is II-1, her father is I-3, and her mother-in-law is I-2. If the trait indeed has a genetic basis, it could be modeled as either a dominant or a recessive trait. Notice that one can infer whether an *A*– individual is *AA* or *Aa* based on the offspring that are produced. Independent of whether the trait is dominant or recessive, about half of the woman's children should be "unreasonable" in this particular situation.

11.36   *Answer:* An uncertainty exists about whether the brother of the man's wife's paternal grandmother had Gaucher's disease. If this distant relative had the disease, a disease allele might have been passed on to the man's wife. Therefore, in a worst-case scenario, consider this distant relative to have had the disease. Under this scenario, the pedigree is as shown on the facing page:

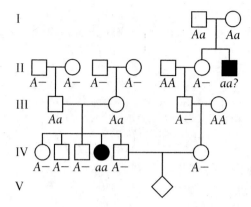

In this pedigree, the man is IV-5, his affected sister is IV-4, his wife is IV-6, and the brother of his wife's paternal grandmother is II-7. Since II-7 is affected but his parents are not, the disease must be a recessive trait and each of his parents must be heterozygous.

To calculate the chance that, if the couple has a child, the child will be affected, one needs to calculate the probability that V-1 can receive an *a* allele from each of its parents. For each parent, this is $\frac{1}{2}$ the chance a parent is *Aa*.

Since we know the parents of IV-5 must be *Aa*, and IV-5 is *A–*, there is a $\frac{2}{3}$ chance that IV-5 is *Aa*. Thus, there is a $\frac{1}{2} \times \frac{2}{3} = \frac{1}{3}$ chance that IV-5 will pass the *a* allele to V-1.

The probability that IV-6 is *Aa* is more complex, and is:

P(III-3 was *Aa and* III-3 passed the *a* allele on to IV-6)

= P[(II-6 was *Aa and* II-6 passed *a* to III-3) *and* (III-3 passed *a* to IV-6)]

= $[(\frac{2}{3} \times \frac{1}{2}) \times \frac{1}{2}] = \frac{1}{6}$.

Thus, there is a $\frac{1}{6} \times \frac{1}{2} = \frac{1}{12}$ chance that IV-6 will pass the *a* allele to V-1. In this worst-case scenario, the chance that both parents will pass on an *a* allele and have an affected child is $\frac{1}{12} \times \frac{1}{3} = \frac{1}{36}$.

If the brother of the wife's paternal grandmother did not have the disease, IV-6 would be *AA*. The child would be *A–* and be phenotypically normal.

11.37 *Answer:* The F_1 cross is $a^+/a\ b^+/b\ c^+/c\ d^+/d \times a^+/a\ b^+/b\ c^+/c\ d^+/d$.

    a. A colorless F_2 individual would result if an individual has an *a/a*, *b/b*, and/or *c/c* genotype. This would consist of many possible genotypes. Rather than identify all of these combinations, use the fact that the proportion of colorless individuals = 1 – the proportion of pigmented individuals. The proportion of pigmented individuals ($a^+/–\ b^+/–\ c^+/–$) is $\frac{3}{4} \times \frac{3}{4} \times \frac{3}{4} = \frac{27}{64}$. The chance of not obtaining this genotype is $1 - \frac{27}{64} = \frac{37}{64}$.

    b. A brown individual is $a^+/–\ b^+/–\ c^+/–\ d/d$. The proportion of brown individuals is $\frac{3}{4} \times \frac{3}{4} \times \frac{3}{4} \times \frac{1}{4} = \frac{27}{256}$.

11.38 *Answer:*

    a. Colorless individuals are *a/a b/b –/–*. The chance of obtaining such an individual from a cross of $a^+/a\ b^+/b\ c^+/c \times a^+/a\ b^+/b\ c^+/c$ is $\frac{1}{4} \times \frac{1}{4} = \frac{1}{16}$.

    b. There are two ways to determine the proportion of red individuals. First, notice that red individuals are obtained either when only one of the a^+ or b^+ functions is present (no matter what genotype is at *c*), or when both a^+ and b^+ functions are present but c^+ is not. Thus, these phenotypes are obtained from the following genotypes: $a^+/–\ b/b\ –/–$, *a/a* $b^+/–\ –/–$, or $a^+/–\ b^+/–\ c/c$. The probability of obtaining one of these genotypes is

$$(\tfrac{3}{4} \times \tfrac{1}{4} \times 1) + (\tfrac{1}{4} \times \tfrac{3}{4} \times 1) + (\tfrac{3}{4} \times \tfrac{3}{4} \times \tfrac{1}{4}) = \tfrac{33}{64}$$

    A second way is to use the information from **(a)** and **(c)**. From **(c)**, one has that $\frac{27}{64}$ individuals are black, so the remaining $\frac{37}{64}$ are either red or colorless. From **(a)**, $\frac{1}{16} = \frac{4}{64}$ are colorless. Thus, there are $(37 - 4)/64 = \frac{33}{64}$ that are red.

    c. Black individuals are formed only if both red pigments are available and are then converted to black pigment. Thus, an individual must be $a^+/- \; b^+/- \; c^+/-$. The chance of obtaining such an individual is $\frac{3}{4} \times \frac{3}{4} \times \frac{3}{4} = \frac{27}{64}$.

11.39   *Answer:*

    a. Since any of the normal alleles a^+, b^+, or c^+ is sufficient to catalyze the reaction leading to color, in order for color to fail to develop, all three normal alleles must be missing. That is, the colorless F_2 must be $a/a \; b/b \; c/c$. The chance of obtaining such an individual is $\frac{1}{4} \times \frac{1}{4} \times \frac{1}{4} = \frac{1}{64}$.

    b. Now, colorless F_2 are obtained if *either* one or both steps of the pathway are blocked. That is, colorless F_2 are obtained in either of the following genotypes: $d/d \; -/- \; -/- \; -/-$ (the first or both steps blocked) or $d^+/- \; a/a \; b/b \; c/c$ (second step blocked). The chance of obtaining such individuals is

$$(\tfrac{1}{4} \times 1 \times 1 \times 1) + (\tfrac{3}{4} \times \tfrac{1}{4} \times \tfrac{1}{4} \times \tfrac{1}{4}) = (64 + 3)/256 = \tfrac{67}{256}$$

11.40   *Answer:*

    a. $\frac{1}{2} \; w/w^+ \; bw/bw^+ \; st/st^+$, fire-red-eyed daughters; $\frac{1}{2} \; w/Y \; bw/bw^+ \; st/st^+$, white-eyed sons

    b. $w/w^+ \; se/se^+ \; bw/bw^+$ and $w^+/Y \; se/se^+ \; bw/bw^+$, all fire-red eyes

    c. $w/w^+ \; v/v^+ \; bw/bw$ and $w^+/Y \; v/v^+ \; bw/bw$, all brown eyes

    d. $\frac{1}{4} \; w^+/w$ or w^+/Y, $bw/bw^+ \; st/st^+$, fire-red eyes; $\frac{1}{4} \; w^+/w$ or w^+/Y, $bw/bw \; st/st^+$, brown eyes; $\frac{1}{4} \; w^+/w$ or w^+/Y, $bw/bw^+ \; st/st$, scarlet eyes; $\frac{1}{4} \; w^+/w$ or w^+/Y, $bw/bw \; st/st$, (the color of 3-hydroxykynurenine plus the color of the precursor to biopterin, or colorless = white)

12

Chromosomal Basis of Inheritance

Chapter Outline

Review of Key Terms, Symbols, and Concepts

In your own words, write a brief, precise definition of each term in the groups below and on the following pages. Check your definitions using the text. Then develop a concept map using the terms in each list.

1	2	3
eukaryote	mitosis	meiosis I, II
diploid	karyokinesis	prophase I, II
haploid	cytokinesis	prometaphase I, II
genome	cell cycle	metaphase I, II
gamete	M, G_1, G_0, S, G_2	anaphase I, II
zygote	sister chromatid, chromatid	telophase I, II
homolog	daughter chromosome	leptonema
homologous chromosome	prophase	zygonema
nonhomologous chromosome	prometaphase	pachynema
sex chromosome	metaphase	diplonema
autosome	anaphase	diakinesis
centromere	telophase	pairing, synapsis
p, q arms	mitotic spindle	crossing-over
metacentric chromosome	tubulin, microtubule	synaptonemal complex
submetacentric chromosome	centriole	bivalent
acrocentric chromosome	kinetochore	tetrad
satellite	metaphase plate	bouquet
telocentric chromosome	aster	chiasma, chiasmata
karyotype	kinetochore, nonkinetochore microtubule	genetic recombination
band	disjunction	recombinant chromosome
G banding	cell plate	pseudoautosomal region (PAR)
ideogram		
chromosome painting		

4	5	6
meiosis	meiosis	chromosome theory
sexual reproduction	angiosperm	sex chromosome
spermatogenesis	gametogenesis	X chromosome
oogenesis	sporogenesis	Y chromosome
spermatozoa	meiospore	homogametic sex
primary spermatogonia	gametophyte	heterogametic sex
primary spermatocytes	sporophyte	sex linkage
meiocyte	stamen	X linkage
secondary spermatocyte	pistil	hemizygous
spermatid	alternation of generations	homozygous
primary oogonia	ovule	crisscross inheritance
secondary oogonia	pollen	reciprocal cross
primary oocyte	anther	X-linked recessive trait
unequal cytokinesis	gametophyte generation	X-linked dominant trait
secondary oocyte	sporophyte generation	Y-linked trait
first polar body	spore	holandric trait
second polar body		
ovum		

7	8
genotypic sex determination	wild type
genic sex determination	mutant allele
Y chromosome sex determination	Mendelian symbolism
X chromosome–autosome balance system	*Drosophila* symbolism
disjunction, nondisjunction	A, a, aa, Aa, AA, aY, AY
segregation	$a^+, a, a^+a^+, a^+a, aa, aY, a^+Y$
chromosome pairing	$A^+, A, AA, A^+A, A^+A^+, AY, A^+Y$
primary nondisjunction	
secondary nondisjunction	
X chromosome nondisjunction	
aneuploidy	
karyotype	
Turner, Klinefelter, XYY syndromes	
dosage compensation	
Barr body	
epigenetic phenomenon	
genetic mosaic	
Lyon hypothesis, lyonization	
testis-determining factor gene	
hermaphroditic	
monoecious, dioecious	
perfect, imperfect flower	
mating type	
$MATa, MAT\alpha$	

Thinking Analytically

The goal of this chapter is for you to learn how to think about gene segregation patterns in terms of chromosomal inheritance patterns. Solving problems is one of the best ways to help you think clearly and precisely about this issue. However, the problems on Mendelian genetics in this chapter are more complicated than those in Chapter 11, and they present more of a challenge to your analytical reasoning skills. Review the "Thinking Analytically" hints in Chapter 11 of this guide, and approach the problems analytically and systematically. After you have arrived at a solution, always go back and test it against the data presented in the problem. Try to avoid falling into a trap: don't look at the answer presented here before you have attempted to solve the problem independently. Being able to understand the answer in this guide is not equivalent to being able to solve the problem independently. You won't have the guide in an exam. By trying to solve problems independently, you will improve your analytical thinking. This will enable you to do better on an exam.

Take care to represent crosses accurately with appropriate symbols. While you can often use Mendelian or normal/abnormal notation (see text Box 12.1, p. 343) equally well, become fluent with both. Geneticists use each type of notation. As you symbolize traits in crosses, consistently use one type of notation, be careful to use a single type of symbol for each gene (e.g., g and g^+ or g and G for green and yellow seed color, not g and Y), and clearly distinguish between X-linked and autosomal traits because these follow different inheritance patterns. For example, when assigning members of a pedigree symbols for genetic traits, use a notation that reflects whether inheritance is autosomal or X-linked. This will make it easier for you to spot patterns as well as infer expected types of offspring. Use aa for a female with an X-linked recessive trait, AY or a^+Y for a male with an X-linked dominant trait, aY for a male with a recessive trait, and Aa or a^+a for an individual with an autosomal trait.

The proof that genes lie on chromosomes came from relating abnormal patterns of trait inheritance to abnormal patterns of chromosome inheritance. Understanding how chromosome behavior during meiosis relates to the segregation and independent assortment of traits in genetic crosses is therefore central to this material. Review the material in this chapter on chromosome pairing and segregation during meiosis and relate it to how autosomal alleles in a heterozygote segregate during the formation of gametes. Then diagram what happens if the alleles are on an X chromosome and there is X chromosome nondisjunction. Are the normal crisscross inheritance patterns altered? Are the results of testcrosses with the progeny altered?

Questions for Practice

Multiple-Choice Questions

1. Which two events occur in leptonema of prophase I?
    a. synapsis and crossing-over
    b. disappearance of the nucleolus and disjunction
    c. synaptonemal complex formation and crossing-over
    d. pairing and chiasma formation
    e. pairing and the beginning of crossing-over

2. Which one of the following statements is *not* true?
    a. Crossing-over begins in leptonema.
    b. Chiasmata are visible manifestations of crossing-over.
    c. Chiasmata are visible in diplonema.
    d. Chiasmata are visible at the time that crossing-over occurs.

3. Which one of the following statements about mitosis is true?
    a. The nucleolus disappears during metaphase.
    b. Nuclear membranes re-form at the end of telophase.
    c. Centromeres are aligned on the metaphase plate at prophase.
    d. The nucleolus re-forms at the end of anaphase.

4. Sister chromatids are
    a. synonymous with homologous chromosomes.
    b. present only in meiosis and not in mitosis.
    c. identical products of chromosome duplication held together by a replicated but unseparated centromere.
    d. visible in interphase just after S phase.

5. The chromosome theory of inheritance holds that
    a. chromosomes are inherited.
    b. the chromosomes contain the hereditary material.
    c. the genes are inherited.
    d. the chromosomes are DNA.

6. Proof that genes lie on chromosomes was obtained by
    a. correlating aneuploids resulting from nondisjunction with inheritance patterns.
    b. showing that some genes appear to be sex linked.
    c. showing that males have an X and a Y, while females have two X's.
    d. showing that in *Drosophila*, males are the heterogametic sex.

7. An individual that produces both ova and sperm
    a. has the XY genotype.
    b. reproduces asexually.
    c. is said to be hermaphroditic.
    d. both b and c above

8. What piece of evidence best indicates that two X chromosomes are required for a normal human female, even though one of the X chromosomes is inactivated into a Barr body?
    a. Turner females are usually infertile and have morphological abnormalities.
    b. XXY individuals show a Klinefelter syndrome.
    c. 47,XXX individuals are almost completely normal females.
    d. Lyonization occurs in 46,XX individuals.

9. The somatic cells of an individual having the karyotype 48,XXXY would have
   a. four Barr bodies.
   b. three Barr bodies.
   c. two Barr bodies.
   d. no Barr bodies.

10. Pedigrees showing X-linked recessive traits typically show
    a. only females being affected.
    b. all daughters of an affected father being affected.
    c. all sons of an unaffected mother being normal.
    d. the trait appearing more frequently in males.

11. In humans, what can be said about genes on a normal male's X chromosome?
    a. They are hemizygous.
    b. They are inactivated when the male's cells form Barr bodies.
    c. They are inherited as autosomal recessive traits.
    d. They are responsible for male sex type.

12. During spermatogenesis in a male fly, there is X chromosome nondisjunction during meiosis I. What types of sperm are produced?
    a. X- and Y-bearing sperm
    b. XX- and YY-bearing sperm
    c. XY- and no-sex-chromosome-bearing sperm
    d. XX-, XY-, X-, and Y-bearing sperm

13. Which of the following is true about organisms where sex type is determined by an X chromosome–autosome balance system?
    a. Sex type is determined by the number of X chromosomes. Organisms with two X chromosomes are female, while organisms with one X chromosome are male, regardless of the number of autosomes.
    b. Sex type is determined by the ratio of X chromosomes to autosomes. The Y chromosome plays no role in sex determination.
    c. A key gene called *SRY* on the Y chromosome determines sex type.
    d. The number of autosomes determines sex type. Organisms with one set of autosomes are male, while organisms with two sets of autosomes are female.

14. As cells develop into gametes during spermatogenesis and oogenesis in an animal cell, they also proceed through stages of meiosis. In which type of cell will meiosis II occur?
    a. primary spermatagonium
    b. secondary spermatagonium
    c. primary spermatocyte
    d. secondary spermatocyte

15. The *yellow* allele is a recessive, X-linked mutation that causes *Drosophila* to have a yellow body color instead of the normal grey body color. How would you represent a wild-type male using *Drosophila* symbolism?
    a. y/Y
    b. y/y
    c. y^+/Y or $+/Y$
    d. y^+/y^+ or $+/+$

Answers: 1e, 2d, 3b, 4c, 5b, 6a, 7c, 8a, 9c, 10d, 11a, 12c, 13b, 14d, 15c

Thought Questions

1. When during meiosis does the chromosomal behavior underlying Mendel's laws occur?
2. What is meant by crisscross inheritance, and what clinical significance does it have in pedigree analysis?
3. Develop a flowchart illustrating the decision-making path you would employ to ascertain whether a pedigree showed autosomal dominant, autosomal recessive, X-linked dominant, X-linked recessive, or Y-linked inheritance.

4. Define the term *lyonization*, give an example of it, and discuss its functional significance.

5. Why do you think most flowering plants are monoecious, whereas in most animals, the sexes are separate?

6. If all mammals have evolved from a common ancestor, how do you account for the variety of chromosome numbers they possess? By what mechanism do you think changes in chromosome number could have occurred? (Consider chromosome number variation resulting from nondisjunction and other accidental changes.)

7. Except for the loci involved with sex determination in mammalian males, there is little clear evidence for genetic loci on the Y chromosome. Why might this be the case, and what might this tell you about the Y chromosome in mammals?

8. What are some of the different mechanisms by which sex type can be determined? Do you think it is significant that so many different mechanisms can be employed?

9. Even though X inactivation occurs in XXY individuals, they do not have the same phenotype as XY males. Similarly, even though X inactivation occurs in XX individuals, they do not have the same phenotype as XO individuals. Why might this be the case?

10. An individual who phenotypically appears to have Klinefelter syndrome has a karyotype of XX,46. An individual who phenotypically appears to have Turner syndrome has a karyotype of XY,46. What common explanation might underlie each of these anomalies?

Thought Questions for Media

After reviewing the media on the *iGenetics* website, try to answer these questions.

1. How are centromeres, centrioles, and centrosomes different in terms of their cellular location and function during mitosis?

2. At what point in the cell cycle are chromosomes replicated? At what point are replicated chromosomes so extended that individual chromatids cannot be seen? When can they first be visualized? When are they maximally condensed?

3. When do centromeres replicate? When do replicated centromeres split apart?

4. During anaphase, chromosomes move to opposite poles and polar and kinetochore microtubules change length. Which type of microtubule shortens, and which type of microtubule elongates?

5. How do the chromosomes of daughter cells produced by mitosis compare with the chromosomes of the parental cell?

6. After which division (meiosis I or meiosis II) are haploid cells produced? At which point are haploid gametes produced?

7. If nondisjunction occurs in meiosis I, how many types of abnormal gametes are produced? Are any normal gametes produced?

8. If nondisjunction occurs in meiosis II, how many types of abnormal gametes are produced? Are any normal gametes produced?

9. The animation illustrates how nondisjunction in either meiosis I or meiosis II can lead to the production of monosomic and trisomic zygotes. How might nondisjunction be involved in generating a nullosomic (none of one type of chromosome) or a tetrasomic (four copies of one kind of chromosome) zygote?

10. In one meiosis in an *Aa Bb* individual, four gametes are produced. How many different genotypes are produced?

11. Based on the animation and considering your answer to question 1, how can four equal frequencies of gametes (¼ *Ab*, ¼ *AB*, ¼ *aB*, ¼ *ab*) be obtained?

12. At what point during meiosis does the chromosome behavior that underlies independent assortment occur?

1. **a.** Why is it important to determine that none of the individuals that have married into Anna's or Jackson's family have a separate family history of deafness?

   b. How would your analysis of the pedigree of Jackson's family change if you learned that individuals II-3, II-5, and III-4 have a history of deafness?

   c. Since both congenital and progressive hearing loss are relatively uncommon traits, when a pedigree analysis is being performed, can you just assume that individuals marrying into the family have no family history of deafness? If not, how would you proceed?

2. What is the chance that if Anna and Jackson have two boys and two girls, they will all have normal hearing?

3. Anna may or may not be a carrier for deafness. Suppose Anna and Jackson indeed have two boys and two girls with normal hearing. Can you conclude anything about whether Anna is a carrier for deafness? If so, what? If not, why not?

Solutions to Text Problems

12.1   *Answer:* c

12.2   *Answer:* G_1 and G_2 are stages of interphase. G_1 is a growth phase during which the cell grows and then prepares for DNA and chromosome replication, which take place during the S stage of interphase. Some cells proceed through G_1 in just a few minutes, while others (such as differentiated adult nerve cells) can spend years in G_1. Other cells exit the cell cycle from G_1 and enter G_0, a quiescent, nondividing state. G_2 is a postsynthesis stage during which the cell prepares for cell division, or M phase. Not all cells proceed through all of each of these phases, because only some cells enter G_0, and those that do will not necessarily proceed through G_2.

12.3   *Answer:* a

12.4   *Answer:* c

12.5   *Answer:*
  a. False. Chromosomes can have different sizes and can have their centromeres positioned differently. For many organisms, this statement will be false. However, in a diploid cell, a pair of homologous chromosomes will be morphologically alike.
  b. True.
  c. False. In meiosis I, only homologous chromosomes will synapse together.

12.6   *Answer:* Try to visualize the events of mitosis dynamically as you solve this problem.

Name of Event		Order of Event
cytokinesis	The cytoplasm divides and the cell contents are separated into two separate cells.	7
metaphase	Chromosomes become aligned along the equatorial plane of the cell.	4
interphase	Chromosome replication occurs.	1
telophase	The migration of the daughter chromosomes to the two poles is complete.	6
prophase	Replicated chromosomes begin to condense and become visible under the microscope.	2
anaphase	Sister chromatids begin to separate and migrate toward opposite poles of the cell.	5
prometaphase	The nuclear envelope breaks down, a developing mitotic spindle enters the former nuclear area, and kinetochores bind to centromeres.	3

12.7   *Answer:*
  a. Yes. If a sexual mating system exists in the species, two haploid cells can fuse to produce a diploid cell that can then go through meiosis to produce haploid progeny. The fungi *Neurospora crassa* and *Saccharomyces cerevisiae* exemplify this life cycle.
  b. No. Meiosis can occur only in a diploid cell. A haploid individual cannot form a diploid cell, so meiosis cannot occur.

12.8   *Answer:* b. Only diploid (2N) cells can undergo meiosis, and haploid cells (N) fuse at fertilization, regenerating the diploid state.

12.9   *Answer:* c. In a haploid organism, gametes and somatic cells are both N. This provides an example of how **(c)** is true.

12.10   *Answer:* e

12.11   *Answer:*
  a. Metaphase: Metaphase in mitosis, metaphase I and metaphase II in meiosis
  b. Anaphase: Anaphase in mitosis, anaphase I and anaphase II in meiosis

12.12   *Answer:*

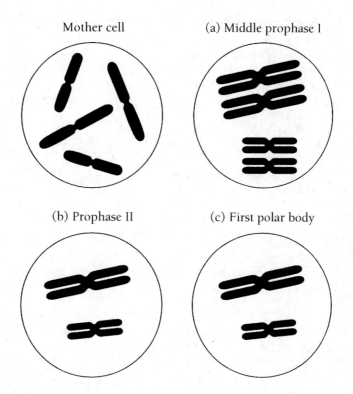

12.13   *Answer:* To reconcile how all the cells illustrated could come from one individual, consider that the cells shown could come from either somatic or germ-line cells. Cell **(a)** shows three pairs of previously synapsed homologs disjoining and must therefore illustrate anaphase I of meiosis. That three pairs of chromosomes are present indicates that the organism has 2N = 6 chromosomes, so that N = 3. Cell **(b)** shows the disjoining of chromatids. Since the organism has 2N = 6 chromosomes, and the daughter cells that will form as a result of this cell division will have 6 chromosomes, **(b)** must illustrate part of mitosis, specifically anaphase. Cell **(c)** also shows the disjoining of chromatids. Since the daughter cells will receive three chromosomes, this must be anaphase II of meiosis. Cell **(d)** shows the pairing of homologs and therefore illustrates metaphase I of meiosis. Because the individual has three pairs of identically appearing chromosomes, there are two identical sex (= X) chromosomes, indicating that the animal is female.

12.14   *Answer:* Meiosis has greater significance. While mitosis generates progeny cells that are genetically identical to a parent cell, meiosis generates gametes that are genetically diverse. Gamete diversity is obtained when nonparental combinations of genes are obtained in two ways: the random assortment of maternal and paternal chromosomes at anaphase I of meiosis I and crossing-over events in prophase I of meiosis I. When gametes from different parents fuse at fertilization, more diversity is obtained. Hence, meiosis provides a means for genetic variation.

12.15 *Answer:*

a. The chance that a gamete would have a particular maternal chromosome is $\frac{1}{2}$. Apply the product rule to determine the chance of obtaining a gamete with all three maternal chromosomes: $P(A \text{ and } B \text{ and } C) = P(A) \times P(B) \times P(C) = (\frac{1}{2})^3 = \frac{1}{8}$.

b. There are two approaches to this question.

1. List all of the possible options to obtain gametes that satisfy the specified condition—that some maternal and paternal chromosomes are present. Use the product rule to determine the probability of each and then, using the sum rule, determine the proportion of the gametes having maternal and paternal chromosomes. Gametes that satisfy the condition that both maternal and paternal chromosomes are present are ABC', AB'C, A'BC, AB'C', A'BC', and A'B'C. For each one of these six gamete types, the chance of obtaining it is $\frac{1}{8}$. This is based on applying the product rule and logic similar to that used in part **(a)** of this question. Apply the sum rule to determine the chance of obtaining one of these types of gametes: $P(\text{ABC' or AB'C or A'BC or AB'C' or A'BC' or A'B'C}) = \frac{1}{8} + \frac{1}{8} + \frac{1}{8} + \frac{1}{8} + \frac{1}{8} + \frac{1}{8} = \frac{6}{8} = \frac{3}{4}$.

2. Realize that the set of gametes with some maternal and paternal chromosomes is composed of all gametes *except* those that have only maternal or only paternal chromosomes. That is, $P(\text{gamete with } both \text{ maternal } and \text{ paternal chromosomes}) = 1 - P(\text{gamete with } only \text{ maternal or only paternal chromosomes})$. From part **(a)**, the chance of a gamete having chromosomes from only one parent is $\frac{1}{8}$. Using the sum rule, $P(\text{gamete with both maternal and paternal chromosomes}) = 1 - (\frac{1}{8} + \frac{1}{8}) = \frac{3}{4}$.

12.16 *Answer:* Since the cells are normal and the cell is diploid, the chromosomes should exist in pairs. The cell could have come from a male mammal with one medium-length pair, one long pair, and a heteromorphic sex chromosome (XY) pair.

12.17 *Answer:* False. Skin cells consist entirely of mitotic, not meiotic, cells.

12.18 *Answer:* False. Genetic diversity in the male's sperm is achieved during meiosis. There is crossing-over between nonsister chromatids as well as independent assortment of the male's maternal and paternal chromosomes during spermatogenesis.

12.19 *Answer:* A female horse has ova with 32 chromosomes, while a male donkey has sperm with 31 chromosomes. A mule has 32 + 31 = 63 chromosomes.

12.20 *Answer:*

a. The red fox will have gametes with 17 chromosomes, and the arctic fox will have gametes with 26 chromosomes. The hybrid will have 17 + 26 = 43 chromosomes. Once the fertilized egg is formed, mitotic division will produce somatic cells with 43 chromosomes.

b. Similar chromosomes pair in meiosis. The pairing pattern seen in the hybrid indicates that some of the chromosomes in the arctic and red foxes share evolutionary similarity, while others do not. Unpaired chromosomes will not segregate in an orderly manner, giving rise to unbalanced meiotic products with either extra or missing chromosomes. This can lead to sterility for two reasons: First, meiotic products that are missing chromosomes may not have genes necessary to form gametes. Second, even if gametes are able to form, a zygote generated from them will not have the chromosome set from either the hybrid, the red, or the arctic fox. The zygote will be an aneuploid with missing or extra genes, causing it to be inviable.

12.21 *Answer:* The chance of getting a particular paternal chromosome is $\frac{1}{2}$. Using the product rule, and logic similar to that in the answer presented for Question 12.15a, the chance of getting all five paternal chromosomes is $(\frac{1}{2})^5 = \frac{1}{32}$.

12.22 *Answer:* The crosses and their progeny are tabulated in the chart on the facing page:

	Mendelian Notation	Drosophila Notation; Long Version	Drosophila Notation; Short Version

a.

	Mendelian Notation	Drosophila Notation; Long Version	Drosophila Notation; Short Version
Allele symbols:	P = normal	p^+ = normal	+ = normal
	p = phenylketo-nuria	p = phenylketonuria	p = phenylketonuria
Cross:	$Pp \times Pp$	$p^+p \times p^+p$	$+p \times +p$
F_1:	$1\,PP : 2\,Pp : 1\,pp$	$1\,p^+p^+ : 2\,p^+p : 1\,pp$	$1\,++ : 2\,+p : 1\,pp$
F_1 phenotypes:	¾ normal, ¼ phenylketonuria		

b.

	Mendelian Notation	Drosophila Notation; Long Version	Drosophila Notation; Short Version
Allele symbols:	C = normal	c^+ = normal	+ = normal
	c = color blind	c = color blind	c = color blind
Cross:	$Cc\,Pp \times CY\,Pp$	$c^+c\,p^+p \times c^+Y\,p^+p$	$+c\,+p \times +Y\,+p$
F_1:	¹⁄₁₆ $CC\,PP$	¹⁄₁₆ $c^+c^+\,p^+p^+$	¹⁄₁₆ $+\,+\,+\,+$
	⅛ $CC\,Pp$	⅛ $c^+c^+\,p^+p$	⅛ $+\,+\,+p$
	¹⁄₁₆ $CC\,pp$	¹⁄₁₆ $c^+c^+\,pp$	¹⁄₁₆ $+\,+\,pp$
	¹⁄₁₆ $Cc\,PP$	¹⁄₁₆ $c^+c\,p^+p^+$	¹⁄₁₆ $+c\,+\,+$
	⅛ $Cc\,Pp$	⅛ $c^+c\,p^+p$	⅛ $+c\,+p$
	¹⁄₁₆ $Cc\,pp$	¹⁄₁₆ $c^+c\,pp$	¹⁄₁₆ $+c\,pp$
	¹⁄₁₆ $CY\,PP$	¹⁄₁₆ $c^+Y\,p^+p^+$	¹⁄₁₆ $+Y\,+\,+$
	⅛ $CY\,Pp$	⅛ $c^+Y\,p^+p$	⅛ $+Y\,+p$
	¹⁄₁₆ $CY\,pp$	¹⁄₁₆ $c^+Y\,pp$	¹⁄₁₆ $+Y\,pp$
	¹⁄₁₆ $cY\,PP$	¹⁄₁₆ $cY\,p^+p^+$	¹⁄₁₆ $cY\,+\,+$
	⅛ $cY\,Pp$	⅛ $cY\,p^+p$	⅛ $cY\,+p$
	¹⁄₁₆ $cY\,pp$	¹⁄₁₆ $cY\,pp$	¹⁄₁₆ $cY\,pp$

F_1 phenotypes: ⅜ normal females   ¹⁄₁₆ phenylketonuria males

⅛ phenylketonuria females   ³⁄₁₆ color-blind males

³⁄₁₆ normal males   ¹⁄₁₆ color-blind phenylketonuria males

c.

	Mendelian Notation	Drosophila Notation; Long Version	Drosophila Notation; Short Version
Allele symbols:	normal eyes = W	normal eyes = w^+	normal eyes = +
	white eyes = w	white eyes = w	white eyes = w
	normal wings = c	normal wings = C^+	normal wings = +
	curled wings = C	curled wings = C	curled wings = C
	normal bristles = s	normal bristles = S^+	normal bristles = +
	stubble bristles = S	stubble bristles = S	stubble bristles = S
Cross:	$ww\,Cc\,ss$	$ww\,CC^+\,S^+S^+$	$ww\,C+\,++$
	$\times$	$\times$	$\times$
	$WY\,cc\,Ss$	$w^+Y\,C^+C^+SS^+$	$+Y\,++\,S+$
F_1 genotypes:	⅛ $Ww\,Cc\,Ss$	⅛ $w^+w\,CC^+SS^+$	⅛ $+w\,C+\,S+$
	⅛ $Ww\,Cc\,ss$	⅛ $w^+w\,CC^+\,S^+S^+$	⅛ $+w\,C+\,++$
	⅛ $Ww\,cc\,Ss$	⅛ $w^+w\,C^+C^+SS^+$	⅛ $+w\,++\,S+$
	⅛ $Ww\,Cc\,ss$	⅛ $w^+w\,C^+C^+\,S^+S^+$	⅛ $+w\,++\,++$
	⅛ $wY\,Cc\,Ss$	⅛ $wY\,CC^+SS^+$	⅛ $wY\,C+\,S+$
	⅛ $wY\,Cc\,ss$	⅛ $wY\,CC^+\,S^+S^+$	⅛ $wY\,C+\,++$
	⅛ $wY\,cc\,Ss$	⅛ $wY\,C^+C^+SS^+$	⅛ $wY\,++\,S+$
	⅛ $wY\,cc\,ss$	⅛ $wY\,C^+C^+\,S^+S^+$	⅛ $wY\,++\,++$

(continued)

	Mendelian Notation	Drosophila Notation; Long Version	Drosophila Notation; Short Version
F_1 phenotypes:	⅛ stubble, curled females	⅛ white, stubble, curled males	
	⅛ curled females	⅛ white, curled males	
	⅛ stubble females	⅛ white, stubble males	
	⅛ normal females	⅛ white males	

d.

	Mendelian Notation	Drosophila Notation; Long Version	Drosophila Notation; Short Version
Allele symbols:	white eye = w	white eye = w	white eye = w
	red eye = W	red eye = w^+	red eye = +
	black body = b	black body = b	black body = b
	grey body = B	grey body = b^+	grey body = +
	normal bristles = S	normal bristles = s^+	normal bristles = +
	tiny bristles = s	tiny bristles = s	tiny bristles = s
	normal size eye = e	normal size eye = E^+	normal size eye = +
	reduced size eye = E	reduced size eye = E	reduced size eye = E
Cross:	$ww\ bb\ ss\ ee$	$ww\ bb\ ss\ E^+E^+$	$ww\ bb\ ss\ ++$
	×	×	×
	$WY\ BB\ SS\ EE$	$w^+Y\ b^+b^+\ s^+s^+\ EE$	$+Y\ ++++\ EE$
F_1 genotypes:	½ $Ww\ Bb\ Ss\ Ee$	½ $w^+w\ b^+b\ s^+s\ EE^+$	½ $+w\ +b\ +s\ +E$
	½ $wY\ Bb\ Ss\ Ee$	½ $wY\ b^+b\ s^+s\ EE^+$	½ $wY\ +b\ +s\ +E$
F_1 phenotypes:	½ eyeless females,	½ white, eyeless males	

12.23 *Answer:* The initial cross is $ww \times w^+Y$, so that the F_1 females are ww^+ and the F_1 males are wY. The second set of crosses are therefore $w^+w \times w^+Y$ and $wY \times ww$. The former will give all brick red females (w^+-) and half white (wY) and half brick red (w^+Y) males. The latter will give only white-eyed males and females (wY and ww).

12.24 *Answer:* Since fathers always give their X chromosome to their daughters, the woman must be heterozygous for the color-blind trait and is c^+c. Her husband received his X chromosome from his mother and has normal color vision, so he is c^+Y. The cross is therefore $c^+c \times c^+Y$. All daughters will receive the paternal X bearing the c^+ allele and have normal color vision. Because sons will receive the maternal X, half will be cY and be color-blind and half will be c^+Y and have normal color vision.

12.25 *Answer:* Let c and c^+ be the color-blind and normal vision alleles, respectively, and let a and a^+ be the albino and normal pigmentation alleles, respectively. Then the cross can be represented as c^+c^+ $aa \times cY\ a^+a^+$. As all the offspring will be a^+a, all will have normal pigmentation. The offspring will be either c^+c or c^+Y and have normal color vision. The daughters will, however, be carriers for the color-blind trait.

12.26   *Answer:*

  a. The initial cross is $ww\ vg^+vg^+ \times w^+Y\ vgvg$. The F_1 consists of $wY\ vg^+vg$ (white, normal-winged) males and $ww^+\ vg^+vg$ (red, normal-winged) females.

  b. The F_2 would be produced by crossing $wY\ vg^+vg$ males and $w^+w\ vg^+vg$ females. In both the male and the female progeny, $\frac{1}{8}$ will be white and vestigial, $\frac{1}{8}$ will be red and vestigial, $\frac{3}{8}$ will be white and normal winged, and $\frac{3}{8}$ will be red and normal winged.

  c. If the F_1 males are crossed back to the female parent, the cross is $wY\ vg^+vg \times ww\ vg^+vg^+$. All the progeny would be white and normal winged. If the F_1 females are crossed back to the male parent, the cross is $ww^+\ vg^+vg \times w^+Y\ vgvg$. Among the male progeny, there would be $\frac{1}{4}$ white, vestigial; $\frac{1}{4}$ red, vestigial; $\frac{1}{4}$ white, normal winged; and $\frac{1}{4}$ red, normal winged. Among the female progeny, half would be red and normal winged and half would be red and vestigial.

12.27   *Answer:* From Question 12.26, we know that w is X-linked while vg is autosomal. This can also be determined by considering just one trait at a time and examining the frequency of progeny phenotypes. The ratio of long-winged to vestigial-winged progeny is 3:1 ($\frac{3}{4}$ to $\frac{1}{4}$) in both sexes, while the ratio of red-eyed to white-eyed progeny is all to none in females and 1:1 in males. This is consistent with vg being autosomal and w being X-linked. The 3:1 ratio of long-winged to vestigial-winged progeny indicates that each parent was heterozygous at the vg locus. Since both parents had red eyes, both had (at least) one w^+ allele. Since half of the sons are white eyed, the mother must have been heterozygous. Therefore, the parents were $w^+w\ vg^+vg$ and $w^+Y\ vg^+vg$.

12.28   *Answer:*

  a. Calico cats are typically female and are genetic mosaics due to X-chromosome inactivation: some cells show the phenotypes of one X chromosome, and the other cells show the phenotypes of the other X chromosome. From the text, calico cats with orange and black patches have the $Oo\ B–$ genotype. The O and o alleles are on the X chromosome and determine whether or not orange coat color is expressed. If O is present, orange coat color is expressed no matter what other genes for coat color are present at the B gene. If O is not present, the alleles at the autosomal B/b gene are not masked and determine the coat color. The B allele specifies black coat color, while the b allele determines brown coat color. Therefore, the orange patches on calico cats arise from cells expressing the O allele when the X chromosome bearing the o allele is inactivated, and the black patches on $Oo\ B–$ calico cats arise from cells expressing the o allele when the X chromosome bearing the O allele is inactivated. Use this information about coat color phenotypes to make inferrences about possible genotypes.

  Since the father of the calico cat is chocolate, he must be $oY\ bb$. Deduce the genotype of his calico daughter by considering her phenotype and what paternal chromosomes she must have received. She has some black pigmentation, so she must also have a dominant B allele, and she received her father's X (with an o allele) and an autosome with a b allele, so she is $Oo\ Bb$. Since the parents of the chocolate male who mates with the calico cat were solid black, that cross was $oo\ Bb \times oY\ Bb$, and their chocolate son is $oY\ bb$. Thus, the cross between the calico female and chocolate male is $Oo\ Bb \times oY\ bb$. The progeny are $\frac{1}{4}$ orange females ($OO\ b–$), $\frac{1}{8}$ calico females with black and orange patches ($Oo\ Bb$), $\frac{1}{8}$ calico females with brown and orange patches ($Oo\ bb$), $\frac{1}{4}$ orange males ($OY\ b–$), $\frac{1}{8}$ black males ($oY\ Bb$), and $\frac{1}{8}$ chocolate males ($oY\ bb$).

  b. Sex-chromosome nondisjunction in meiosis I and II produces XXY, XO, XXX, and XYY animals. In the table on page 220, the parenthetical terms refer to the feline phenotypes corresponding to the Klinefelter, Turner, triplo-X, and XYY human phenotypes.

Paternal Gametes

Maternal Gametes	Nondisjunction in Meiosis I		Nondisjunction in Meiosis II	
	oY b	nullo-X *b*	*oo b*	YY *b*
O B	*OoY Bb* "Klinefelter" male, calico with black and orange patches	*O Bb* "Turner" female, orange	*Ooo Bb* "Triplo-X" female, calico with black and orange patches	*OYY Bb* "XYY" male, orange
O b	*OoY bb* "Klinefelter" male, calico with chocolate and orange patches	*O bb* "Turner" female, orange	*Ooo bb* "Triplo-X" female, calico with chocolate and orange patches	*OYY bb* "XYY" male, orange
o B	*ooY Bb* "Klinefelter" male, black	*o Bb* "Turner" female, black	*ooo Bb* "Triplo-X" female, black	*oYY Bb* "XYY" male, black
o b	*ooY bb* "Klinefelter" male, chocolate	*o bb* "Turner" female, chocolate	*ooo bb* "Triplo-X" female, chocolate	*oYY bb* "XYY" male, chocolate

12.29   *Answer:*

   a. In poultry, sex type is determined by a ZZ (male) and ZW (female) system. The cross can be depicted as *bb* (nonbarred cock) $\times$ *BW* (barred hen). The F_1 progeny will be *b*W (nonbarred) hens and *Bb* (barred) cocks.

   b. The cross can be represented as *b*W $\times$ *bb*. All the progeny will be nonbarred.

   c. The cross can be represented as *Bb* $\times$ *BW*. The progeny will be $\frac{1}{2}$ barred cocks ($\frac{1}{4}$ *BB*, $\frac{1}{4}$ *Bb*), $\frac{1}{4}$ barred hens (*BW*), and $\frac{1}{4}$ nonbarred hens (*bW*).

12.30   *Answer:* Notice that the trait is transmitted from the father to his daughters, indicating crisscross inheritance. This is typical of an X-linked trait. Since the man marries a normal woman and all of their daughters have the trait, the trait must be dominant. The man's X chromosome bearing the defective tooth enamel allele is inherited by all of his daughters and none of his sons. All of his daughters would therefore have defective tooth enamel and be heterozygous for the defective enamel allele. These daughters would transmit the defective enamel allele half of the time, giving rise to 50% of their children being affected.

12.31   *Answer:* Since the inability to taste the substance is recessive, the nontaster child must be homozygous for the recessive allele, and each of his parents must have given the child a recessive allele. Since both parents can taste, they must also bear a dominant allele. Let *T* represent the dominant (taster) allele, and *t* represent the recessive (nontaster) allele [Note: Mendelian notation is used here for convenience, but also because there is no value in assigning a normal (+) and abnormal allele.] Then the cross can be written as *Tt* $\times$ *Tt*. The chance that their next child will be a taster is the chance that the child will be *TT* or *Tt*, or $\frac{3}{4}$.

12.32   *Answer:*

   a. Since the disease is autosomal recessive, and unaffected parents have affected offspring, both parents must be heterozygous. Let c^+ represent the normal allele and *c* represent the disease allele. Then the parental cross can be represented as $c^+c \times c^+c$, and there is a $\frac{1}{4}$ chance that any conception will produce a *cc* (affected) child.

   b. If a child is not affected, the child is either c^+c^+ ($P = \frac{1}{3}$) or c^+c ($P = \frac{2}{3}$). Thus, there is a $\frac{2}{3}$ chance that a nonaffected child is heterozygous.

12.33 *Answer:* Let H represent the disease allele, and let h represent the normal allele. Since just one of Woody's parents died of the disease, we may assume that only one parent had the disease allele. Thus, Woody must have been Hh. His children are the progeny of a cross that can be represented as $Hh \times hh$. Each will have a 50% chance of receiving the H allele.

12.34 *Answer:*

a. Since only a single trait is being followed, consider just part of the cross: $AA \times a$Y. The progeny will be either AY or Aa, and all are $A-$. Thus, the chance of obtaining an $A-$ individual in the F_1 is 1.

b. As shown in (a), there is no chance ($P = 0$) of obtaining an aY individual in the F_1.

c. The F_1 progeny will be $A- Bb\ Cc\ Dd$. Half will be female, so $P = \frac{1}{2}$.

d. Two, $Aa\ Bb\ Cc\ Dd$ (females) and AY $Bb\ Cc\ Dd$ (males).

e. For the X chromosome trait, the F_1 cross is AY $\times Aa$. Half of the female offspring ($\frac{1}{4}$ of the total) will be heterozygous Aa individuals. For each of the autosomal traits, $\frac{1}{2}$ of the offspring will be heterozygous (e.g., $Bb \times Bb$ gives $\frac{1}{2}$ Bb individuals). Thus, the chance that an F_2 individual will be heterozygous at all four traits is $\frac{1}{4} \times \frac{1}{2} \times \frac{1}{2} \times \frac{1}{2} = \frac{1}{32}$.

f. Before determining the probabilities, consider that at any autosomal gene, there is a $\frac{1}{4}$ chance of obtaining either type of homozygote (e.g., BB, bb) and a $\frac{1}{2}$ chance of obtaining a heterozygote. At the A gene, the cross is AY $\times Aa$, so there is a $\frac{1}{4}$ chance of obtaining an AY male, a $\frac{1}{4}$ chance of obtaining an aY male, a $\frac{1}{4}$ chance of obtaining an Aa female, and a $\frac{1}{4}$ chance of obtaining an AA female (there will be a $\frac{1}{2}$ chance of obtaining an $A-$ female). Then the chance of obtaining (1) an $A-bb\ CC\ dd$ (female) is $P = (\frac{1}{2} \times \frac{1}{4} \times \frac{1}{4} \times \frac{1}{4}) = \frac{1}{128}$; (2) an aY $BB\ Cc\ Dd$ (male) is $P = (\frac{1}{4} \times \frac{1}{4} \times \frac{1}{2} \times \frac{1}{2}) = \frac{1}{64}$; (3) an AY $bb\ CC\ dd$ (male) is $P = (\frac{1}{4} \times \frac{1}{4} \times \frac{1}{4} \times \frac{1}{4}) = \frac{1}{256}$; and (4) an $aa\ bb\ Cc\ Dd$ (female) is $P = (0 \times \frac{1}{4} \times \frac{1}{2} \times \frac{1}{2}) = 0$.

12.35 *Answer:*

a. In humans, sex type is determined by the presence or absence of a Y chromosome. The testis-determining factor gene present on the Y chromosome causes individuals with a Y to become males. In both *Drosophila melanogaster* and *Caenorhabditis elegans*, sex type is determined by the ratio of the number of X chromosomes to the sets of autosomes. In *Drosophila*, animals with an X : A ratio of 2:2 are female while animals with an X : A ratio of 1:2 are male. In *C. elegans*, animals with an X : A ratio of 2:2 are hermaphrodites, while animals with an X : A ratio of 1:2 are males.

b. In humans, X-linked gene dosage is equalized by inactivating all but one X chromosome to form a Barr body. Consequently, normal XX females have one Barr body, as do Klinefelter XXY males. In flies, transcription of X-linked genes in males is higher than that in females so as to equal the sum of the expression levels of the two X chromosomes in females. In worms, genes on both of the X chromosomes of an XX hermaphrodite are transcribed at half the rate as the same gene on the single X chromosome in an XO male.

12.36 *Answer:*

a. In *C. elegans*, XX animals are hermaphroditic and XO animals are male. Even though hermaphrodites are capable of self-fertilization, a mating between an XX hermaphrodite and an XO male produces equal frequencies of XX hermaphrodites and XO males because the male's sperm have a competitive advantage in fertilization. Let + represent the normal, dominant allele at *unc-115*, and determine the types of offspring using a Punnett square, as shown here.

		Gametes of *unc-115* Male	
		$\frac{1}{2}$ *unc-115* (X)	$\frac{1}{2}$ O
Gametes of *unc-115* + Hermaphrodite	$\frac{1}{2}$ *unc-115* (X)	$\frac{1}{4}$ *unc-115 unc-115* (XX) uncoordinated, hermaphrodite	$\frac{1}{4}$ *unc-115* (XO) uncoordinated male
	$\frac{1}{2}$ + (X)	$\frac{1}{4}$ *unc-115* + (XX) coordinated hermaphrodite	$\frac{1}{4}$ + (XO) coordinated male

b. When progeny are produced by self-fertilization in *C. elegans*, XO males are produced 0.2% of the time via nondisjunction. These males would obtain the X chromosome bearing the *unc-115* allele 50% of the time, and the X chromosome bearing the + allele 50% of the time. So, there will be 0.1% *unc-115* (uncoordinated) XO males and 0.1% + (coordinated) XO males. The remaining 99.8% of the offspring will be hermaphrodites that result from the fertilization of an X-bearing egg by an X-bearing sperm. Since the hermaphroditic parent is heterozygous, these hermaphrodites will be $\frac{1}{4}$ *unc-115 unc-115* (uncoordinated) homozygotes, $\frac{1}{2}$ *unc-115* + (coordinated) heterozygotes, and $\frac{1}{4}$ + + (coordinated) heterozygotes. Therefore, the expected offspring are 0.1% uncoordinated males, 0.1% coordinated males, 24.95% uncoordinated hermaphrodites, and 74.85% coordinated *hermaphrodites*.

c. Since *unc-26* is autosomal, a cross that involves *unc-26* + and *unc-26 unc-26* genotypes will produce $\frac{1}{2}$ *unc-26 unc-26* and $\frac{1}{2}$ + *unc-26* offspring. All *unc-26 unc-26* animals will be uncoordinated even if they have a + allele at the *unc-115* gene, just as all *unc-115 unc-115* (XX) hermaphrodites and *unc-115* (XO) males will be uncoordinated even if they have a + allele at the *unc-26* gene. The following branch diagram uses this information and the result from part **(a)** to show that the cross between these double mutants will produce $\frac{1}{8}$ coordinated hermaphrodites, $\frac{1}{8}$ coordinated males, $\frac{3}{8}$ uncoordinated hermaphrodites, and $\frac{3}{8}$ uncoordinated males.

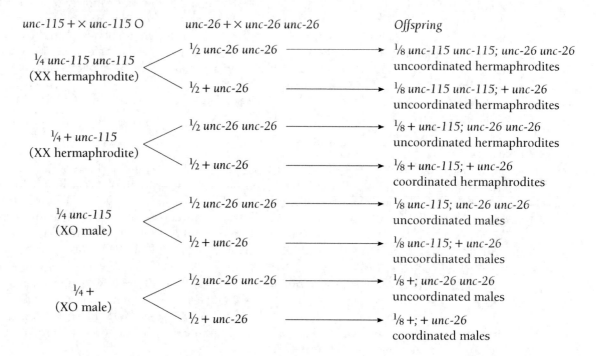

12.37 *Answer:* First consider what kinds of animals will be produced in the "engineered" cross. Primary nondisjunction of sex chromosomes in the meiosis of a female will result in eggs that have either zero or two X chromosomes. Thus, the eggs will either lack the *w* allele or be *ww*. Sperm from a red-eyed male will either bear a Y chromosome or bear the w^+ allele. Upon fertilization then, four classes of embryos will be obtained: Y only, w^+O, *ww*Y, and w^+*ww*. Animals with either zero or three X chromosomes are inviable, and so only w^+ (red, XO males) and *ww*Y (white, XXY females) animals will be obtained.

Now consider the backcrosses. The "engineered" red males will be sterile because they lack a Y chromosome needed for male fertility. Hence, the only backcross that will give progeny is the mating between the *ww*Y females and the w^+Y males. The sex chromosome constitution of the female's gametes is dependent on the pairing and disjunction of the two X chromosomes and the Y chromosome during meiosis. If there is normal pairing and disjunction of the two X chromosomes and the Y chromosome assorts independently of them, XY (*w*Y) and X (*w*) eggs will be produced. If, as described in the text, less frequent secondary nondisjunction occurs, XX-bearing (*ww*) and Y-bearing eggs will be produced. The zygotes produced when these eggs are fertilized by sperm from a w^+Y male are shown in the following Punnett square:

		Normal Disjunction		Secondary Nondisjunction	
		wY	w	ww	Y
Gametes of w^+Y Male	w^+	w^+wY (XXY) red female	w^+w (XX) red female	w^+ww (XXX) inviable	w^+Y (XY) red male
	Y	wYY (XYY) white male	wY (XY) white male	wwY (XXY) white female	YY inviable

*(table heading above: **Gametes of wwY Female**)*

12.38 *Answer:* The cross that gave rise to the wild-type F_1 female can be denoted as $X^{bb} X^{bb} \times X^{bb+} Y^{bb+}$. Nondisjunction in meiosis of the $X^{bb} X^{bb}$ female would produce an $X^{bb} X^{bb}$ egg. Fertilization by a Y^{bb+}-bearing sperm would produce a bb^+ ($X^{bb} X^{bb} Y^{bb+}$) female. We want to know what progeny result when this female is mated to a bb ($X^{bb} Y^{bb}$) male. Normal disjunction (which occurs about 96% of the time) in this female will produce $X^{bb} Y^{bb+}$ and X^{bb}-bearing eggs. If these eggs are fertilized by sperm from a bb male (i.e., either X^{bb} or Y^{bb}), half bb^+ ($X^{bb} X^{bb} Y^{bb+}$ and $X^{bb} Y^{bb+} Y^{bb}$) males and females and half bb ($X^{bb} X^{bb}$ and $X^{bb} Y^{bb}$) males and females will be produced. If secondary nondisjunction occurs (about 4% of the time), then $X^{bb} X^{bb}$ and Y^{bb+} eggs will be produced. When these eggs are fertilized by sperm from a bb male, the only viable progeny will be bb females ($X^{bb} X^{bb} Y^{bb}$) and bb^+ males ($X^{bb} Y^{bb+}$). This is diagrammed as follows:

		Normal Disjunction 1/m—96%		Secondary Nondisjunction—4%	
		48% $X^{bb} Y^{bb+}$	**48% X^{bb}**	**2% $X^{bb} X^{bb}$**	**2% Y^{bb+}**
Gametes of $X^{bb}Y^{bb}$ Male	50% X^{bb}	$X^{bb} X^{bb} Y^{bb+}$ bb^+ female 24%	$X^{bb} X^{bb}$ bb female 24%	$X^{bb} X^{bb} X^{bb}$ inviable 1%	$X^{bb} Y^{bb+}$ bb^+ male 1%
	50% Y^{bb}	$X^{bb} Y^{bb+} Y^{bb}$ bb^+ male 24%	$X^{bb} Y^{bb}$ bb male 24%	$X^{bb} X^{bb} Y^{bb}$ bb female 1%	YY inviable 1%

*(table heading above: **Gametes of $X^{bb} X^{bb} Y^{bb+}$ Female**)*

Among the viable progeny there will be $^{24}/_{98} = 24.5\%$ normal females, $^{24}/_{98} = 25.5\%$ bobbed females, $^{24}/_{98} = 25.5\%$ normal males, and $^{24}/_{98} = 24.5\%$ bobbed males.

12.39 *Answer:* None. Turner syndrome individuals are XO. They have only one X, so no X is inactivated.

12.40 *Answer:* All but one X chromosome is inactivated. An XXY individual, having two X chromosomes, has one inactivated.

12.41 *Answer:* Epigenetic phenomena are heritable changes in gene expression that occur without a change in DNA sequence. In female mammals, the inactivation of one of the two X chromosomes into a Barr body is an example of an epigenetic phenomenon: genes on the inactivated X chromosome are not expressed, and this change in gene expression is heritable within a somatic cell lineage once lyonization has occurred. Therefore, you can distinguish between genetic and epigenetic phenomena by determining whether or not a heritable change in gene expression is associated with a change in DNA sequence.

a. Epigenetic. Patch color in calico cats depends on which X has been inactivated, not a *de novo* DNA-based change. If the X bearing the *O* allele in an *Oo* individual has not been inactivated, the patch is orange, while if it has been inactivated, the patch is black.

b. Epigenetic. X-linked gene transcription in a *Drosophila* male increases relative to that in a female to provide for dosage compensation.

c. Genetic. The first curly-winged male has a new mutation. The trait is heritable and autosomal dominant, since crossing the curly-winged male to a normal female produces a 1:1 ratio of curly-winged and normal males and females.

d. Epigenetic. Since diethylstilbestrol is not positive in the Ames test, it does not increase tumor frequency by inducing DNA mutations.

e. Epigenetic. The *in utero* hormonal environment, not a DNA-based change, activates a pattern of gene expression in the XX animal that leads to male sexual characteristics.

f. Genetic. The cinnamon-colored-stripe phenotype shows crisscross inheritance, indicating that it is inherited as a sex-linked trait. The first cinnamon female has a new Z-linked recessive mutation.

12.42 *Answer:* This problem raises the issue that the precise mode of inheritance of a trait often cannot be determined when a pedigree is small and the frequency of the trait in a population is unknown. For example, Pedigree A could easily fit an autosomal dominant trait (*AA* and *Aa* = affected): The affected father would be heterozygous for the trait (*Aa*), the mother would be unaffected (*aa*), and half of their offspring would be affected. However, if the trait were autosomal recessive (i.e., *aa* = affected individuals) and the mother were heterozygous (*Aa*) and the father homozygous (*aa*), half of the offspring would still be affected. One could also fit the pedigree to an X-linked recessive trait: the mother would be heterozygous *Aa*, the father hemizygous *a*Y, and half of the progeny would be affected (either *aa* or *a*Y). An X-linked dominant trait would not fit the pedigree, because it would require all the daughters of the affected father to be affected (since they all receive their father's X) and not allow a son to be affected (since he does not receive his father's X). Pedigrees B and C can be solved by similar analytical reasoning.

	Pedigree A	Pedigree B	Pedigree C
Autosomal recessive	Yes	Yes	Yes
Autosomal dominant	Yes	Yes	No
X-linked recessive	Yes	Yes	No
X-linked dominant	No	No	No

12.43 *Answer:* If the trait were X-linked recessive, then II-5 should be affected because he would receive his mother's X chromosome. Therefore, the correct answer is **(c)**, II-5.

12.44 *Answer:*

a. Since unaffected parents have affected offspring, the trait shown in the pedigree must be recessive. Since only males and no parents are affected, Duchenne muscular dystrophy fits best to an X-linked recessive trait.

b. Since the trait is X-linked, heterozygous individuals must be female. Sons always receive their X chromosome from their mothers, so females who are heterozygous can have affected sons. Therefore, females who have affected sons must be heterozygous. I-1, II-2, and II-7 must be heterozygous.

c. For III-1 and III-2 to have an affected child, three events must occur: III-2 must be heterozygous ($P = 1/2$); III-2 must transmit the X bearing the Duchenne muscular dystrophy mutation ($P = 1/2$); and the child must be a male (the child receives a Y, and not a normal X, from the father, $P = 1/2$). Using the product rule, $P = (1/2)^3 = 1/8$.

d. $P = 0$, since neither parent carries the disease allele (assume that III-5 is homozygous for the normal allele).

12.45 *Answer:* Y-linked inheritance can be excluded because females are affected. X-linked recessive inheritance can also be excluded, because an affected mother (I-2) has a normal son (II-5). Autosomal recessive inheritance can also be excluded, because in such a case two affected parents, such as II-1 and II-2, could only have affected offspring, which they do not.

12.46   *Answer:*

    a. The trait must be recessive, since unaffected parents (I-1 and I-2, II-1 and II-2) have affected offspring. It also must be autosomal, since affected female daughters are born to unaffected fathers.

    b. Given the answer to **(a)**, individuals I-1 and I-2, as well as individuals II-1 and II-2, must be heterozygous. Also, individuals III-4 and III-5 must be heterozygous since they have an affected, homozygous mother.

    c. One can denote the parents of III-2 as $Aa \times Aa$. We know individual III-2 is $A-$, so she is either AA ($P = \frac{1}{3}$) or Aa ($P = \frac{2}{3}$).

    d. By the same reasoning described in **(c)**, individual III-3 has a $\frac{2}{3}$ chance of being Aa. The chance that he will contribute an a allele to his offspring is thus $\frac{2}{3} \times \frac{1}{2} = \frac{1}{3}$. The chance that individual III-4 will contribute an a allele to her offspring is $\frac{1}{2}$, since she is heterozygous. Thus, the chance that progeny of III-3 and III-4 will be affected is $\frac{1}{3} \times \frac{1}{2} = \frac{1}{6}$.

12.47   *Answer:* In complex pedigrees, an appropriate strategy is to ask initially whether the trait is Y-linked, then if it is dominant or recessive, and finally whether it is autosomal or X-linked. Proceeding logically through these choices helps limit the options. Before concluding, it is important to verify that the phenotype of every member of the pedigree fits the inferred inheritance pattern. Often, there may be only a single individual that can be used to distinguish one type of inheritance pattern from another.

    Pedigree A: Clearly, the trait is not Y-linked, because males are not the sole transmitters of the trait. The most striking aspect of this pedigree is that the trait skips generations (i.e., unaffected parents have affected offspring). This indicates that the trait must be recessive. Now, one is left to determine if it is autosomal or X-linked. It does not fit an X-linked pedigree, because two affected females have normal (albeit heterozygous) fathers. For X-linked recessive pedigrees, both parents must contribute an abnormal allele, so that affected daughters must have affected fathers. The trait is therefore autosomal recessive. (Check by assigning appropriate genotypes to each pedigree member.)

    Pedigree B: This pedigree also shows that the trait is not Y-linked, and must be recessive, because twice there are unaffected parents who have affected offspring. The preponderance of affected males suggests that it might be X-linked. To determine this for certain, try to assign genotypes to see if such an inheritance mode fits. It does. Could the trait be autosomal recessive? This would be a possibility if the trait were relatively common, since one would have to suppose that the individuals who married into the family in generation II were heterozygotes. This may be the case, because several homozygotes do marry into the family in generation III. What is the best guess then? X-linked recessive is the most likely, partly because of the frequency of affected males, but mostly because the homozygous female in generation III has three affected male offspring.

    Pedigree C: The trait is expressed in every generation, making it a good candidate for a dominant trait. It is expressed equally by males and females, making it a good candidate for an autosomal trait. Indeed, it must be autosomal, for two reasons: First, individuals III-5 and III-6 have unaffected daughters, which would not be possible if the trait were X-linked and dominant. Second, individual IV-2, a male, has an affected male offspring, which would not be possible if the trait were X-linked. Thus, the trait is autosomal dominant.

12.48   *Answer:* Answer **(a)** is untrue because if the affected father is heterozygous, only half of his offspring should be affected. Answer **(b)** is untrue because if the mother is heterozygous, half of her offspring, regardless of sex type, should be affected. Answer **(c)** is untrue because if the parents are each heterozygous, $\frac{1}{4}$ of their offspring should be homozygous recessive and normal. Answer **(d)** is the most likely. Note, however, that if the mutation was new in either the child or his or her parents, his or her grandparent could have been unaffected.

12.49   *Answer:* Answer **(a)** is true because two affected individuals will always have affected children ($aa \times aa$ can give only aa offspring). Answer **(b)** is untrue because an autosomal trait is inherited independent of sex type. Answer **(c)** need not be true, because the trait could be masked by normal dominant alleles through many generations before two heterozygotes marry and produce affected, homozygous offspring. Answer **(d)** could also be true. If the trait is rare, then it is likely that an unaffected individual marrying into the pedigree is homozygous for a normal allele. Since the trait is recessive, and the children receive the dominant, normal allele from the unaffected parent, the children will be normal. Answer **(d)** would not be true if the unaffected individual was heterozygous. In this case, half of the children would be affected.

12.50   *Answer:* The only untrue statement is **(d)**. Since daughters receive an X chromosome from each of their parents, they can inherit an X-linked dominant disease from either their mother or father.

12.51   *Answer:* Since hemophilia is an X-linked trait, the most likely explanation is that random inactivation of X chromosomes (lyonization) produces individuals with different proportions of cells with a functioning allele. Normal clotting times would be expected in females with a functional h^+ allele (i.e., females whose h-bearing X chromosome was very frequently inactivated). Clinical hemophilia would be expected in females without a functional h^+ allele (i.e., females whose h^+-bearing X chromosome was very frequently inactivated). Intermediate clotting times would be expected to be proportional to the amount of h^+ function, which is related to the frequency of inactivation of the h^+-bearing X chromosome.

12.52   *Answer:* Draw out the pedigree of the patient and try to assign genotypes to the relevant individuals. Let h represent the Hurler syndrome Type I allele. Then the patient is hh. Since we are told that Hurler syndrome patients virtually never reproduce, neither of her parents is expected to be hh. Still, in order for the patient to be hh, her parents must have both been Hh. (The cross was $Hh \times Hh$.) Since her brother is normal, he is $H-$, with a $\frac{2}{3}$ chance of being Hh. The brother's daughter has a half chance of receiving either of the brother's (H or h) alleles. Thus, the chance that the brother's daughter has an h allele is $\frac{2}{3} \times \frac{1}{2} = \frac{1}{3}$. Since the trait is extremely rare, it is likely she will marry an HH individual and have $H-$ children. Therefore, there is no chance the brother's daughter will have affected children, because her husband most likely will provide a dominant, normal H allele. Since Type I is autosomal, there will be no sex differences.

13

Extensions of and Deviations from Mendelian Genetic Principles

Chapter Outline

Review of Key Terms, Symbols, and Concepts

In your own words, write a brief, precise definition of each term in the groups below. Check your definitions using the text. Then develop a concept map using the terms in each list.

1	2	3
multiple alleles	dominance	extranuclear inheritance, gene
multiple allelic series	epistasis, epistatic	non-Mendelian inheritance, gene
wild-type allele	hypostasis, hypostatic	uniparental inheritance
complete dominance	dihybrid cross	maternal inheritance
complete recessiveness	dominant epistasis	paternal inheritance
incomplete dominance	recessive epistasis	biparental inheritance
semidominance	duplicate dominant epistasis	nuclear genotype
partial dominance	duplicate recessive epistasis	mitochondria
codominance	duplicate gene interaction	chloroplast
intermediate phenotype	complementary gene action	maternal effect
essential gene	complementation test	maternal effect gene
lethal allele	cis-trans test	dextral, sinistral coiling in
recessive lethal allele	modifier gene	*Limnaea peregra*
dominant lethal allele	suppressor gene	[poky] in *Neurospora crassa*
ABO blood group	9:3:3:1	protoperithecia
glycosyltransferases	9:6:1	cytohet
Bombay blood type	9:3:4	heteroplasmon, heteroplasmy
blood typing	9:7	Leber's hereditary optic
cellular antigen	12:3:1	neuropathy
antibody	13:3	Kearns–Sayre syndrome
agglutination	9:6:1	myoclonic epilepsy and ragged
universal donor, recipient	15:1	red fiber (MERRF) disease
H antigen, locus		heterosis
haplosufficient		heterozygote superiority
		genic, cytoplasmic male
		sterility
		controlled cross
		restorer of fertility (Rf) gene
		barnase, barnstar

4		
penetrance	hereditary trait	sex-influenced trait
expressivity	nature vs. nurture	sex-linked gene
population	norm of reaction	autosomal gene
individual	sex-limited trait	

Thinking Analytically

While the reasoning methods used in this chapter are not very different from those used in the earlier chapters on Mendelian genetics, there is much more information to consider. In this chapter, you learn how phenotypes are affected by multiple alleles, modifications of dominance relationships, gene interactions, internal and external environmental influences, maternal effects, modifier genes, and extranuclear inheritance. Hints about which factors contribute to a phenotype come from the analysis of inheritance patterns, so as you consider the text examples of each of these factors, consider how each reveals itself in the inheritance of a phenotype. In many situations, more than one factor influences a phenotype. Therefore, it is important to be able to recognize how factor influences a phenotype and how it is manifested in an inheritance pattern. If you suspect that different factors could contribute to a phenotype, start by *analyzing just one aspect of the phenotype*. Generate hypotheses about what factors could contribute to that phenotype, and evaluate whether the hypothesis is supported by the observed inheritance pattern.

Maternal effects are sometimes confused with extranuclear inheritance patterns, so it is important to keep the distinctions between them clear. Unlike extranuclear inheritance patterns that are controlled by extranuclear genes, maternal effects are controlled by nuclear genes. Extranuclear inheritance patterns show non-Mendelian inheritance. Usually, they are due to the extranuclear inheritance of mitochondrial or chloroplast genomes and show well-defined patterns of inheritance. In general, they follow from the cytoplasmic contributions of one (usually female) parent to the offspring. If you think that a maternal effect might be involved in the inheritance of a trait, diagram the generations of a cross and identify whether maternal contributions in the parental generation are important for the development of the phenotype in the progeny. Several of the problems in this chapter will help you discover how to distinguish a maternal effect from an extranuclear, maternally inherited trait.

Mutations at different genes can produce the same phenotype, so once a set of mutations with a particular phenotype has been identified, it is important to identify how many genes are affected in that set of mutations. This can be determined by using complementation tests. In a complementation test, two mutations with the same phenotype are crossed and the phenotype of the progeny is observed. If the two mutations affect different genes, complementation occurs and the progeny are wild type. In this case, the progeny are heterozygous for each mutation and the normal allele at each gene ensures wild-type progeny. If the mutations affect the same gene, no normal allele is present, the mutations will not complement each other, and the progeny will have a mutant phenotype. Complementation tests are elegant and quick ways to organize sets of mutations by the genes they affect: cross pairs of mutants and observe the phenotype of their progeny.

This chapter introduces many terms describing phenotypes that are applied contextually. As geneticists discover additional factors that affect a phenotype, the phenotype is often described in different, more revealing ways. For example, when a disease is first observed, it may be described only in terms of its inheritance pattern—say, as a dominantly inherited trait. As more is learned about the disease, its phenotype will be reassessed in light of the new knowledge. Consequently, as more is understood, different labels will be applied to the disease phenotype. These labels will indicate the kind and degree of interaction that occurs within a set of alleles at one gene (e.g., the types of dominance relationships), between several alleles at more than one gene (e.g., the types of epistasis or the effects of modifier genes), and between genetic and environmental influences (e.g., the level of penetrance and/or expressivity). Although complex, these labels are very useful: they quickly convey a coherent, informative description of the phenotype.

The major message of this chapter is that phenotypes can be affected by many factors. These factors include the set of alleles an organism inherits as well as the environment(s) in which it develops and lives.

Questions for Practice

Multiple-Choice Questions

1. In clover leaves, chevron pattern (a light-colored triangular leaf pattern) is controlled by seven different alleles at a single gene. From this information alone, what can be said about this trait?
   a. Alleles at this gene show incomplete dominance.
   b. There is a multiple allelic series with seven alleles that controls chevron pattern.
   c. This gene shows epistasis.
   d. One allele at this gene must be completely dominant.

2. The phenotype associated with a wild-type allele of a particular gene is
   a. the phenotype that is always found in nature.
   b. a reference phenotype used by geneticists for comparison.
   c. a special mutant phenotype.
   d. the most common phenotype seen.

3. In general, extranuclear genes show
   a. dominance.
   b. Mendelian inheritance.
   c. maternal effects.
   d. maternal inheritance.

4. Neurofibromatosis is a dominantly inherited disease that can show mild, moderate, or severe symptoms. Every individual that inherits the dominant allele shows at least mild symptoms. This means that the disease allele shows
   a. variable penetrance and complete expressivity.
   b. variable expressivity and complete penetrance.
   c. variable penetrance and variable expressivity.
   d. complete penetrance and complete expressivity.

5. Two alleles at the *white* locus in *Drosophila melanogaster* are $w^{apricot}$, which has orange-colored eyes, and w^{coral}, which has pink-colored eyes. This is an example of
   a. codominance.
   b. a multiple allelic series.
   c. penetrance.
   d. epistasis.

6. One difference between epistasis and dominance is that
   a. epistasis occurs between two different genes while dominance occurs between alleles at one gene.
   b. only epistasis is influenced by environmental interactions.
   c. dominant traits are completely penetrant, while epistatic interactions may not be.
   d. dominant traits may show variable penetrance, while epistatic interactions may not.

For questions 7, 8, 9, and 10, choose the form of inheritance that best explains the data. Explain your choices.
   a. recessive lethal allele
   b. dominant lethal allele
   c. incomplete dominance; two allelic pairs
   d. duplicate recessive epistasis; two allelic pairs
   e. dominant epistasis; two allelic pairs

7. When crossed, two pure-breeding varieties of white kernel corn yield progeny with purple kernels. When these purple progeny are selfed, a count of the kernels in the F_2 yields an average of 270 purple kernels : 210 white kernels per ear.

8. When pure-breeding wheat with red kernels is crossed to the pure-breeding white variety, the progeny have pink kernels. One hundred F_2 plants exhibit the following phenotypes: 6 red, 25 dark pink, 38 pink, 25 light pink, 6 white.

9. Yellow mice crossed to pure-breeding agouti mice produce a 50:50 ratio of yellow to agouti offspring. Crosses between yellow mice never produce 100% yellow progeny, but rather yield 36 yellow and 15 agouti offspring.

10. At age 52, a man begins to show the symptoms of Huntington disease. Like his mother before him, he eventually dies from the disease. His wife is normal and there is no history of the disease in his wife's family or his father's family. Two of his four children also die from the disease, albeit not until late in their lives.

11. Which one of the following statements about complementation is *true*?
   a. Two mutants that complement each other affect the same gene.
   b. In a complementation test, two mutants are crossed together and the progeny phenotype is assessed. If the progeny phenotype is normal, the two mutants complement each other.
   c. Complementation tests can be used to determine whether dominant mutations affect the same function.
   d. Alleles at the same gene will complement each other.

12. Six independently isolated mutations (*a–f*) all result in yellow tomatoes and are recessive to the normal red color. When different pairs of homozygous mutants are crossed, all produce plants bearing yellow tomatoes except for pairs involving mutation *c*. When *cc* plants are crossed to any of the other strains, progeny plants produce red tomatoes. Based on these observations, which one of the following statements is *not* true?
    a. The six mutations affect six different genes.
    b. Mutations *a, b, d, e,* and *f* are alleles at the same gene.
    c. A complementation test was performed.
    d. Mutation *c* affects a different gene than do mutations *a, b, d, e,* and *f.*
    e. Mutations *a, b, d, e,* and *f* are members of a multiple allelic series at one gene.

13. DNA is found in
    a. the nucleus of eukaryotes.
    b. mitochondria.
    c. chloroplasts.
    d. all subcellular organelles.
    e. a, b, and c only

14. Which of the following is *not* a typical characteristic of extranuclear traits?
    a. They show uniparental inheritance.
    b. They cannot be mapped relative to nuclear genes.
    c. They show non-Mendelian segregation in crosses.
    d. They are affected by substitution of a nucleus with a different genotype.

15. Two brothers have a hereditary disease associated with a particular lesion in mitochondrial DNA. One brother is more severely affected than the other. Which of the following is *not* a plausible explanation for this observation?
    a. The brothers have different degrees of heteroplasmy.
    b. The brothers have different proportions of two mitochondrial types.
    c. The brothers do not have identical nuclear genomes.
    d. Different mitochondrial genes are affected in the two brothers.

16. Which of the following crosses is most useful for generating hybrid seed?
    a. female [*CMS*] *rf/rf* × male [*CMS*] *Rf/rf*
    b. male [*CMS*] *rf/rf* × female [*CMS*] *Rf/rf*
    c. female [*CMS*] *Rf/Rf* × male [*CMS*] *rf/rf*
    d. male [*CMS*] *Rf/Rf* × female [*CMS*] *rf/rf*

Answers: 1b, 2b, 3d, 4b, 5b, 6a, 7d, 8c, 9a, 10b, 11b, 12a, 13e, 14d, 15d, 16a

Thought Questions

1. Distinguish between dominance and epistasis and between epistasis and multiple alleles.
2. How would you distinguish whether a complex mutant phenotype was caused by one gene or alleles at several genes? (Hint: Review independent assortment.)
3. Tay–Sachs disease is fatal due to a lack of the enzyme hexoaminidase A. Phenotypically normal heterozygotes have about half as much enzyme activity as do homozygotes for the normal allele. In what sense do alleles at the gene affected in Tay–Sachs disease show incomplete dominance, codominance, and recessive lethality?
4. A sex-linked gene controls coat color in cats. One allele determines black coat color while another allele determines orange coat color. A separate set of genes determines where color is produced (i.e., where white patches are). Use this information to explain why most calico (black-, orange-, and white-patched) cats are female. How do rare calico males arise? Do you expect them to be fertile?
5. In a very large natural population, could you ever presume to know all the allelic variants in a multiple allelic series? (Hint: Could new variants appear at any time?)
6. Devise a situation in which a multiple allelic series shows elements of codominance as well as dominant lethality.
7. Could a lethal allele, either dominant or recessive, be incompletely penetrant? (Hint: Consider small variations in the timing of events during development.)

8. As we discussed in Chapter 9, single nucleotide polymorphisms (SNPs) are very common, about one per several hundred base pairs of DNA. What does this tell you about the number of alleles that exist at one gene in a population? Do you expect the allelic differences to always show clear patterns of dominance or recessiveness relative to a "wild-type" allele?

9. Some traits are influenced by many genes as well as by the environment. How might you identify genes influencing such a trait? How would you then analyze the epistatic relationships between the genes influencing such a trait?

10. What different explanations are there for a trait to be incompletely penetrant? What approaches can be devised to test these explanations?

11. How might molecular methods be employed to analyze a maternal line of descent? (See text Box 13.1, p. 387.) How might this be useful to trace movements of populations over time? Do any significant complications arise because of paternal contributions to mtDNA inheritance?

12. Distinguish between biparental and uniparental inheritance. Which organisms have organelles that show biparental inheritance?

13. Why is it useful to develop male-sterile crops? How does the strategy for developing these types of plants using CMS differ from a strategy that employs nuclear transgenes?

14. How do you account for the maternal effect in shell coiling in the snail *Limnaea peregra*? What features of this phenomenon indicate that it is controlled by a maternal effect and not by extranuclear inheritance?

Thought Questions for Media

After reviewing the media on the *iGenetics* website, try to answer these questions.

1. Based on viewing the animation on incomplete dominance and codominance, give an example where neither of two alleles at a gene is dominant or recessive. Using the alleles of your example, write the genotypes of a cross whose progeny show identical genotypic and phenotypic ratios. What type of dominance relationship is shown by these two alleles?

2. Correct the following false statement: "In incomplete dominance, a heterozygous individual exhibits the phenotype of both homozygotes."

3. Based on viewing the animation on incomplete dominance and codominance, give an example of a situation where two dominant alleles are fully expressed at the same time. Using the alleles of your example, write the genotypes of a cross whose progeny show identical genotypic and phenotypic ratios. What type of dominance relationship is shown by these two alleles?

4. Suppose you are able to show that a cross of two heterozygotes gives progeny in 1:2:1 genotypic and phenotypic ratios. What additional information do you need to distinguish between incomplete dominance and codominance?

5. In the animation describing maternal effects, dextral (right-handed) coiling is dominant to sinistral (left-handed) coiling. However, the coiling pattern is determined by the maternal contribution, not the genotype of the zygote. Suppose you had a population of *Dd* dextral snails.
   a. What crosses would you do to obtain a *Dd* sinistral snail? (Remember that you can determine only the coiling phenotype in progeny and must infer progeny genotypes by testcrossing or selfing!)
   b. What crosses would you do to obtain a *dd* sinistral snail?
   c. Could you ever obtain a *DD* sinistral snail?

6. How does maternal effect differ from maternal inheritance, since both can involve cytoplasmic contributions from the mother?

1. In the modern courtroom, blood type tests can be used to exclude paternity, but it has become more difficult to use them convincingly to demonstrate paternity.
   a. Should the blood type tests have excluded Charlie Chaplin from paternity of Carol Ann? Why or why not?
   b. Suppose a defendant who is the alleged father takes a blood type test that does not exclude him from paternity consideration. What arguments might the lawyer of the defendant make in a modern courtroom to support the exclusion of the test results as "compelling" evidence? (Assume the tests are done correctly.)

   c. As mentioned in the iActivity *Was She Charlie Chaplin's Child?*, an individual of type A blood can be either homozygous or heterozygous. Suppose a blood typing test allowed these two genetic conditions to be distinguished. Based on what you inferred about the ABO blood types of Joan and Carol Ann Berry in the iActivity, and supposing that you could identify their exact blood types, can you now predict the exact blood type of the father?

2. Why is it helpful to use both the M-N and the ABO blood group tests, instead of just one alone? Would a third blood type test be even more useful, or are two enough?

3. The iActivity on mitochondrial DNA and human disease provided data indicating that individuals with MERFF show one or more symptoms that can include hearing loss, dementia, muscle jumps, seizures, unsteadiness, vision problems, and loss of cognitive skills.

   a. How would you characterize MERFF in terms of penetrance and expressivity?

   b. Based on what you know about the mode of inheritance of MERFF, what hypotheses can you form to explain its symptomatic variability?

   c. How could you use methods similar to those presented in the iActivity to test your hypotheses?

4. The iActivity on mitochondrial DNA and human disease presented data that allowed you to distinguish between heteroplasmic maternal inheritance and autosomal dominant inheritance with variable expressivity.

   a. What methods were used in the iActivity to distinguish between these modes of inheritance?

   b. Would it ever be possible to distinguish these modes of inheritance based on pedigree analysis alone?

   c. What challenges does mitochondrial inheritance present for the analysis of pedigrees?

5. Suppose a MERFF-like disorder was caused by a mutation in a nuclear gene whose product was imported into the mitochondrion. What types of inheritance might be associated with this disorder?

Solutions to Text Questions and Problems

13.1   *Answer:*

a. All agouti

b. ¾ agouti, ¼ chinchilla

c. ¾ agouti, ¼ albino

d. ½ agouti, ½ Himalayan

e. ½ agouti, ½ Himalayan

13.2   *Answer:* Six genotypes are possible: w/w, w/w^1, w/w^2, w^1/w^1, w^1/w^2, w^2/w^2.

13.3   *Answer:*

a. Yes, if both parents were $I^A i$.

b. Yes, if the A parent were $I^A i$ and the B parent were $I^B i$.

c. No, as neither parent has an I^B allele.

d. No, since an O child must obtain an i allele from each parent, and one parent is $I^A I^B$.

e. Yes, providing that the B parent is $I^B i$ (and the child is $I^A i$).

13.4   *Answer:* d. If both parents are M, an MN child is impossible because neither has an N allele. An A child is possible if the mother contributes I^A and the father contributes i.

13.5   *Answer:* First determine the genotypes of the parents. The mother is type AB, so she must have the genotype $I^A I^B$. The father is type A, so he must have at least one I^A allele. The grandfather was type O, so he only had i alleles. Therefore the cross must be $I^A I^B \times I^A i$. The four equally likely genotypes ($I^A I^A$, $I^A i$, $I^B I^A$, $I^B i$) give rise to three phenotypes: A ($P = ½$), AB ($P = ¼$), or B ($P = ¼$).

a. The chance that two children will both be group A is $½ \times ½ = ¼$.

b. There is no chance of producing an O child, so $P = 0$.

c. The chance of a male AB child is $½ \times ¼ = ⅛$. The chance of a male B child is $½ \times ¼ = ⅛$. Therefore the chance of both events happening is $⅛ \times ⅛ = 1/64$. The first event is independent of the second, so this is the chance of the events happening in the order specified.

13.6   *Answer:*

a. The cross is $C^R C^R \times C^W C^W$; the F_1 are all $C^R C^W$ and are pink.

b. The F_2 will be 1 $C^R C^R$: 2 $C^R C^W$: 1 $C^W C^W$ and be 1 red : 2 pink : 1 white.

c. $C^R C^W \times C^R C^R$ produces ½ $C^R C^R$ (red) and ½ $C^R C^W$ (pink) progeny.

d. $C^R C^W \times C^W C^W$ produces ½ $C^R C^W$ (pink) and ½ $C^W C^W$ (white) progeny.

13.7   *Answer:* A cross between two roan cattle can be denoted as $C^R C^W \times C^R C^W$. The progeny will be ¼ $C^R C^R$, ½ $C^R C^W$, and ¼ $C^W C^W$. Thus, half will be roan progeny.

13.8   *Answer:* The initial cross can be diagrammed as $L- C^Y C^W \times ll\ C^W C^W$. As a long-haired cream baby ($ll\ C^Y C^W$) is produced, one can infer that the short-haired parent must have been Ll. The backcross can be diagrammed as $ll\ C^Y C^W \times Ll\ C^Y C^W$. There will be ⅛ short-haired yellow, ¼ short-haired cream, ⅛ short-haired white, ⅛ long-haired yellow, ¼ long-haired cream, and ⅛ long-haired white progeny.

13.9   *Answer:* The cross can be diagrammed as $S^L/S^L\ C^R/C^R \times S^S/S^S\ C^W/C^W$. The F_1 will be oval and purple ($S^L/S^S\ C^R/C^W$). The F_2 consists of $1/16$ long red ($S^L/S^L\ C^R/C^R$), ⅛ oval red ($S^L/S^S\ C^R/C^R$), $1/16$ round red ($S^S/S^S\ C^R/C^R$), ⅛ long purple ($S^L/S^L\ C^R/C^W$), ¼ oval purple ($S^L/S^S\ C^R/C^W$), ⅛ round purple ($S^S/S^S\ C^R/C^W$), $1/16$ long white ($S^L/S^L\ C^W/C^W$), ⅛ oval white ($S^L/S^S\ C^W/C^W$), and $1/16$ round white ($S^S/S^S\ C^W/C^W$).

14.24 *Answer:*

    a. $a\,b^+\,c$ and $a^+\,b\,c^+$ (least frequent).

    b. $a^+\,b\,c$ and $a\,b^+\,c^+$ (most frequent).

    c. locus c (see solution to Question 14.22 for a method to determine the middle locus).

14.25 *Answer:* The differential appearance of the traits in males and females indicates that the traits are sex-linked (i.e., they are X-linked). The female progeny are normal, since they received their father's X chromosome, which was $a^+\,b^+\,c^+$. Because they are phenotypically normal, they are not helpful in a mapping analysis. The male progeny received an X chromosome from the mother, and therefore they can be used to analyze the results of recombination in the mother.

    The most frequent progeny classes in the males are $a^+\,b\,c$ and $a\,b^+\,c^+$. These are the parental-type chromosomes. The least frequent classes (the double-crossover classes) are $a^+\,b^+\,c^+$ and $a\,b\,c$. Comparison of these two classes indicates that gene a is in the middle, and the correct order is $b\text{–}a\text{–}c$ (or $c\text{–}a\text{–}b$) (see solution to Question 14.22). The parental cross (with the correct gene order) was $c\,a^+\,b/c^+\,a\,b^+$ (female) $\times$ $a^+\,b^+\,c/Y$ (male). Now analyze the data to determine which progeny classes result from crossing-over in each gene interval and calculate the recombination frequencies in each interval (sco = single crossover; dco = double crossover).

Gamete Genotype	Number	Class
$c\ a^+\ b$	839	parental
$c^+\ a\ b^+$	825	parental
$c^+\ a\ b$	86	sco ($a - b$)
$c\ a^+\ b^+$	90	sco ($a - b$)
$c\ a\ b^+$	81	sco ($c - a$)
$c^+\ a^+\ b$	75	sco ($c - a$)
$c\ a\ b$	1	dco ($a - b, c - a$)
$c^+\ a^+\ b^+$	3	dco ($a - b, c - a$)
Total	2,000	

    Note that, since recombination cannot be scored in the female progeny, and only the 2,000 male progeny are being considered, the total that is used as the divisor in the calculation of recombination frequency (RF) is 2,000.

$$\text{RF } (a - b) = [(86 + 90 + 1 + 3)/2{,}000] \times 100\% = 9.0\%$$
$$\text{RF } (c - a) = [(81 + 75 + 1 + 3)/2{,}000] \times 100\% = 8.0\%$$

With this information, draw the following map:

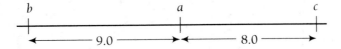

To calculate the coefficient of coincidence (c.o.c.), compare the frequency of actual double crossovers to that expected based on the crossover frequency observed in each interval.

    c.o.c = observed dco frequency/expected dco frequency

        = $[(3 + 1)/2{,}000]/(0.09 \times 0.08)$

        = $0.002/0.0072$

        = 0.28

14.26 *Answer:*

    a. There are 20 map units between j and b, so there will be 20% recombinant-type and 80% parental-type gametes. In a $J\,B/j\,b$ parent, $j\,b$ gametes are half of the parental-type gametes, or 40% of the total gametes.

b. There are 65 map units between *A* and *M,* so these loci will show independent assortment because the frequency of recombinant-type gametes cannot exceed 50%. In an *a M/A m* parent, the *A M* gametes are half of the recombinant-type gametes. There will be 25% *A M* gametes.

c. In a *j B d/J b D* individual, *J B D* gametes are produced by a double crossover: a crossover in the interval *j – b* and a crossover in the interval *b – d*. Since there are 20 map units between *j* and *b* and 10 map units between *b* and *d,* the frequency of double crossovers is expected to be 0.20 × 0.10 × 100% = 2%. *J B D* gametes are half of the double crossovers produced, so will be seen 1% of the time.

d. In a *j B d/J b D* individual, *J B d* gametes are one-half of the gametes produced by a single crossover in the interval *j – b*. Since there are 20 map units between these genes, 10% of the gametes will be *J B d*.

e. By the reasoning in **(c)**, *j b d* gametes will be seen 1% of the time in a *j B d/J b D* individual. To obtain a *j b d/j b d* genotype, one must obtain such gametes from both parents. The frequency of this is (0.01 × 0.01) × 100% = 0.01%.

f. Based on the map distances, one expects 10% recombination between *a* and *k* and 50% recombination between *k* and *f*. (Again, note that even though *k* and *f* are more than 50 map units apart, one observes only 50% recombination between these two genes.) In an *A K F/a k f* individual, an *A k F* gamete results from a double crossover: one crossover between *a* and *k* (10% chance) and one crossover between *k* and *f* (50% chance). The chance of both crossovers occurring simultaneously is 0.10 × 0.50 = 0.05, or 5%. Since *A k F* gametes are half of the double crossovers produced, they will be 2.5% of the total.

14.27   *Answer:* First, consider what happens when a female that is heterozygous for an X-linked lethal is crossed to a normal male. One can diagram such a cross as:

P: *l/l⁺* female × *l⁺/Y* male

F₁: females: *l/l⁺* and *l⁺/l⁺* (phenotypically normal)
       males: *l⁺/Y* (normal) and *l/Y* (dead, not recovered)

In such a cross, one-half of the male progeny are not recovered due to the presence of the lethal allele. Only progeny bearing the *l⁺* allele are recovered. Thus, the 499 males that are recovered in this cross are half of the expected male progeny.

Second, consider that the lethal-bearing chromosome can be recovered in the female progeny. Since the lethal allele is a recessive mutation, it is "rescued" by the normal *l⁺* allele contributed to the female progeny by the father's X chromosome. However, because the father's X chromosome bears the + alleles of each gene, the females are phenotypically normal and are not helpful in a recombination analysis.

Now, analyze the phenotypes of the male progeny that are recovered to infer map distances and the gene order. Since one-half of the male progeny are not recovered, each of the four classes seen represents one of the two reciprocal classes of progeny recovered in a three-point cross. Include the third (*l/l⁺*) locus and assign each genotype to a progeny class based on its frequency:

Male progeny:	405	*a b⁺ l⁺* parental type
	44	*a⁺ b l⁺* single crossover
	48	*a⁺ b⁺ l⁺* single crossover
	2	*a b⁺ l⁺* double crossover

Comparison of the parental and double-crossover classes indicates that *b* is in the middle, and the correct order is *a–b–l* (see solution to Question 14.22 for determining the middle locus). Since one of the parental-type chromosomes was *a b⁺ l⁺,* the other must have been *a⁺ b l,* the reciprocal. The heterozygous female was therefore *a b⁺ c⁺/a⁺ b l.*

The 44 *a⁺ b l⁺* progeny are obtained from gametes arising from single crossovers between *b* and *l*. They are half of the total single crossovers in that interval. The other half were not recovered, because they bore the *l* allele. Similarly, the 48 *a⁺ b⁺ l⁺* progeny are half of the single crossovers in the interval $a - b$. This information can be used to calculate recombination frequencies (RF) and draw a map.

$$RF\ (a - b) = [(48 + 2)/499] \times 100\% = 10\%$$
$$RF\ (b - l) = [(44 + 2)/499] \times 100\% = 9.2\%$$

14.28   *Answer:* Since the male parent is triply recessive, the phenotypes associated with the female parent's gametes will be evident equally in males and females. The map distances between the loci give the frequency of recombinants (i.e., crossovers) in each gene interval. There will be 14% recombinants in the $a - c$ interval (7% each of $a\ c$ and $a^+\ c^+$), and 12% recombinants in the $c - b$ interval (6% each of $c^+\ b$ and $c\ b$). These recombinants will be distributed between both single- and double-crossover classes.

The coefficient of coincidence gives the percentage of expected double crossovers that are observed. The expected double crossovers can be calculated based on the recombination frequency in each of the two gene intervals, and is $(0.12 \times 0.14) \times 100\% = 1.68\%$. Since the coefficient of coincidence is 0.3, only 30% of the expected double crossovers are observed, or $1.68\% \times 30\% = 0.50\%$ (0.25% each of $a\ c\ b$ and $a^+\ c^+\ b^+$).

The remaining recombinants will be single-crossover classes. This can be calculated by considering that some of the crossovers in each gene interval contribute to the double-crossover classes, and each double crossover has a crossover in each gene interval. This means the frequency of single crossovers in each gene interval is equal to the difference between the frequency of crossovers in that interval and the frequency of double crossovers. Consequently, there will be $14\% - 0.5\% = 13.5\%$ single crossovers in the $a - c$ interval (6.75% each $a\ c\ b^+$ and $a^+\ c^+\ b$), and $12\% - 0.5\% = 11.5\%$ single crossovers in the $c - b$ interval (5.75% each $a\ c^+\ b^+$ and $a^+\ c\ b$).

The remaining progeny $[100\% - (13.5\% + 11.5\% + 0.5\%) = 74.5\%]$ will be parental types (37.25% $a\ c^+\ b$ and 37.25% $a^+\ c\ b^+$). The types or progeny are therefore:

Genotype	Percent	Number
$a\ c^+\ b$	37.25	745
$a^+\ c\ b^+$	37.25	745
$a\ c\ b^+$	6.75	135
$a^+\ c^+\ b$	6.75	135
$a\ c^+\ b^+$	5.75	115
$a^+\ c\ b$	5.75	115
$a\ c\ b$	0.25	5
$a^+\ c^+\ b^+$	0.25	5

14.29   *Answer:* The crosses under consideration are:

P: $h\ le\ Ch/h\ le\ Ch \times H\ Le\ ch/H\ Le\ ch$

F_1: $h\ le\ Ch/H\ Le\ ch \times h\ le\ ch/h\ le\ ch$

To be profitable, the farmer needs 25% of the progeny to be either $h\ le\ ch/h\ le\ ch$ or $H\ le\ ch/h\ le\ ch$. Hence, he is concerned with the probability of obtaining an $h\ le\ ch$ or an $H\ le\ ch$ gamete from an $h\ le\ Ch/H\ Le\ ch$ individual. Gametes that are $h\ le\ ch$ arise from a single crossover between le and ch. Since there are 32 mu between le and ch, there will be 16% $h\ le\ ch$ individuals (one-half of the recombinants between le and ch). Gametes that are $H\ le\ ch$ arise from a crossover in each interval. Since there is no interference, their frequency will be half of the expected double-crossover frequency, or $(0.5 \times 0.32 \times 0.26) \times 100\% = 4.16\%$. The expected frequency of $h\ le\ ch$ and $H\ le\ ch$ gametes is $4.16\% + 16\% = 20.16\%$. The farmer should stop breeding and cut his losses.

14.30   *Answer:* Since all of the genes have a dominant phenotype, and crosses are made to a homozygous recessive strain, the data can be analyzed as a series of two-point testcrosses as shown in the following table:

Cross	Genes Involved	# Recombinants Total	Recombination Frequency (%)	Apparent Map Distance
1	*Fu, Ki*	2/200	1	1 mu
2	*Fu, H-2*	8/200	4	4 mu
3	*T, H-2*	300/2,500	12	12 mu
4	*Fu, T*	24/300	8	8 mu

Two maps are consistent with these data.

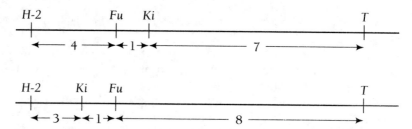

14.31   *Answer:*

a.   Approach this problem by considering two genes at a time. Then one has:

Gene Pair	# Parental-Type Progeny	# Recombinant-Type Progeny	Recombination Frequency (%)	Linked?
a,b	902	98	9.8	yes
a,c	973	27	2.7	yes
a,d	957	43	4.3	yes
a,e	497	503	50.0	no
b,c	875	125	12.5	yes
b,d	945	55	5.5	yes
b,e	497	503	50.0	no
c,d	930	70	7.0	yes
c,e	498	502	50.0	no
d,e	496	504	50.0	no

The genes *a, b, c,* and *d* are linked, while *e* is unlinked to the other four genes. Use the smallest distances as the most accurate map distances. One has:

b.   Rewrite the parental cross using the correct gene order:

$$\frac{b^+ \; d \;\; a^+ \; c}{b \;\; d^+ \; a \;\; c^+} \;\; \frac{e}{e^+} \;\; \times \;\; \frac{b\,d\,a\,c}{b\,d\,a\,c} \;\; \frac{e}{e}$$

To obtain a $b^+ \; d^+ \; a^+ \; c^+$ fly, there must be crossovers between *b* and *d, d* and *a,* and *a* and *c.* Two reciprocal crossovers will be found: one-half of the progeny will be $b^+ \; d^+ \; a^+ \; c^+$ and one-half of the progeny will be *b d a c.* Among these progeny, one-half will be e^+ and one-half will be *e.*

$$P(b^+ \; d^+ \; a^+ \; c^+ \; e^+) = P(\text{triple crossover}) \times 1/2 \times 1/2$$
$$= (0.055 \times 0.043 \times 0.027) \times 0.25$$
$$= 1.6 \times 10^{-5}.$$

14.32 *Answer:*

a. The cross is $w\ cho^+/w\ cho^+$ (white female) $\times\ w^+\ cho^+/Y$ (chocolate male), and the F_1 females are $w\ cho^+/w^+\ cho$ (red). Since the w and cho genes are 11.5 map units apart, the F_1 females will have 11.5% recombinant-type gametes (5.75% each $w^+\ cho^+$ and $w\ cho$) and 88.5% parental-type gametes (44.25% each $w\ cho^+$ and $w^+\ cho$). When these gametes are combined with those of wild-type (50% each $w^+\ cho^+$ and Y) or white-eyed (50% each $w\ cho^+$ and Y) males, one obtains the progeny shown in the following branch diagrams.

Cross: $w\ cho^+/w^+\ cho \times w^+\ cho^+/Y$

Gametes of		
$w\ cho^+/w^+\ cho$	$w^+\ cho^+/Y$	Progeny

0.4425 $w\ cho^+$
- 0.5 $w^+\ cho^+$ ⟶ 0.22125 $w\ cho^+/w^+\ cho^+$ (red female)
- 0.5 Y ⟶ 0.22125 $w\ cho^+/Y$ (white male)

0.4425 $w^+\ cho$
- 0.5 $w^+\ cho^+$ ⟶ 0.22125 $w^+\ cho/w^+\ cho^+$ (red female)
- 0.5 Y ⟶ 0.22125 $w^+\ cho/Y$ (chocolate male)

0.0575 $w^+\ cho^+$
- 0.5 $w^+\ cho^+$ ⟶ 0.02875 $w^+\ cho^+/w^+\ cho^+$ (red female
- 0.5 Y ⟶ 0.02875 $w^+\ cho^+/Y$ (red male)

0.0575 $w\ cho$
- 0.5 $w^+\ cho^+$ ⟶ 0.02875 $w\ cho/w^+\ cho^+$ (red female)
- 0.5 Y ⟶ 0.02875 $w\ cho/Y$ (white male)

Result: 50% red females   2.875% red males
25% white males
22.125% chocolate males

Cross: $w\ cho^+/w^+\ cho \times w\ cho^+/Y$

Gametes of		
$w\ cho^+/w^+\ cho$	$w\ cho^+/Y$	Progeny

0.4425 $w\ cho^+$
- 0.5 $w\ cho^+$ ⟶ 0.22125 $w\ cho^+/w\ cho^+$ (white female)
- 0.5 Y ⟶ 0.22125 $w\ cho^+/Y$ (white male)

0.4425 $w^+\ cho$
- 0.5 $w\ cho^+$ ⟶ 0.22125 $w^+\ cho/w\ cho^+$ (red female)
- 0.5 Y ⟶ 0.22125 $w^+\ cho/Y$ (chocolate male)

0.0575 $w^+\ cho^+$
- 0.5 $w\ cho^+$ ⟶ 0.02875 $w^+\ cho^+/w\ cho^+$ (red female)
- 0.5 Y ⟶ 0.02875 $w^+\ cho^+/Y$ (red male)

0.0575 $w\ cho$
- 0.5 $w\ cho^+$ ⟶ 0.02875 $w\ cho/w\ cho^+$ (white female)
- 0.5 Y ⟶ 0.02875 $w\ cho/Y$ (white male)

Result: 25% red females   2.875% red males
25% white females   25% white males
22.125% chocolate males

b. The initial cross is $w\ cho^+/Y;\ st^+/st^+ \times w^+\ cho/w^+\ cho;\ st/st$ with F_1 females being $w\ cho^+/w^+\ cho;$ st^+/st. These trihybrid females will have eight types of gametes: 88.5% will be parental types [22.125% each of $(w\ cho^+;\ st^+)$, $(w\ cho^+;\ st)$, $(w^+\ cho;\ st^+)$, $(w^+\ cho;\ st)$], and 11.5% will be recombinants between w and cho [2.875% each of $(w^+\ cho^+;\ st^+)$, $(w^+\ cho^+;\ st)$, $(w\ cho;\ st^+)$, $(w\ cho;\ st)$]. The results obtained when the F_1 female is crossed to a true-breeding scarlet male [with $(w^+\ cho^+;\ st)$ and $(Y;\ st)$ gametes] are shown in the following branch diagrams:

Cross: $w\ cho^+/w^+\ cho;\ st/st^+ \times w^+\ cho^+/Y;\ st/st$

Gametes of

$w\ cho^+/w^+\ cho;\ st/st^+$	$w^+\ cho^+/Y;\ st/st$	Progeny
0.2215 $w\ cho^+;\ st^+$	0.5 $w^+\ cho^+;\ st$	0.110625 $w\ cho^+/w^+\ cho;\ st^+\ st$ (red female)
	0.5 $Y;\ st$	0.110625 $w\ cho^+/Y;\ st^+\ st$ (white male)
0.2215 $w\ cho^+;\ st$	0.5 $w^+\ cho^+;\ st$	0.110625 $w\ cho^+/w^+\ cho;\ st/st$ (scarlet female)
	0.5 $Y;\ st$	0.110625 $w\ cho^+/Y;\ st/st$ (white male)
0.2215 $w^+\ cho;\ st^+$	0.5 $w^+\ cho^+;\ st$	0.110625 $w^+\ cho/w^+\ cho^+;\ st^+\ st$ (red female)
	0.5 $Y;\ st$	0.110625 $w^+\ cho/Y;\ st^+\ st$ (chocolate male)
0.2215 $w^+\ cho;\ st$	0.5 $w^+\ cho^+;\ st$	0.110625 $w^+\ cho/w^+\ cho^+;\ st/st$ (scarlet female)
	0.5 $Y;\ st$	0.110625 $w^+\ cho/Y;\ st/st$ (white male)
0.02875 $w^+\ cho^+;\ st^+$	0.5 $w^+\ cho^+;\ st$	0.014375 $w^+\ cho^+/w^+\ cho^+;\ st^+\ st$ (red female)
	0.5 $Y;\ st$	0.014375 $w^+\ cho^+/Y;\ st^+\ st$ (red male)
0.02875 $w^+\ cho^+;\ st$	0.5 $w^+\ cho^+;\ st$	0.014375 $w^+\ cho^+/w^+\ cho^+;\ st/st$ (scarlet female)
	0.5 $Y;\ st$	0.014375 $w^+\ cho^+/Y;\ st/st$ (scarlet male)
00.02875 $w\ cho;\ st^+$	0.5 $w^+\ cho^+;\ st$	0.014375 $w\ cho/w^+\ cho^+;\ st^+\ st$ (red female)
	0.5 $Y;\ st$	0.014375 $w\ cho/Y;\ st^+\ st$ (white male)
0.02875 $w\ cho;\ st$	0.5 $w^+\ cho^+;\ st$	0.014375 $w\ cho/w^+\ cho^+;\ st/st$ (scarlet female)
	0.5 $Y;\ st$	0.014375 $w\ cho/Y;\ st/st$ (white male)

Result: 25% red females   1.4375% red males
           25% scarlet females   1.4375% scarlet males
                                      36.0625% white males
                                      11.0625% chocolate males

14.33   *Answer:* First, use the chi-square test to evaluate the hypothesis that there is no relationship between chestnut coat color and class. Further investigation into the potential linkage of this coat color gene and a hypothetical class gene is warranted if we can reject this hypothesis. The assumptions in this initial chi-square test involve the genotypes of the horses bred to Sharpen Up, as stated in the problem, and the hypothesis of the chi-square test, that chestnut coat color and class are unrelated.

From the initial hypothesis of *no relationship between class and chestnut coat color*, the likelihood of Sharpen Up siring a classy horse is uniform with regard to its coat color. There were 83 classy horses produced from a total of 627 (367 + 260) progeny, so the chance of Sharpen Up siring a classy horse, independent of its coat color, is 83/627 = 13.24%. To perform the chi-square test, we need to compare the expected and observed number of classy chestnut and classy bay horses.

Assumption I: Sharpen Up is mated equally frequently to homozygous bay, heterozygous bay/chestnut, and homozygous chestnut mares. Chestnut is recessive to bay, so let *c* represent chestnut and *C* represent bay. Sharpen Up is chestnut (*cc*), so the crosses and their progeny are (1) $cc \times CC \rightarrow$ all $C-$ (bay); (2) $cc \times Cc \rightarrow \frac{1}{2} Cc$ (bay), $\frac{1}{2} cc$ (chestnut); and (3) $cc \times cc \rightarrow$ all cc (chestnut). If each cross is equally likely ($P = \frac{1}{3}$), the expected number of chestnut offspring, rounding up or down to the nearest whole horse, is $627 \times [(\frac{1}{3} \times 0) + (\frac{1}{3} \times \frac{1}{2}) + (\frac{1}{3} \times 1)] = 314$. The remaining $627 - 314 = 313$ offspring are expected to be bay. Using assumption I and assuming that the frequency of classy offspring is uniform (13.24%) with respect to their coat color, the expected number of classy chestnut progeny is $314 \times 0.1324 = 42$, and the expected number of classy bay progeny is $313 \times 0.1324 = 41$. The observed numbers of classy horses were 45 chestnut and 38 bay. For these values, $\chi^2 = [(45 - 42)^2/42 + (38 - 41)^2/41] = 0.43$, df = 1, $0.50 < P < 0.70$. Under assumption I, then, the hypothesis that chestnut coat color and class are unrelated is accepted as possible.

Assumption II: Sharpen Up is mated equally frequently to heterozygous bay/chestnut and chestnut mares. These crosses and their progeny are (1) $cc \times Cc \rightarrow \frac{1}{2} Cc$ (bay), $\frac{1}{2} cc$ (chestnut); and (2) $cc \times cc \rightarrow$ all cc (chestnut). If each cross is equally likely ($P = \frac{1}{2}$), the expected number of chestnut offspring is $627 \times [(\frac{1}{2} \times \frac{1}{2}) + (\frac{1}{2} \times 1)] = 470$. The expected number of bay offspring is $627 - 470 = 157$. Using assumption II and assuming that the frequency of classy offspring is uniform (13.24%) with respect to their coat color, the classy progeny are expected to be $470 \times 0.1324 = 62$ chestnut and $157 \times 0.1324 = 21$ bay. The observed numbers of classy horses were 45 chestnut and 38 bay. For these values, $\chi^2 = [(45 - 62)^2/62 + (38 - 21)^2/21] = 18.4$, df = 1, $P < 0.001$. Under assumption II, then, the hypothesis that chestnut coat color and class are unrelated is rejected as being unlikely. It would be reasonable to consider the hypothesis that a gene closely linked to chestnut/bay coat color might contribute to class.

Notice that the evidence for a relationship between chestnut coat color and class hinges on knowing what alleles at the chestnut/bay gene were present in the mares bred to Sharpen Up. This information is available (although not in this problem). Additional assumptions required to specifically test for linkage to a class gene might include assumptions about the number of alleles in the population of horses, the dominance relationships between them, and which alleles reside on the same homolog with the chestnut allele.

14.34 *Answer:* A physical exchange between two loci during meiosis will produce two recombinant and two nonrecombinant gametes. If 14% of meioses have physical exchanges, about 7% of the gametes will be recombinants, $a^+ b$ or $a b^+$.

14.35 *Answer:* In lod score analyses, the logarithm of the odds of linkage (lod) score is calculated for a pair of loci at each of a set of recombination frequencies (θs) between 0.0 and 0.5. If the lod score is greater than 3.0, there is evidence for linkage. An estimate of the distance between the loci is given by the recombination frequency that gives the maximum lod score. Here, a graph of θ versus lod score reveals a maximum lod score of 4.01 at a θ of 0.25. This corresponds to a map distance of about 25 mu. Since the lod score is greater than 3, the marker is linked to a *waf* gene. However, the marker is not closely linked. Using the estimate that 1 mu corresponds on average to 1 Mb, the marker is about 25 Mb away from a *waf* gene.

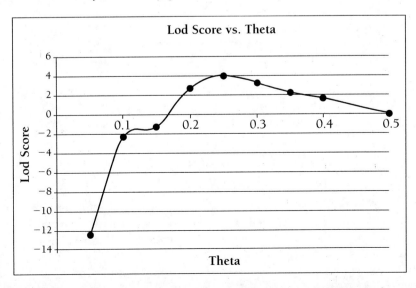

14.36   *Answer:* In answering this problem, remember that males have just one X chromosome, which they receive from their mother, while females have two X chromosomes, one from their mother and one from their father. Trace the inheritance of the markers by following the inheritance of the X chromosomes. As you do so, keep in mind that mothers, but not fathers, can transmit recombinant X chromosomes. Therefore, as you follow the inheritance of the chromosomes, identify whether a chromosome transmitted by a mother is recombinant.

   a. **i.** Males have just one X chromosome, so they have only one allele at each X-linked STR locus. Females with just one STR allele are homozygous for that STR allele. Females with two STR alleles are heterozygotes.

      ii. Individual II-1 received an X from her father (I-2) with $A^4 B^9 C^2$. To account for her genotype, her mother (I-1) must have given her an X with $A^6 B^7 C^1$, so she is $A^4 B^9 C^2/A^6 B^7 C^1$.

     iii. The paternal X chromosome with $A^4 B^9 C^2$ (from I-2) is a nonrecombinant chromosome since males have just one X, and crossing-over requires two homologous chromosomes. We cannot tell whether the maternal X chromosome with $A^6 B^7 C^1$ (from I-1) is recombinant or not, because we do not know what combinations of alleles were given to I-1 by each of her parents.

  iv, v. The cross between II-1 and II-2 is $A^4 B^9 C^2/A^6 B^7 C^1 \times A^6 B^8 C^1/Y$. Two individuals received recombinant X chromosomes from II-1. The X chromosome of individual III-2 ($A^6 B^7 C^2$) was produced by a crossover between B and C. Individual III-11 is $A^6 B^8 C^1/A^4 B^7 C^1$. A crossover between A and B produced her maternal X chromosome ($A^4 B^7 C^1$). There were no double crossovers.

   b. The observed recombination frequency between A and B, and between B and C, is 1/11 = 9.1%. This gives the following map:

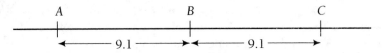

   c. The sample size is quite small, so the map may not be very accurate. To increase the sample size and build a more accurate map, analyze these markers in additional three-generation pedigrees.

   d. Average rate of recombination = [2/11) × 100] mu/1 mB = 18.8 mu/mB.

14.37   *Answer:*

   a. The chromosomal sequence coordinates of the STR loci are known, so when deCODE Genetics tracked the transmission of the 5,136 STR loci through 1,257 meioses, they could determine how often recombination occurred in the intervals between adjacent STR loci and construct a genetic map. That map could be compared to the physical map to identify how the rate of recombination varies along the length of human chromosomes, and it can serve as a reference in future mapping studies.

        If the 5,136 STR loci were evenly distributed over 2.85 billion DNA base pairs, there would be

$$2.85 \times 10^9 \text{ bp}/5{,}136 \text{ STRs} = 5.55 \times 10^5 \text{ bp between adjacent STRs.}$$

   b. In text Figure 14.B, p. 427, it appears that the rate of recombination for most regions of Xq is about 1 cM/Mb. This may also be close to the average rate of recombination on Xq. However, there are extended regions where there is much less recombination—the recombination rate is close to 0 cM/Mb in a 10-Mb interval around sequence coordinate 80 Mb. There also are smaller intervals where there is much more recombination—there are much greater recombination rates near sequence coordinates 112, 124, 131, 134, 150, 140–145, and 150 Mb.

   c. Recall that map distances are defined as

$$\text{mu (cM)} = \frac{\text{number of recombinants}}{\text{total number of progeny}} \times 100\%$$

Since Figure 14.B plots cM/Mb, a region with a higher rate has a greater number of recombinants in a similarly sized interval. Therefore, the interval between sequence coordinates 149 and 150 Mb that has a recombination rate over 8 cM/Mb has a greater average number of crossovers per Mb of DNA.

d. Two genes that lie 500,000 bp apart are more likely to be separated by crossing-over when the recombination rate is higher. They are more likely to be separated in a region with a recombination rate of 8 cM/Mb.

e. To ascertain the recombination rate in a region, one must analyze the products of meioses for recombination in that region, that is, identify recombinant and nonrecombinant chromosomes. Therefore, one would need to follow the transmission of linked STR markers through meioses and determine when alleles at adjacent STR markers recombine. The following figure shows an idealized depiction of the transmission of two hypothetical, linked STR markers to illustrate how this could be done.

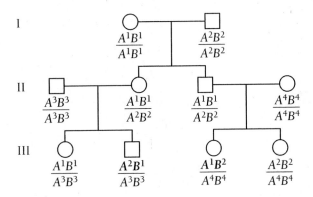

In the pedigree shown, A and B are linked STR loci. There are four alleles at each locus (A^1–A^4 and B^1–B^4) indicated by superscripts. In this pedigree, individuals I-1, I-2, II-1, and II-4 have been made homozygous to more easily follow the transmission of their chromosomes into offspring. Because they are homozygous, we can infer the arrangement of the STR alleles on each of the chromosomes in individuals II-2 and II-3, who are dihybrids. Knowledge of the arrangement of the STR alleles in II-2 and II-3 allows us to determine whether their offspring received recombinant or nonrecombinant chromosomes. The mating of II-1 and II-2 produces two individuals that we can use to determine whether recombination occurred during meiosis in the *mother*: III-1 is nonrecombinant and III-2 is recombinant. The mating of II-3 and II-4 produces two individuals that we can use to determine whether recombination occurred during meiosis in the *father*: III-4 is nonrecombinant and III-3 is recombinant. (Note that we cannot tell if recombination occurred in I-1, I-2, II-1, and II-4 because these individuals are homozygous at both STR loci.) Therefore, to ascertain whether the recombination rate in an autosomal region differs between males and females, reanalyze the results obtained in the 1,257 meioses to identify whether the recombinant and nonrecombinant chromosomes were produced during meiosis in a male or a female, and calculate recombination rates using the separate datasets.

f. A genomic sequence map is a physical map. Here, the genomic sequence map reveals the chromosome and sequence coordinates of the 5,126 STR markers. It does not describe how often different alleles are separated by recombination during meiosis. In constrast, a genetic map does describe this because it is based on recombination frequency. The two maps are colinear, but the relative distances between a specific pair of STR loci in the two maps are not always the same. In the example using chromosome Xp, there are some regions that appear contracted in the genetic map when compared to the genomic sequence map (e.g., the region where STRs map to sequence coordinates between about 75 and 85 Mb) and other regions that appear expanded in the genetic map when compared to the genomic sequence map (e.g., the region where STRs map to sequence coordinates between about 140 and 150 Mb).

14.38 *Answer:*

a. The lod score gives the odds of linkage at a particular recombination frequency, or distance, from the disease locus. The expected number of recombinants will vary depending on the map distance between the marker and disease locus, so lod score calculations to assess the likelihood of linkage must consider a range of potential distances between the marker and disease locus. If the marker locus shows linkage to a disease locus, the distance that gives a maximum lod score indicates whether the two loci are closely linked.

b. The increase in lod scores means that the likelihood of linkage increases. The disease locus is more likely to be close to those markers.

c. In the following figure, which displays lod score values at the sequence map position of each STR marker as a function of θ, notice that the lod scores reach a maximum value in the interval between about 31 and 47 Mb, and that within this interval, lod scores increase as θ decreases (maximal lod scores are seen for θ = 0.001 or 0.1% recombination).

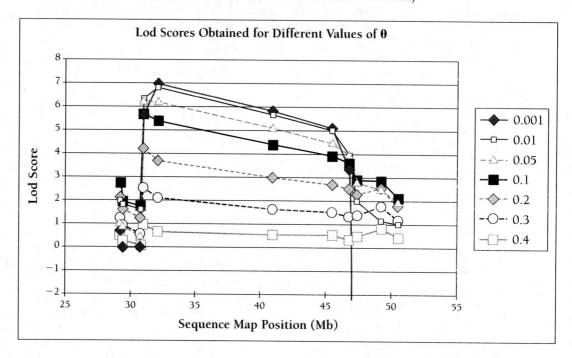

The lod score for some markers increases as θ decreases because the likelihood of linkage is increasing. If the lod score is sufficiently high, it suggests that the marker and disease locus are linked. If the lod score decreases as θ continues to decrease, the marker and the disease locus are not likely to be closely linked.

d. Markers AFMB041XB9 (at 30.9756 Mb), AFM296YG5 (at 32.1160 Mb), AFMB283XH5 (at 40.9934 Mb), AFM122XF6 (at 45.5229 Mb), and AFMB314YH5 (at 46.7925 Mb) all have lod scores above three and show evidence of linkage to this disease locus.

e. Marker AFM296YG5 shows the highest lod score of 6.97 at θ = 0.001. This indicates that there is a $10^{6.97}$:1 = 9,332,542:1 chance that the disease locus is linked to this marker at a distance of 0.1% recombination. Put another way, it is very likely that the disease locus and this marker locus are closely linked.

f. The interval containing all of the markers noted in part **(d)** corresponds to the cytological interval between 12p11.21 and 12q13.11. It spans the centromere and has a genetic map distance of 11.35 cM and a physical distance of 15.8169 Mb. The markers AFM296YG5, AFMB283XH5, and AFM122XF6 define a subinterval where maximal lod scores are seen at θ = 0.001. Still substantial, this interval corresponds to cytological positions 12p11.21 to 12q13.11, includes the centromere, spans a genetic map distance of 8.25 cM, and has a physical distance of 13.4069 Mb.

It may seem puzzling that a broad interval shows similarly high lod scores and there is not a small interval with a dramatic lod-score peak. To understand this, consider that when testcrosses are used in *Drosophila* or other experimental organisms, the accuracy with which a locus is mapped depends on the number of offspring examined in the testcross. A population of offspring is being sampled for recombinants, and so as more offspring are sampled, more products of meioses are evaluated for being recombinant or nonrecombinant. This leads to an increase in the accuracy of the map position being determined. In a similar way, the size of the region defined by lod score analysis depends on the size of the pedigrees being assessed, since this determines how many products of meioses are analyzed. Here, the interval remains substantial in size. If additional pedigrees were analyzed, additional recombinants in this interval might be seen, and these could narrow the interval to a smaller region of chromosome 12.

15

Genetics of Bacteria and Bacteriophages

Chapter Outline

Review of Key Terms, Symbols, and Concepts

In your own words, write a brief, precise definition of each term in the groups below. Check your definitions using the text. Then develop a concept map using the terms in each list.

1	2	3
transfer of genetic material	transduction, cotransduction	bacteriophage cross
conjugation	phage vectors	turbid, clear plaques
plating	transductants	permissive host
colony	phage lysate	nonpermissive host
minimal medium	titer	bacterial lawn
complete medium	virulent vs. temperate phage	host range property
auxotroph	lysogenic pathway	intergenic mapping
prototroph	prophage	"beads-on-a-string" view
nutritional, auxotrophic mutant	lysogeny	intragenic mapping
replica plating	lytic cycle	fine-structure mapping
transconjugants, exconjugant	generalized transduction	homoallelic mutations
sex factor	specialized transduction	heteroallelic mutations
F^-, F', Hfr, F^+ strains	transducing phage	deletion mapping
plasmid, episome	specialized transducing phage	point, deletion, revertant
F-duction (sexduction)	filterable agent	mutations
merodiploid	low-frequency, high-frequency	hot spot
interrupted mating	transducing lysate	*cis-trans* test
donor vs. recipient	helper phage	complementation test
F-pili (sex-pili)	λ*d gal*$^+$ phage	cistron
F-factor origin	selected, unselected marker	gene as a unit of function
	transformation	
	competent cells	
	natural, engineered	
	transformation	
	electroporation	
	heteroduplex DNA	
	cotransformation	

Thinking Analytically

While this chapter focuses on the genetics of bacteria and bacteriophages, many of the core concepts introduced here are used throughout the study of genetics. Of particular importance are the genetic principles that underlie selection, recombination, and complementation. These have had a major impact on how we think about gene structure and function: Geneticists working in many different research areas are concerned with how to *select* for or against specific phenotypes; analysis of recombination within a gene (*intragenic* recombination) formed a foundation for our current understanding of gene structure; the concept of a gene as a unit of function was developed by using complementation tests to measure whether two mutants affect the same function. It is therefore essential to thoroughly understand these genetic principles as they are developed using bacterial and phage systems in this chapter.

Having stressed the importance of the concepts presented in this chapter, it is also important to be forewarned that much of the material used to develop these concepts is complicated and will not necessarily be intuitive. For example, there are many refinements of bacteria and phage types and special characteristics that are associated with one or another aspect of bacterial or phage growth and mating. Carefully read the chapter sections that describe these characteristics until you thoroughly understand them. The names are quite descriptive, and once you use them a few times in solving problems, you will become adept at using them. Approach using the terms with more than rote memorization. Use them in context until you fix upon what is practically a visual image of them.

As with the preceding chapters, carefully read the statements and conditions of a particular problem so that you gain a clear understanding of what it asks and what data it gives you to work with. Then organize and reorganize the data, and sometimes reorganize again, using scratch paper and pencil until you can see how to use the data to solve the problem. If you still get stuck, try representing the processes that are used in the problem with diagrams, and ask yourself how the data fit into the biological process you've drawn out.

The problems in this chapter are especially organized to help you build up your understanding of the material. Work through each of them sequentially to fully develop your understanding and analytical skills.

Questions for Practice

Multiple-Choice Questions

1. A strain, such as a strain of *E. coli,* that requires nutritional or other kinds of supplements for growth and/or survival is known as
   a. a prototroph.
   b. a heterotroph.
   c. a pleiotroph.
   d. an auxotroph.

2. A conjugating bacterial cell that typically transfers only part of its *F* factor and some chromosomal genes is
   a. F^+.
   b. F'.
   c. *Hfr*.
   d. F^-.

3. The process by which cells take up genetic material from the extracellular environment and incorporate it into their genetic complement is called
   a. transduction.
   b. transformation.
   c. translocation.
   d. DNA transfusion.

4. In bacteria, conjugation involves
   a. the union of two bacterial genomes.
   b. the fusion of two cells of opposite mating types.
   c. a virus-mediated exchange of DNA.
   d. the transfer of DNA from one cell into another.

5. A self-replicating genetic element found in the cytoplasm of bacteria is a
   a. sex pilus.
   b. plasmid.
   c. viral capsid.
   d. contransductant.

6. Which of the following statements is *true* of cells possessing *F* factors?
   a. In both F^+ and *Hfr* cells, fertility genes are transferred first.
   b. In both F^+ and *Hfr* cells, genes are transferred through sex pili.
   c. In *Hfr* cells, bacterial genes closest to the origin are transferred first.
   d. In F' cells, only *F*-factor genes are transferred.

7. Phages that can grow using either a lytic or lysogenic pathway are called
    a. virulent.
    b. temperate.
    c. intemperate.
    d. transductant.

8. Recombination that occurs between two alleles at one gene is
    a. not possible.
    b. known as intergenic recombination.
    c. known as intragenic recombination.
    d. more frequent than recombination between two closely linked genes.

9. A complementation test measures
    a. whether two mutants undergo intergenic recombination.
    b. whether two mutants undergo intragenic recombination.
    c. whether two mutants are linked.
    d. whether two mutants affect the same function.

10. *E. coli K12(λ)* cells will only support the growth of T4 phage that are r^+. If two different mutant *rII* phage coinfect an *E. coli K12(λ)* cell and lysis occurs,
    a. intragenic recombination must have occurred.
    b. complementation must have occurred.
    c. the two *rII* phage must have mutations in different cistrons.
    d. a and b only
    e. b and c only
    f. a, b, and c

11. How can you distinguish between a point mutation and a deletion mutation?
    a. Point mutations can't be seen cytologically; deletion mutations can be seen.
    b. Point mutations can be reverted; deletion mutations can't be reverted.
    c. A deletion mutation will complement a point mutation in the same gene.
    d. Point mutations can be transduced; deletion mutations can't be transduced.

12. Which of the following statements is (are) *true* of episomes and plasmids?
    a. An episome is a plasmid that can integrate into the host chromosome.
    b. A plasmid is a circular extrachromosomal element.
    c. An *F* factor is a plasmid that is also an episome.
    d. All episomes are *F* factors, but not all *F* factors are plasmids.
    e. a, b, and c only
    f. a, b, c, and d

Answers: 1d, 2c, 3b, 4d, 5b, 6c, 7b, 8c, 9d, 10e, 11b, 12e

Thought Questions

1. Explain why two genes that are close together on a chromosome show a high frequency of cotransduction and cotransformation.
2. Compare the life cycles of T4, P1, and λ. Which is (are) temperate? Which is (are) virulent? Which can undergo lysogeny?
3. Contrast the features and/or conditions of generalized transduction and specialized transduction.
4. What is the significance of bacterial transformation and conjugation in relation to the rapidity with which certain infectious organisms adapt to changing environmental conditions or factors, such as antibiotics? (Hint: Sexual reproduction promotes genetic variability. How do parasexual systems compare?)
5. Explain how intragenic recombination is different from complementation.
6. Deletion mapping as used by Benzer in T4 was important in defining the location of point mutations at the *rII* locus. What might it mean for recessive mutations to be "uncovered" by deletions in eukaryotes? Diagram how you might use a set of nested deletions to localize a *Drosophila* point mutant. (*Drosophila* has polytene chromosomes in which deletion breakpoints can be mapped cytologically.)
7. Consider how we may select for prototrophic and drug-resistant bacterial strains. Can you think of clever (or even not so clever) ways to attempt to select for (a) a pesticide-resistant strain of beetles,

(b) bacteria that are able to degrade a toxic chemical, (c) extra-sweet sweet corn, and (d) a strain of cats that doesn't respond to catnip?

8. When two true-breeding white-flowered sweet peas are crossed, a purple F_1 is produced. When the F_1 is selfed, the F_2 is 9 purple : 7 white. As described in Chapter 13, pp. 383–384, the 9:7 ratio is characteristic of duplicate recessive epistasis. Why is duplicate recessive epistasis also called complementary gene action?

9. Suppose a linear piece of DNA with genes (in order) $a^+ b^+ c^+$ enters a bacterial cell that is $a^- b^-$ and c^-. How many crossovers are required to convert the bacterial cell to (a) $a^+ b^+ c^+$, (b) $a^+ b^+ c^-$, (c) $a^+ b^- c^+$, (d) $a^- b^+ c^-$? How would your answers change if the DNA was circular? In each case, which would be the most frequent and the least frequent event?

10. P1 and λ phage have been modified to serve as cloning vectors by removing selected genes (thereby making room for DNA inserts) and introducing specific mutations to remove some functions. Carefully consider their life cycles, and speculate on what features of their life cycles it might be useful to retain in a cloning vector and what features it might be necessary to remove.

Thought Questions for Media

After reviewing the media on the *iGenetics* website, try to answer these questions.

1. The *Mapping Bacterial Genes by Conjugation* animation shows that the leu^+ and thr^+ genes are transferred about 8 minutes after conjugation begins but that we can't tell which one is transferred first. What does this tell you about the limits of resolution of mapping by using the interrupted mating technique?

2. What are the units used to relate the distance between two bacterial genes mapped by interrupted mating? Do you expect these units to be proportional to the number of DNA base pairs between the two loci?

3. Could you perform an interrupted mating experiment between an F^+ strain and an F^- strain? Why or why not?

4. Why is it necessary to use diploids to perform a complementation test?

5. Suppose you had two true-breeding mutant lines of deaf rabbits. How would you determine if the cause of deafness in each line was the same?

6. To assess if two genes complement each other, is it important to obtain recombinants between them?

1. Suppose that in the initial cross between the prototrophic strain to the F^- strain that was leu^-, arg^-, his^-, and trp^-, the media used for selection of leu^+ recombinants was prepared incorrectly. On plate A, streptomycin was mistakenly left out of the medium, and only supplemental arginine, histidine, and tryptophan were added. On plate B, streptomycin was added, but leucine was mistakenly added along with the other supplements (arginine, histidine, and tryptophan). Compared to all of the other plates used to select for recombinants at the other loci, you observe a much larger number of colonies on plates A and B.
   a. Why are there so many more colonies on plates A and B, compared to the others?
   b. Suppose you picked several dozen individual colonies from each of plates A and B. Would you expect the genotypes of all of the colonies from both plates to be the same? Would you expect the genotypes of all of the colonies from just one of the plates to be the same?
   c. Could any of the colonies on plates A and B be recombinants?
   d. What would you expect their genotype(s) to be?
   e. How could you experimentally address your answers to (c) and (d)?

2. As presented in the iActivity, multiple *Hfr* strains are used to map the relative location of genes distributed throughout the *E. coli* chromosome.
   a. Does each *Hfr* strain have one or more than one *F* factor inserted in its *E. coli* chromosome?
   b. If, in an *Hfr* strain, a bacterial gene is far from the *F* factor site of insertion, will it be transferred frequently to an F^- strain?
   c. Why are multiple *Hfr* strains needed to map genes distributed throughout the *E. coli* chromosome?
   d. When maps are being constructed, why doesn't it matter if the F factors in the different *Hfr* strains are inserted in opposite directions (relative to each other) in the *E. coli* chromosome?

Solutions to Text Questions and Problems

15.1 *Answer:* The frequency with which a recipient is converted to a donor reflects the frequency with which a complete F factor is transferred. In $F^+ \times F^-$ crosses, only the F factor is transferred, and this occurs relatively quickly. In $Hfr \times F^-$ crosses, transfer starts at the origin within the F element and then must proceed through the bacterial chromosome before reaching the F factor. For the entire F factor to be transferred, the whole chromosome would have to be transferred. This would take about 100 minutes, and usually the conjugal unions break apart before then.

15.2 *Answer:*

a. i. In the cross *Hfr* (resistant) $\times$ F^- (sensitive), the *Hfr* cell is donating DNA to the F^- cell. DNA transfer starts at the F-factor origin of replication and proceeds unidirectionally from that point. For an antibiotic resistance gene to be transferred reliably, it would need to be located near the F-factor origin and on the side of it that is transferred early during conjugation. In the following figure, the antibiotic resistance gene *ant^R* would be transferred reliably because it is replicated and transferred early, but the *b* gene would not be transferred reliably because it is transferred only after most of the bacterial chromosome is transferred, and matings rarely last this long.

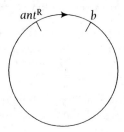

ii. In the cross F^+ (resistant) $\times$ F^- (sensitive), the F^+ cell only donates its F factor to the F^- cell. Since the F factor is small, it is transferred quickly and in its entirety to the recipient cell. Therefore, for an antibiotic resistance gene to be transferred reliably, it should be on the F factor.

b. The cross F^+ (resistant) $\times$ F^- (sensitive) would be more efficient at spreading antibiotic resistance between cells because the cells that receive the antibiotic resistance gene also are converted to F^+ donor cells. The F^- (sensitive) cells are converted to F^+ (resistant) cells that can transfer antibiotic resistance to other sensitive cells. This allows for the efficient spread of antibiotic resistance. In the cross *Hfr* (resistant) $\times$ F^- (sensitive), even if the F^- cell becomes resistant to the antibiotic, it will not become an *Hfr* or F^+ cell, and so it will not spread antibiotic resistance to other cells.

c. Two hypotheses are that: (1) F factors bearing the antibiotic resistance genes were released into the environment when *Shigella* was lysed and other bacteria took up these F factors by transformation; (2) interspecies conjugation occurred between a resistant *Shigella* F^+ cell and a sensitive F^- cell of another bacterial species.

15.3 *Answer:* The diagram here shows the gene sequence in the original F^+ strain and the relative location and orientation of the four different F factor insertions. (Note that only one insertion exists in a particular *Hfr* strain.)

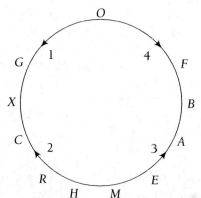

15.4   *Answer:*

   a. **i.** True. The graph indicates that a^+ is transferred last, starting about 16 minutes after conjugal pairing. The genes are transferred linearly in the order h^+ (starting at 0 minutes), e^+ (starting at 2 minutes), b^+ (starting at 9 minutes), g^+ (starting at 12 minutes), and then a^+.

       ii. False. The data show that a^+ took the longest time to be transferred and so was the last gene to be received. The correct order of gene transfer was h^+ (first), e^+, b^+, g^+, and a^+ (last).

     iii. False. In order for the recipient cell to be converted to F^+ or *Hfr*, it must receive a complete copy of the F factor. Since only part of the F factor is transferred at the beginning of conjugation, and e^+ is transferred quite quickly after conjugal pairing, most e^+ str^R recombinants will have only a small part of the donor chromosome. The remaining part of the F factor is transferred only after the entire bacterial chromosome is transferred. Because of turbulence, the conjugal pairing is almost always disrupted before transfer of an entire chromosome is completed. Hence, the chance that complete transfer will occur is quite remote.

     iv. True. The graph shows that a^+ is not transferred until after about 16 minutes have elapsed.

   b.

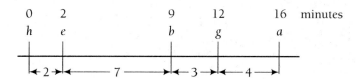

15.5   *Answer:*

    Mixture A: Leaving out histidine from an otherwise complete medium will select for his^+ cells, since they can synthesize their own histidine. To select for *his* cells, plate cells on medium with histidine where both *his* and his^+ cells grow. Then check individual colonies for their ability to grow on medium without histidine (use replica plating). Colonies able to grow on medium with histidine but not on medium without histidine are *his*.

    Mixture B: Adding sodium azide to complete medium will select for azi^R cells. To select for azi^S cells, plate cells on medium with sodium azide and then check individual colonies for their ability to grow on medium with sodium azide (use replica plating). The azi^S colonies will not grow on medium with sodium azide.

    Mixture C: Using lactose as the sole sugar in the medium will select for lac^+ cells. To select for *lac* cells, plate cells on medium with a sugar other than lactose (e.g., glucose), where both *lac* and lac^+ cells can grow. Then assess whether individual colonies can grow on medium with lactose as the sole sugar. Colonies unable to grow on this medium are *lac*.

    Mixture D: Since *pcsA* cells are cold sensitive, incubating plated cells at 30°C will select for $pcsA^+$ cells. To select for *pcsA* cells, incubate plated cells at 37°C and then test individual colonies for their ability to grow at 30°C. Cells unable to grow at 30°C but able to grow at 37°C are *pcsA*.

15.6   *Answer:*

   a. To initially select for c^+ str^R recombinants, plate the progeny on minimal medium without compound C, but supplemented with streptomycin and compounds A, B, D, E, F, G, and H. To assess the complete genotype of the c^+ str^R recombinants, replica plate them onto different minimal media supplemented with streptomycin and all but two of the compounds (compound C and one other). For example, to test if a c^+ str^R colony was also a^+, replica-plate it onto a medium that lacked compound A, but was supplemented with streptomycin and B, D, E, F, G, and H. If the colony were able to grow on this medium, it would be a^+ c^+ str^R. If it were unable to grow, it would be a c^+ str^R.

   b. Strain *1:* Since no c^+ recombinants are ever obtained, strain *1* is unable to transfer c^+. This means it is either (1) F^-; (2) *Hfr*, but with the F factor inserted either far from c^+, or close to it but in an orientation so that genes are transferred in a direction opposite to c^+; (3) F', with c^+ in the bacterial chromosome. It should not be F^+, because then, at a very low frequency, some c^+ recombinants would be obtained.

     Strain *2:* Since c^+ recombinants are obtained at 6 minutes, and g^+, h^+, a^+, and b^+ recombinants are obtained at subsequent time intervals, strain *2* is *Hfr*. The genes are transferred in the following order: c^+, g^+, h^+, a^+, and b^+. From the times of their transfer, the map position of the genes is: origin $(0) - c^+ (6) - g^+ (8) - h^+ (11) - a^+ (14) - b^+ (16)$. The location of genes d^+, e^+, and f^+ cannot be precisely determined; since they are not transferred in an $Hfr \times F^-$ cross, they are either far away from the F-factor insertion site or close to it but near the fertility genes, which are only rarely transferred by an Hfr strain. When the recombinants obtained from the strain $2 \times F^-$ mating at the 16-minute time period are crossed to an $amp^R F^-$ strain, c^+ is not transferred. If these recombinants cannot conjugate with F^-, this indicates that although strain 2 is fertile, it did not transfer a complete F factor. It therefore must be Hfr.

Strain 3: Strain 3 transfers c^+ within 1 minute and g^+ by 3 minutes. From analysis of the strain $2 \times F^-$ cross, we knew that these genes are 2 minutes apart. This data supports this conclusion. Since no other recombinants are obtained, no other genes are transferred. This suggests that strain 3 is F', and that the segment of DNA containing c^+ and g^+ is in the F' factor. If this is the case, the complete F factor will be transferred in a strain $3 \times F^-$ cross if the mating is allowed to proceed long enough. This is observed: c^+ recombinants from the strain $3 \times F^-$ cross obtained at 16 minutes are able to transfer c^+ to an $F^- amp^R$ strain. Therefore, strain 3 is F'.

c. Information known with certainty is diagrammed below. The location of genes in strains 1 and 3 is inferred from crosses with strain 2. The location of genes d^+, e^+, and f^+ is unknown.

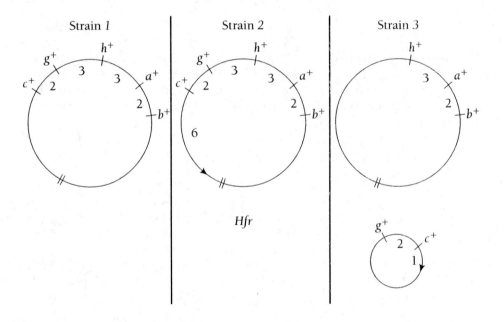

15.7   *Answer:* Strain A is $thy^- leu^+$, while strain B is $thy^+ leu^-$. To test if DNA from A can transform B, determine whether the leu^- allele of B can be transformed to leu^+ by DNA from A. Add DNA from strain A to a leucine-fortified culture of B. Incubate long enough for transformation to occur, then plate out the potentially transformed B cells on minimal medium or on medium supplemented only with thymine. As shown in the table below, one can select for transformants by plating on such media since growth on such media requires leu^+.

| | | Medium Type | | |
Strain	Minimal	Plus Leucine	Plus Thymine	Plus Thymine and Leucine
$leu^+ thy^+$	+	+	+	+
$leu^+ thy^-$	–	–	+	+
$leu^- thy^+$	–	+	–	+
$leu^- thy^-$	–	–	–	+

15.8   *Answer:*

a. Prepare a set of bacterial plates with five different media, each containing minimal media supplemented with ampicillin and all but one of leucine, arginine, lysine, purine, and biotin. Mix the *Hfr* strain with the *F⁻* strain. After, say, 2 minutes and 5 minutes, remove some of the bacteria from the mating, violently shake them, and plate them on each of the media. This will select for growth of *amp*^R recombinants that are able to grow in the absence of one supplement. For example, plating on medium with ampicillin, leucine, arginine, lysine, and purine will select for *bio⁺ amp*^R recombinants. Incubate the plates to let colonies grow, and identify the plate that has the most colonies after the shortest mating interval. This will identify the prototrophic gene transferred first, and so identify the gene closest to the origin of replication of the F factor. If, say, only plates lacking leucine have growth after 2 minutes, then *leu⁺* is closest to the *F*-factor origin of replication.

b. The *str*^R gene could be far from the origin of replication of the *F* factor in the *Hfr* chromosome. Alternatively, the *str*^R gene might be on a separate plasmid unable to be transferred to the *F⁻* cell (perhaps it is a defective *F* factor).

15.9   *Answer:* Start to analyze the information in this question by diagramming the sequence of treatments and matings that the question describes so that you can determine: (1) the point at which mutations were induced by the mutagen; (2) what type of DNA (chromosomal or *F*-factor) was transferred in each type of mating; and (3) what genotypes were selected for and against after each mating.

a. The cells that are treated with the mutagen MMS are *F⁻ leu arg str*^R cells. They can be recipient, but not donor cells. Since they were treated with MMS, the colonies that are picked and plated into the grid-like pattern have randomly induced mutations. The medium on which they were plated in a grid-like pattern contained leucine, arginine, and streptomycin, so this media selects for *str*^R cells, but allows *leu* and *leu⁺*, and *arg* and *arg⁺* cells to grow. Plating a mixture of mutant *F⁻ str*^R and *Hfr leu⁺ arg⁺ str*^S cells on minimal medium with streptomycin selects for *leu⁺ arg⁺ str*^R exconjugants: growth will occur only if the *Hfr* strain donates DNA containing the *leu⁺* and *arg⁺* genes to the *F⁻ leu arg str*^R cells via conjugation and that DNA is incorporated into the genome of the mutant *F⁻* cell. Since nearly all of the 5,000 mixtures produced growth, the *leu⁺* and *arg⁺* genes are transferred relatively early from the *Hfr* strain. They must lie close to the *F*-factor origin of replication and reside in the region that is transferred early.

b. To identify what mutations were induced by MMS that prevented some exconjugants from growing, consider the molecular events that accompany DNA transfer. After the *Hfr* cell transfers a single strand of DNA to the *F⁻* cell during conjugation, DNA polymerase synthesizes a complementary strand, and a double crossover leads to the incorporation of linear donor DNA into the circular recipient chromosome. *F⁻* mutants unable to synthesize the complementary strand or recombine the double-stranded DNA into their chromosome would not produce exconjugants. Since the mutant *F⁻* cell can divide on medium supplemented with arginine and leucine, the mutation is unlikely to affect chromosomal DNA synthesis. Most mutants unable to generate *leu⁺ arg⁺* exconjugants probably affect genes needed for recombination of the donor DNA into the recipient chromosome.

15.10   *Answer:*

a. The question describes a set of matings between an *F′* cell that is sensitive to streptomycin and whose *F′* element bears either a *metC⁺* or *metD⁺* gene and an *F⁻* cell auxotrophic for one of four *met* mutations that is also resistant to streptomycin. In each, the *F′* cell transfers its *F′* element with the *met⁺* gene to the *F⁻* cell. Exconjugants are selected on medium without methionine but containing streptomycin. Using medium without methionine selects for exconjugants that are *met⁺* and against those that are *met*. Using medium with streptomycin selects for *str*^R exconjugants and against the *F′* donors. If colonies are recovered when *metC⁺* is transferred to a particular *met* mutation, then complementation has occurred at the *metC* gene: the *metC⁺* gene can provide for the deficit in methionine synthesis that results from the *met* mutation, and so that *met* mutation must affect the function of *metC*. Similarly, if colonies are recovered when *metD⁺* is transferred to a particular *met* mutation, then complementation has occurred at the *metD* gene: that *met* mutation must affect the function of *metD*. Therefore, *met1*, *met3*, and *met4* affect *metD*, and *met2* affects *metC*. We can therefore think of *met1*, *met2*, *met3*, and *met4* as mutations that affect specific sites in the *metC* and *metD* loci.

b. In each of the interrupted matings in this part of the problem, an *Hfr* strain that is *lac⁺*, sensitive to streptomycin, and bears a particular *met* mutant is mated to an *F⁻* strain that is *lac*, resistant to streptomycin, and bears a different *met* mutant. The matings are interrupted after 6 minutes, and exconjugants are plated on medium A that contains lactose as the sole carbon source, methionine, and streptomycin. This medium selects for *lac⁺ str^R* cells and against *lac str^S* cells. However, it does not select for or against *met* or *met⁺* cells since the presence of methionine allows both types of cells to grow. Therefore, we do not know (yet) whether the *met* mutant present in the donor was also transferred. Since the mating was interrupted after 6 minutes, only part of the *Hfr* chromosome was transferred, and the exconjugants remain *F⁻* cells. Therefore, the exconjugants that grow on medium A are either *F⁻ lac⁺ str^R met* or *F⁻ lac⁺ str^R met⁺*.

Replica-plating the exconjugants onto medium B, which has lactose as the sole carbon source and is supplemented only with streptomycin, selects for cells that could grow without supplemental methionine—*met⁺* cells. Since the parental *Hfr* and *F⁻* strains are *met*, *met⁺* exconjugants can only arise when an *Hfr* chromosomal segment bearing one *met* mutation is transferred to an *F⁻* cell having a chromosome with a second *met* mutation, and recombination occurs to produce a *met⁺* chromosome. To understand how recombination between two different *met* mutations can give rise to a *met⁺* chromosome, it is helpful to sketch how the *met* mutant sites might be arranged relative to each other and *lac⁺*, keeping in mind that *lac⁺* is always transferred (since all of the exconjugants are *lac⁺*). The following figure illustrates how crossing-over (shown by a dotted line) between DNA fragments that bear two different *met* mutations, *metX* and *metY*, can produce a *met⁺ lac⁺ F⁻* chromosome. In the figure, the order is *metX–metY–lac*, interval 1 lies between *metX* and *metY*, interval 2 lies between *metY* and *lac*, and two types of crosses are shown. In cross A, the *Hfr* chromosome (in grey) bears *metX* and a normal *metY⁺* site, and the *F⁻* chromosome (in black) bears *metY* and a normal *metX⁺* allele. In cross B, the *Hfr* chromosome bears *metY* and a normal *metX⁺* site, and the *F⁻* chromosome bears *metX* and a normal *metY⁺* allele.

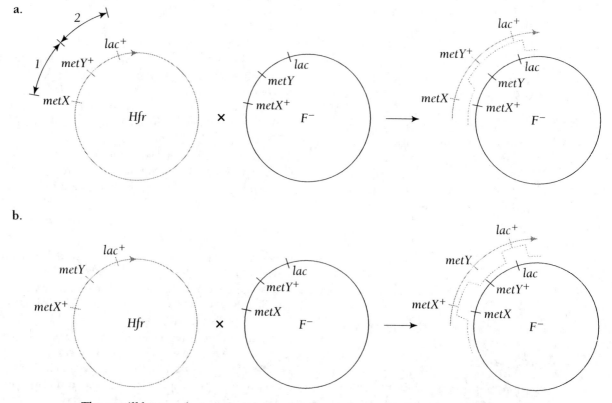

There will be two factors that determine how often recombination will occur. The first is the distance between two different *met* mutations. The closer together they lie, the less likely a crossover will occur between them. The second is the order of the two *met* mutations relative to the *lac* locus. As the figure shows in cross A, when the normal *met* allele on the **Hfr** chromosome is closer to the *lac* locus than the *met* mutation (when *metY*⁺ is closer to *lac* than *metX*), only two crossovers are required to obtain a *met*⁺ *lac*⁺ chromosome. One crossover must be between the origin and *lac*, and the second crossover must be between *metX* and *metY*. As the figure shows in cross B, if the *met* mutation on the *Hfr* chromosome (*metY*) is closer to the *lac* locus than the normal *met* allele (*metX*⁺), four crossovers are required to obtain a *met*⁺ *lac*⁺ chromosome: crossovers must occur between the origin and *lac*, *lac* and *metY*, *metY* and *metX*, and past *metX*. Since two crossovers are more likely than four crossovers, situations like that in cross A will produce a greater number of *met*⁺ *lac*⁺ recombinants. In this problem, all possible pairwise combinations of crosses were done. Therefore, we can tell the relative order of the different *met* mutants relative to *lac* and to each other by identifying which cross between a particular pair of *met* mutants produces more *met*⁺ *lac*⁺ exconjugants. In that cross, only two crossovers were required, and the cross is like that diagrammed in cross A: the normal *met*⁺ allele on the *Hfr* chromosome is closer to *lac* than the mutant *met* allele.

For example, consider the results of the following two crosses:

1. *Hfr met1 lac*⁺ *str*ˢ × *F*⁻ *met2 lac*⁻ *str*ᴿ   No *lac*⁺ exconjugants are *met*⁺.
2. *Hfr met2 lac*⁺ *str*ˢ × *F*⁻ *met1 lac*⁻ *str*ᴿ   0.018 of *lac*⁺ exconjugants are *met*⁺.

For clarity, we can rewrite the crosses to indicate the alleles at each of the sites defined by *met1*, *met2*, *lac* and *str* as:

1. *Hfr met1 met2*⁺ *lac*⁺ *str*ˢ × *F*⁻ *met1*⁺ *met2 lac*⁻ *str*ᴿ
2. *Hfr met1*⁺ *met2 lac*⁺ *str*ˢ × *F*⁻ *met1 met2*⁺ *lac*⁻ *str*ᴿ

Cross 2 produces more *lac*⁺ *met*⁺ exconjugants than cross 1 does. Therefore, cross 2 is like cross A of the figure, and the normal *met* allele on the *Hfr* chromosome, *met1*⁺, is closer to *lac*⁺ than the mutant *met* allele on the *Hfr* chromosome, *met2*. This tells us that the relative order of these mutations is *met2–met1–lac*. Use this approach to infer the relative order of pairs of *met* mutations. The result is:

met2–met1–lac
met3–met1–lac
met1–met4–lac
met2–met3–lac
met2–met4–lac
met3–met4–lac

These inferences are consistent with those from the solution to part **(a)** of this question. From part **(a)**, we know that *met2* is a mutation at *metC* while *met1*, *met3*, and *met4* are mutations at *metD*. Since *met2* is to the left of each of *met1*, *met3*, and *met4*, the order of the *metC*, *metD*, and *lac* loci is *metC–metD–lac*. By comparing the order of pairs of mutations, we can determine that the relative order of the four *met* mutations and *lac* from these crosses is *met2–met3–met1–met4–lac*.

Since the frequency of recombination between two mutant sites depends on the distance between them, we can use the fraction of exconjugants that are *met*⁺ *lac*⁺ to estimate the distances between the loci. In cross A of the figure, this fraction arises from crossovers in interval 2, while in cross B, this fraction arises from double crossovers in intervals 1 and 2. Therefore, the fraction of *lac*⁺ *met*⁺ exconjugants from cross A can be used to estimate the distance between a pair of *met* mutants, and with this information, the fraction of exconjugants from cross B can be used to estimate the distance between those mutants and *lac*. Notice that in the figure, only one of the two products of recombination is shown. If you draw in the reciprocal product, you will see that it does not produce *lac*⁺ exconjugants. Therefore, the recombination frequency is this fraction multiplied by two. Using the fraction of exconjugants from crosses like cross A to estimate the distance between pairs of *met* mutants, we have:

$RF(met1, met2) = 2 \times 0.180 = 0.360$
$RF(met1, met3) = 2 \times 0.020 = 0.040$
$RF(met1, met4) = 2 \times 0.015 = 0.030$
$RF(met2, met3) = 2 \times 0.160 = 0.320$
$RF(met2, met4) = 2 \times 0.185 = 0.370$
$RF(met3, met4) = 2 \times 0.035 = 0.070$

To estimate the distance from *met4* to *lac*, consider the cross *Hfr met4 lac⁺ str^S × F⁻ met1 lac⁻ str^R*. In this cross, 0.003 of the *lac⁺* recombinants were also *met⁺* recombinants. They arose from a double crossover, one between *met1* and *met4* and one between *met4* and *lac*. Since half of the double recombinants are not recovered, the fraction of double recombinants is 2 × 0.003 = 0.006. Since the expected frequency of double recombinants is the product of the frequency of single recombinants in each interval,

0.006 = RF(*met1, met4*) × RF(*met4, lac*)
0.006 = 0.300 × RF(*met4, lac*)
RF(*met4, lac*) = 0.006/0.030 = 0.200

In principle, data from any pair of *met* mutants can be used to calculate the distance between *lac* and the closest *met* mutant. Indeed, similar frequencies are obtained in all of the cases except when *met2* is present in the *F⁻* recipient. However, in all crosses involving an *F⁻ met2 lac⁻ str^R* recipient, no double recombinants are ever recovered. To identify why this might be, consider that the matings were interrupted at 6 minutes, and *met2* is furthest from the origin on the *Hfr* chromosome. This could reflect the distance of *met2⁺* from the origin in the *Hfr* donor strain. If *met2⁺* was not transferred by 6 minutes, no *met⁺* recombinants would be ever recovered in these types of crosses. The following map is drawn using the recombination frequencies between adjacent sites.

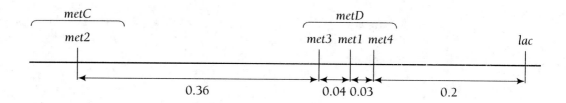

15.11   Answer:

a. In the cross *Hfr leu⁺ arg⁺ str^S × F⁻ leu arg str^R*, the *Hfr* donates genes at a high frequency to the *F⁻* recipient. Most conjugations do not last long enough for an entire F factor to be transferred. So, for an *F⁺ leu⁺ arg str^R* cell to be produced, an intact F factor and *leu⁺* must have been transferred to the *F⁻* recipient. This could happen if an *F′ (leu⁺)* element had formed in a cell of the *Hfr* strain when the F factor looped out of the host chromosome as shown in text Figure 15.6, p. 434, and that element was transferred to the *F⁻* recipient. In this case, the events would have occurred in an *Hfr* donor cell, and the *F⁺ leu⁺ arg str^R* exconjugant would really be a *F′ (leu⁺) str^R* cell. It would transfer fertility as well as *leu⁺* to recipients. If the *F⁺ leu⁺ arg str^R* exconjugant is truly an *F⁺* cell, then two events probably occurred, one in the donor and one in the recipient cell. In the *Hfr* donor, an *F′ (leu⁺)* element was formed by outlooping as just described. Upon transfer to the *F⁻* recipient, the *F′ (leu⁺)* element was integrated into the host chromosome (converting its *leu* gene to *leu⁺*) and then the F factor was precisely excised. In this case, the *F⁺ leu⁺ arg str^R* exconjugant would transfer fertility, but not *leu⁺*, at a high frequency. It would exhibit a low frequency of transfer of *leu⁺* since some cells in a population will have the F factor integrated nearby the *leu⁺* gene.

b. If the *F⁺ leu⁺ arg str^R* cell is really an *F′ (leu⁺) str^R* cell, then it will transfer *leu⁺* and fertility at a high frequency. Assuming that it is sensitive to another antibiotic such as ampicillin (*amp^S*), perform an interrupted mating experiment with *F⁺ leu⁺ arg str^R amp^S* and *F⁻ leu (arg or arg⁺) amp^R* cells and plate the exconjugants on medium without leucine that contains ampicillin. This will select for *leu⁺ amp^R* cells and against the parents. If abundant colonies are seen when the matings are interrupted even after a few minutes, then the donor strain is *F′ (leu⁺) str^R*. If no or only a few colonies are seen at any time, then the donor strain is *F⁺ leu⁺ arg str^R* and *leu⁺* is part of the host chromosome. Such colonies would arise at a low frequency when the F factor integrates near the *leu⁺* gene in a small number of cells in the donor cell population and transfers *leu⁺* to a recipient cell.

15.12 *Answer:*

    a. GT

    b. ST

    c. ST

    d. GT

    e. GT

    f. B

    g. B

    h. B

    i. N

15.13 *Answer:* The notation *aceF* represents a specific insertion site for an *F* factor. This table shows that cells selected for transduction of F^+ were isolated and then tested for the cotransduction of *dhl* or *leu*. It shows that in one experiment, of the $aceF^+$ transductants that were isolated, 88% were also transduced with the *dhl* marker. In another experiment, of the $aceF^+$ transductants that were isolated, only 34% were also transduced with the *leu* marker.

    In order to obtain a transductant, a double crossover must occur between the transduced, donor DNA, and the host chromosome. The closer two loci are together on the same chromosome, the greater the probability that they will both be included within the limits of a double crossover. Therefore, two loci that are closer together will show a greater frequency of cotransduction: *dhl* is closer to $aceF^+$ than *leu*.

15.14 *Answer:* The frequency of cotransduction gives an indication of the closeness of each pair of genes: the higher their cotransduction frequency, the closer the two genes. The *pryD* and *cmlB* genes show the highest cotransduction frequency and are the closest together. This eliminates **(c)** as a possibility. The genes *aroA* and *pyrD* show the lowest cotransduction frequency, and so they are the farthest apart. This eliminates **(b)** as a possibility. The *aroA* and *cmlB* genes show an intermediate cotransduction frequency, as would be expected if *cmlB* were between *aroA* and *pyrD*. Thus, the correct answer is **(a)**.

15.15 *Answer:* Notice that in this cross, by selecting for trp^+ one selects for recombinants. The frequency of the different classes of recombinants can be affected by two factors: the distance between genes and the number of crossovers that are needed to obtain a particular genotype. Since the bacterial chromosome is circular, recombinants are obtained only by either two or some multiple of two crossovers. Obtaining four crossovers will be less common than obtaining two crossovers, and so a genotype that requires four crossovers to be produced is likely to be the least common. The parents are $trp^+ pry^+ qts$ and $trp\ pyr\ qts^+$. To produce the least frequent $trp^+ pyr\ qts$ class by a quadruple crossover, the gene order must be *trp–pyr–qts*. The other three transductant classes can be generated by double crossovers. Try drawing this out.

15.16 *Answer:* The higher the frequency of cotransduction, the closer the loci. Thus, the relative proximity of the loci to each other is:

        cheB–eda   closest together

        cheA–eda $\downarrow$

        cheA–supD $\downarrow$

        cheB–supD $\downarrow$

        eda–supD   farthest apart

    A gene order that is consistent with these relationships is *eda–cheB–cheA–supD*.

15.17 *Answer:*

    a. When the F^- *gal* cells were treated with mutagen, random mutations were introduced. That is, the mutations that were introduced could lie in any region of the chromosome. Since the mutagenized cells were plated on a rich medium, auxotrophic mutations (including the original *gal* mutation) would not be selected against. Colonies that grow at 37°C but not 41°C have temperature-sensitive mutations. Since the 20 colonies that were picked grow at 37°C but not 41°C, they have temperature-sensitive mutations.

When phage λ is grown on wild-type *E. coli* and a lysate is produced, the lysate mostly contains normal λ phage. However, some of the time, λ will integrate into the host near the *gal*⁺ locus and abnormal outlooping leads to imprecise excision. If this occurs, a λd *gal*⁺ chromosome can form. This chromosome has part of the λ chromosome and the *gal*⁺ gene (see text Figure 15.14, p. 444). If such a lysate is mixed with a *gal* mutant, as is done here, and the λd *gal*⁺ phage infects the *gal* cell, two outcomes are possible. As shown in Figure 15.14, one possibility is that a λd *gal*⁺ and a λ chromosome integrate. This produces an unstable transductant that is a double lysogen. When λ is induced in this type of transductant, a high-frequency transducing (HFT) lysate is produced that has about equal numbers of λd *gal*⁺ and normal λ phage. The

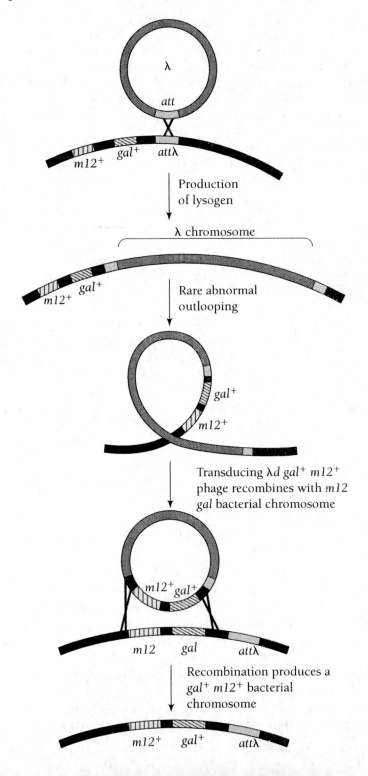

other outcome is to produce a stable transductant. This occurs when a single λd gal^+ phage chromosome integrates into the bacterial chromosome. Integration would introduce gal^+ and any other genes present on the λd gal^+ phage into the bacterial chromosome.

Here, the lysate is mixed with each of 20 different temperature-sensitive mutants, and the mixtures are plated on medium with galactose as the sole carbon source and incubated at 41°C. Only one sample, sample 12, produced colonies. If we call the mutation in this sample $m12^{ts}$, the original sample has the genotype gal $m12^{ts}$. For a transductant to be able to grow under these conditions, the gal $m12^{ts}$ cell must have been infected by a λd gal^+ phage that contains $m12^+$ and gal^+ and integration of the phage led to the formation of a stable $m12^+$ gal^+ transductant. The other 19 samples did not grow because wild-type alleles ($m1^+$, $m2^+$, etc.) able to complement their temperature-sensitive mutations were not introduced by a λd gal^+ phage.

b. The following diagram illustrates the production how a λd gal^+ $m12^+$ phage can be produced by a rare abnormal outlooping of a lambda lysogen, and how recombination between a gal $m12$ bacterial chromosome and the λd gal^+ $m12^+$ phage can produce a stable gal^+ $m12^+$ transductant.

c. The temperature-sensitive mutation ($m12$) present in sample 12 must be in or nearby the gal locus, since a λd gal^+ transducing phage is a specialized transducing phage and only can carry DNA at or near the gal locus. It is likely to be recessive, since the insertion of the $m12^+$ gene in the stable transductant is able to complement the $m12^{ts}$ mutation.

d. One approach to map the sites of the remaining temperature-sensitive mutations is to use generalized transduction. Let m^{ts} represent one of the temperature-sensitive mutations. When a generalized transducing phage infects an m^{ts} gal mutant, it will package random chromosomal DNA segments and produce a lysate. A phage containing the m^{ts} mutation will also contain wild-type alleles at neighboring genes. To identify the location of the mutation, collect a set of auxotrophic strains having mutations that map to known different regions of the *E. coli* chromosome. Infect each strain individually with the phage lysate, plate each mixture on minimal medium, and grow the culture at 37°C. Colonies will be seen if the auxotrophic strain was transduced with the wild-type allele for the auxotrophic mutation. Now, replica-plate these colonies onto minimal media and grow the cultures at 41°C. Growth will not occur if the cell was also cotransduced with the m^{ts} mutation. Therefore, compare the patterns of growth at 37°C and 41°C, and identify the location of the auxotrophic mutants unable to grow at 41°C. In some of colonies unable to grow at 41°C, the m^+ allele and the wild-type allele for the auxotrophic mutation will have been transduced in the same phage. Test this possibility by evaluating the frequency of cotransduction in a separate experiment. If the m^{ts} mutation lies close to the site of a gene for a specific auxotrophic mutation, there should be a high frequency of cotransduction.

You could also map the m^{ts} mutations by conjugation if you construct a set of Hfr m^{ts} strains that have F factors integrated into different chromosomal locations and an appropriate antibiotic resistance marker.

15.18   *Answer:* The plaques produced on *E. coli K12*(λ) are r^+, while those on *E. coli B* may be either r^+ or r^-. Thus, the total number of progeny can be inferred from the number of plaques formed on *E. coli B*. Since *E. coli B* is coinfected with $rIIx$ and $rIIy$, the only way to obtain an r^+ progeny phage is to have a crossover within the rII locus. The progeny resulting from a crossover would be half r^+ and half $rIIxy$ recombinants. The number of recombinant phage is twice the number of r^+ phage, which can be assayed for by growth on *E. coli K12*(λ).

$$\text{\# recombinant progeny in 1 mL} = 2 \times (\text{number of } r^+ \text{ phage/mL})$$
$$= 2 \times (470/0.2)$$
$$= 4,700/\text{mL}$$

$$\text{total \# of progeny in 1 mL} = (\text{dilution factor}) \times (\text{\# progeny phage/mL})$$
$$= 1,000 \times (672/0.1)$$
$$= 6.72 \times 10^6/\text{mL}$$

$$\text{RF} = [4,700/(6.72 \times 10^6)] \times 100\%$$
$$= 0.07\%$$

The map distance between $rIIx$ and $rIIy$ is 0.07 mu.

15.19   *Answer:* Recall that, as discussed in Chapter 14, the most accurate map distances are those obtained over the shortest intervals.

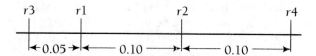

15.20   *Answer:* Analyze the data as you would a set of two-factor crosses:

Cross	Number of Progeny	# Recombinants	mu
c mi⁺ × c⁺ mi	2,577	159	6.2
c s⁺ × c⁺ s	1,413	39	2.8
co mi⁺ × co⁺ mi	12,324	652	5.3
mi s⁺ × mi⁺ s	1,270	121	9.5

Two maps are compatible with these data:

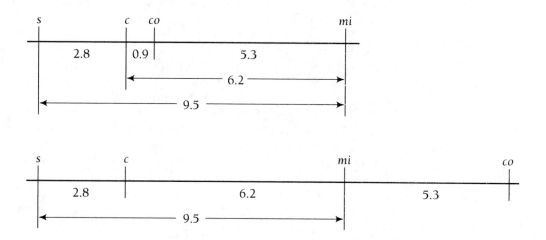

15.21   *Answer:* Between any two *rII* mutants *rIIx* and *rIIy* there are two products of intragenic recombination: *r⁺* (wild type) and *rIIxy* (a double mutant). Thus, the frequency of wild-type recombinants is half the total recombinant frequency. These data give the following map:

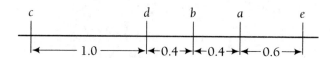

15.22   *Answer:* If no *r⁺* recombinants are obtained, the deletion removes the site of the point mutant. If *r⁺* recombinants are obtained, the site of the point mutation is not within the boundaries of the deletion. To determine the deleted region then, define the region that includes all of the point mutations unable to recombine with the deletion. Check your answer by verifying that all of the point mutations outside of this region do recombine with the deletion.

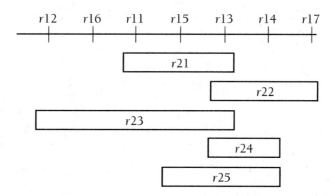

15.23   *Answer:* First define where the point mutants lie using a systematic approach that utilizes two facts: (1) If a point mutant is *able* to recombine with a deletion mutant, it must lie *outside* of the deleted region; and (2) if a point mutant is *unable* to recombine with a deletion mutant, it must lie *within* the deleted region. This means that a point mutant must lie within a region remaining intact in each of the deletions with which it does recombine, and, conversely, it must lie in a deleted region that is shared by each of the deletions with which it does not recombine. Employ both of these inferences to define the region in which the point mutant lies.

Then determine the positions of the *A* and *B* cistrons. Use the fact that if two mutants are unable to grow on *E. coli* K12(λ) ("0"), the mutants cannot together provide the functions to complete the *rII* pathway. Either the *rIIA* or *rIIB* function is missing. Consequently, both mutants must be defective in the same function. In other words, the mutants do not complement each other. For example, if a mutant does not complement a known *rIIA* mutant (i.e., there is no growth on *E. coli* K12(λ), ("0"), then the mutation is in the *A* cistron. Note that deletions can affect both the *A* and *B* cistrons, while point mutations can only affect one or the other cistron.

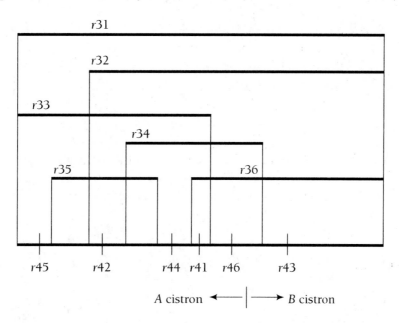

15.24   *Answer:* When two haploid strains mate to form a diploid cell, each contributes its genome. Consequently, there are two sets of genes in a diploid cell, and complementation between two mutants can be observed. If two mutations are in the same unit of function (i.e., the same gene), then they will not complement when together in a diploid cell and the mutant phenotype will be exhibited. If two mutations are in different genes, they will complement each other in a diploid cell and the wild-type phenotype will result.

In the data presented here, mutations 1 and 3 and mutations 1 and 4 complement each other, indicating that mutations 1 and 3 are in different genes and mutations 1 and 4 are in different genes.

On the other hand, mutations 1 and 2 and mutations 3 and 4 fail to complement each other. Thus, mutations 1 and 2 are in one gene, while mutations 3 and 4 are in a different gene. There are two genes.

15.25   *Answer:* Specialized transduction by λ occurs when a portion of the *E. coli* chromosome near the site of the λ chromosome insertion (*att*) is transduced into the recipient cell. See text Figure 15.14, p. 444. The *gal* and *bio* genes are near the *att* site, so portions of these genes can be transduced. If a transducing phage can recombine with a mutant to give a wild-type phenotype, the transducing phage must carry normal DNA that can recombine with and replace the mutant site. This information lets you deduce the relative order of the mutants *a–e* and identify the regions of the *gal* locus that are transduced by the five λ*d gal* phage. For example, λ*d gal* phage 5 can recombine only with mutant *c*, so must contain DNA for the mutant *c* site, but not any of the other mutant sites. Therefore, λ*d gal* phage 5 carries the least amount of DNA for the *gal* locus, and mutant *c* is the closest to the *att* site where the λ chromosome recombines into *E. coli*. In contrast, λ*d gal* phage 2 can recombine with all of the mutants, so it must contain DNA for all of their sites. Therefore, λ*d gal* phage 2 contains the most DNA of the *gal* locus and extends furthest into the *gal* locus. By similar reasoning, λ*d gal* phage 3 covers the *c* and *d* mutants, λ*d gal* phage 1 covers the *c*, *d*, and *e* mutants, and λ*d gal* phage 4 covers the *c*, *d*, *e*, and *b* mutants. This gives the mutant order: *(gal) a–b–e–d–c–att–bio*.

During specialized transduction, an abnormal outlooping occurs in which λ gains part of the *E. coli* chromosome and loses part of its own chromosome. The second set of data shed light on how much of the λ chromosome is lost. Using the same reasoning as before, a λ*d gal* phage will recombine with a λ mutant if it has DNA for the mutant site in λ. No λ*d gal* phage recombines with λ mutant *n* and so none of the phage have DNA containing this site. In contrast, λ*d gal* phage 1 can recombine with λ mutants *j, l, k,* and *m,* and so has DNA for all of these sites. By similar reasoning, λ*d gal* phage 5 covers mutant sites *k, l,* and *j,* λ*d gal* phage 3 covers mutant sites *l* and *j,* λ*d gal* phage 4 covers mutant site *j,* and λ*d gal* phage 2 covers no mutant sites. This gives the order of λ mutant sites as: *j–l–k–m–n.*

These data can be summarized in the following map:

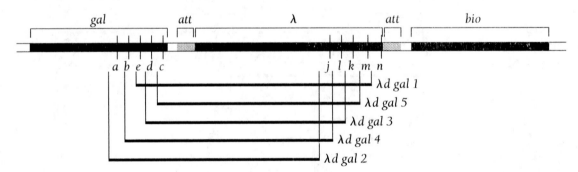

15.26   *Answer:*

a. If DNA transduced into a particular *leu* mutant recombines with its chromosome to produce a *leu*⁺ recombinant, the transduced DNA must contain a wild-type site that can replace the mutated *leu* site. Therefore, pairs of mutants that produce *leu*⁺ recombinants affect different sites, while pairs of mutants unable to produce *leu*⁺ recombinants affect one or more common sites. The sites may be single or multiple base-pair regions. Mutants that affect more than one site must be deletions. Deletions can be recognized by identifying mutants unable to produce *leu*⁺ recombinants with pairs of mutants that lie in different sites. For example, mutants 3 and 8 can recombine to produce *leu*⁺ recombinants, so they lie in different sites. Mutant 7 cannot recombine with either mutant 3 or mutant 8, so it must delete both sites. Using this logic, mutants 2, 4, and 7 must be deletions. In the map below, these deletions are shown by open boxes.

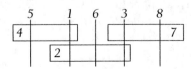

b. A site may be one or more base pairs. To address if a site is a point mutation, check if a mutant can be reverted. Point mutants, but not deletions, can be reverted.

c. This analysis does not address how many cistrons are present in this region. For this, complementation tests are needed.

15.27   *Answer:*

a. True. In the cross $w_1/w_1 \times w_2/w_2$, the offspring are $w_1 \, w_2$. That they are white-eyed indicates that w_1 and w_2 are mutations in the same function (i.e., the same gene). Thus, w_1 and w_2 are allelic genes.

b. False. If the genes were nonallelic, each mutation would be in a different function. The two mutations would each be in different steps of a pathway, with each mutant retaining the function of a different step. Since the progeny obtain a set of genes from each mutant parent, they would have the function of both steps and have red eyes. Since they have white eyes, this statement is false.

c. True.

d. True. A complementation test examines whether two mutations affect the same function.

e. True. The F_1 is a *trans*-heterozygote.

f. True. If two genes affect the same function, they are allelic.

   The complementation test indicates that the two mutations affect the same function and are therefore alleles at the same gene. However, it does not indicate whether they are *identical* alleles or not. To evaluate if two allelic mutations lie in exactly the same position in a gene, one needs to assess whether recombination can occur between them. If two alleles are identical and lie in the same site, *intragenic* recombination between them cannot occur. If they lie in different sites, intragenic recombination can occur, giving rise to wild-type recombinant chromosomes. The appearance of wild-type F_2 progeny results from intragenic recombination, as illustrated here.

If w_1 and w_2 lie in different sites in the same gene, the cross and the F_1 progeny can be written as

$$\text{P:} \quad \frac{w_1 +}{w_1 +} \times \frac{+ \, w_2}{+ \, w_2} \qquad \text{F}_1\text{:} \quad \frac{w_1 +}{+ \, w_2}$$

A rare intragenic crossover between the two mutant sites can be diagrammed as follows:

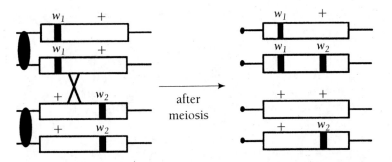

This crossover gives rise to gametes that are $w_1 \, w_2$ and $+ \, +$. The $w_1 \, w_2$ gamete would not be detected ($w_1 \, w_2 \, /w_1 \, +$ and $w_1 \, w_2/ + w_2$ flies are white eyed, as are their noncrossover siblings), but a $+ \, +$ gamete would give rise to a red-eyed offspring that has a genotype of $+ \, + /w_1 \, +$ or $+ \, +/ + \, w_2$. It is interesting to note that from the frequency of the white-eyed progeny, one can determine the recombination frequency (RF) between the two point mutants, just as in Benzer's *cis-trans* tests in the *rII* region of T4.

RF (w_1, w_2) = [(2 × 10)/20,010] × 100% = 0.1%.

The w_1 and w_2 mutation sites are 0.1 mu apart.

15.28   *Answer:* First think about why the parents might be white and have mostly white offspring. Presumably, the parents are white because they lack a functional gene that makes a product (an enzyme, perhaps) that produces black pigment. If the parents were white because they lacked the function of two *different* genes needed for black pigment production, a cross between them would produce black, and not white, offspring. Since most of their offspring are white, it is likely that they each lack an identical function needed for black pigment production. Consider the options for how this could occur and then consider how a black offspring might arise under each option.

Option 1: Each parent is homoallelic at a gene that results in white and not black pigmentation. In this case, denote the cross as $a^1a^1 \times a^2a^2$, all progeny are a^1/a^2. Since the parents are homoallelic, no intragenic recombination will occur. In this case, an a^+ allele could arise by a rare, new mutation (a reversion mutation), which would restore the function of the gene in the black pigment pathway. The offspring would be $a^{++}/(a^1$ or $a^2)$, and be black.

Option 2: At least one parent is heteroallelic at a gene that results in white and not black pigmentation. In this case, one can denote the cross as $a^1/a^2 \times a^-/a^-$, where a^- represents any mutant, nonfunctional allele at this gene (the two a^- alleles need not be identical). In the heteroallelic parent a^1/a^2, a rare intragenic crossover between the sites of the a^1 and a^2 mutations will result in a^+ and $a^{1,2}$ alleles, so that an a^+/a^- offspring will be produced. This offspring will have a^+ gene function and so it will be black.

15.29   *Answer:* There are at least two options. First, the enzyme could be composed of multiple polypeptide subunits. The mutants are at different genes, each of which encodes a polypeptide that is part of the multimeric enzyme. Second, the enzyme is composed of just one type of polypeptide but the polypeptide is modified before it becomes active as an enzyme. One mutant is at a gene that encodes the polypeptide that will be modified to become the enzyme; the second mutant is at a gene that encodes a protein that modifies the enzymatic polypeptide and that is required to make it functional (e.g., it could be a protease that cleaves a proenzyme, making it active as an enzyme; it could be a kinase that phosphorylates a nonactive form of the enzyme, making it active).

15.30   *Answer:* Use the nutrition and accumulation data to infer where each mutant is blocked. Mutant 1 accumulates ornithine and can grow only if citrulline or arginine is added. Hence, Mutant 1 is blocked in the conversion of ornithine to citrulline. Mutants 2 and 3 are blocked in the conversion of citrulline to arginine. Mutant 4 is more complex. It can grow only if supplemented with arginine, but accumulates ornithine. Mutant 4 must be a double mutant and is blocked in the conversion of ornithine to citrulline as well as from citrulline to arginine. This gives the following pathway:

$$\text{precursor} \xrightarrow{\hspace{1.5cm}} \text{ornithine} \xrightarrow{1,\,4} \text{citrulline} \xrightarrow{2,\,3,\,4} \text{arginine}$$
$$\text{Enzyme:} \qquad\quad A \qquad\qquad\qquad B \qquad\qquad\quad C$$

Use the complementation test data to determine whether two mutants affect the same function. Diploids constructed from two mutants that are able to grow on minimal media indicate that the mutants complement each other: One provides a function missing in the other. Failure to grow indicates no complementation: both are missing the same function. Mutants 2 and 3 complement 1, so 2 and 3 affect a different step than 1. Mutants 2 and 3 fail to complement each other, so they affect the same step. Mutant 4 fails to complement 1, 2, or 3 and affects both steps. This is consistent with the deduced pathway: Mutants 1 and 4 affect enzyme B, and 2, 3, and 4 affect enzyme C.

Start analyzing the recombination data by assigning symbols to the genes and writing out the genotypes and crosses. Let b^+ encode enzyme B and c^+ encode enzyme C. Then $1 = b^1 c^+$, $2 = b^+ c^2$, $3 = b^+ c^3$, and $4 = b^4 c^4$. The prototrophic ascospres produced in the crosses 1×2, 1×3, and 2×3 are $b^+ c^+$ and are half of the recombinant progeny (e.g., in 1×2, parental types are $b^1 c^+$ and $b^+ c^2$, recombinant types are $b^+ c^+$ and $b^1 c^2$). The results can be tabulated as:

Cross	Genotypes	$b^+ c^+$ Spores
1×2	$b^1 c^+ \times b^+ c^2$	25.0%
1×3	$b^1 c^+ \times b^+ c^3$	25.0%
1×4	$b^1 c^+ \times b^4 c^4$	$< 1 \times 10^{-6}$
2×3	$b^+ c^2 \times b^+ c^3$	0.002%
2×4	$b^+ c^2 \times b^4 c^4$	0.001%
3×4	$b^+ c^3 \times b^4 c^4$	$< 1 \times 10^{-6}$

Use the recombination frequencies to infer whether the *b* and *c* genes are linked and whether two alleles at one gene affect the same site or are separable by recombination and affect different sites. Crosses 1 × 2 and 1 × 3 give 25% prototrophs (show 50% recombination), so *b* and *c* are unlinked. Cross 2 × 3 produces very few prototrophs, since they can only arise from rare, intragenic recombination. The 0.002% prototrophs (= half the recombinants) indicate that c^2 and c^3 are 0.004 mu apart. Mutant 4 fails to recombine with 1 or 3, indicating that b^4 and b^1 affect the same site, and that c^4 and c^3 affect the same site. The 0.001% prototrophs from 2 × 4 arise when a c^+ allele is obtained after intragenic recombination between c^2 and c^4 *and* the b^+ allele (in mutant 2) assorts with it into the ascospore. When c^+ assorts with b^4 (half the time), a prototrophic ascospore is not obtained. This is why only 0.001% prototrophs are recovered from 2 × 4, instead of the 0.002% prototrophs recovered from 2 × 3. This results in the following map:

a. Three distinct mutational sites exist based on the recombination analysis: one in the *b* gene and two in the *c* gene.

b. Two polypeptide chains are affected based on the complementation analysis: one encoded by the *b* gene and one encoded by the *c* gene.

c. The genotypes are as given in the table above.

d. There are 0.004 mu between the two mutant sites in the *c* gene identified by c^2 and c^3. The *b* and *c* genes are unlinked.

e. The *b* and *c* genes assort independently of one another. Thus, strain 1, 2, or 3, when mated with the wild type, will give 50% prototrophs and 50% auxotrophs. As strain 4 is a double mutant, it will give only 25% prototrophs. Four equally frequent genotypes would be expected from the cross $b^4 c^4 \times b^+ c^+$. Only one of the four will be $b^+ c^+$.

15.31   *Answer:*

a. Since all nine very early mutants can be reverted, all are point mutants.

b. All nine very early mutants fail to complement each other (none produce enough virus in pairwise coinfections to be considered positive), so they affect one function.

c. Eight of the mutants (*B2, B21, B27, B28, B32, 901, LB2, D*) are able to recombine with each other and so affect different sites. Mutant *c75* fails to recombine with mutant *D*, so these two mutants may affect the same site.

d. Mutant *c75* may be a mutant affecting multiple sites. It reverts at a lower frequency than the others and shows inconsistent recombination relative to the other mutants.

e. The mutants incompletely block viral growth, so some virus is produced by each mutant. *I* compares the amount of virus produced by coinfection of two mutants to the sum of the amounts produced by individual infections. If two viruses are blocked in the same function, a coinfection should produce low amounts of virus similar to the sum of two separate infections, and *I* will be about 1.0. If two mutants are blocked in different functions, coinfection allows for complementation because the function blocked in one mutant is provided by the other mutant. Substantial viral growth will occur, and *I* should be much larger than 1.

At the restrictive temperature of 39°C, neither parent nor doubly mutant recombinants can grow. Only wild-type recombinants can grow. These are half of the recombinants, so doubling the amount of virus produced at 39°C will estimate the number of recombinants between the two mutant sites. At the permissive temperature of 34°C, mutant and wild-type virus can grow, so the amount of virus produced at 34°C measures the total amount of virus produced by coinfecting the two mutant strains. RF is calculated by doubling the amount of virus produced by coinfecting two mutants at 39°C and then dividing this number by the amount of virus produced by coinfecting the mutants at 34°C, so RF estimates recombination between two mutants.

f.

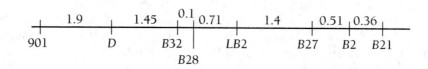

g. Mutant *c75*'s reversion rate is less than that of the other mutants, suggesting that it is more complex than a simple point mutant. If it affected multiple sites, it would have recombination data inconsistent with the other mutants.

15.32 *Answer:*

a. Cross each mutation to the wild-type, brick red strain and observe the phenotypes of the progeny. A dominant mutation, by definition, is one that appears in a heterozygote. If the progeny show brick red eyes, the mutation must be recessive. If the progeny show brownish eyes, the mutation is dominant.

b. Set up pairs of crosses between the mutants to perform complementation tests. Mutations that affect the same gene function will produce brown-eyed progeny when crossed and belong to the same complementation group. Mutations that affect different functions will produce brick red-eyed progeny when crossed and belong to different complementation groups. Counting the number of different complementation groups will give the number of genes that are affected.

c. Allelic mutations are those that are members of the same complementation group, as determined in **(b)**.

d. One could assess if a particular mutant is allelic to a known eye color gene by performing complementation tests between it and mutants at all known eye color genes. This would involve crossing the mutant to mutants from a collection of strains with known eye color mutations and observing the progeny of each cross. If the progeny have a mutant eye color, one would infer that the mutations carried in the two strains are allelic. However, this would be a tremendous amount of work. There are many eye color mutations, and this would require a large number of crosses. It would be faster to first determine which of the six mutations are allelic and then choose a representative allele from each complementation group and identify its chromosomal location using a set of two- and/or three-point mapping crosses. Once this is done, examine published genetic maps of the *Drosophila* genome (e.g., at http://www.flybase.org) and ask if any known eye color mutations lie in the same region. Then obtain strains with these eye color mutations and perform complementation tests between these mutant strains and a representative mutant from each complementation group identified with the new eye color mutations.

15.33 *Answer:*

a. Start by performing complementation tests. Cross a rosy-eyed mutant (call it *x*) to a known mutation, *ry*, at the *rosy* locus, and observe the phenotype of the offspring. If the progeny have wild-type (brick red) eyes, the mutations complement each other, suggesting that *x* is not an allele at the *rosy* locus. This can be verified by mapping mutant *x* using two- and three-point testcrosses. If mutant *x* maps to a different locus, it can be excluded from further consideration. However, if *x* is tightly linked to the *rosy* locus, *x* and the known *ry* mutation may lie in different cistrons at the *ry* locus. If *x* does not complement *ry*, then *x* affects the same cistron as the known *ry* mutant.

b. Intragenic recombination can be evaluated by observing whether the progeny of heterozygotes bearing different *ry* alleles (e.g., ry^1/ry^2) receive an ry^+ allele. Using a logic similar to that of Benzer, intragenic recombination in ry^1/ry^2 heterozygotes will generate ry^+ and $ry^{1,2}$ chromosomes. If the heterozygotes are crossed to *ry/ry* males, recombinant offspring that are $ry^{1,2}/ry$ will have rosy eyes, while recombinants that are ry^+/ry will have brick red eyes. Therefore, set up these types of crosses (females heterozygous for different *ry* alleles crossed to *ry/ry* males) and count the number of offspring with brick red eyes. The recombination frequency is given by (2 × # brick red-eyed progeny)/(total progeny). Since recombination within a gene is rare, very few recombinants are expected (0.01% < RF < 0.3% based on Benzer's findings) and so this process could be tedious.

Since intragenic recombination is rare, it is important to verify that the brick red-eyed progeny result from intragenic recombination and not reversion of one of the ry mutations. If the crosses were set up so that one of the ry chromosomes had flanking markers, intragenic recombination could be verified by checking for flanking marker exchange. For example, suppose the cross was $kar \; ry^1 \; l(3)26/kar^+ \; ry^2 \; l(3)26^+$ (females) $\times \; ry^3/ry^3$ (males), that there was intragenic recombination between the sites of ry^1 and ry^2, and that the relative order of the mutant sites was $kar–ry^1–ry^2–l(3)26$. Then the resulting ry^+ recombinant would be $kar^+ \; ry^+ \; l(3)26/ry^3$ (demonstrate this by drawing it out). Flanking marker exchange associated with crossing-over between ry^1 and ry^2 could be verified by testcrossing the brick red-eyed fly to a $kar \; ry^+$ $l(3)26/kar^+ \; ry \; l(3)26^+$ individual and counting the number of progeny phenotypes. In this case, flanking marker exchange should be associated with a 2 ry^+ : 1 ry ratio due to the recessive lethality of the $l(3)26$ mutation. If the order of the mutant sites was $kar–ry^2–ry^1–l(3)26$, then the resulting ry^+ recombinant would be $kar \; ry^+ \; l(3)26^+$, and flanking marker exchange would be associated with a 3 kar^+ : 1 kar progeny ratio.

c. One way to efficiently select for intragenic recombinants is to use supplemental purines in the diet to eliminate all ry progeny. Estimate the number of progeny (by counting the number of eggs laid, for example) and then raise the offspring on media rich in purines. Only ry^+ progeny would survive, and so this method would select for intragenic recombinants (and unintentionally, ry^+ revertants). This would make the process much less tedious because it wouldn't be necessary to look at the eye color of tens of thousands of flies.

d. Based on Benzer's work, one would expect that intragenic recombination is rare, that mutations can be mapped to sites within the ry locus, that some "hot spots" (sites where mutations are more prevalent) may exist, that some mutations will be unable to recombine with others (because they are deletions), and that there will be a minimum map distance between the closest ry alleles (corresponding to the recombination frequency between mutants affecting neighboring DNA base pairs). A complementation analysis will reveal if the ry locus has multiple cistrons (functional units).

16

Variations in Chromosome Structure and Number

Chapter Outline

Review of Key Terms, Symbols, and Concepts

In your own words, write a brief, precise definition of each term in the groups below. Check your definitions using the text. Then develop a concept map using the terms in each list.

1	2
chromosomal mutation, aberration	euploid
deletion	aneuploid
duplication	polyploid
translocation	monoploid
inversion	diploid, triploid, tetraploid
position effect	haploid
epigenetic phenomenon, epigenetics	nullisomy
karyotype	monosomy
polytene chromosomes, bands and interbands	trisomy
chromocenter	tetrasomy
larval salivary gland	double monosomic, tetrasomic
endoreduplication	autopolyploidy
pseudodominance	allopolyploidy
deletion mapping	allotetraploid
tandem, terminal tandem, reverse tandem duplication	odd-number polyploidy
multigene family	even-number polyploidy
unequal crossing-over	seedless fruit
pericentric vs. paracentric inversion	chromosome
dicentric bridge, acentric fragment	centromere
intra-, interchromosomal translocation	distal to/from
reciprocal vs. nonreciprocal translocation	promixal to/from
alternate, adjacent-1, adjacent-2 segregation	Down syndrome
semisterility	trisomy-21, -13, -18
fragile sites	Patau syndrome
triplet repeat amplification	Edwards syndrome
premutation	Turner syndrome
normal transmitting male	Klinefelter syndrome
cri-du-chat syndrome	familial Down syndrome
Prader–Willi syndrome	Robertsonian translocation
Drosophila Bar mutation	
Philadelphia chromosome	
Burkitt lymphoma	
chronic myelogenous leukemia	
proto-oncogene	
oncogenes, *c-abl, c-myc*	
fragile X syndrome, mental retardation	
FMR-1	

Thinking Analytically

In this chapter, it is crucial to be able to visualize the physical structure of chromosomes in the context of cellular processes such as meiosis and gene expression. Start by developing mental images of chromosomal aberrations. Practice drawing inversions, transpositions, translocations, duplications, and deletions.

To understand fully the impact of chromosomal mutations on gene expression and inheritance of traits, you will need a solid grasp of cellular processes involving chromosome movement. Review how chromosomes move and align during meiosis. Then consider how chromosomal aberrations and mutations affecting chromosome number alter the behavior of chromosomes during meiosis and thereby affect the inheritance of traits. The disruptions in meiosis that result from a particular chromosomal aberration are best understood by drawing out the chromosomal mutation as it proceeds through meiosis. As you do the problems, take the time to draw out the consequences of crossing-over in inversion and translocation heterozygotes. To understand how chromosome aberrations affect gene expression and gene function, consider what happens when the structure of a gene is rearranged and broken into two separate parts by a chromosomal aberration. Ask yourself, What are the possible consequences if a rearrangement breakpoint is in the amino acid-coding region of the gene, if it is in the promoter or other regulatory region, if it rearranges the gene nearby the enhancer of a different gene, or if it fuses two unrelated genes in their intronic regions?

Aneuploidy and polyploidy have direct effects on gene dosage: A normal phenotype requires proper gene dosage. As you examine the consequences of different types of aneuploidy and polyploidy, consider how the different phenotypes that arise result from altering gene dosage.

Questions for Practice

Multiple-Choice and True-False Questions

1. The number of polytene chromosomes in dipterans, such as *Drosophila*, is characteristically
   a. twice the diploid number.
   b. hundreds or more times the diploid number.
   c. half the diploid number.
   d. the same as the diploid number.

2. The chromosomes that become polytene chromosomes are
   a. somatically paired.
   b. genetically inert.
   c. uniformly pycnotic.
   d. acentric.

3. Nonhomologous chromosomes that have exchanged segments are the products of a
   a. double deletion.
   b. reciprocal translocation.
   c. pericentric inversion.
   d. paracentric inversion.

4. The abbreviated karyotype 2N − 1 describes
   a. nullisomy.
   b. monosomy.
   c. trisomy.
   d. haploidy.

5. The abbreviated karyotype 2N + 1 + 1 describes
   a. double trisomy.
   b. tetrasomy.
   c. double monosomy.
   d. none of the above

6. All known monosomics in humans have been
   a. lethal.
   b. semilethal.
   c. treatable.
   d. deletion heterozygotes.

7. The cultivated bread wheat *Triticum aestivum,* although a polyploid, is fertile because it
  a. has an odd number of chromosome sets.
  b. has an even multiple of chromosome sets.
  c. is a double hybrid.
  d. is propagated by grafting.
8. Cultivated bananas and Baldwin apples are
  a. double diploids.
  b. tetraploids.
  c. double haploids.
  d. triploids.
9. Down syndrome is associated with
  a. an inversion.
  b. a Robertsonian translocation.
  c. trisomy-21.
  d. both b and c
10. Gene expression can be altered by
  a. an inversion.
  b. a duplication.
  c. a transposition.
  d. any of the above

Decide whether each of the following statements is true or false.
11. In terms of severity of symptoms found in infants, trisomies for chromosomes 13, 18, and 21 are all about equally severe.
12. All deletions are cytologically visible.
13. A dicentric chromosome has two arms.
14. Crossing-over within the inverted region of a pericentric inversion, in an inversion heterozygote, produces gametes with duplications and deletions.
15. The Philadelphia chromosome (a specific translocation between chromosomes 9 and 22) found in chronic myelogenous leukemia fuses two genes, resulting in an oncogene.
16. The semi-sterility seen in individuals heterozygous for chromosomal rearrangements such as inversions and translocations always results from the production of aneuploid gametes following crossing-over.
17. Duplications can result in dominant phenotypes if the duplication includes a dose-sensitive region.
18. Pericentric inversions occur on one arm of a chromosome.
19. Polytene chromosomes are chromosomes that have replicated without nuclear division.
20. In contrast to triploid animals, which usually die, triploid plants usually live (but are sterile).

Answers: 1c, 2a, 3b, 4b, 5a, 6a, 7b, 8d, 9d, 10d, 11F, 12F, 13F, 14T, 15T, 16F, 17T, 18F, 19T, 20T

Thought Questions

1. Identify and describe five examples of changes in chromosome structure that alter gene expression.
2. A chromosomal inversion in the heterozygous condition seems to act as a suppressor of crossing-over. Why might this be the case? How might such chromosomes be important for keeping a laboratory stock of three linked recessive mutations?
3. What are two causes of Down syndrome? Why might one be more frequent than the other? If a normal female has a sibling with Down syndrome, what information would be critical in the assessment of the chances that she might have a child with Down syndrome? How would the assessment be different if the assessed individual were a normal male whose sibling had Down syndrome?
4. Consider the data presented in Table 16.2. Given these data, how do you account for the fact that most children with Down syndrome are born to women under 25 years of age? Does this alter the need for caution and prenatal diagnosis in women over 35 years of age?

5. How do you account for the fact that polyploidy is significantly more common in plants than in animals? (Hint: What basic difference between sexual and asexual reproduction might be significant here?)

6. What might be the significance of the following in the evolutionary process of speciation? (1) autopolyploidy, (2) allopolyploidy, (3) inversions, (4) translocations. Provide an explanation that considers how animals might be affected differently than plants.

7. Many small deletions, when heterozygous, display a normal phenotype. Others display a mutant phenotype. For example, a small deletion that removes just the *Notch* gene in *Drosophila*, when heterozygous with a normal chromosome, displays a mutant phenotype of notched (nicked) wings. A nearby deletion that removes just the *white* gene, when heterozygous with a normal chromosome, displays the wild-type phenotype of deep-red eyes. Speculate why some heterozygous deletions might show a phenotype while others do not.

8. Which, if any, of the chromosomal aberrations discussed in this chapter are able to revert to a normal phenotype?

Thought Questions for Media

After reviewing the media on the *iGenetics* website, try to answer these questions.

1. After viewing the *Crossing-over in an Inversion Heterozygote* animation, consider the following two situations.

   I. No crossovers occur in the inverted region of a pericentric inversion in an inversion heterozygote.

   II. A single crossover occurs in the inverted region of a pericentric inversion in an inversion heterozygote.

   a. What different types of *viable* gametes are produced in these two situations?

   b. Are the ratios of different types of *viable* gametes are produced in these situations the same or different?

   c. Are *inviable* gametes produced in either of these situations? If so, how are they produced and why are they inviable?

2. In the *Meiosis in a Translocation Heterozygote* animation, the chromosomes in a reciprocal translocation heterozygote were depicted as N_1, N_2, T_1, and T_2 N_1 and N_2 were the normal ordered, nonhomologous chromosomes. T_1 and T_2 were the chromosomes in which a reciprocal translocation occurred. N_1 and T_1 have homologous centromeres, as do N_2 and T_2. In the animation, homologous regions of these chromosomes paired during meiosis I and aligned in a crosslike figure. They were arranged with N_1 in the upper left-hand corner, N_2 in the lower right-hand corner, T_1 in the lower left-hand corner, and T_2 in the upper right-hand corner, as follows:

   $$N_1 \rightarrow T_2$$
   $$T_1 \rightarrow N_2$$

   Use this illustration as you answer the following questions:

   a. The animation illustrated three different patterns of segregation of these chromosomes during meiosis I called alternate, adjacent-1, and adjacent-2 segregation. Which chromosomes go to each pole in the different types of segregation?

   b. Which two types of segregation are most frequent? Which one type of segregation is rare?

   c. Which type(s) of segregation pattern produces balanced gametes? Which type(s) produces inviable gametes?

   d. Why are individuals with a reciprocal translocation semi-sterile?

1. Suppose Sonia and Ramon conceive a fetus that has the T(14;21) translocation. Can you tell, from this information alone, whether the child will have Down syndrome or be healthy? If not, what additional information about the karyotype would you need to know? If the child has Down syndrome, what can you infer about the chromosomes carried by the sperm used in fertilization?

2. Suppose Sonia and Ramon, having had one normal child, are interested in having a second child. They seek genetic counseling for advice. What advice should the counselor give them, and how, if at all, would it differ from any advice they might have received when attempting to have their first child?

3. What is the chance that Sonia and Ramon will have a child with the same karyotype as Ramon? With the same karyotype as Sonia?

Solutions to Text Questions and Problems

16.1 *Answer:*
   a. pericentric inversion (inversion of D–o–E–F)
   b. nonreciprocal translocation (B–C moved from left to right arm)
   c. tandem duplication (E–F duplicated)
   d. reverse tandem duplication (E–F duplicated)
   e. deletion (C deleted)

16.2 *Answer:* A pericentric inversion is an inversion that includes the centromere, while a paracentric inversion lies wholly within one chromosomal arm. See text Figure 16.7, p. 468.

16.3 *Answer:* Deletions, whether just a few bases or large segments of DNA, are unable to be reverted. Point mutations that affect only a single base can be reverted. If a recessive mutation is able to be reverted to a wild-type phenotype, it cannot be a deletion.

16.4 *Answer:*
   a. Paracentric inversion, because the centromere is not included in the inverted DNA segment

   b.

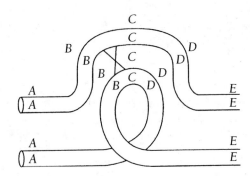

   c. A crossover between B and C results in the following chromosomes:

   A B C D E   (normal order)

   A B C D A   (dicentric, duplication for A, deletion for E)

   E B C D E   (acentric, duplication for E, deletion for A)

   A D C B E   (inverted order)

16.5   *Answer:* If a two-strand double crossover occurs within a paracentric inversion, the four products of meiosis have a complete set of genes, without duplications or deletions. No acentric or dicentric fragments are formed. Consequently, all four meiotic products are viable. This is illustrated in the following example:

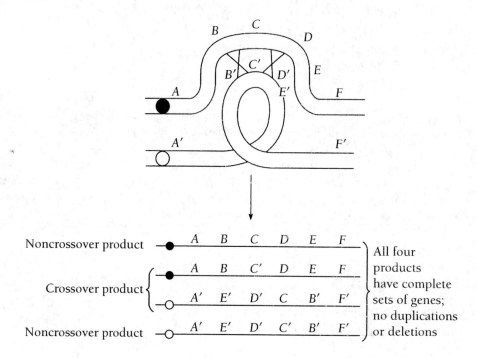

16.6   *Answer:* Diagrammed below is a four-strand double crossover, where the crossover between *c* and *d* involves strands 2 and 4, and the crossover between *e* and *f* involves strands 1 and 3. The bridge strands will break at anaphase I as the centromeres move toward opposite poles of the cell.

Synapsis:

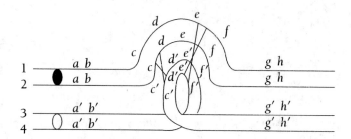

First Anaphase:

16.7   *Answer:* One series of sequential inversions is:

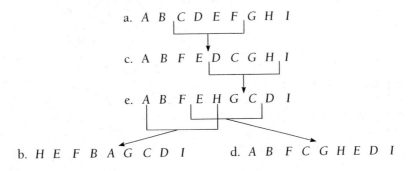

The regions inverted in each step are illustrated here.

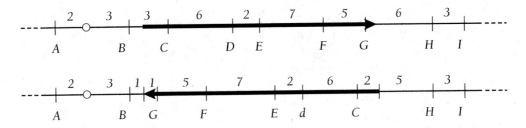

16.8   *Answer:* The following figure, in which the inverted region is depicted by an arrow, depicts the chromosomes in the heterozygote.

a. If no crossovers occur in the inversion heterozygote or if a crossover occurs outside of the inverted region, the *d*-bearing chromosome contributed by the inversion heterozygote will be inverted. If one crossover occurs, inviable deletion products would result (see text Figure 16.8, p. 470). Therefore, for zero or one crossover, no *dd* offspring will have chromosomes with only wild-type arrangements.

b. A two-strand double crossover could produce a normal-ordered, *d*-bearing homolog (see the solution to Question 16.5). To produce a *d*-bearing homolog, one crossover must occur between the proximal (toward the centromere) breakpoint of the inversion and the *d* locus, and a second crossover involving the same pair of chromatids must occur between the *d* locus and the distal (toward the telomere) breakpoint of the inversion. There are 15 map units between the proximal breakpoint and *d*, and 8 map units between the *d* and the distal breakpoint. Assuming that there is no crossover interference, *P* (double crossover) = 0.15 × 0.08 = 0.012. Two-strand double crossovers are ¼ of the possible double crossovers (see text Figure 14.4, p. 411), so *P* (desired event) = ¼ × 0.012 = 0.003.

c. Most of the time, mutations within an inversion will be transmitted with that inversion and not with the normal ordered chromosome. Over time, additional genetic differences will accumulate in the inverted region. These will not usually be shared with individuals having normal ordered chromosomes. Therefore, the inversion contributes to the maintenance of genetic differences between subpopulations of a species.

16.9   *Answer:*

a. The following diagram shows a normal chromosome bearing w^+, the w^{M4}-associated inversion, and a second inversion found in a w^+ revertant. The genes *a, b, c,* and *d* are inserted nearby the breakpoints of the different inversions to help visualize the inverted regions. Euchromatin is represented by a thin line, centromeric heterochromatin by a thick line, and the centromere by an open circle. The brackets delineate inverted regions.

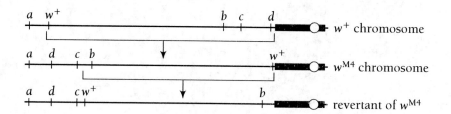

The mottled-eye phenotype is associated with chromosomal rearrangements induced on a w^+-bearing chromosome that place the w^+ gene near heterochromatin. When a rearrangement is heterozygous with a w allele, only the w^+ gene on the rearranged chromosome can provide for normal eye pigmentation. The mottled appearance of the eye indicates that it functions in some but not all cells. This suggests that the *white* gene's DNA sequence is unaltered. It is more likely an epigenetic phenomenon caused by a position effect, a phenotypic change due to inactivation of the w^+ allele by neighboring heterochromatin.

b. The second inversion that occurs on the w^{M4} chromosome repositions the w^+ gene to a euchromatic location. This supports the view that the mottled-eye phenotype is caused by a position effect.

16.10 *Answer:*

a. Parents of Rec(8) individuals are heterozygous for a pericentric inversion with breakpoints at 8p23.1 and 8q22.1. Rec(8) offspring with 8q-duplication and 8p-deletion probably arose from a single crossover within the pericentric inversion. Such an event is diagrammed in text Figure 16.9, p. 471.

b. As shown in text Figure 16.9, a single crossover between two nonsister chromatids in an inversion heterozygote results in four products: two have the noncrossover chromosomes (one is normal ordered and one is inverted) and two are duplication/deletion products. Here, the product with 8q-duplication and 8p-deletion contribute to a viable zygote with Rec(8) syndrome. The product with 8q-deletion and 8p-duplication is not discussed in the problem. It may be that zygotes with this product do not survive. In this case, $\frac{1}{3}$ of the surviving zygotes have Rec(8) syndrome. Of the $\frac{2}{3}$ normal zygotes, $\frac{1}{2}$ carry the chromosome 8 inversion.

c. The phenotypes of Rec(8) individuals could vary for one or a combination of reasons.
   (1) There could be several different chromosome 8 inversions in the population that vary slightly in their inversion breakpoints. The Rec(8) individuals resulting from single crossovers in inversion heterozygotes would differ symptomatically due to variation in genes that are duplicated and deleted or due to differences in gene activation or gene inactivation.
   (2) There may be a position effect.
   (3) The genetic background could vary. The phenotypic effects of gene deletion or duplication could depend on genetic interactions with other genes in the genome. In this case, alleles inherited from the father that are different from those inherited from the mother and grandmother could contribute to the phenotype.
   (4) Environmental effects could exacerbate the effects of the deleted and duplicated region. These effects may not be uniform, and so could contribute to the observed phenotypic variability. Since many of the symptoms associated with Rec(8) syndrome are developmental abnormalities, variation of the environment during fetal development may contribute to phenotypic variability.
   (5) There may be other, cytologically invisible mutations associated with the Rec(8) individuals that could strongly affect their phenotype.

d. The child has the chromosome 8 inversion, but not the duplication/deletion chromosome that results from a single crossover in an inversion heterozygote; she is an atypical Rec(8) individual. There are several explanations for why some of her symptoms overlap with those of Rec(8) syndrome. She may have an additional mutation near one of the Rec(8) breakpoints, in a region that is duplicated or deleted in Rec(8) syndrome, or in a gene that interacts with genes in the duplicated or deleted regions. Alternatively, it is possible that the inversion disrupts the function of a gene or genes at one or both breakpoints, and that normally, the inversion is an asymptomatic condition. In this case, the inversion chromosome (in her mother and grandmother) would bear a recessive mutation. If she had a new allelic mutation, or her paternally contributed chromosome had an allelic mutation, she would be affected. This could also explain why she has only some of the symptoms of Rec(8) syndrome; she would have fewer genes affected than most Rec(8) individuals.

Small deletions would be cytologically invisible, as would point mutations. Thus, the explanations given above could not be evaluated solely by karyotype analysis. DNA marker and/or DNA sequence analyses (see text Chapters 8 and 10) could be used to evaluate the integrity of the chromosomal regions near the breakpoints.

16.11 *Answer:*

a. The irradiated chromosome has a paracentric inversion (i.e., an inversion within one of its arms). Dicentric chromosomes and fragments arise as the result of single crossovers within paracentric inversions, and dicentric chromosomes with two bridges and two fragments result from a four-strand double crossover within paracentric inversions. An example of such a chromosome is diagrammed here.

$$a \quad b \quad c \quad \bullet \quad d \quad e \quad f \quad g \quad h \quad i \qquad \text{normal order}$$

$$a \quad b \quad c \quad \bullet \quad d \quad h \quad g \quad f \quad e \quad i \qquad \text{paracentric inversion}$$

b. The bridge chromosome would arise by a single crossover within an inversion loop during meiosis. In the above example, the crossover would occur between d and i. See text Figure 16.8, p. 470, for an illustration of such a crossover.

16.12 *Answer:* Since the crosses are three-point testcrosses, the progeny phenotypes are specified by the genotypes of the gametes of the trihybrid parent. In each case, it helps to diagram the two chromosomes of the trihybrid and then consider the different types of gametes that can be produced by crossovers in the trihybrid parent. Since an inversion is present in parts **(b)**, **(c)**, and **(d)** of this question, some recombinant gametes will not be viable due to the aneuploidy that results when crossovers of this question occur within the inverted region. As discussed below, this will alter the proportions of gamete genotypes relative to those seen in trihybrids with normal-ordered chromosomes.

a. The chromosomes can be diagrammed as:

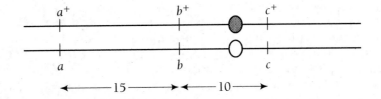

The trihybrid has no inversion, and its gametes will be exactly those expected from a trihybrid testcross. Since there are 15 mu between a and b, and 10 mu between b and c, 15% of the gametes will be single or double recombinants with crossovers between a and b, and 10% of the gametes will be single or double recombinants with crossovers between b and c. The remaining [100 − (10 + 15)] = 75% of the gametes will be parental types. This gives a frequency of 37.5% each of $a^+ b^+ c^+$ and $a\,b\,c$. Assuming that there is no interference, the expected frequency of double recombinants in the a–c interval is $0.10 \times 0.15 = 0.015$, or 1.5%. This gives a frequency of 0.75% each of $a^+ b\,c^+$ and $a\,b^+ c$. The remaining recombinants will result from single crossovers. There will be $15 − (1.5/2) = 14.25\%$ single recombinants in the a–b interval, giving 7.125% each of $a^+ b\,c$ and $a\,b^+ c^+$. There will be $10 − (1.5/2) = 9.25\%$ single recombinants in the b–c interval, giving 4.625% each of $a^+ b^+ c$ and $a\,b\,c^+$.

b. Here, nearly the entire region between a^+ and b^+ is inverted. The chromosomes can be diagrammed as indicated here, using a thick line with an arrowhead to represent the inverted region.

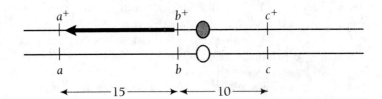

The inverted region is a paracentric inversion. As shown in text Figure 16.8, p. 470, a single crossover within a paracentric inversion results in a dicentric bridge that produces deletion-bearing chromosomes. Gametes that receive these chromosomes are not viable. If this region were not inverted, nearly 15% of the gametes would be recombinant for the a–b interval. However, because of the inversion, these recombinants will not be recovered. As a consequence, the frequency of the remaining recombinant and parental gametes will not be the same as these gamete types in a trihybrid parent with normal-ordered chromosomes. Relative to a trihybrid parent with normal-ordered chromosomes, the frequency of the remaining recombinant and parental gametes will be increased by a factor of $[1/(1.00 - 0.15)] = 1.176$.

The only viable recombinant gametes from this trihybrid parent are those that result from crossovers between b and c. In a normal-ordered chromosome, since there are 10 mu between b and c, 10% of the gametes will be recombinant in this interval. Since 15% of the gametes are not seen in this trihybrid parent, there will be $1.176 \times 10\% = 11.76\%$ recombinants in the b–c interval. The remaining gametes $[1.176 \times 90\% = 88.24\%]$ will be parental types. This gives 5.88% $a^+ b^+ c$, 5.88% $a b c^+$, 44.12% $a^+ b^+ c^+$, and 44.12% $a b c$.

c. Here, nearly the entire region between a^+ and c^+ has been inverted. The chromosomes can be diagrammed as shown below, using a thick line with an arrowhead to show the inverted region.

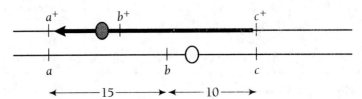

The inverted region is a pericentric inversion. As shown in text Figure 16.9, p. 471, the only viable gametes that are produced from a meiosis with a single crossover within the inverted region are parental types (either normal-ordered or inversion-bearing chromosomes). Gametes with either of the two types of duplication/deletion-bearing chromosomes resulting from a single crossover are not viable. Thus, single crossovers occurring in nearly the entire a–c interval will not produce recombinant gametes.

Crossovers that occur simultaneously in each of the a–b and b–c intervals (double crossovers) may produce viable recombinants, depending on whether they are two-strand, three-strand, or four-strand double crossovers. As shown in the answer to Question 16.5, a two-strand double crossover will produce viable gametes. Half of the gametes from such a meiosis are double recombinants ($a b^+ c$ and $a^+ b c^+$). As shown in the answer to Question 16.6, a four-strand double crossover will not produce any viable gametes. There are two possible types of three-strand double crossovers (see text Figure 14.4, p. 411). These are diagrammed for an inversion heterozygote in the figure here.

I.

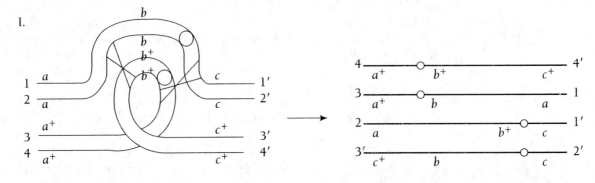

II.

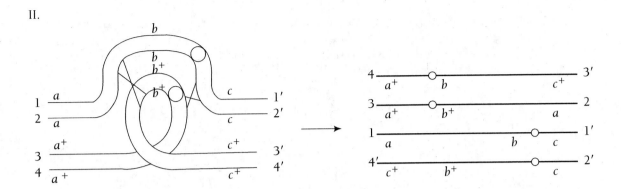

The three-strand double crossover shown in part I will produce the doubly recombinant chromosome $a\ b^+\ c$, two duplication/deletion chromosomes, and the parental-type chromosome $a^+\ b^+\ c^+$. The three-strand double crossover shown in part II will produce the doubly recombinant chromosome $a^+\ b\ c^+$, two duplication/deletion chromosomes, and the parental-type chromosome $a\ b\ c$. Thus, in a meiosis with either type of three-strand double crossover, two gametes will not be viable (the duplication/deletion-bearing gametes) and two gametes will be viable (one parental and one recombinant gamete). The results of meioses with each type of double crossover are summarized in the table here:

Type of Double Crossover	Nonviable Gametes	Viable Gametes		
		Recombinants	Parentals	Total
Two-strand	0	2	2	4
Three-strand (I)	2	1	1	2
Three-strand (II)	2	1	1	2
Four-strand	4	0	0	0

If each of the four types of double-crossover meioses occur equally frequently in a trihybrid with a heterozygous inversion, on average these meioses will produce 1/2 viable gametes and 1/4 doubly recombinant gametes. By comparison, double-crossover meioses in a trihybrid with normal-ordered chromosomes will produce on average all viable gametes and half doubly recombinant gametes. Thus, the pericentric inversion reduces both the number of gametes and the number of double recombinants by half. Since this pericentric inversion spans nearly the entire $a–c$ interval, the observed number of double recombinants will be very close to half of the expected number of double recombinants in a normal-ordered trihybrid parent. From **(a)**, a normal-ordered trihybrid parent has 1.25% doubly recombinant gametes, so here there will be $1/2 \times 1.25\% = 0.625\%$. This gives $(100 - 0.625)/2 = 49.6875\%$ each of $a^+\ b^+\ c^+$ and $a\ b\ c$, and 0.3125% each of $a^+\ b\ c^+$ and $a\ b^+\ c$.

d. Here, the inversion is only slightly larger than that in **(c)**, because the inverted region extends distally just past a and c. The trihybrid chromosomes can be diagrammed as shown here, using a thick line with an arrowhead to show the inverted region.

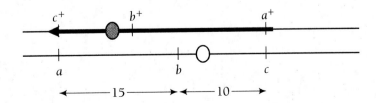

The frequency of progeny phenotypes will be very close to those observed in **(c)**, since the inversion is very similar in size.

16.13   *Answer:*

    a. Mr. Lambert is heterozygous for a pericentric inversion of chromosome 6. Relative to the centromere of the normal chromosome 6, one of the breakpoints is within the fourth light band up from the centromere, while the other is in the sixth dark band below the centromere. Mrs. Lambert's chromosomes are normal.

    b. When Mr. Lambert's number 6 chromosomes paired during meiosis, they formed an inversion loop that included the centromere. Crossing-over occurred within the loop and gave rise to the partially duplicated, partially deficient chromosome 6 that the child received.

    c. The child is not phenotypically normal because the duplications and deletions for different parts of chromosome 6 lead to severe abnormalities. The child has three copies of some and only one copy of other chromosome 6 regions. The top part of the short arm is duplicated, and there is a deficiency of the distal part of the long arm.

    d. Most future conceptions by this couple will produce an abnormal fetus. This is because the inversion covers more than half of the length of chromosome 6, and so the majority of meioses will have a crossover within the inverted region. A normal child will be produced in a minority of meioses where there is a two-strand double crossover inside the loop, where crossing-over occurs outside the loop, or where a crossover has occurred within the loop but the child receives a noncrossover chromosome. There is significant risk of abnormality, so fetal chromosomes should be monitored.

16.14   *Answer:*

    a. Mr. Simpson has a paracentric inversion in the long arm of one of his number 12 chromosomes. Moving downward (distally) from the centromere of the normal chromosome, the breakpoints are in the first dark band and in the sixth light band.

    b. Crossing-over within the inversion loop will produce dicentric chromatids that will form anaphase bridges. These chromatin bridges joining the two chromatin masses at the beginning of anaphase I will be visible in the testicular biopsy.

    c. The inversion is large, so the frequency of crossing-over within it will be significant. Consequently, bridges will be formed in the majority of meioses. Cells in which bridges form do not complete meiosis or form sperm in mammals.

    d. Nothing can be done to increase Mr. Simpson's sperm count. This might be an instance to consider *in vitro* fertilization.

16.15   *Answer:*

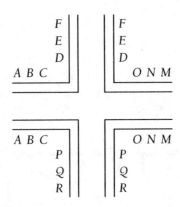

16.16   *Answer:* The following figure illustrates the pairing behavior of the translocation heterozygote.

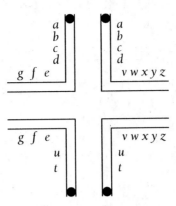

Text Figure 16.11, p. 473, shows the three types of segregation that can occur at anaphase I: alternate (~50% of the time), adjacent-1 (~50% of the time) and adjacent-2 (uncommon). In alternate segregation, alternate centromeres migrate to the same pole. Assuming that there is no crossing over, gametes will have either *abcdefg* and *utvwxyz* chromosomes or *abcdvwxyz* and *utefg* chromosomes. In adjacent-1 segregation, adjacent nonhomologous centromeres migrate to the same pole. Gametes will have *abcdefg* and *utefg* chromosomes or *abcdvwxyz* and *utvwxyz* chromosomes. In adjacent-2 segregation, adjacent homologous centromeres migrate to the same pole. Gametes will have *abcdefg* and *abcdvwxyz* chromosomes or *utefg* and *utvwxyz* chromosomes.

16.17   *Answer:*

  a. Mr. Denton has normal chromosomes. Mrs. Denton is heterozygous for a balanced reciprocal translocation between chromosomes 6 and 12. Most of the short arm of chromosome 6 has been reciprocally translocated onto the long arm of chromosome 12. The breakpoints appear to be in the first thick, dark band just above the centromere of 6 and in the third dark band below the centromere of 12.

  b. The child received a normal 6 and a normal 12 from his father. In prophase I of meiosis in Mrs. Denton, chromosomes 6 and 12 and the reciprocally translocated 6 and 12 paired to form a cruciform-like structure. Segregation of adjacent, nonhomologous centromeres to the same pole ensued, so that the child received a gamete containing a normal 6 and one of the translocation chromosomes. See text Figure 16.11, p. 473, for an illustration of adjacent-1 segregation.

  c. The child has a normal 6 and a normal 12 chromosome from Mr. Denton. The child also has a normal 6 chromosome from Mrs. Denton. However, the child also has one of the translocation chromosomes from Mrs. Denton. With this chromosome, the child is partially trisomic as well as partially monosomic. It has three copies of part of the short arm of chromosome 6 and only one copy of most of the long arm of chromosome 12. This abnormality in gene dosage is the cause of its physical abnormality.

  d. Segregation of adjacent homologous centromeres to the same pole is relatively rare. The segregation pattern seen in this child (adjacent-1 segregation) and alternate segregation (see text Figure 16.11) are more common. About half of the time, when alternate segregation occurs, the gamete will have a complete haploid set of genes, and the embryo should be normal. However, half of the gametes resulting from alternate segregation will be translocation heterozygotes.

  e. Prenatal monitoring of fetal chromosomes could be done, and given the severity of the abnormalities (high probability of miscarriage and multiple congenital abnormalities), therapeutic abortion of chromosomally unbalanced fetuses would be a consideration.

16.18   *Answer:* Mature sperm bear either an X or a Y chromosome, not both. For X-Y translocations to be obtained, both chromosomes must be present in the same sperm cell.

16.19   *Answer:*

a. The following figure shows how the translocation will pair with the normal chromosome 2.

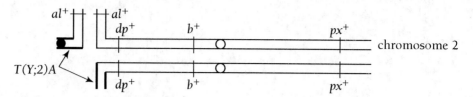

b. In *Drosophila* males, the Y and X chromosome centromeres normally segregate from each other. Though the X chromosome is not shown in the drawing in part **(a)**, keep this in mind as you identify what chromosomes are present in gametes.

In most meioses, the two chromosome 2 centromeres will segregate from each other. If the chromosomes segregate using alternate segregation, one type of gamete will contain the two fragments of $T(Y;2)A$ and the other type of gamete will contain the normal ordered chromosome 2 and the Y chromosome. Both gametes will be euploid. If the chromosomes segregate using adjacent-1 segregation, one type of gamete will contain the translocation fragment bearing the Y-chromosome centromere and the al^+ locus (hereafter referred to as $Y^{Cen}\ al^+$) and the normal ordered chromosome 2. It is aneuploid because it has a duplication for the region of chromosome 2 bearing the al^+ locus and is missing part of the Y chromosome. The other type of gamete will contain the X chromosome and the translocation fragment with the remaining portion of the Y chromosome and the portion of chromosome 2 containing the dp^+, b^+, and px^+ genes (hereafter referred to as $Y^{noCen}\ dp^+b^+px^+$). It is also aneuploid because it is missing part of the Y chromosome and the distal tip of chromosome 2. Adjacent-2 segregation is rare and produces inviable, aneuploid gametes. In adjacent-2 segregation, one type of gamete will have the normal ordered chromosome 2 and $Y^{noCen}\ dp^+b^+px^+$—it will have nearly two complete copies of chromosome 2 but only a fragment of the Y and no X chromosome. If it fertilizes a normal egg, the zygote will be nearly trisomic for chromosome 2 and be inviable. The other type of gamete will be missing most of chromosome 2 and will have the X chromosome and $Y^{Cen}\ al^+$. If it fertilizes a normal egg, the zygote will be nearly monosomic for chromosome 2 and be inviable.

c. **i.** Since no mutations involve the X or Y chromosome in this cross, equal numbers of viable males and females will be produced. They will be $^1/_4$ *Del(2)al/al$^+$ dp$^+$ b$^+$ px$^+$* (normal), $^1/_4$ *Del(2)al (dp$^+$ b$^+$ px$^+$) /al dp b px* (aristaless), $^1/_4$ *al$^+$ dp$^+$ b$^+$ px$^+$/al dp b px* (normal), and $^1/_4$ *al$^+$ dp$^+$ b$^+$ px$^+$/al$^+$ dp$^+$ b$^+$ px$^+$* (normal). So the progeny will be 3 normal : 1 aristaless.

ii, iii. Since adjacent-2 segregation in the $T(Y;2)A/+$ male is rare and produces inviable offspring, it need not be considered further. The table on the facing page gives the types of offspring produced when alternate or adjacent-1 segregation occur in the $T(Y;2)A/al^+\ dp^+\ b^+\ px^+$ male and the male is mated to either a *al dp b px/al$^+$ dp$^+$ b$^+$ px$^+$* or *Del(2)al/al$^+$ dp$^+$ b$^+$ px$^+$* female (crossovers are ignored).

16.20   *Answer:* Trisomy-21, -13, and -18 are the only trisomies seen in live births, and infants with these trisomies survive for differing lengths of time. Trisomy-21 occurs at a frequency of 3,510 per 1 million conceptions but is only seen in 1,430 per 1 million live births (14.3 in 10,000 live births), indicating that about 59% of conceptions with trisomy-21 do not survive until birth. Infants with trisomy-21 have Down syndrome, which is characterized by such abnormalities as low IQ, epicanthal folds, short and broad hands, and below-average height. Only some survive to adulthood.

Trisomy-13 occurs at a frequency of 2 in 10,000 live births and results in Patau syndrome. Characteristics of individuals with trisomy-13 include cleft lip and palate, small eyes, polydactyly, mental and developmental retardation, and cardiac anomalies. Most infants die before the age of 3 months.

Trisomy-18 occurs at a frequency of about 2.5 in 10,000 live births and results in Edwards syndrome. About 80% of infants with Edwards syndrome are female. Individuals with trisomy-18 are small at birth and have multiple congenital malformations affecting nearly all of the organs of the body, clenched fists, an elongated skull, low-set malformed ears, and mental and developmental retardation. Ninety percent of infants with Edwards syndrome die within 6 months, often from cardiac problems.

Gametes of *T(Y;2)A*, *al⁺dp⁺b⁺px⁺/al⁺dp⁺b⁺px⁺* male		Gametes of XX; *al dp b px/al⁺dp⁺b⁺px⁺* Female		Gametes of XX; *Del(2)al/al⁺dp⁺b⁺px⁺* Female	
		X; *al dp b px*	X; *al⁺dp⁺b⁺px⁺*	X; *Del(2)al*	X; *al⁺dp⁺b⁺px⁺*
Alternate Segregation	*T(Y;2)A*, *al⁺dp⁺b⁺px⁺*	X; *T(Y;2)A*, *al⁺dp⁺b⁺px⁺/ al dp b px* normal male	X; *T(Y;2)A*, *al⁺dp⁺b⁺px⁺/ al⁺dp⁺b⁺px⁺* normal male	X; *T(Y;2)A*, *al⁺dp⁺b⁺px⁺/ Del(2)al* normal male	X; *T(Y;2)A*, *al⁺dp⁺b⁺px⁺/ al⁺dp⁺b⁺px⁺* normal male
	X; *al⁺dp⁺b⁺px⁺*	XX; *al dp b px/ al⁺dp⁺b⁺px⁺* normal female	XX; *al⁺dp⁺b⁺px⁺/ al⁺dp⁺b⁺px⁺* normal female	XX; *Del(2)al/ al⁺dp⁺b⁺px⁺* normal female	XX; *al⁺dp⁺b⁺px⁺/ al⁺dp⁺b⁺px⁺* normal female
Adjacent-1 Segregation	Y^Cen *al⁺*; *al⁺dp⁺b⁺px⁺*	X Y^Cen *al⁺*; *al dp b px/ al⁺dp⁺b⁺px⁺* sterile male	X Y^Cen *al⁺*; *al⁺dp⁺b⁺px⁺/al ⁺dp⁺b⁺px⁺* sterile male	X Y^Cen *al⁺*; *Del(2)al/ al⁺dp⁺b⁺px⁺* sterile male	X Y^Cen *al⁺*; *al⁺dp⁺b⁺px⁺/ al⁺dp⁺b⁺px⁺* sterile male
	X; Y^noCen *dp⁺b⁺px⁺*	X X Y^noCen; *al dp b px/ dp⁺b⁺px* fertile *aristaless* female	X X Y^noCen; *al⁺dp⁺b⁺px⁺/ dp⁺b⁺px* fertile female	X X Y^noCen *Del(2)al/ dp⁺b⁺px⁺* fertile *aristaless* female	X X Y^noCen; *al⁺dp⁺b⁺px⁺/ dp⁺b⁺px* fertile female

16.21   *Answer:*

  a. The known risk factors for having a child with Down syndrome are: (1) maternal age (see text Table 16.2, p. 479); (2) paternal age if the mother is 35 years or older; (3) smoking if the mother is under 35 years of age; (4) oral contraceptive use if the mother is under 35 years of age and also smokes. Where a person lives, social class, and race have no influence on the chance of having a baby with Down syndrome.

  b. One genetic cause of trisomy-21 is the nondisjunction of chromosome 21 during meiosis. This produces a gamete with two copies of chromosome 21. A zygote with trisomy-21 is produced when that gamete fuses with a normal gamete having one copy of chromosome 21. A second genetic cause of trisomy-21 is the centric fusion of the long arms of chromosomes 14 (or 15) and 21. This results in a Robertsonian translocation. A carrier parent—an individual with the Robertsonian translocation and one normal copy of each of chromosomes 14 and 21—can produce several different types of gametes (see text Figure 16.19, p. 480). When some (if they contain chromosome 21 but not 14, if they contain chromosome 14 but not 21, or if they contain the translocation and chromosome 14), are fused with a normal gamete, inviable offspring are produced. A gamete with the translocation and a normal copy of chromosome 21, when fused with a normal gamete, will produce a zygote with three copies of the long arm of chromosome 21 who has Down syndrome. A gamete with just the translocation, when fused with a normal gamete, will produce a normal, carrier zygote. A gamete with normal chromosomes 14 and 21, when fused with another normal gamete, will produce a normal individual.

  c. It would be helpful first to know the karyotype of the couple's Down syndrome child. If the child has three copies of chromosome 21 and does not have a Robertsonian translocation involving chromosome 21 and chromosome 14 (or 15), then it is likely that the parents are not carriers of such a translocation. In this case, it does not seem as important that the parents have their own karyotypes examined. However, if the child carries a Robertsonian translocation, then the parents should have their own karyotypes examined before conceiving another child. If the parents are chromosomally normal, then the Robertsonian translocation arose *de novo* (new) during meiosis in one of them. However, if either of the parents has a Robertsonian translocation, then it is also reasonable that the karyotype of that parent's siblings be assessed if their siblings are interested in having offspring. Information from this analysis would indicate if the translocation was present in and transmitted from a member of the grandparental generation to multiple members of the parental generation.

16.22 *Answer:*

a. A reciprocal (interchromosomal) translocation results from the exchange of segments between two chromosomes without a gain or loss of genetic material. In a reciprocal translocation, part or all of one arm of one chromosome is exchanged for part or all of an arm of a second chromosome (see text Figure 16.10c, p. 470). In contrast, a Robertsonian translocation occurs when two nonhomologous acrocentric chromosomes break near their centromeres and the long arms become attached to a single centromere. The short arms join to form the reciprocal product but are lost after a few cell divisions.

b. The zygote has 45 chromosomes: 23 from the mother; and a Y, 20 normal autosomes, and the Robertsonian translocation from the father.

c. Since chromosomes 13, 14, 15, 21, and 22 are acrocentric, they can be involved in Robertsonian translocations. Offspring inheriting a Robertsonian translocation involving two of these chromosomes from one parent and normal chromosomes from the other parent could be phenotypically normal if the short arms of the two chromosomes lack genes that are essential in two copies.

d. Different patterns of chromosome segregation during meiosis in the translocation-bearing male can give rise to offspring who are chromosomally normal, are translocation-bearing carriers, have Down syndrome, or are inviable. If the male donates normal chromosomes 14 and 21 or the translocation, he will produce phenotypically normal offspring. If he donates the translocation with his normal copy of chromosome 21, the offspring will have trisomy-21 and so have Down syndrome. If he donates the translocation with his normal copy of chromosome 14 (giving rise to trisomy-14), or if he donates only one copy of chromosome 14 or 21 (giving rise to monosomy-14 or monosomy-21), the offspring will be inviable. The following figure diagrams the pairing of the Robertsonian translocation during male meiosis, his gametes and zygotes that will be produced if he mates with a normal female. The thick grey lines represent chromosome 14, and the thick black lines represent chromosome 21.

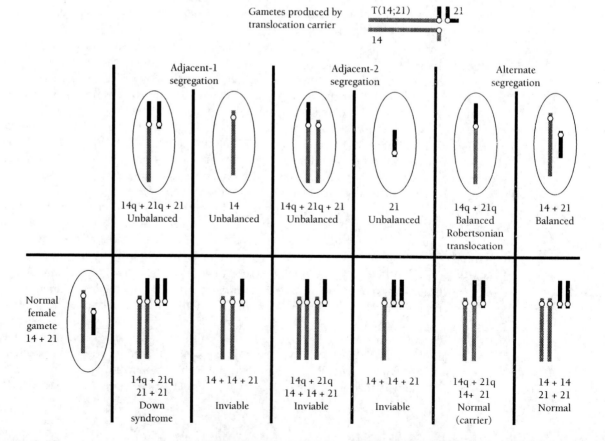

16.23   *Answer:*

a.   First, the pedigree is consistent with an X-linked recessive trait such as fragile X syndrome. Second, in fragile X-syndrome, normal transmitting males carry a premutation that is passed to their daughters, and the sons of these daughters frequently show mental retardation. Here, individual I-1's daughters (II-3, II-8, II-11) all have sons who have mental retardation, but neither I-1 nor the children of his sons (the children of II-1, II-5, and II-9) show mental retardation. Therefore, individual I-1 could have an X chromosome bearing a premutation that is passed to his daughters (but not his sons, since his sons receive his Y chromosome). During DNA replication in his daughters, the CGG triplet repeat in the *FMR-1* gene can be amplified to generate a full mutation. Mental retardation is seen in their offspring when the X-chromosome bearing the full mutation is transmitted.

b.   Culture cells from the affected individuals, and examine chromosomes cytologically to determine whether a fragile site is present. Also, use PCR with primers that flank the CGG repeat in the *FMR-1* gene to evaluate the size of the repeat. Individuals with fragile X syndrome will exhibit a fragile site at Xp27.3, and have 200 to 1,300 copies of the CGG repeat.

c.   **i.**   I-1, II-3, II-8, II-11

 ii.   I-1

 iii.   I-1, II-3, II-8, II-11, III-5, III-6, III-13, III-14, IIII-15, III-21

 iv.   III-7, III-8, III-20, III-26, III-27

d.   In females, one X chromosome is inactivated. In some cells, the fragile X chromosome will be inactivated while the other X chromosome will have a normal *FMR-1* gene. This could underlie the less severe phenotype seen in females.

16.24   *Answer:* An aneuploid cell or organism is one in which there is not an exact multiple of a haploid set of chromosomes, or one in which part or parts of chromosomes have been duplicated or deleted. It is one that does not have a *euploid* number of chromosomes. It is a general term used to describe a typically abnormal individual with an "unbalanced" chromosomal set.

A monoploid cell or individual has only one set of chromosomes. In humans, a monoploid cell would have 23 chromosomes instead of the normal diploid number of 46. In this case, a monoploid cell is also a haploid cell. A haploid number of chromosomes is typically the number of chromosomes in a gamete. Thus, in diploid individuals, a haploid gamete is also a monoploid cell. This is not always the case for nondiploid individuals. For example, in a hexaploid plant that has 36 chromosomes, a gamete will have 18 chromosomes (haploid number = 18), but the monoploid number will be 6.

A polyploid cell or individual has multiple sets of chromosomes. It is euploid, having multiple *complete* sets of chromosomes.

16.25   *Answer:*

a.   2N − 2 (two copies of the same chromosome are missing)

b.   2N − 1 (missing one chromosome)

c.   2N − 1 − 1 (one copy of each of two different chromosomes are missing)

d.   2N + 2 (two extra copies of one chromosome)

e.   2N + 1 + 1 (an extra copy of each of two different chromosomes)

f.   4N

g.   6N

16.26   *Answer:*

a.   45

b.   47

c.   23

d.   69

e.   48

16.27   *Answer:* b

16.28   *Answer:*

a. The cross can be written as $c^+ + c^+ \times c/Y$. Turner syndrome children are XO. If the child is color blind, it received its father's c allele via a chromosomally normal X-bearing sperm. Therefore, the egg that was fertilized must have lacked an X, and nondisjunction occurred in the mother.

b. If the child has normal vision, it must have received its mother's normal X bearing c^+ amd is c^+/O. To be XO, this must be the only X the embryo received, so that the egg must have been fertilized by a nullo-X, nullo-Y sperm. Nondisjunction occurred in the father.

16.29   *Answer:* The *pal* mutation causes the loss of paternally contributed chromosomes. Following chromosome loss, one daughter nucleus has a normal diploid set of chromosomes, while the other is monosomic for one chromosome. This problem considers what happens when a chromosome is lost at the very first mitotic division (and only at that division).

a. The cross is y/y *pal$^+$/pal$^+$* ♀ $\times$ y^+/Y *pal/pal* ♂, with progeny y/y^+ *pal/pal$^+$* (daughters) and y/Y *pal/pal$^+$* (sons). The paternally contributed X is only found in the y/y^+ *pal/pal$^+$* daughter, so we only need to consider the consequence of its loss in daughters. If a paternally contributed X chromosome (y^+) is lost during the first mitotic division in a y/y^+ *pal/pal$^+$* zygote, one daughter cell will lose an X chromosome and be y *pal/pal$^+$*. The other daughter cell will have two X chromosomes and be y/y^+ *pal/pal$^+$*. The cell with two X chromosomes would be female (XX) and produce nonyellow cells (y/y^+), while the cell with one X chromosome would be male (XO) and produce yellow cells (y). The animal will be a mosaic with cells of two sex chromosome compositions that are marked by yellow (male) or grey (female) cuticle.

b. The cross is *pal$^+$/pal$^+$* *eye/eye* ♀ $\times$ *pal/pal* *eye$^+$/eye$^+$* ♂, with progeny *pal/pal$^+$* *eye/eye$^+$* (daughters and sons). The paternally contributed fourth chromosome is *eye$^+$*. If it is lost during the first mitotic division in a *pal/pal$^+$* *eye/eye$^+$* zygote, one daughter cell will lose a fourth chromosome and be *pal/pal$^+$* *eye*. The other daughter cell will have two fourth chromosomes and be normal, while the cell with one fourth chromosome will be *eye*. The animal will be a mosaic with some cells that are haploid for the fourth chromosome and some cells that are diploid for the fourth chromosome. If a patch of haplo-4 cells forms an eye during development, the eye will be reduced in size.

c. The cross is *pal$^+$/pal$^+$* *e/e* ♀ $\times$ *pal/pal* *e$^+$/e$^+$* ♂, with progeny *pal/pal$^+$* *e/e$^+$*. The paternally contributed third chromosome is *e$^+$*. If it is lost during the first mitotic division in a *pal/pal$^+$* *e/e$^+$* zygote, one daughter cell will lose a third chromosome, and be *pal/pal$^+$* *e*. This cell is inviable and so will not be recovered in the organism, should the organism survive. Consequently, if the organism survives, it will be phenotypically normal (*pal/pal$^+$* *e/e$^+$*).

16.30   *Answer:*

a. If the new mutant is not on chromosome 10, the cross can be written as $x/x \times x^+/x^+$ (considering only the chromosome carrying the x gene). The progeny will be x/x^+, and the backcross will be $x/x^+ \times x/x$. A 1:1 ratio of x/x (recessive mutant) to x/x^+ (normal) individuals will be seen.

b. If the new mutant is on chromosome 10, the cross can be written as $x/x \times x^+/x^+/x^+$. Trisomic progeny will be $x/x^+/x^+$, and the backcross can be written as $x/x^+/x^+ \times x/x$. In the trisomic $x/x^+/x^+$ individual, there will be four kinds of gametes produced depending on how chromosome 10 segregates during meiosis. In $\frac{1}{3}$ of the meioses, x and x^+/x^+ gametes will be produced, giving $\frac{1}{6}x$ and $\frac{1}{6}$ x^+/x^+ gametes. In $\frac{2}{3}$ of the meioses, x^+ and x/x^+ gametes will be produced, giving $\frac{1}{3}$ x/x^+ and $\frac{1}{3}$ x^+ gametes. When such gametes fuse with an x-bearing gamete (from the xx parent) at fertilization, $\frac{1}{6}$ of the progeny will have the mutant phenotype (i.e., be x/x) and $\frac{5}{6}$ will be normal (i.e., $x^+/x^+/x$, $x^+/x/x$, x/x^+). The phenotypic ratio would be 5 dominant:1 recessive mutant.

16.31   *Answer:* Polyploids with even multiples of the chromosome set can better form chromosome pairs in meiosis I than can polyploids with odd multiples. Triploids, for example, will generate an unpaired chromatid pair for each chromosome type in the genome, so that chromosome segregation to the gametes is irregular and the resulting zygotes will not be euploid.

16.32 *Answer:* A general approach to answering this question is to model the appearance of males in the cleft species after a known sex-determination mechanism. Since there are multiple mechanisms for sex determination, this question has multiple solutions, each of which can be very instructive. The solution provided here models the appearance of males after mammalian sex determination mechanisms. Recall that in organisms that use chromosomal sex determination mechanisms, such as mammals and birds, sex chromosomes appear to have evolved from different autosome pairs, and that in humans, male sex determination results from the expression of the Y-linked testis-determining factor gene (see Chapter 12). Using this framework, hypothesize that the original cleft females had pairs of autosomes, but no sex chromosomes, and developed as females due to a default sex-determination pathway until a chromosomal mutation occurred to generate a sex chromosome able to direct male sex determination. One scenario for this would be a nonreciprocal interchromosomal translocation between two different medium-sized chromosomes that produced a small Y-like chromosome and a larger X-like chromosome. If the translocation breakpoint affected the expression of a gene on the small Y-like chromosome that was already involved in sex determination, then some features of human sex determination would be in place. For example, we can hypothesize that altered expression of the gene would lead to an altered hormonal milieu and that this would initiate a male sex-determination pathway.

Explore whether this chromosomal mutation could explain the "increasingly frequent" birth of males by following the inheritance of the translocation products. For this purpose, hypothesize that cleft females reproduce parthenogenetically, that they are diploids who produce haploid eggs, and that the diploid number is restored in a developing egg when its first nuclear division proceeds without cytokinesis. During meiosis in a diploid organism, the products of a nonreciprocal interchromosomal translocation pair with the chromosomes they derived from, and they undergo alternate, adjacent-1, or adjacent-2 segregation (see text Figure 16.11, p. 473). The following figure illustrates the meiotic pairing of two acrocentric chromosomes A (black line) and B (grey line) with the products of a nonreciprocal interchromosomal translocation between them, T(A,B) and B', and gametes that this produces.

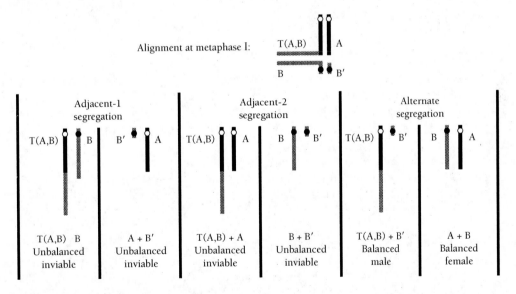

Only two gametes would be viable: the gamete having the A+B chromosomes would have only autosomes and so develop as a female; the gamete having the T(A,B) + B' chromosomes would develop as a male due to the new B' chromosome. While this explains the appearance of one or a few males from a single cleft female, it does not explain the appearance of males with increasing frequency in a population of cleft females. Males would be seen with increasing frequency only if there were transfer of genetic information between cleft females (which does not happen), if the same translocation occurred nearly simultaneously in multiple cleft females (which is unlikely), or if the translocation-bearing cleft females mated with the newly produced males (which does not happen initially). To explain how multiple cleft females produce male offspring, we must modify our speculation about the male sex-determination gene on the B' chromosome. Now suppose that all the T(A,B) + B' individuals were initially females and that a male sex determination gene on the B'

chromosome evolved only later, after the T(A,B) + B′ individuals had become more common in the population. If at that point the expression of a sex-determination gene on the B′ chromosome were altered, say, by a heritable genetic alteration such as the expansion of an unstable trinucleotide repeat, and this alteration in expression led to male development, then males would begin to appear in the offspring of multiple females.

If males mated with translocation-bearing females, males and females would be produced in a 1:1 ratio. Balanced male gametes have T(A + B) + B′ and A + B, and translocation-bearing females produce A + B gametes. Zygotes would be half T(A + B) + B′ + A + B males and half A + A + B + B females. (To explore how the T(A + B) chromosome might eventually take on the role of the human X chromosome, consider the consequences to zygotes if the B′ element is lost during male meiosis.)

16.33   *Answer:* To form the initial alloploid, gametes from each species fused, so that the initial alloploid had 11 + 19 = 30 chromosomes. A fertile, allotetraploid plant was produced by the doubling of this chromosome set, so that the allotetraploid plant has 60 chromosomes, two sets of 11 and two sets of 19. Thus Statement II is true, but Statement I is not. The allotetraploid has 60 chromosomes and 30 linkage groups (30 pairs of homologs). Answer **(c)** is correct.

16.34   *Answer:*

a. The F_1 will be *AA aa*.

b. If we label the four alleles in the F_1 as A^1, A^2, a^1, and a^2, there are six possible gamete genotypes: A^1A^2, A^1a^1, A^1a^2, A^2a^1, A^2a^2, a^1a^2. This the F_1 gametes will be ⅙ *AA*, 4/6 *Aa*, and ⅙ *aa*. As shown in the following Punnett square, selfing the F_1 gives a phenotypic ratio of 35 *A*– : 1 *aa*.

	⅙ **AA**	4/6 **Aa**	⅙ **aa**
⅙ *AA*	1/36 *AAAA*	4/36 *AAAa*	1/36 *AAaa*
4/6 *Aa*	4/36 *AAAa*	16/36 *AAaa*	4/36 *Aaaa*
⅙ *aa*	1/36 *AAaa*	4/36 *Aaaa*	1/36 *aaaa*

16.35   *Answer:* Label the four alleles of the *AAaa* plant as A^1, A^2, a^1, and a^2. As in Question 16.34, these four alleles can segregate into gametes in six ways: A^1A^2, A^1a^1, A^1a^2, A^2a^1, A^2a^2, a^1a^2 giving ⅙ *AA*, 4/6 *Aa*, and ⅙ *aa* gametes. When these gametes fuse with *aa* gametes at fertilization, the testcross progeny will be ⅙ *AAaa*, 4/6 *Aaaa*, and ⅙ *aaaa*. The phenotypic ratio will be 5 *A*:1 *a*.

16.36   *Answer:* The somatic cells of an autotetraploid plant have four identical sets of chromosomes. Because root tip cells are mitotically dividing somatic cells, they, too, have four identical sets of chromosomes. Therefore, the gametes of the diploid from which this plant was derived had 12 chromosomes.

16.37   *Answer:* Plants with 56, 70, and 84 chromosomes have gametes that have 28, 35, and 42 chromosomes, respectively. If these plants are fertile polyploids, they should have an even number of chromosome sets. This would be the case if the monoploid number of these plants is 7, and the 56, 70, and 84 chromosome plants have 8, 10, and 12 times the monoploid number of chromosomes. A plant with 28 chromosomes would therefore be tetraploid, and should be fertile.

16.38   *Answer:* The initial allopolyploid will have 17 chromosomes. After doubling, the somatic cells will have 34 chromosomes.

16.39   *Answer:* The C plants are allotetraploids, containing a diploid chromosome set from each of species A and species B. These plants should be fertile, since they will have no abnormal chromosome pairing or unpaired chromosomes. They should be able to produce gametes with 9 chromosomes (the 4 of species A and the 5 of species B) and can either be selfed or crossed to other C plants to produce fertile seed.

17

Regulation of Gene Expression in Bacteria and Bacteriophages

Chapter Outline

The *lac* Operon of *E. coli*
Lactose as a Carbon Source for *E. coli*
Experimental Evidence for the Regulation of *lac* Genes
Jacob and Monod's Operon Model for the Regulation of *lac* Genes
Positive Control of the *lac* Operon
Molecular Details of *lac* Operon Regulation

The *trp* Operon of *E. coli*
Gene Organization of the Tryptophan Biosynthesis Genes
Regulation of the *trp* Operon

The *ara* Operon of *E. coli*: Positive and Negative Control

Regulation of Gene Expression in Phage Lambda
Early Transcription Events
The Lysogenic Pathway
The Lytic Pathway

Review of Key Terms, Symbols, and Concepts

In your own words, write a brief, precise definition of each term in the groups below. Check your definitions using the text. Then develop a concept map using the terms in each list.

1	2	3
regulated genes	*lac, trp, ara* operons	lambda (λ) phage
constitutive genes	*lacA, -Z, -Y, -I* genes	lytic pathway
inducible, repressible genes, operons	P_{lacI}, P_{lac}, *lacO*	lysogenic pathway
inducers and effectors	*trpA-E, trpL, trpR* genes	genetic switch
controlling site	P_{trp}, *trpO*	lambda repressor
housekeeping genes	*araC, -B, -A, -D* genes	*cro* gene, Cro protein
induction	$araO_2$, P_C, P_{BAD}, $araI_1$, $araI_2$	*recA* gene, RecA protein
coordinate induction	negative, positive control	antiterminator
structural gene cluster	lactose, allolactose	P_R, P_{RE}, $\boldsymbol{P_{RM}}$, P_L, P_I
operon	isomerization	O_R, O_L
polycistronic mRNA	β-galactosidase	antitermination
polygenic mRNA	lactose permease, M protein	integrase
read-through transcription	β-galactoside transacetylase	*cI, cII, cIII* genes
repressor gene, molecule	partial diploids	Q, N, O, P proteins
promoter	*cis*-dominance	induction by UV light
polarity	*trans*-dominance	
polar effects	O^c, I^-, I^s, I^{-d}, I^Q, I^{SQ}, P_{lac} mutations	
polar mutations	constitutive expression	
missense mutation	superrepressor	
nonsense mutation	allosteric shift	
	catabolite repression	
	effector molecule	
	glucose effect	
	operator CAP–cAMP complex	
	CAP protein, site	
	adenylate cyclase	
	III^{Glc}	
	effector	
	aporepressor	
	attenuation	
	attenuator site (*att*)	
	pause, termination of transcription signals	
	antitermination, antitermination signal	
	feedback inhibition	
	allosteric shift	
	inducible, repressible operon	

Thinking Analytically

This chapter presents how the expression of bacterial and bacteriophage genes is regulated. While the regulation of a particular set of genes can be complex, it is invariably based on a general paradigm: The structural organization of a set of genes is related to both their induction by effector molecules and subsequent expression (as diagrammed in text Figure 17.1). As you study the regulation of each set of genes, keep this general principle in mind. Reconsider it with each of the operons; analyze how it is used and elaborated upon.

Once you have a solid understanding of the general principle underlying prokaryotic gene expression, the challenge is to understand and retain the complex details of the regulatory circuitry. It will help first to study the text figures and then diagram (eventually, from memory) the structure of each operon and the role of regulatory factors within it. This is especially valuable when considering the regulation of genes in phage λ. This will take time since it requires repeated practice and comparative review.

You can strengthen your understanding of the principles underlying prokaryotic gene expression and your detailed knowledge of the regulatory circuitry of operons by examining the consequences of mutations in different operon elements. First, address why mutations in regulatory elements such as the promoter or operator will be *cis*-dominant. Second, address why some mutations in the genes for diffusible regulatory factors *can* be *trans*-dominant. Third, consider how the properties of different mutations in a specific operon can provide you with a basis to develop a model of its structure. Fourth, identify whether the operon is under negative control, positive control, or both. Finally, relate the regulation of the operon to how it functions within a biochemical or growth pathway.

Questions for Practice

Multiple-Choice Questions

1. Genes that respond to the needs of a cell or organism in a controlled manner are known as
   a. inducer genes.
   b. effector genes.
   c. regulated genes.
   d. constitutive genes.

2. A mutation that causes a gene always to be expressed, irrespective of what the environmental conditions may be, is known as a(n)
   a. inducer mutation.
   b. effector mutation.
   c. regulator mutation.
   d. constitutive mutation.

3. A gene that is stimulated to undergo transcription in response to a particular molecular event that occurs at a controlling site near that gene is said to be
   a. inducible.
   b. constitutive.
   c. a promoter.
   d. an inducer.

4. An operon that is inducible may be under
   a. positive control only.
   b. negative control only.
   c. constitutive control only.
   d. both positive and negative control.

5. The effector molecule that induces the *lac* protein-coding genes is
   a. lactose.
   b. allolactose.
   c. glucose.
   d. β-galactosidase.

6. Before transcription of the *lac* operon can occur, RNA polymerase must bind strongly to the promoter. This happens when
   a. CAP binds to the CAP site in the promoter.
   b. a CAP–cAMP complex binds to the CAP site in the promoter.
   c. catabolite repression occurs.
   d. *lacI⁺* is mutated to *lacI⁻*.

7. Which of the following is an example of an effector molecule acting via positive control?
   a. lactose inducing the *lac* operon
   b. glucose causing catabolite repression
   c. tryptophan attenuating the *trp* operon
   d. the λ cI gene product, at a certain cellular level, favoring the lysogenic pathway

8. Bacterial operons containing protein-coding genes for the synthesis of amino acids, such as the tryptophan operon, are customarily classified as
   a. negatively controlled.
   b. positively controlled.
   c. repressible operons.
   d. inducible operons.

9. Ultraviolet light induces integrated phage λ to enter the lytic pathway by
   a. cleaving repressor monomers.
   b. initiating transcription of the *cro* gene.
   c. converting the RecA protein to a protease.
   d. all of the above, directly or indirectly.

10. Which of the following is *not* critical to the genetic switch controlling the choice between the lysogenic and lytic pathways in phage λ?
    a. the competition between the products of the *cI* gene and the *cro* gene
    b. transcription of the genes *J, K, L,* and *M*
    c. the concentration of λ repressor protein dimers
    d. whether RNA polymerase binds to P_{RM} or P_R

11. Attenuation at the *trp* operon of *E. coli* will be greatest when
    a. tryptophan is highly abundant.
    b. tryptophan is available in limited quantities.
    c. the cell is starved for tryptophan.

Answers: 1c, 2d, 3a, 4d, 5b, 6b, 7b, 8c, 9d, 10b, 11a

Thought Questions

1. What three proteins are synthesized when lactose is the sole carbon source in *E. coli*? What does each do?

2. What are the roles of *lacA, lacI, lacO, lacY,* and *lacZ* in *E. coli* carbohydrate metabolism? In what order are they arranged in the DNA molecule?

3. Describe the sequence of events that occurs in the *lac* operon when *E. coli* is grown in the presence of both glucose and lactose.

4. Distinguish between *cis*-dominant mutations and *trans*-dominant mutations. Why is *lacO^c cis*-dominant but *lacI^s trans*-dominant? Would a mutation that led to constitutive expression of the *cI* gene be *cis*- or *trans*-dominant?

5. How is attenuation related to the coupling of transcription and translation in prokaryotes?

6. What are the fundamental differences between the *lac, trp,* and *ara* operons in *E. coli*?

7. How do structural changes in DNA or RNA conformation play a role in:
   a. catabolite repression by glucose and CAP–cAMP?
   b. antitermination and termination in attenuation of the *trp* operon?

8. What is catabolite repression?

9. In what different or similar ways are allosteric shifts used in the regulation of inducible and repressible operons?

10. Speculate as to what phenotype each of the following λ mutations would have: (a) a mutation in the *cI* gene that resulted in repressor molecules that bound O_L and O_R less well; (b) a mutation in the *cro* gene that resulted in no Cro protein being produced; (c) a mutation in O_R that resulted in decreased affinity for repressor molecules.

Thought Questions for Media

After reviewing the media on the *iGenetics* website, try to answer these questions.

1. In the *lac* operon is the operator wholly within, wholly outside of, or partially within the promoter?
2. How could you distinguish between promoter and operator mutations?
3. An operon is defined as a cluster of genes along with an adjacent promoter and operator that controls the transcription of those genes.
   a. Must all operons be polycistronic?
   b. Must all of the genes in one operon be transcribed together?
4. How does lactose mediate de-repression of the *lac* operon? Does it act directly?
5. Which type of mutation in the *lac* operon causes the production of β-galactosidase whether or not lactose is present?
6. Why does it make sense for *E. coli* to transcribe the *lac* operon at a very slow rate in the presence of glucose? (Consider the products of β-galactosidase enzymatic activity.)
7. What phenotype would you expect of a mutation in the CAP site in the *lac* promoter?

1. In the iActivity, the strain containing the O^c mutation ($I^+ O^c Z^+$) showed constitutive expression both by itself and as a merozygote of the form $I^+ O^c Z^+/F' I^+ O^+ Z^+$. Would the phenotype be different if the merozygote had a genotype that was either $I^+ O^c Z^+/F' I^+ O^+ Z^-$ or $I^+ O^c Z^+/F' I^- O^+ Z^+$? For each case, why or why not?
2. In the iActivity, the strain containing the I^s mutation ($I^s O^+ Z^+$) showed repressed expression both by itself and as a merozygote of the form $I^s O^+ Z^+/F' I^+ O^+ Z^+$. Would the phenotype be different if the merozygote had a genotype that was either $I^s O^+ Z^+/F' I^+ O^+ Z^-$ or $I^s O^+ Z^+/F' I^- O^+ Z^+$? For each case, why or why not?
3. In the iActivity, you analyzed data showing that the *lac* operon was inducible and under negative control.
   a. In theory, if you can experimentally demonstrate that an operon is inducible, must it also be under negative control?
   b. Can an inducible operon be under both negative and positive control?
   c. Can an inducible operon be under only positive control?

Solutions to Text Questions and Problems

17.1   *Answer:* Genes that are always active in growing cells are constitutive, or housekeeping genes. Thus, constitutive gene expression refers to gene expression that is constantly present, while regulated gene expression refers to gene expression that is controlled in response to the needs of a cell or organism. We tend to think of genes that show constitutive gene expression as also having a fixed, unchanging level of expression, although this may not always be true. In fact, all genes are regulated at some level. A mutation that causes constitutive expression of a protein that normally shows regulated expression is likely to lie in a site that contributes to the regulation of that protein's gene. In bacterial operons, a mutation in an operator could prevent the binding of a transcriptional repressor. Alternatively, a mutation in the gene for the repressor could prevent the repressor from binding to the operator. Both types of mutation would lead to constitutive expression.

17.2   *Answer:* Allolactose and tryptophan are effector molecules that regulate the *lac* and *trp* operons, respectively. Effectors cause allosteric shifts in repressor proteins to alter their affinity for operator sites in DNA. When allolactose binds to the *lac* repressor, it loses its affinity for the *lac* operator, inducing transcription at the *lac* operon. When tryptophan interacts with the *trp* aporepressor, it is converted to an active repressor that can bind the *trp* operator, repressing transcription at the *trp* operon.

17.3   *Answer:* Polygenic mRNAs contain coding information for more than one protein. These mRNAs are transcribed from operons that contain several genes encoding related functions, such as catalyzing steps of a biosynthetic pathway. One advantage conferred by utilizing such mRNAs is that cells can regulate all of the steps of a pathway coordinately. By using a polygenic mRNA, the synthesis of each of a set of enzymes acting in one pathway can be produced by a single regulatory signal.

17.4   *Answer:* The addition of lactose to *E. coli* cells brings about a rapid synthesis of these three enzymes by the induction of a single promoter that lies upstream from the genes for these three enzymes. The three genes are part of a *lac* operon that is transcribed as a single unit. When lactose is added, it is metabolized (isomerized) to allolactose, which binds to a repressor protein. Without bound allolactose, the repressor protein blocks transcription from the *lac* promoter. Hence, the *lac* operon is normally under a negative control mechanism. When allolactose is bound, the repressor protein is inactivated and is unable to bind to the operator site to block transcription. As a result, RNA polymerase binds to the promoter and initiates transcription of a single mRNA that encodes all three proteins.

One of the enzymes that is synthesized, β-galactosidase, cleaves lactose to produce glucose and galactose (which is converted to glucose in a subsequent enzymatic step). Consequently, if glucose is present in the medium, it is redundant to induce the *lac* operon. Glucose blocks induction of the *lac* operon by utilizing a positive control mechanism. In this catabolite repression, glucose causes a great reduction in the amount of cAMP in the cell. For normal induction of the *lac* operon, cAMP must complex with a CAP (catabolite gene activator protein) that in turn binds to a CAP site upstream of the *lac* promoter and activates transcription. In the absence of cAMP, the cAMP–CAP complex is absent, and so transcription cannot be activated.

17.5   *Answer:* There are two possibilities. First, the repressor protein bound by the inducer could be unable to bind to the operator (i.e., the repressor is nonfunctional and the strain is I^-), so that its presence or absence makes no difference. Second, there could be base-pair alterations in the operator region that make it unrecognizable by the repressor protein (i.e., the operon is constitutively expressed and the strain is O^c).

17.6   *Answer:* Answering this question requires you to consider the difference between an operon's structural and regulatory genes and then differentiate between the loss-of-function phenotypes in the structural and regulatory genes. A *lac* phenotype is defined by the inability of a cell to grow on a particular substrate—medium with lactose as the sole carbon source. Since a cell with a *lac* phenotype cannot utilize lactose, it is most likely the result of a loss of a particular function (e.g., an enzyme) needed to take up or metabolize lactose. In contrast, the phenotype of a loss-of-function mutation in a regulatory gene that controls the transcription of the *lac* operon will depend on how that gene regulates transcription. If it normally represses transcription of structural genes, its loss could result in constitutive expression of the structural genes. If it normally activates transcription of the structural genes, its loss could result in the inability of those genes to be transcribed.

   a. Since *lacA*, *lacY*, and *lacZ* are structural genes, loss-of-function mutations in them would prevent the bacterium from taking up and metabolizing lactose and show a *lac* phenotype. Since loss-of-function mutations in *lacI* would eliminate Lac repressor synthesis and allow synthesis of the structural genes even when lactose was not present (but in the absence of glucose), this mutation would not show a *lac* phenotype. Loss-of-function mutations in *lacI* should show constitutive expression of the structural genes.

   b. Loss-of-function mutations in the structural genes *trpA*, *trpB*, *trpC*, and *trpD* would show a *trp* phenotype while such mutations in *trpR*, which encodes the Trp aporepressor protein, would not. Without aporepressor sythesis, the *trp* operon would be transcribed even if tryptophan were present, though transcription would not be at maximal levels due to attenuation. Loss-of-function mutations in *trpR* should show constitutive, low-level expression of the structural genes in the presence of even high levels of tryptophan.

   c. Loss-of-function mutations in the structural genes *araB*, *araA*, and *araD* would show an *ara* phenotype because the proteins needed to metabolize arabinose would not be synthesized. A loss-of-function mutation in *araC* would eliminate synthesis of the regulatory protein AraC. AraC plays two roles: it serves as a repressor of the operon when arabinose is absent, and it serves as an activator when arabinose is present. In an *araC* loss-of-function mutation, the activator function would be absent, so the structural genes needed to metabolize arabinose would not be synthesized, and the mutation would show an *ara* phenotype.

17.7   *Answer:* The use of partial diploids allowed observation of the consequences of placing sequences in *trans* and in *cis*. Partial diploids were used to show that some regulatory sequences must lie in *cis* to *lacZ* (the *lacO* region upstream of the *lacZ* gene) to exert a regulatory effect. For example, O^c mutations are *cis*-acting: They cause constitutive activation of the *lac* promoter that they lie upstream from, but do not activate any other promoter. Partial diploids also were used to show that the *lacI* gene encoded a *trans*-acting factor (a diffusible product that could bind to the *lacO* region) and that promoter function did not require a diffusible substance. For example, a $lacI^+$ gene on a plasmid could function in *trans* to regulate a *lac* promoter in *cis* to a $lacI^-$ gene.

17.8   *Answer:* To observe such a phenotype, there are three requirements: (1) a functional *lacZ* and a nonfunctional *lacY* gene must both lie downstream from a functional operator and promoter; (2) a nonfunctional *lacZ* and a functional *lacY* gene must lie downstream from an inducible (i.e., O^+) promoter; and (3) a functional repressor gene must be present in the cell (I^+). A genotype that satisfies these requirements is the partial diploid $lacI^+\ lacO^c\ lacP^+\ lacZ^+\ lacY^-/lacI^+\ lacO^+\ lacP^+\ lacZ^-$ $lacY^+$. Only one $lacI^+$ gene is required, so one may be $lacI^-$.

17.9   *Answer:* P_{lac} mutants are promoter mutants—they affect the sequence recognized by RNA polymerase and do not affect the coding region of a gene. The effect of P_{lac} mutations is confined to the genes that the promoter controls on the same DNA strand. Since the mutations only affect transcription of genes downstream of the promoter, they are *cis*-dominant.

   a. Mutants that are $lacO^c$ are mutants in the operator region that is normally bound by the repressor protein. The $lacO^c$ mutants result from a DNA alteration that precludes the repressor protein from binding the operator. Since the repressor normally blocks transcription initiation from a downstream promoter, $lacO^c$ mutants result in constitutive transcription at that promoter. Since the operator acts only on an adjacent, and not any other, promoter, mutations in the operator are only *cis*-dominant. The *lacO*^{c} has no effect on other lactose operons in the same cell because *lacO*^{c} does not code for a product that could diffuse through the cell and affect other DNA sequences.

b. In wild-type strains, *lacI* encodes a repressor that can block transcription at the *lac* operon by binding to an operator region. By binding the operator, the repressor blocks RNA polymerase from binding to the promoter. This activity of the repressor can be altered if allolactose is present, which binds to the repressor and inhibits it from binding the operator. The superrepressor (*lacI*^{s}) mutation results in a repressor protein that can bind the operator, but cannot bind allolactose. Once it binds to the operator, it cannot leave the operator, and transcription is always blocked. This results in a dominant mutation, since even if normal repressor molecules (made by *lacI*$^+$) are present, the superrepressor molecules do not vacate the operator region, and the operon cannot be induced. Unlike the *lacI*^{S} mutations that produce repressors which are always bound to the operator and so always block production of the *lac* enzymes, the *lacI*$^{-d}$ mutations produce nonfunctional repressor that result in constitutive expression of the *lac* enzymes. The *lacI*$^{-d}$ mutations are *trans*-dominant because the polypeptides they produce prevent the formation of functional repressors even when normal polypeptides produced by a *lacI*$^+$ allele are present. The Lac repressor protein is a tetramer consisting of four identical polypeptides. In *lacI*$^{-d}$ mutations, the repressor subunits do not combine normally, so no functional repressor tetramer is formed and no operator-specific binding is possible. In *lacI*$^{-d}$/*lacI*$^+$ diploids, the mixture of normal and mutant polypeptides combine randomly to form repressor tetramers, and just one defective polypeptide subunit is enough to block normal binding to the operator. Since there are only about a dozen repressor molecules in the cell, there is a good chance that no normal repressor tetramers will be produced. This results in a *trans*-dominant, constitutive enzyme phenotype. On the other hand, *lacI*$^-$ mutants either do not make repressor protein or make repressor that is unable to bind to the operator. In a partial diploid that has both *lacI*$^-$ and *lacI*$^+$ genes, repressor proteins are made (by *lacI*$^+$) and are capable of diffusing to any *lac* operator region to regulate a *lac* operon. Hence, *lacI*$^-$ is recessive to *lacI*$^+$ because the defect caused by the absence of the repressor proteins in *lacI*$^-$ mutants can be overcome by the synthesis of diffusible repressor protein from the *lacI*$^+$ gene.

c. The *lacI* gene is constitutively expressed at a low level. Mutations in the repressor gene promoter result in either an increase or a decrease in the level of expression of the repressor gene. They will not affect the structure of the repressor molecule, but will affect its cellular concentration. If the mutation causes a complete loss of expression of the repressor protein, it would have the same phenotype as an I^- mutant, since no functional repressor would be produced. These mutants would result in constitutive expression of *lacZ*, *lacY*, and *lacA* and be recessive to I^+ in partial diploids. If the promoter mutation only partially decreases transcription below normal levels, there will be increased expression of *lacZ*, *lacY*, and *lacA* in the absence of inducer. If the promoter mutation increases transcription above normal levels (the *lacI*^{Q} and *lacI*^{SQ} mutations presented in the text), a large number of repressor molecules will be produced. Such mutants will reduce the efficiency of induction of the *lac* operon by allolactose, and will be *trans*-dominant.

17.10   *Answer:* The answer is given in the following table.

		Inducer Absent		Inducer Present	
	Genotype	β-Galactosidase	Permease	β-Galactosidase	Permease
a.	$I^+ P^+ O^+ Z^+ Y^+$	−	−	+	+
b.	$I^+ P^+ O^+ Z^- Y^+$	−	−	−	+
c.	$I^+ P^+ O^+ Z^+ Y^-$	−	−	+	−
d.	$I^- P^+ O^+ Z^+ Y^+$	+	+	+	+
e.	$I^S P^+ O^+ Z^+ Y^+$	−	−	−	−
f.	$I^+ P^+ O^c Z^+ Y^+$	+	+	+	+
g.	$I^S P^+ O^c Z^+ Y^+$	+	+	+	+
h.	$I^+ P^+ O^c Z^+ Y^-$	+	−	+	−
i.	$I^{-d} P^+ O^+ Z^+ Y^+$	+	+	+	+
j.	$\dfrac{I^- P^+ O^+ Z^+ Y^+}{I^+ P^+ O^+ Z^- Y^-}$	−	−	+	+
k.	$\dfrac{I^- P^+ O^+ Z^+ Y^-}{I^+ P^+ O^+ Z^- Y^+}$	−	−	+	+
l.	$\dfrac{I^S P^+ O^+ Z^+ Y^-}{I^+ P^+ O^+ Z^- Y^+}$	−	−	−	−
m.	$\dfrac{I^+ P^+ O^c Z^- Y^+}{I^+ P^+ O^+ Z^+ Y^-}$	−	+	+	+
n.	$\dfrac{I^- P^+ O^c Z^+ Y^-}{I^+ P^+ O^+ Z^- Y^+}$	+	−	+	+
o.	$\dfrac{I^S P^+ O^+ Z^+ Y^+}{I^+ P^+ O^c Z^+ Y^+}$	+	+	+	+
p.	$\dfrac{I^{-d} P^+ O^+ Z^+ Y^-}{I^+ P^+ O^+ Z^- Y^+}$	+	+	+	+
q.	$\dfrac{I^+ P^- O^c Z^+ Y^-}{I^+ P^+ O^+ Z^- Y^+}$	−	−	−	+
r.	$\dfrac{I^+ P^- O^+ Z^+ Y^-}{I^+ P^+ O^c Z^- Y^+}$	−	+	−	+
s.	$\dfrac{I^- P^- O^+ Z^+ Y^+}{I^+ P^+ O^+ Z^- Y^-}$				
t.	$\dfrac{I^- P^+ O^+ Z^+ Y^-}{I^+ P^- O^+ Z^- Y^+}$	−	−	+	−

17.11   *Answer:* The CAP, in a complex with cAMP, is required to recruit RNA polymerase binding to the *lac* and *ara* promoters. RNA polymerase binds each promoter only in the absence of glucose. For the *lac* promoter, it occurs only if the operator is not occupied by repressor (i.e., lactose is present). For the *ara* promoter, it occurs only if AraC is not bound to the inducer site, $araI_1$ (i.e., arabinose is present). A loss-of-function mutation in the *CAP* gene, then, would render both the *lac* and *ara* operons incapable of expression because RNA polymerase would be unable to recognize the promoter. A constitutive mutation in the *CAP* gene would not affect the expression of these operons for two reasons. First, it is the binding of the CAP–cAMP complex, not CAP alone, that facilitates RNA polymerase binding to a promoter. In the presence of glucose, no new cAMP is produced, so the operons will still be subject to catabolite repression. Second, unless lactose (for the *lac* operon) or arabinose (for the *ara* operon) is present, the CAP–cAMP complex binding will be blocked by repressor molecules.

17.12   *Answer:* Whether the form of control is positive or negative reflects whether transcription is stimulated or repressed. Catabolite repression is considered a form of positive control because in the absence of glucose, CAP–cAMP is produced and binds to the *lac* promoter to stimulate transcription of the *lac* operon. In contrast, the *lac* repressor is considered a form of negative control because when lactose is absent, the repressor binds the *lac* operator and blocks transcription.

17.13   *Answer:*

    a. A DNase protection experiment is an *in vitro* method to identify DNA sites that are bound by a protein. After a purified protein is allowed to bind a DNA segment, the complex is treated with DNase and sequences unprotected by protein binding are digested. Then, the sequence of the protected region is determined. DNase protection experiments defined the location of the operator, promoter, and CAP–cAMP-binding site.

    b. See text Figure 17.14, p. 503.

    c. **i.** This deletion disrupts the operator, so the operon would be expressed constitutively.

        ii. A −12 transversion alters the −10 promoter consensus sequence, possibly decreasing the efficiency of transcription initiation. The operon may still be coordinately induced, but there will be diminished levels of β-galactosidase, permease, and transacetylase activity.

        iii. A −69 transversion alters the consensus sequence for the CAP-binding site. If CAP–cAMP is unable to bind the CAP site, RNA polymerase will not be recruited to the promoter and the operon will not be coordinately induced.

        iv. A +28 transition alters the Shine–Dalgarno sequence and, by affecting translation initiation, could result in diminished or absent β-galactosidase and, due to polar effects, diminished or absent expression of permease and transacetylase.

        v. A +9 transition alters the operator. It could either have no effect, cause the repressor to have more affinity for the operator (preventing coordinate induction in a *cis*-dominant manner), or cause the repressor to have less affinity for the operator (leading to constitutive expression).

    d. None of the mutants will prevent catabolite repression.

17.14   *Answer:* First consider the data in general terms. Mutations in genes *A* or *B* result in a loss of one, but not both, enzyme activities. These are likely to be structural genes for the enzymes (*B* = enzyme 1, *A* = enzyme 2). The mutations in genes *C* and *D* result in loss or constitutive expression of both enzyme activities, suggesting that these genes or regions regulate or affect both genes.

    a. Gene *B* is likely to be the gene for enzyme 1, since only a mutation in gene *B* produced a loss of enzyme 1 activity with no effect on enzyme 2 activity. (By similar logic, gene *A* codes for enzyme 2.)

    b. **i.** False. A mutation in *D* leads to the constitutive synthesis of both enzymes 1 and 2, so *D* cannot be a structural gene for either enzyme.

        ii. True. *D* could encode a repressor. Suppose the repressor acted as the *lac* repressor does in the *lac* operon. If mutations in *D* inactivated the repressor, then an absence of repressor would lead to constitutive activation of the operon. In this model, D^- mutants would be recessive to D^+ mutants, which is seen in the analysis of partial diploids ($A^- B^+ C^+ D^+/A^+ B^- C^+ D^-$ shows inducible activity of both A^+ and B^+).

iii. False. If D was needed to induce the *sug* operon, D^- mutants should produce no enzymes. This is not observed.

iv. False. One does see that D^- mutants are constitutive, as would be expected if a D^- operator region could not be bound by a repressor to repress transcription. However, not all of the results support this view. If D was an operator, consider what phenotype would be expected in the partial diploid $A^- B^+ C^+ D^+/A^+ B^- C^+ D^-$. If D^- was a defective operator, this partial diploid would express the A^+ gene (enzyme 2) constitutively, in a *cis*-dominant manner, and not in an inducible manner. This is not seen. What is seen is a *trans*-dominant effect where the A^+ gene is inducible. Thus, D is not an operator.

v. False. Since the products of genes A and B are not inducible in C^- mutants, one might speculate that gene C produced a cytoplasmic product that was required to induce genes A and B. However, consider the partial diploid data. In two of the partial diploids ($A^+ B^- C^- D^+/A^- B^+ C^+ D^+$ and $A^- B^+ C^- D^+/A^+ B^- C^+ D^+$), the wild-type genes on the C^- chromosome are not expressed, even though a C^+ gene is on another chromosome. This indicates that C shows *cis*-dominance and not *trans*-dominance. If C^+ encoded a cytoplasmic factor, it would diffuse and be capable of acting in a *trans*-dominant fashion. Since it does not, C does not encode a cytoplasmic, *trans*-acting factor.

vi. True. The *cis*-dominant effects that C^- mutants show in partial diploids could be explained if the mutations were in the controlling end of the *sug* operon, in a region such as the promoter.

17.15 *Answer:* Both inducible and repressible operons allow sensitive control of transcription. They differ from each other in the details of how such control is achieved. In the *lac* operon, a repressor protein bound to an operator blocks transcription unless lactose is present. Thus, if lactose is absent, the system is OFF. When lactose is added, it is converted to allolactose and acts as an effector molecule to release the repressor from the operator, so that RNA polymerase can transcribe the operon. In the *trp* operon, the control strategy is the opposite. When tryptophan is abundant in the medium, the operon is turned off because it is unnecessary to synthesize the enzymes needed to build tryptophan. Tryptophan also acts as an effector molecule. It binds to an aporepressor protein and converts it into an active repressor. This repressor is capable of binding the *trp* operator to reduce transcription of the *trp* operon protein-coding genes by RNA polymerase. Transcription of the *trp* operon is reduced by about 70% in the presence of tryptophan, while the aporepressor has no affinity for the operator in the absence of tryptophan.

The *trp* operon also can be regulated by attenuation, a mechanism that controls the ratio of the transcripts that include the five structural genes to those that are terminated before the structural genes. Under conditions where some tryptophan is present in the medium, short 140-bp transcripts are produced, and transcription is attenuated. Under conditions of tryptophan starvation or limitation, full-length transcripts are produced. A model for how attenuation occurs is described in text Figures 17.16, p. 505 and 17.17, p. 506.

17.16 *Answer:*

a. When the cell has an abundance of tryptophan, the aporepressor interacts with tryptophan and becomes an active repressor able to repress transcription of the *trp* operon by about 70-fold. Attenuation can further reduce transcription of the *trp* operon by a factor of 8 to 10.

There are at least three possible reasons that the active repressor could be unable to completely repress transcription at the *trp* operon: (1) it may not be very abundant in the cell; (2) it may not have a very high affinity for the operator and so may not be bound to it constantly (transcription initiation could occur when it is not bound); and/or (3) it may have a relatively low affinity for tryptophan (which it must bind to become and remain an active repressor).

Tryptophan is an amino acid present in many proteins, and it is very likely to be present in the enzymes used for its own biosynthesis. If transcription at the *trp* operon were completely silenced when tryptophan is abundant, a cell growing in the presence of tryptophan would cease to make even low levels of the biosynthetic enzymes needed to produce tryptophan. Over time, the biosynthetic enzymes would be degraded (assuming they have a set half-life). Should tryptophan levels become depleted, such a cell would be unable to synthesize new enzymes for tryptophan biosynthesis (since the tryptophan needed for incorporation into the polypeptide chain of the enzyme would be unavailable) and also be unable to synthesize any other protein containing tryptophan. This would lead to the cell's death. By allowing some transcription of the *trp* operon, the cell ensures that it can survive should tryptophan ever become unavailable, since it retains an ability to synthesize tryptophan.

b. In the *trp* operon, the mRNA transcript of the leader region includes a sequence that can be translated into a short polypeptide. Just prior to the stop codon in this transcript are two adjacent codons for tryptophan. Transcription is coupled to translation during the synthesis of the *trp* operon, so that RNA polymerase is synthesizing the *trp* mRNA just ahead of a ribosome that is translating it. If enough tryptophan is present in the cell for the ribosome to translate the two Trp codons, the ribosome continues to the stop codon for the leader peptide. In doing so, it covers part of the newly synthesized mRNA and allows an attenuator structure to form (the 3:4 structure shown in text Figure 17.17b, p. 506). This structure terminates transcription. If very few tryptophan molecules are present, the amount of Trp–tRNA molecules is very low and the ribosome translating the leader transcript stalls at the tandem Trp codons. This allows an antitermination structure to form (the 2:3 pairing shown in text Figure 17.17a, p. 506) so that RNA polymerase can continue and transcribe the structural genes. In this way, transcription of the structural genes of the *trp* operon is dependent on translation.

17.17   *Answer:* For a wild-type *trp* operon, the absence of tryptophan results in antitermination; that is, the structural genes are transcribed and the tryptophan biosynthetic enzymes are made. This occurs because a lack of tryptophan results in the absence of, or at least a very low level of, Trp–tRNA.Trp. In turn, this causes the ribosome translating the leader sequence to stall at the Trp codons (see text Figure 17.17a, p. 506). When the ribosome is stalled at the Trp codons, the RNA being synthesized just ahead of the ribosome by RNA polymerase assumes a particular secondary structure. This favors continued transcription of the structural genes by the polymerase. If the two Trp codons were mutated to stop codons, then the mutant operon would function constitutively in the same way as the wild-type operon in the absence of tryptophan. The ribosome would stall in the same place, and antitermination would result in transcription of the structural genes.

For a wild-type *trp* operon, the presence of tryptophan turns off transcription of the structural genes. This occurs because the presence of tryptophan leads to the accumulation of Trp–tRNA.Trp, which allows the ribosome to read the two Trp codons and stall at the normal stop codon for the leader sequence. When stalled in that position, the antitermination signal cannot form in the RNA being synthesized; instead, a termination signal is formed, resulting in the termination of transcription. In a mutant *trp* operon with two stop codons instead of the Trp codons, the stop codons cause the ribosome to stall, even though tryptophan and Trp–tRNA.Trp are present. This results in an antitermination signal and transcription of the structural genes.

In sum, in both the presence and the absence of tryptophan, the mutant *trp* operon will not show attenuation. The structural genes will be transcribed in both cases, and the tryptophan biosynthetic enzymes will be synthesized.

17.18   *Answer:*

1:   If the aporepressor cannot bind to tryptophan, it will not be converted to an active repressor when tryptophan is present. This will lead to constitutive expression of tryptophan synthetase: in medium without tryptophan, expression will be the same as in the wild type; in medium with tryptophan, expression will be reduced only through attenuation, and so it will be about 70-fold more than in the wild type.

2:   The *trp* operon will exhibit constitutive expression, so mutant *2* will show the same expression patterns as mutant *1*.

3:   The *trpE* gene is the first gene transcribed in the *trp* operon (see text Figure 17.15, p. 504). A nonsense mutation could have a polar effect, leading to diminished or absent translation of *trpB* and *trpA*, which encode tryptophan synthetase. Therefore, in a medium without tryptophan where the operon is not repressed, mutant *3* would produce diminished levels of tryptophan synthetase compared to wild-type cells. In a medium with tryptophan, the levels will be the same as in wild-type cells (very low).

4: Trp-tRNA.Trp molecules are needed to attenuate transcription at the *trp* operon. Therefore, if the levels of Trp-tRNA.Trp are always low, transcription of the *trp* operon will not be attenuated even when tryptophan levels are high. Therefore, in medium with tryptophan, mutant *4* will have about 8- to 10-fold higher levels of tryptophan synthetase than will wild-type cells. In medium without tryptophan, attenuation does not occur, so mutant *4* will have levels of tryptophan synthetase that are similar to the wild type.

5: In mutant *5*, the 3:4 attenuator structure shown in Figure 17.17, p. 506, will not form, so attenuation will not occur when tryptophan levels are high. Tryptophan synthetase levels will be the same as in mutant *4*.

17.19   *Answer:* If the products of the *ilvGMEDA* operon were required for the synthesis of the branched chain amino acids leucine, isoleucine, and valine, then it would make sense that attenuation of the operon is relieved by low levels of Leu–tRNA, Ile–tRNA, or Val–tRNA. Use attenuation at the *trp* operon as a model to hypothesize how this could occur. One hypothetical mechanism is that the mRNA leader sequence containing multiple codons for leucine, isoleucine, and valine forms a set of secondary structures that control the rate of transcription and whether transcripts are terminated in this region. During transcription of the leader sequence, regions within it pair to form a secondary structure—a pause signal—that causes RNA polymerase to pause. This pause allows the ribosome to load onto the mRNA and begin translating the leader peptide in close proximity to RNA polymerase. If the cells are starved for one or more of the three amino acids, levels of their aminoacyl tRNAs will be low and the ribosome will pause at the codons for one or more of these amino acids. The pausing of the ribosome leads the mRNA to adopt a secondary structure that serves as an antitermination signal allowing RNA polymerase to transcribe past the attenuator and transcribe the operon's structural genes. If leucine, isoleucine, and valine are present in high enough amounts so that a paucity of Leu–tRNA, Ile–tRNA, or Val–tRNA does not cause the ribosome to pause in the region of the leader peptide, the mRNA adopts a different secondary structure that attenuates transcription by serving as a signal for transcription termination.

Evidence supporting this hypothesis would come from the analysis of mutants that failed to attenuate the expression of structural genes within the *ilvGMEDA* operon. If the hypothesis is correct, these mutations should destabilize the secondary structures predicted to form by base pairing within the leader transcript. Additional evidence would come from DNA manipulations in which the DNA sequences for each of the Leu, Ile, or Val codons within the leader peptide mRNA were changed to other amino acids. If the hypothesis is correct, the *ilvGMEDA* operon would now be attenuated by changing the levels of the amino acid(s) now specified by the altered set of codons and not by leucine, isoleucine, or valine.

17.20   *Answer:* Mutations that cause the loss of activity in just one enzyme are mutations in structural genes, similar to *lacZ* and *lacY* mutations. Mutations that cause loss of all seven enzymes could be mutations in the promoter, similar to $P_{lac}-$ mutations.

17.21   *Answer:* When λ infects a cell and its genome circularizes, phage growth begins when RNA polymerase binds the λ early operon promoters P_L and P_R and transcribes mRNA for the *N* and *cro* genes, respectively. N acts as a transcription antiterminator and extends RNA synthesis to other genes that include the gene *cII*. The cII protein turns on *cI*, the gene for the λ repressor, as well as genes *O* and *P*, whose products are needed for DNA replication, and gene *Q*, whose product is needed for transcription of the late genes used in lysis and to produce phage particle proteins. Once the λ repressor and Cro are produced, there is competition between them to set a genetic switch that determines whether a lysogenic or a lytic pathway will be taken. A lysogenic pathway is taken if the λ repressor dominates, while a lytic pathway is taken if Cro dominates. The events that occur under Cro or repressor domination are diagrammed in text Figure 17.22, p. 511.

In a cell that will undergo lysogeny, the cII protein (stabilized by the cIII protein) will stimulate transcription of mRNA from P_{RE} and from P_I. This results in synthesis of repressor and of integrase. The λ repressor binds to two operators: O_R and O_L. This binding blocks transcription from P_R and P_L and so blocks production of Cro and N. It also stimulates transcription from P_{RM} and the production of additional λ repressor molecules. The stable repression of transcription from P_R together with the integrase-catalyzed integration of the λ chromosome into the *E. coli* host chromosome leads to the establishment of lysogeny. If the λ repressor is not present in high enough concentration or is cleaved and inactivated, the absence of repressor at O_R leads to the binding of RNA polymerase at P_R and transcription of the *cro* gene. When the Cro protein is produced in increasing amounts, it acts to decrease transcription from P_R and P_L, which reduces synthesis of the cII protein and blocks synthesis of repressor from P_{RM}. By this means, an increase in Cro protein blocks production of the λ repressor. It allows enough transcription from P_R for Q proteins to accumulate and stimulate the late gene transcription that is needed for starting the lytic pathway. In this way, the competition between the Cro and λ repressor proteins for the operator sites determines how the genetic switch is set.

17.22   *Answer:* The λ repressor binds to the operator O_R. When the λ repressor is bound, it stimulates synthesis of more repressor mRNA from the promoter P_{RM}. Eventually, however, at very high concentrations of λ repressor, O_R will be bound by the λ repressor in a way that blocks further transcription from the promoter P_{RM}. This maintains repressor concentrations in the cell. In the absence of repressor binding to O_R, RNA polymerase transcribes *cro* mRNA from the promoter P_R. As the concentration of Cro protein produced from this mRNA increases, Cro binds to the operator O_R and decreases synthesis from P_R and P_L. Not only does this serve to block synthesis of λ repressor mRNA from P_{RM}, but it will eventually block synthesis of *cro* mRNA as well. Thus, just as the λ repressor regulates the ability of RNA polymerase to transcribe its own *cI* gene from P_{RM}, Cro regulates the ability of RNA polymerase to transcribe *cro* from P_R. See text Figure 17.22, p. 511.

17.23   *Answer:* The *cI* gene product is a repressor protein that acts to keep the lytic functions of the phage repressed when λ is in the lysogenic state. A *cI* mutant strain would lack the repressor and be unable to repress lysis, so that the phage would always follow a lytic pathway.

17.24   *Answer:* CAP functions as a positive regulator; the *lacI*, *cI*, and *trpR* gene products function as negative regulators; and the *araC* gene product can function as both. Only CAP interacts directly with RNA polymerase. A CAP dimer bound to cAMP serves to positively regulate operons related to the catabolism of sugars other than glucose by binding to a CAP site in DNA and recruiting RNA polymerase to promoters. The *lacI*, *cI*, and *trpR* genes all produce repressor molecules that bind to operators near promoters. When bound to the operator sequences, they block the binding of RNA polymerase. The Lac repressor binds to the *lac* operator blocking RNA polymerase from binding the *lac* promoter. The product of the *cI* gene encodes a repressor that binds to two operator regions, O_L and O_R, in phage λ. These overlap the P_L and P_R promoters, and so repressor binding prevents the transcription of phage λ early operons from these promoters. The *trpR* gene produces an aporepressor protein. When tryptophan is present, it acts as an effector molecule to convert the aporepressor to an active Trp repressor. The active repressor binds to the *trp* operator and prevents transcription initiation. At the *ara* operon, AraC can serve as a negative regulator (repressor) or a positive regulator (activator) depending on whether arabinose is present. In the absence of arabinose, one subunit of AraC binds to the inducer site, $araI_1$, while the other subunit binds to the operator, $araO_2$. This causes the DNA to form a loop that blocks cAMP–CAP from binding to the CAP site so transcription cannot be initiated. AraC can also serve as a positive regulator because it undergoes an allosteric shift when bound by arabinose. In this form, the subunit of AraC bound to $araO_2$ is released and binds instead to $araI_2$ while the other subunit remains bound to $araI_1$. DNA no longer forms a loop, so cAMP–CAP can bind the CAP site to recruit RNA polymerase for transcription of the *ara* operon.

17.25   *Answer:*
   a. Intact LexA binds to DNA sequences within promoters to block transcription, so it functions as a negative regulatory protein.
   b. Binding of the sequence by LexA controls the transcription of a nearby gene, so the sequence functions as an operator sequence.

   c. Since the gene affected by mutant A lacks a consensus sequence able to bind LexA, it will be transcribed constitutively. Though it will be active and provide its "normal" function during an SOS response, it will not be repressed after the severe DNA damage is repaired by the SOS response. Since the SOS response is itself a mutagenic response, the constitutive expression of an SOS-response function in mutant *A* could cause it to show a mutator phenotype (see text Chapter 7).

      When the SOS response is triggered, RecA activation results in the LexA protein cleaving itself. Since cleaved LexA cannot bind DNA, and since the equilibrium between bound and unbound LexA is determined by the affinity of LexA for its binding sites, LexA self-cleavage leads to the additional release of DNA-bound LexA. This allows RNA polymerase access to the promoters of the genes repressed by LexA. In mutant *B*, LexA has a greater affinity to a LexA-binding site. It will be released from the gene more slowly during an SOS response, and RNA polymerase will not gain access to the gene's promoter as readily as it normally would. This would delay the implementation of the SOS response. If this delay contributed to the cell's inability to recover from severe DNA damage, the cell would die.

   d. Since the mutant LexA binds DNA more tightly than the normal LexA protein, it will replace normal LexA at its binding sites. Since the mutant LexA does not undergo self-cleavage, the genes normally activated in the SOS response would remain repressed following severe DNA damage. Therefore, the mutant would act as a dominant suppressor of the SOS response and show increased sensitivity to mutagenic agents such as UV light.

17.26   *Answer:*

   a. No. The repressor is necessary to keep the lytic function of the phage repressed and allow the phage to enter lysogeny. In the presence of a c_i mutation, only the lytic pathway can be taken.

   b. Yes. A normal repressor will be made from the wild-type c^+ gene. This repressor is diffusible and will act in a *trans*-dominant manner to repress lytic growth.

   c. No. UV irradiation of lysogenic bacteria destroys repressor function, which in turn leads to induction, including excision of λ and lytic growth. In a c^{IN} mutant, the repressor would not be destroyed following UV irradiation, so that the prophage would not be excised and lysogeny would be retained.

17.27   *Answer:*

   a. An antiterminator protein is a protein that allows RNA transcription to proceed past certain transcription terminators. In the λ life cycle, the transcription of *N* from P_L produces the *N* antiterminator protein that allows transcription from P_L to proceed past *N* to include *cII, O, P,* and *Q* (see text Figure 17.22, p. 511; N allows transcription leftward of *N*). The presence of N also allows transcription from P_R to proceed past *cro* (rightward in text Figure 17.22) to include all of the early genes, including the gene for integrase that is needed for integration of the λ chromosome into the host chromosome in a lysogenic cycle, two genes for DNA replication, and the *Q* gene, another antiterminator gene needed for the transcription of late genes that function in the lytic pathway. The N antiterminator protein is unstable, so if transcription of *N* (and that of *cro*) is blocked by the λ repressor to O_L and O_R, whose sequences overlap with P_L (and P_R), then its concentration will drop dramatically, Q protein will not accumulate, and a lysogenic pathway will be taken. If it is not blocked (which involves additional events; see text pp. 509–512) and Q accumulates, Q will act as an antiterminator to allow for late gene transcription and a lytic pathway.

   b. i. The N protein is needed for antitermination at the early promoters P_L and P_R. If *E. coli* is infected with N^{ts} λ and immediately shifted to the restrictive temperature, transcription from P_L will terminate after the *cro* gene is transcribed. The *cII, O, P,* and *Q* genes will not be transcribed. Since cII is required to turn on two genes critical for the lysogenic pathway, *cI* (which encodes the λ repressor needed to establish and maintain lysogeny) and *int* (which encodes the integrase required for integrating the lambda chromosome into the host chromosome during the lysogenic pathway), the lysogenic pathway cannot proceed. Since Q is used as an antiterminator to allow transcription of late genes needed for the lytic pathway, that pathway will also not proceed. Therefore, this type of infection will not produce either a lytic or lysogenic pathway, and no λ progeny will be obtained.

The Q protein is a positive regulator of late gene transcription used in the lytic pathway: it stimulates the transcription of structural genes whose products are needed to package DNA into new phage particles and for cell lysis. Therefore, if *E. coli* is infected with Q^{ts} λ and immediately shifted to the restrictive temperature, these genes could not be transcribed and a lytic pathway will be blocked. However, the lysogenic pathway is unaffected, and so a λ lysogen could still be obtained.

Since the N protein acts prior to the Q protein in a λ infection, if *E. coli* were infected with N^{ts} Q^{ts} λ and immediately shifted to the restrictive temperature, the phenotype associated with N^{ts} λ would be seen. Neither a lytic nor lysogenic pathway would be followed, and no λ progeny would be obtained.

ii.   Under normal conditions, the irradiation of a λ lysogen with UV light will induce a lytic pathway. However, as described in the answer to part (i), late gene synthesis required during lytic growth cannot occur without functional N and/or Q proteins. Therefore, a lytic pathway will not be induced in any of these circumstances.

17.28   Answer:

Mutant	Molecular Phenotype	Lytic Growth	Lysogenic Growth	Inducible by UV Light
1	The Cro protein is unable to bind DNA.	no	yes	no
2	The N protein does not function.	no	no	no
3	The cII protein does not function.	yes	no	yes
4	The Q protein does not function.	no	yes	no
5	P_{RM} is unable to bind RNA polymerase.	yes	no	yes

18

Regulation of Gene Expression in Eukaryotes

Chapter Outline

Review Of Key Terms, Symbols, and Concepts

In your own words, write a brief, precise definition of each term in the groups below and on the following page. Check your definitions using the text. Then develop a concept map using the terms in each list.

1	2	3
mRNA transcriptional control	mRNA transcriptional control	mRNA translation control
general transcription factor (GTF)	combinatorial gene regulation	mRNA degradation control
activator	activator	protein processing control
activation domain	*GAL1, GAL3, GAL4, GAL7,*	protein degradation control
structural motif	*GAL10, GAL80, MIG1* genes	stored mRNA
DNA-binding domain	Gal1p, Gal3p, Gal4p, Gal7p,	polyadenylation
helix-turn-helix, zinc finger,	Gal10p, Gal80p, Mig1p	deadenylation
leucine zipper motifs	UAS$_G$, URS$_G$	cytoplasmic polyadenylation
heterodimer	steroid hormone	adenylate/uridylate (AU)-rich
homodimer	polypeptide hormone	element (ARE)
coactivator	signal transduction pathway	deadenylation-dependent,
Mediator complex	steroid hormone receptor,	-independent decay pathway
enhancer	response element	yeast *PAN1, DCP1, XRN1*
promoter	chaperone	genes
silencer	effector molecule	decapping
repressor	*even-skipped* (*eve*), *bicoid,*	5'-to-3' exonuclease
corepressor	*hunchback, giant, Kruppel,*	endonuclease
combinatorial gene regulation	*fushi-tarazu* genes	proteolysis
core promoter	segment, parasegment	ubiquitin
promoter-proximal region	maternal-effect gene	proteosome
regulatory promoter element	segmentation gene	N-end rule
	gap gene	RNA interference (RNAi)
	pair-rule gene	posttranscriptional gene
		silencing (PTGS)
		microRNA (miRNA)
		short interfering RNA (siRNA)
		primary miRNA transcript
		(pri-miRNA)
		guide, passenger strands
		Argonaute protein family
		antisense RNA
		Drosha, Pasha, Dicer, Loq,
		Ago1, Ago2, Slicer
		RISC, pre-miRISC, pre-siRISC
		P body
		trans-acting RNA regulatory
		molecule

4	5	6
transcriptional control	RNA processing control	transcriptional control
gene silencing	mRNA transport control	chromatin remodeling
epigenetic phenomenon	alternative polyadenylation	DNase I hypersensitive site,
constitutive, facultative	alternative splicing	region
heterochromatin	differential splicing	histone acetyl transferase
genomic imprinting	protein isoform	(HAT)
telomere position effect	*CALC*, calcitonin gene	lysine (K) acetyl transferase
Sir silencing complex	CGRP	(KAT)
Rap1p, Sir2p, Sir3p, Sir4p	*Dscam* gene	histone deacetylase (HDAC)
RAP1, SIR2, SIR3, SIR4 genes		nucleosome remodeling
DNA methylation		complex
DNA methyltransferase (DNMT)		slide, restructure, transfer a
5-methylcytosine (5^{m}C)		nucleosome
*Hpa*II, *Msp*I		SWI/SNF
CpG island		
histone deacetylase		
insulator		
Igf2, H19 genes		
Beckwith–Wiedemann,		
Prader–Willi, Angelman		
syndromes		

Thinking Analytically

The goal of this chapter is to provide you with an understanding of the mechanisms used to regulate the expression of eukaryotic genes. A prerequisite for comprehending this information is a solid grasp of the packaging of eukaryotic DNA into chromatin, the structure of eukaryotic genes, and the processes used by eukaryotes to synthesize functional gene products. Ensure that you have a firm understanding of this information by reviewing the material in text Chapters 2, 5, and 6.

While gene regulation in eukaryotes occurs at many more levels than in prokaryotes, some of the fundamental principles of prokaryotic gene regulation are retained: promoter sequences vary to specify the rate of transcription initiation; regulatory sequences determine the response of a gene to effector molecules; and gene transcription is controlled using both activators and repressors having specific DNA-binding domains that interact with regulatory sequences. As you examine the strategies used by eukaryotes to regulate their gene expression, analyze the strategies to determine whether a parallel situation exists in prokaryotes and, if it does, how the mechanism used by eukaryotes differs.

It is helpful initially to focus on one level of regulation. Solidify your understanding of each level of regulation by referring to the text figures and redrawing them. Then, analyze the chapter material to see how different levels of gene regulation are integrated. For example, a gene can be regulated at the level of transcriptional activation, posttranscriptionally, and posttranslationally. Start by analyzing how its organization, regulatory factors, and alterations in chromatin structure are important in the activation or silencing of its transcription. Then analyze how subsequent aspects of its expression are regulated by distinct sets of regulatory RNAs and proteins.

Eukaryotes control gene expression using far more regulatory strategies than do prokaryotes, so the regulation of gene expression in eukaryotes is more complex than in prokaryotes. Identifying the factors that contribute to this complexity will help you think more clearly about the different levels of eukaryotic gene regulation. Here are some of key differences between eukaryotes and prokaryotes that contribute to the complexity of eukaryotic gene regulation:

1. Eukaryotic cells are compartmentalized into subcellular compartments. The packaging of eukaryotic genetic material into a nucleus separates the processes of transcription and translation, which provides additional levels for regulating the expression of protein-coding genes. The targeting of proteins to different subcellular organelles for processing or degradation also provides additional levels for regulating gene function.

2. Eukaryotic DNA is packaged into chromatin. In eukaryotes, this establishes a new basis for the regulation of gene expression: unless the transcription machinery can access DNA, genes are not transcribed. Thus, the remodeling of chromatin structure is an important factor to consider when thinking about how eukaryotes regulate gene expression.

3. The organization of eukaryotic and prokaryotic genes is different. While prokaryotic genes are organized into operons that produce polycistronic mRNAs, eukaryotic genes are not generally organized in this manner. Eukaryotic genes having related functions typically are dispersed throughout the genome, even when they are regulated coordinately.

4. Unlike prokaryotic genes, eukaryotic genes produce primary transcripts that are extensively processed by addition of a 5' cap, a 3' poly(A) tail, and splicing to remove introns. This allows them to be regulated at additional levels including transcript processing, transport, translation, and degradation.

5. Eukaryotes use additional types of RNAs, such as miRNAs, to control gene expression.

6. Eukaryotic cells are involved in substantially more cellular interactions than are prokaryotic cells. Eukaryotic cells interact during development and differentiation, and these interactions lead to different patterns of gene expression. The temporal and spatial variation in gene expression within an organism is obtained using combinatorial gene regulation.

Questions for Practice

Multiple-Choice Questions

1. In eukaryotes, cell- and tissue-specific gene expression is achieved via
   a. the use of operons.
   b. a cell- and tissue-specific set of activators and repressors.
   c. DNase I sensitivity.
   d. selective deletion of genes not active in differentiated cells.

2. Transcription in eukaryotes is activated if activators are bound to
   a. enhancer elements.
   b. promoter elements.
   c. the operator.
   d. both a and b

3. Histones act in eukaryotic gene regulation primarily as
   a. enhancers of gene expression.
   b. repressors of gene expression.
   c. promoters.
   d. proteins preventing DNase I digestion.

4. A gene lying in chromatin that is actively transcribed by RNA polymerase II is likely to
   a. have DNase I-hypersensitive sites upstream from the protein-coding region.
   b. have DNase I-hypersensitive sites within the protein-coding region.
   c. be relatively insensitive to DNase I.
   d. be heavily methylated.

5. The receptors for steroid hormones
   a. lie on the cell surface and act via second messengers.
   b. lie on the cell surface and when bound by hormone are transported into the nucleus and bind response elements to activate transcription.
   c. lie in the cytoplasm and act via second messengers.
   d. lie in the cytoplasm and when bound by hormone are transported into the nucleus and bind response elements to activate transcription.

6. Receptors bound by polypeptide hormones can alter gene expression by
   a. acting through a second messenger such as cAMP.
   b. directly binding DNA sequences in the 5′ end of genes.
   c. directly binding DNA sequences in the 3′ end of genes.
   d. affecting signal transduction.
   e. both a and d
   f. both b and c

7. Both miRNAs and siRNAs can posttranscriptionally silence gene expression. What is the difference between them?
   a. Both are RNA regulatory molecules, but miRNAs are *trans*-acting while siRNAs are *cis*-acting.
   b. miRNAs are much larger than siRNAs.
   c. siRNAs are produced by the processing of long dsRNA molecules while miRNAs derive from RNA transcripts about 70 nt long.
   d. Members of the Argonaute protein family are involved in producing miRNAs but not siRNAs.

8. How is ATP hydrolysis used in chromatin remodeling?
   a. to catalyze histone acetylation by HATS so that chromatin forms a looser structure
   b. to catalyze histone deacetylation by HDACs so that chromatin forms a tighter structure
   c. to methylate DNA
   d. to alter the position of nucleosomes by nucleosome remodeling complexes

9. What is the relationship between activators and coactivators?
   a. Activators bind DNA with the assistance of coactivators.
   b. Activators activate transcription by interacting with coactivators, which in turn interact with transcription factors.
   c. Coactivators prevent repressors from binding DNA so that activators can bind DNA.
   d. Coactivators bind DNA using helix-turn-helix, zinc-finger, and leucine-zipper domains. Activators bind to the coactivators and interact with transcription factors to activate transcription.

10. The *GAL1, GAL7,* and *GAL10* genes are located near each other and are coordinately expressed. How is their expression prevented by the Gal80p protein?
    a. In the absence of an inducer, Gal80p binds to the Gal4p activation domain and prevents it from activating transcription.
    b. Gal80p blocks transcription by binding to an operator in the GAL operon.
    c. In the absence of an inducer, Gal80p binds a silencer near these genes.
    d. In the presence of galactose, an inducer is formed that binds to Gal80p. The inducer-bound Gal80p binds to Gal4p and prevents it from binding to the UAS_G operator. This allows RNA polymerase to bind the promoter.

11. Which type of histone modification is able to prevent the spreading of heterochromatin?
    a. deacetylation
    b. acetylation
    c. demethylation
    d. methylation

12. Which of the following could be most readily explained by genomic imprinting?
    a. the transcriptional silencing of only the paternal copy of a gene
    b. the liver-specific transcriptional activation of both alleles of a gene
    c. the silencing of a gene containing an expanded CpG island near its promoter
    d. the activation of a gene containing a HRE in the presence of a steroid hormone

13. When a cDNA library is screened using a probe from a single-copy gene, two different cDNAs are isolated. When their sequences are analyzed, two different, unrelated ORFs are identified. Based on this observation, which of the following types of gene regulation might occur at this gene?
    a. alternative polyadenylation
    b. alternative splicing
    c. mRNA degradation control
    d. alternative protein phosphorylation
    e. both a and b
    f. all of the above

14. What role does RISC have in RNAi?
    a. RISC cleaves double-stranded RNA into 21–23-bp fragments having 3′ overhangs.
    b. RISC binds short double-stranded RNA, unwinds it, pairs one strand with a complementary mRNA, and then cleaves that mRNA.
    c. RISC binds short double-stranded RNA, unwinds it, pairs one strand with a complementary mRNA, and, in doing so, blocks transcription.
    d. RISC amplifies the interference signal.
    e. b, c, and d only

Answers: 1b, 2d, 3b, 4a, 5d, 6e, 7c, 8d, 9b, 10a, 11d, 12a, 13e, 14e

Thought Questions

1. Suppose you have cloned gene X. (a) Design an experiment to determine if gene X *is available for transcription* in liver and in brain tissue. (b) Now design an experiment to determine if gene X *is transcribed* in liver and/or in brain tissue. How do these experiments differ?

2. Present evidence that argues for or against the following statement: Histone and nonhistone proteins function as repressors of gene expression in eukaryotic cells.

3. What is the evidence that methylation plays a role in transcriptional control in some eukaryotes? What evidence is there that methylation does not entirely determine the transcriptional activity of some genes?

4. Consider how hormones act. (a) Since hormones are diffusible, why are certain cells, but not others, targets of a particular hormonal signal? (b) How is the response of a cell to a peptide hormone fundamentally different from the response of a cell to a steroid hormone? (c) Propose a hypothesis to explain why it is that steroid hormone receptors are located inside the target cells, whereas the receptors for peptide hormones are located on the surfaces of target cells.

5. The primary transcripts of many genes undergo tissue-specific alternative mRNA splicing. Indeed, about 15% of human disease mutations are associated with mRNA splicing alterations. (a) For genes that are alternatively spliced, do you expect the proteins that are produced to have identical functions? Why or why not? (b) How might spliceosomes process primary mRNAs differently in different tissues to achieve alternative mRNA processing?

6. What is the mechanism that underlies the ability of a short double-stranded RNA molecule to block gene expression? What different roles does an activated RISC complex have in this process?

7. How are the cellular processing of miRNAs and siRNAs similar? How are they different? How do the biological functions carried out by miRNAs and siRNAs differ?

8. Why is it important to regulate the degradation of proteins? In what different ways can protein degradation be regulated?

9. In text Chapter 6, we saw that the 5′ cap was important for translation initiation. How is it also important in mRNA stability and degradation?

10. Mammalian cells have between 10,000 and 100,000 SHR molecules. Why might so many SHR molecules be necessary?

Thought Questions for Media

After reviewing the media on the *iGenetics* website, try to answer these questions.

1. In neuronal cells, the calcitonin/CGRP transcript is cleaved and polyadenylation occurs at the site called pA_2, producing a pre-mRNA with exons 1, 2, 3, 4, and 5. In the thyroid gland, a transcript with exons 1, 2, 3, and 4 is produced and calcitonin, a functional peptide hormone encoded by exon 4, is produced. Why is calcitonin not produced in neurons?

2. What role do chaperones play in hormone receptor activation?

3. Where is the GRE found, and what is its role in triggering a specific transcriptional response to the presence of glucocorticoids?

4. Why is the transcriptional response to glucocorticoid exposure cell-type specific?

1. Explain, in general terms, how the regulatory networks affected by a specific gene can be identified by comparing the gene expression profiles in normal cells and in cells where that gene's function has been knocked out.

2. In these types of experiments, can we infer whether the gene acts directly to activate or repress the expression of genes in a regulatory network?

Solutions to Text Questions and Problems

18.1   *Answer:* The contention that prokaryotes and eukaryotes use fundamentally different mechanisms to control gene expression has some merit. However, there are similarities between certain aspects of eukaryotic and prokaryotic gene regulation. In both types of organisms, promoter sequences vary to specify the rate of transcription initiation, regulatory sequences determine the response of a gene to effector molecules, and regulatory proteins—both activators and repressors—with specific DNA-binding domains interact with regulatory sequences to control transcription.

The merit in the contention comes from considering the many differences in gene regulation between prokaryotes and eukaryotes. One key difference is that prokaryotic promoters are transcribed unless they are silenced by the binding of repressors that block transcription initiation. For example, RNA polymerase can initiate transcription of the *lac* operon whenever a repressor protein is not bound to the *lac* operator. Prokaryotic genes can be transcribed without altering how they are packaged—they are accessible for transcription. In eukaryotes, the nucleosome organization of chromosomes has a generally repressive effect on gene expression—it impedes the transcription machinery from accessing genes. For a eukaryotic gene to be activated, the chromatin structure must be remodeled nearby the core promoter. Histones generally repress gene activity, and actively transcribed genes have DNAse I hypersensitive sites or regions indicating that they are packaged more loosely. To activate transcription, chromatin must be remodeled by acetylating or deacetylating histones using HATs (KATs) or by using nucleosome remodeling complexes. Genes can also be silenced by DNA methylation, which leads to chromatin remodeling. These aspects of eukaryotic gene regulation are fundamentally different from the regulation of gene expression in prokaryotes.

Eukaryotic gene expression is regulated at many additional levels than is prokaryotic gene expression. In eukaryotes, gene expression is regulated not only at the level of gene transcription but also at the level of transcript processing, transport, translation and degradation, and protein processing and degradation. Gene transcription is combinatorially controlled using multiple activator and repressor proteins. Transcripts can undergo alternative polyadenylation and splicing to produce different protein isoforms. They are subject to translational control using cytoplasmic polyadenylation, to silencing using small regulatory RNAs (miRNAs, siRNAs), and to degradation control using deadenylation-dependent and deadenylation-independent decay pathways. The degradation of proteins by the proteosome is also tightly controlled, so that some proteins have a short half-life while others have a long half-life. These levels of regulation over gene expression exist in eukaryotes and, for the most part, do not exist in prokaryotes. This provides some support for the contention that prokaryotes and eukaryotes use fundamentally different mechanisms to control gene expression.

18.2   *Answer:*

   a. Promoters and enhancers are DNA elements that bind specific regulatory proteins. Promoter elements are located just upstream from the site at which transcription begins, while enhancers are usually some distance away, either upstream or downstream. Some promoter elements—those in the core promoter—are required for transcription to begin, while others—those in the promoter proximal region—are specialized for the gene they control and determine whether transcription can occur. In contrast to promoter elements that are crucial for determining whether transcription can occur, enhancer elements ensure maximal transcription of the gene. Specific regulatory proteins bound to enhancer elements can activate transcription through their interaction with multiprotein complexes interacting with proteins bound to the promoter elements.

   b. General transcription factors (GTFs) are proteins that are required for basal levels of transcription but are unable, by themselves alone, to influence the rate of transcription. TBP and TFIID, which bind to core promoter elements, are examples of GTFs. Activators (also known as *trans*-activators) influence transcription at a distance. They bind to enhancers and simulate transcription through interactions with coactivators. Coactivators are multiprotein complexes that interact both with activators and with transcription factors. The coactivators do not bind DNA directly, but rather mediate interactions between activators and transcription factors, the proteins that do bind to DNA. Interactions between activators and a coactivator complex, between a coactivator complex and RNA polymerase II, and between RNA polymerase II and the GTFs cause the DNA to loop back upon itself and lead to the activation of transcription. Repressors are similar to activators in that they bind to both DNA elements and coactivators. However, they quench transcription rather than stimulate it. For this reason, DNA sites bound by repressors are referred to as silencers.

c. Activators have two functional domains. One domain is a DNA-binding domain that binds to an enhancer. This domain has a structural motif important for DNA binding such as a helix-turn-helix, zinc finger, or leucine zipper motif. The second domain is a transcription activation domain that stimulates transcription by recruiting a coactivator protein complex.

d. Repressors in eukaryotes are unlike those in prokaryotes in that they do not directly bind to DNA to prevent RNA polymerase from binding a promoter. Unlike the situation in prokaryotes, in eukaryotes, the packaging of DNA by nucleosomes establishes a repressed state that must be overcome by activators. Eukaryotic repressors counteract the action of activators to block transcription. Like activators, they have two domains, in this case a DNA-binding domain and a repressor domain. Repressors can work in several different ways: (1) They can bind to DNA sites near an activator's binding site and block the action of the activator's activation domain through their repressor domain; (2) they can bind to a DNA site that overlaps the site bound by the activator and prevent the activator from binding; and (3) they can recruit a histone deacetylase complex to bring about chromatin compaction.

e. Whether a particular DNA sequence serves to stimulate or quench transcription depends first on the type of regulatory protein bound to it. If it is bound by an activator that stimulates transcription, the sequence serves as an enhancer; while if it is bound by a repressor that quenches transcription, it acts as a silencer. The magnitude of its effect on transcription also depends on the strength of that protein's effect compared with that of regulatory proteins bound to other DNA elements in the gene. Therefore, the function of a DNA element able to bind a regulatory protein depends on the type of regulatory proteins present in a cell and the types of other DNA elements present in the gene.

f. Transcriptional specificity is generated through the combinatorial use of a set of GTFs, activators, and repressors. Some of these are common to many cells, while others have a more restricted spatial and/or temporal distribution. The transcription of defined subsets of genes in different cells at different times is controlled by the constellation of regulatory proteins present in a eukaryotic cell at a particular time.

18.3   *Answer:* To answer this question, recall that the galactose utilization genes in yeast are subject to both positive and negative regulation. Three genes, *GAL1*, *GAL7*, and *GAL10*, encode enzymes needed to utilize galactose as a source of carbon. If glucose is not present, the addition of galactose causes the rapid production of the enzymes encoded by these three genes because of positive regulation through the activity of the activator protein Gal4p. Gal4p, which is expressed only in the absence of glucose, binds as a homodimer to upstream activator sequences (UAS_G) for each of the *GAL1*, *GAL7*, and *GAL10* genes. However, another protein, Gal80p, functions as a negative regulatory protein—a repressor. It binds to the activation domain of Gal4p and prevents it from activating transcription. To activate transcription at the *GAL1*, *GAL7*, and *GAL10* genes, an inducer must be present. The inducer is produced in the absence of glucose and the presence of galactose by the action of Gal3p. When it binds to Gal80p, Gal80p changes its position on Gal4p, exposing the Gal4p activation domain. This leads to the transcriptional activation of the *GAL1*, *GAL7*, and *GAL10* genes.

In this question, the cells have a temperature-sensitive Gal80p protein that functions only at the permissive temperature. If at the permissive temperature, galactose but not glucose is present, the inducer is produced, Gal80p binds the inducer, Gal80p changes its position on Gal4p, and the activation domain of Gal4p is exposed. This results in transcription of the *GAL1*, *GAL7*, and *GAL10* genes. If the same cells are shifted to the restrictive temperature, Gal80p will not function. Presumably the activation domain of Gal4p remains exposed, so the *GAL* genes continue to be transcribed and a shift to the restrictive temperature does not change their expression.

If neither galactose nor glucose is present, the inducer is not produced, so it is not present to bind to Gal80p. At the permissive temperature for Gal80p, Gal80p will repress transcription of the *GAL1*, *GAL7*, and *GAL10* genes. At the restrictive temperature, the Gal80p protein will not function, and so transcription at the *GAL1*, *GAL7*, and *GAL10* genes will not be repressed (as long as glucose is absent; see the following paragraph). Indeed, as long as glucose is absent and even if galactose and the inducer are absent, the *GAL1*, *GAL7*, and *GAL10* genes will be constitutively transcribed at the restrictive temperature. Therefore, if the cells are shifted from the permissive to the restrictive temperature and glucose and galactose are absent, there will be a net increase in the transcription of the *GAL1*, *GAL7*, and *GAL10* genes.

Since glucose is yeast's preferred carbon source, the presence of glucose leads to the repression of the *GAL1*, *GAL7*, and *GAL10* genes. They are not transcribed in the presence of glucose because the repressor protein, Mig1p, is activated when glucose is present. Activated Mig1p binds to an upstream repressing sequence (URS_G) within the *GAL* gene promoters and blocks the activation of their transcription by Gal4p. Therefore, whenever glucose is present, and independent of the functional status of Gal80p, *MIG1* but none of the *GAL* genes will be transcribed.

Use this information to fill in the table as shown.

Gene	Glucose and Galactose	Glucose Only	Galactose Only	Neither Glucose nor Galactose
MIG1	no change (on)	no change (on)	no change (presumably on)	no change (presumably on)
GAL1	no change (off)	no change (off)	no change (on)	increases (previously off)
GAL4	no change (off)	no change (off)	no change (on)	no change (on)
GAL7	no change (off)	no change (off)	no change (on)	increases (previously off)
GAL10	no change (off)	no change (off)	no change (on)	increases (previously off)

18.4   *Answer:*

a. A hormone is typically a chemical messenger possessing a low molecular weight that is synthesized in low concentrations in one tissue or cell and transmitted in body fluids to another part of the organism. Hormones act as effector molecules to produce specific effects after binding to a receptor in target cells that may be remote from the hormone's point of origin. Hormones function to regulate gene activity, physiology, growth, differentiation, or behavior.

b, c. Steroid hormones and peptide hormones employ two fundamentally different mechanisms to regulate gene expression. Steroid hormones traverse the cell membrane and bind to a cytoplasmic steroid hormone receptor (SHR). SHRs have three domains, a DNA-binding domain, an activation or repression domain, and a specific, steroid hormone binding domain. When the steroid hormone is absent the SHR is inactive, and the SHR complexes with chaperones to maintain its funtionality. After the steroid hormone enters the cell, it complexes with the SHR and displaces Hsp90, a chaperone. The complex of the hormone and SHR then enters the nucleus and acts directly to regulate gene expression. The DNA-binding domain of the SHR binds to specific steroid hormone response elements (HREs) near genes to regulate their transcription.

Polypeptide hormones, such as insulin and certain growth factors, bind to receptors that reside on cell surfaces. The activated, bound receptor then transduces a signal via a second messenger system inside the cell. Some activated receptors increase the activity of the membrane-bound enzyme adenylate cyclase, which results in an increase in cAMP levels. Increased intracellular levels of cAMP send an intracellular signal (a second messenger) to activate other cellular processes that ultimately lead to an alteration in patterns of gene expression.

d. Each hormone acts on specific target cells that have receptors capable of recognizing and binding that particular hormone. Polypeptide hormones bind to receptors on the cell surface, while steroid hormones bind to receptors inside the cell. Two distinct cell types that possess receptors for a hormone can be activated by the same hormone signal, while a third cell type that lacks receptors for the hormone will fail to respond. However, even the two cell types that possess hormone receptors may respond in different ways. Though the cells have the same SHR, they may differ in the types of other regulatory proteins they have. Since the pattern of genes that is activated by the hormone is dependent on the array of other regulatory proteins that are present, two receptor-bearing cell types may respond differently to the same hormone signal.

18.5 *Answer:*

a. The disappearance of the 4-kb band indicates that the promoter region has a DNase I hypersensitive site—a less highly coiled site where DNA is more accessible to DNase I for digestion. Since DNase I digestion produces a 2-kb band, the site lies near the middle of the 4-kb *Eco*RI fragment. The 3-kb band does not diminish in intensity except at the highest DNase I concentration, so the region of the gene containing the 3-kb *Eco*RI fragment is more highly coiled by nucleosomes.

b. Following the ecdysone pulse, increased concentrations of DNase I lead to the disappearance of both the 4- and 3-kb bands, indicating that DNase I has increased access and the gene is less tightly coiled during transcription. The appearance of low-molecular-weight digestion products indicates that DNase I cannot access some regions of the 4- and 3-kb *Eco*RI fragments. These regions may be bound by proteins such as general transcription factors.

18.6 *Answer:*

a. Histones repress gene expression, so if they are present on DNA, promoter-binding proteins cannot bind promoters and transcription cannot occur.

b. Histones will compete more strongly for promoters than will promoter-binding proteins, so transcription will not occur.

c. If promoter-binding proteins are already assembled on promoters, nucleosomes will be unable to assemble on these sites, so transcription will occur.

d. Enhancer-binding proteins will help promoter-binding proteins to bind promoters even in the presence of histones, so transcription will occur.

18.7 *Answer:*

a. Histone acetyl transferases (HATs) and histone deacetylases (HDACs) modify nucleosomes by acetylating or deacetylating core histones. As positively charged acetyl groups are added to the negatively charged histones by HATs, the histones slowly lose their affinity for negatively charged DNA, and the 30-nm chromatin fiber loses histone H1 and changes conformation to a 10-nm chromatin fiber. This makes promoters more accessible for the activation of transcription. Conversely, as HDACs remove acetyl groups from histones, the histones will slowly gain more affinity for DNA. The 30-nm chromatin fiber will reform and make promoters less accessible for the activation of transcription.

b. Chromatin can also be remodeled using ATP-dependent nucleosome remodeling complexes. They use the energy of ATP hydrolysis to alter nucleosome position or structure and facilitate the binding of the transcription machinery to the core promoter. See text Figure 18.10b, p. 530.

c. Mutants in which a protein involved in chromatin remodeling fails to function will exhibit marked decreases in the expression of many genes in different, unrelated pathways. They are likely to grow very slowly and may be unable to complete some cellular processes altogether. See the text discussion (p. 530) of the discovery of the SWI/SNF genes that affect mating-type switching in yeast.

18.8 *Answer:* The data indicate that the synthesis of ovalbumin is dependent upon the presence of the hormone estrogen. These data do not address the mechanism by which estrogen achieves its effects. Theoretically, it could act (1) to increase transcription of the ovalbumin gene by binding to an intracellular receptor that, as an activated complex, stimulates transcription at the ovalbumin gene; (2) to stabilize the ovalbumin precursor mRNA; (3) to increase the processing of the precursor ovalbumin mRNA; (4) to increase the transport of the processed ovalbumin mRNA out of the nucleus; (5) to stabilize the mature ovalbumin mRNA once it has been transported into the cytoplasm; (6) to stimulate translation of the ovalbumin mRNA in the cytoplasm; or (7) to stabilize (or process) the newly synthesized ovalbumin protein. Experiments in which the levels of ovalbumin mRNA were measured have shown that the production of ovalbumin mRNA is primarily regulated at the level of transcription.

18.9   *Answer:* In some organisms, DNA methylation results in the transcriptional silencing of specific DNA sequences. One example illustrating how DNA methylation can affect gene expression is the abnormal methylation associated with an expanded triplet repeat in the *FMR-1* gene. This results in transcriptional silencing at *FMR-1* and the development of fragile-X syndrome.

A second example is DNA imprinting. In DNA imprinting, specific DNA sequences are methylated in just one parent prior to their inheritance. The methylation imprint is maintained following DNA replication in zygotic cells so that the paternally and maternally contributed chromosomes of the zygote retain their different methylation patterns. Therefore, imprinting results in different patterns of gene silencing on maternally and paternally contributed chromosomes. An illustration of this for the linked *Igf2* and *H19* genes is shown in text Figure 18.13, p. 533. A single enhancer downstream from both genes controls their expression. However, an activator bound to this enhancer activates the upstream *Igf2* gene only if its action is not blocked by the binding of the CTCF protein to an insulator element lying in between the genes. If the CTCF protein binds the insulator element, only the downstream *H19* gene is transcribed. Methylation of the paternally contributed chromosome—imprinting—alters this situation. Methylation of the insulator element and the *H19* promoter in the paternally contributed chromosome prevents binding of the insulator by the CTCF protein and transcription of the *H19* gene. Consequently, the paternal copy of the *Igf2* gene, but not the *H19* gene, is expressed. In contrast, the maternally contributed chromosome is not methylated in this region. Thus, the insulator element functions, allowing expression of the maternal *Igf2* gene and preventing expression of the maternal *H19* gene.

18.10   *Answer:* Epigenetic mechanisms that lead to gene silencing involve changes in chromatin structure to produce heterochromatin, methylation of cytosines in the promoter region upstream of a gene, and genomic imprinting associated with the inheritance of specific methylated sequences from one parent. In each case, chromatin remodeling leads to a promoter-inaccessible conformation so that a gene or zone of genes can no longer be transcribed. Heterochromatin formation is controlled by the acetylation and deacetylation of core histones and by ATP-dependent nucleosome remodeling complexes. Methylation of cytosines within CpG islands results in transcriptional repression via the recruitment of histone deacetylases to cause chromatin remodeling. Genomic imprinting is associated with the inheritance of specific methylated DNA sequences from one parent. Chromatin remodeling of the region containing the methylated DNA sequences blocks gene expression, so that only the gene inherited from the other parent is expressed.

18.11   *Answer:*

a. For an abnormal phenotype to be associated with imprinting, the phenotype must be seen when a nonfunctional imprinted allele is inherited and a functional normal allele is not inherited. Here, offspring inheriting a deletion from the male but not the female parent exhibit an abnormal phenotype. Therefore, in a normal individual the paternally contributed allele of a gene within the deletion must function while the maternally contributed allele must be imprinted.

b. Imprinting is associated with the methylation of DNA sequences that results in gene silencing. It occurs during the formation of gametes—during spermatogenesis and oogenesis.

c. There are two possibilities that must be considered before determining whether an imprinted gene will show dominant or recessive inheritance. First, consider a situation like that described in this problem and a mouse that has normal (non-deletion bearing) chromosomes in this region of chromosome 2. A normal mouse will receive an imprinted copy of a gene in this region from its mother and a nonimprinted functional copy of the gene from its father. If a mutation in the father results in the zygote's paternally donated gene to be imprinted, that zygote will not have a functional copy of the gene; it will display a mutant phenotype. Since the mutant phenotype is inherited as a single allele from the father, the phenotype is transmitted as a dominant trait.

Second, consider a region in which neither the paternal nor maternal copies of a zygote's genes are normally imprinted. If a mutation in one parent results in a zygote receiving one imprinted copy of a gene, the zygote will be heterozygous for what we can consider a loss-of-function mutation. In most situations, this will not cause a phenotype, because in most cases a single normal copy of a gene is sufficient to provide for a normal phenotype—most loss-of-function mutations are recessive. If the imprinted allele is transmitted as an imprinted allele to subsequent generations, then a phenotype would be observed when both copies of the gene received by a zygote are imprinted. In this case, the mutation will be recessive.

   d. The DNA polymorphism lies in an expressed region of the gene, so the polymorphism can be evaluated in cDNAs made from *Neuronatin* mRNA by using RT-PCR-RFLP—isolate mRNA from the tissue where the *Neuronatin* gene is normally expressed, prepare cDNA by reverse transcription, and use PCR-RFLP to characterize the polymorphism. RT-PCR-RFLP allows us to determine if one or both alleles of the *Neuronatin* gene are expressed. Contrast this with PCR-RFLP using a genomic DNA template, which would tell us about the genotype of an individual—whether they are homozygous or heterozygous. Based on the reasoning in (a), we can hypothesize that the maternally contributed copy of the *Neuronatin* gene is imprinted and the paternally contributed copy of the gene is expressed. Suppose that a normal male homozygous for one polymorphism is crossed to a normal female homozygous for another polymorphism. Under the imprinting hypothesis, RT-PCR-RFLP using mRNA prepared from the offspring should identify the polymorphism present in the father and not the mother. If the hypothesis is incorrect and both the maternal and paternal alleles are expressed—the *Neuronatin* gene is not imprinted—then RT-PCR-RFLP should identify the polymorphisms present in each parent. Whether or not the gene is imprinted, PCR-RFLP used with a genomic DNA template should reveal that the individual is heterozygous for the polymorphism. If we use RT-PCR-RFLP to examine the hemizygous individuals described in the problem and the *Neuronatin* gene is imprinted, we should find that the affected, deletion-bearing offspring produced from a cross of a deletion-bearing male with a normal female do not express the *Neuronatin* gene. The only copy of the gene they received—the one from their mother—is imprinted. In contrast, the normal offspring produced from a cross of a deletion-bearing female with a normal male should express only the paternal allele.

18.12 *Answer:*

   a. The goals of the Human Epigenome Project (HEP) are to identify, catalogue, and interpret genome-wide DNA methylation patterns of all human genes in all major tissues. DNA methylation patterns can alter whether genes are expressed and may be influenced by genetic factors, disease, and environment. One anticipated benefit of understanding the pattern of genome-wide methylation in different tissues is to provide a reference for assessing the role of DNA methylation patterns in the etiology of human disease. Identifying the patterns of differentially methylated cytosines that are associated with a tissue type and how they are altered in a disease state would provide epigenetic markers that can aid in our understanding and diagnosis of human disease.

   b. The methylation pattern at one gene can vary between tissues, and so its methylation pattern in one tissue is not indicative of its methylation pattern in another tissue. Since the goal of the HEP is to understand how methylation patterns at each gene change with respect to tissue, environment, and disease, methylation patterns must be assessed in different tissues.

   c. Genomic DNA is isolated from a particular tissue and treated with bisulphite. This chemical treatment converts all nonmethylated cytosines to uracils. Gene segments are then amplified using PCR and bisulfite-specific primers and the PCR products are sequenced. Since nonmethylated cytosines are converted to uracil by treatment with bisulfite, nonmethylated CpG sites in the genomic DNA are amplified as TpG while methylated CpG sites in the genomic DNA are amplified as CpG. Therefore, comparison of the PCR-amplified DNA to the known sequence of the gene allows identification of methylated and nonmethylated sites.

18.13 *Answer:*

   a. In fragile X syndrome, the expanded CGG repeat results in hypermethylation and transcriptional silencing. A CAG codon specifies glutamine, so in Huntington disease, the expanded CAG repeat results in the inclusion of a polyglutamine stretch within the Huntington protein. This causes it to have a novel, abnormal function.

b. A heterozygote with a CGG repeat expansion near one copy of the *FMR-1* gene will still have one normal copy of the *FMR-1* gene. The normal gene can produce a normal product, even if the other is silenced. (The actual situation is made somewhat more complex by the process of X inactivation in females, but in general one would expect that a mutation that caused transcriptional silencing of one allele would not affect a normal allele on a homolog.) In contrast, a novel, abnormal protein is produced by the CAG expansion in the disease allele in Huntington disease. Since the disease phenotype is due to the presence of the abnormal protein, the disease trait is dominant.

c. Transcriptional silencing may require significant amounts of hypermethylation, and so require more CGG repeats for an effect to be seen. In contrast, protein function may be altered by a stretch of more than 36 glutamines.

18.14 *Answer:* Two mechanisms by which distinct protein isoforms can be produced from the same primary transcript are alternative polyadenylation and alternative splicing. Alternative polyadenylation can lead to the inclusion of different exons in the region near the 3'-end of an mRNA, producing protein isoforms with different C-terminal regions. Alternative splicing can lead to mature mRNAs having different exons that produce different protein isoforms. Alternative polyadenylation can be independent of alternative splicing.

The human calcitonin gene (*CALC*) is regulated by both alternative polyadenylation and alternative splicing (see text Figure 18.14, p. 535). In thyroid tissue, alternative polyadenylation occurs at the polyadenylation site next to exon 4, while in neuronal cells, a polyadenylation site next to exon 5 is used. The pre-mRNAs are then alternatively spliced. The pre-mRNA in thyroid tissue is spliced to remove three introns and bring together exons 1, 2, 3, and 4, while the pre-mRNA in neuronal tissue is spliced to remove introns and bring together exons 1, 2, 3, and 5. The two processed transcripts produce different protein products that are then proteolytically cleaved to produce different functional hormones: calcitonin is produced in thyroid tissue while CGRP (calcitonin gene-related peptide) is produced in neuronal tissue.

Estimates in humans suggest that three-quarters of genes are alternatively spliced, so alternative splicing is a common regulatory mechanism in some organisms. The number of protein isoforms produced by alternative splicing of a pre-mRNA can be very large. One extreme example is that of the *Drosophila Dscam* gene, which encodes proteins required for the formation of neuronal connections. This gene produces 38,016 different protein isoforms by alternative splicing.

18.15 *Answer:*

a. Four different protein isoforms differing in their C-terminus are produced.

b. The cDNA structures indicate that alternative mRNA splicing is used to generate the different protein isoforms. Specifically, alternative 5' splice sites are used: the last exon of cDNA 4 contains a 5' splice site that is used by cDNAs 1, 2, and 3; the last exon of cDNA 1 contains a splice site that is used by cDNAs 2 and 3; and the last exon of cDNA 2 contains a 5' splice site that is used by cDNA 3.

c. Use short interfering RNAs (siRNAs) to posttranscriptionally silence each of the different transcripts. Synthesize short, double-stranded RNAs targeted to regions specific to each of the cDNAs. Inject these individually into the (model) organism and examine the organism for phenotypic alterations. Phenotypes caused by the injection of a short double-stranded RNA targeted to a specific mRNA isoform most likely arise because of the posttranscriptional gene silencing of that mRNA and a decrease in the synthesis of the protein it encodes.

18.16 *Answer:*

a. MicroRNAs are 21–23 nt-long noncoding ssRNA regulatory molecules. They derive from RNA transcripts encoded by genes within the genomes of all multicellular eukaryotes, as well as from some genes in unicellular eukaryotes. In humans, about 5,000 miRNA genes are scattered throughout all of the chromosomes except the Y. About 30% are located in intergenic regions, are transcribed by RNA polymerase II, and lead to capped, polyadenylated transcripts. Some are located in transposons. The remaining miRNAs are located within other genes, and they are found in introns of protein-coding genes or in introns and exons of non-protein-coding genes. For most of these, the miRNA sequence is transcribed as part of the transcript of the "host" gene. Some intron-located miRNA genes are transcribed by RNA polymerase II.

Like miRNAs, short interfering RNAs are about 22 nt long, function as noncoding ssRNA regulatory molecules, and are found in eukaryotes throughout the phylogenetic spectrum. Unlike miRNAs, they are produced by the processing of cytoplasmic dsRNA molecules that can be hundreds to thousands of base pairs long. The dsRNA molecules that will be processed into siRNAs derive from intermediates in the replication of viruses with RNA genomes, naturally generated molecules from complementary or partially complementary sense and antisense transcripts from regions of the genome, and transcripts that fold into long, extended hairpins.

b. A miRISC ribonucleoprotein complex that can silence gene expression is produced as follows (see text Figure 18.15a, p. 538). First, a hairpin structure about 70 nt long that contains the miRNA and lies within the transcribed primary miRNA transcript (pri-miRNA) is excised by Drosha, a dsRNA-specific endonuclease, complexed to an accessory protein. Once Drosha makes staggered cuts in the pri-miRNA that leave a ~2 nt 3' single-stranded overhang, the excised hairpin is exported rapidly to the cytoplasm. There, another dsRNA-specific endonuclease, Dicer, complexed to an accessory protein, makes additional staggered cuts in the pre-miRNA to release a short miRNA:miRNA* dsRNA. This dsRNA consists of two imperfectly paired RNA strands from some of the former paired sides of the hairpin. The miRNA, or guide strand, is the mature miRNA strand that subsequently functions in the cell for RNA silencing, while the miRNA*, or the passenger strand, is its partial complement and does not function in RNA silencing. Then, the dsRNA, Dicer, and accessory protein bind to Ago1 and other proteins to form the pre-microRNA-induced silencing complex, or pre-miRISC. Ago1, also called Slicer, is a member of the Argonaute family of proteins and functions as an RNA endonuclease to make a single cut with the miRNA* passenger strand. A helicase that is part of the pre-miRISC then unwinds the two pieces from the miRNA guide strand so that they dissociate from the complex. This produces the mature miRISC, the ribonucleoprotein complex that can silence gene expression.

A siRISC complex is produced in a similar manner to the miRISC complex (see text Figure 18.15b). First, the long cytoplasmic dsRNA is processed by a Dicer–protein complex into many ~22-nt duplexes, each with a 2-nt 3' single-stranded overhang. One strand of each duplex is the siRNA guide strand that will carry out RNA silencing, while the complementary strand is the passenger strand that will be discarded. The dsRNA–Dicer–protein complex binds to Ago2, another member of the Argonaute family, and other proteins to form the pre-siRNA-induced silencing complex, or pre-siRISC. A mature siRISC complex is produced using steps that parallel those used to generate a mature miRISC from the pre-miRISC complex.

c. A distinguishing feature of miRNAs compared to siRNAs is that the miRNA in the miRISC, unlike the siRNA in the siRISC, acts as a *trans*-acting regulatory molecule: it targets mRNAs that are not the same as the RNA molecules from which the miRNA is derived. A miRISC silences gene expression by binding to a target mRNA through complementary base pairing involving the miRNA, usually to short sequences in the 3' UTR of the mRNA. In animals, binding of most miRISCs to their target mRNAs involves imperfect pairing between the miRNA and the 3' UTR of the mRNA. This pairing triggers translational repression. The translationally repressed mRNA with its associated miRISC (or miRISCs, if multiple miRNAs target a particular mRNA) are then sequestered from the translation machinery by becoming, or moving into a P body. A P body is a cytoplasmically located aggregate of translationally repressed mRNAs complexed with proteins, and proteins for mRNA decapping and for mRNA degradation. The mRNAs in P bodies may be degraded using the mRNA degradation machinery in the P body, or they may be stored in ribonucleoprotein complexes. Stored mRNAs can be returned to translation at a later time. In plants, binding of most miRISCs to their target mRNAs involves perfect or near-perfect pairing between much of the miRNA and the 3' UTR of the mRNA. This triggers mRNA degradation rather than translational repression.

The siRISC functions in posttranscriptional gene silencing by recognizing ssRNAs that are complementary to one strand or the other of the dsRNAs from which the siRNAs were produced. The siRNA in the siRISC pairs to the target RNA with perfect base pairing, and Ago2 cleaves the target RNA into two. The two RNA pieces are then degraded in a P body.

d. MicroRNAs and siRNAs serve different roles in the cell. MicroRNAs play central roles in controlling gene expression in a variety of cellular, physiological, and developmental processes. The 3' UTR of one gene can have one or more sequences to which the same miRNA can bind, and/or it may have several sequences to which several different miRNAs can bind. Thus, one gene can be regulated by various combinations of miRNAs. In contrast, siRNAs function in an RNA-directed immune system: they target the RNA of a viral genome or viral transcript and lead to inhibition of the viral life cycle.

18.17   *Answer:*

a. Inactive stored mRNAs have shorter poly(A) tails (15–90 As), while actively translated mRNAs have longer poly(A) tails (100–300 As).

b. At least some of the mRNAs that will be stored prior to translation are initially processed with a longer poly(A) tail of 300–400 As. Their poly(A) tail is rapidly de-adenylated to a length of 40–60 As in the mature stored message, and later, when activated for translation, increased in length by about 150 A nucleotides by a cytoplasmic polyadenylation enzyme.

c. A sequence in the 3' UTR, the adenylate/uridylate (AU)-rich element (ARE, UUUUUAU), that lies upstream from the polyadenylation sequence (AAUAAA) provides a signal for deadenylation and polyadenylation.

d. In addition to the rapid deadenylation pathway discussed above, mRNAs can undergo a default, slow decrease in poly(A) length. If the poly(A) tails are de-adenylated and become too short (5–15 As) to bind PAB (poly(A) binding protein), the 5' cap is removed enzymatically (decapping) and the mRNA is degraded from the 5' end by a 5'-to-3' exonuclease. This deadenylation-dependent pathway is one of two major mRNA decay pathways. In the other major pathway, decapping and 5'-to-3' degradation or internal endonuclease cleavage occurs without de-adenylation.

18.18   *Answer:*

a. The *cortex* and *grauzone* mutants affect how much protein is produced by the maternally deposited *bicoid* and *toll* mRNAs, so they most likely affect how efficiently ribosomes select these mRNAs for translation. The translation of maternally deposited mRNAs increases significantly following fertilization. Prior to fertilization, proteins bind to the mRNAs to protect them and inhibit their translation. Subsequent to fertilization, translation is regulated by controlling an increase in the length of the poly(A) tail of maternally deposited mRNAs. Maternally deposited mRNAs generally have shorter poly(A) tails (15–90 As) than do actively translated mRNAs (100–300 As). If the *cortex* and *grauzone* genes encoded proteins that functioned in protecting and limiting translation of the *bicoid* and *toll* mRNAs, deficits in *cortex* and *grauzone* would most likely result in either decreased amounts of these mRNAs or their increased translation. In contrast, if the *cortex* and *grauzone* genes function in the post-fertilization lengthening poly(A) tails, mutations in these genes would lead to decreased protein synthesis from mRNAs deposited with shorter poly(A) tails. Therefore, one hypothesis is that *cortex* and *grauzone* function to elongate poly(A) tails of maternally deposited mRNAs following fertilization.

b. The efficient translation of *nanos* mRNAs does not require lengthening of its poly(A) tail using the functions provided by *cortex* and *grauzone*. This could be because *nanos* mRNAs are deposited into the embryo with longer poly(A) tails, or because the post-fertilization poly(A) tail elongation of *nanos* mRNAs is accomplished using functions provided by other genes.

c. In wild-type embryos, the *bicoid* and *toll* mRNAs would have short poly(A) tails (15–90 As) prior to fertilization and longer poly(A) tails (100–300 As) after fertilization. The mRNAs produced by *nanos* would have the same poly(A) tail length before and after fertilization (presumably long, 100–300 As). In *cortex* and *grauzone* embryos, the *bicoid*, *toll*, and *nanos* mRNAs would have the same poly(A) tail length before and after fertilization. The mRNAs of *bicoid* and *toll* would be short (15–90 As) while the mRNAs of *nanos* would (presumably) be long (100–300 As).

d. Similar amounts of Bicoid protein will be produced in i, ii, and iii; in ii, the poly(A) tail can be lengthened by wild-type *cortex* and *grauzone* functions; in iii, the poly(A) tail can be efficiently translated without further lengthening. Less Bicoid protein will be produced in iv, since the *bicoid* mRNA has a short poly(A) tail that cannot be lengthened due to a deficit in *cortex* function.

18.19 *Answer:*

a. From text Figure 18.9d, p. 529, the transcriptional repressors Giant and Krüppel are expressed in a pattern that is nearly the opposite to that of *eve* stripe-2 transcription. They are present at very low levels in parasegment 3 where the *eve* stripe-2 enhancer drives *eve* transcription, but the levels of Giant rise in parasegments 1 and 2, and the levels of Krüppel rise in parasegments 4 and 5, where *eve* is not transcribed.

b. From text Figure 18.9d, p. 529, the expression of the transcriptional activator Hunchback reaches a high level and then plateaus within parasegment 3, where the *eve* stripe-2 enhancer drives *eve* transcription. The transcriptional activator Bicoid is also expressed in parasegment 3, though its level is diminishing posteriorly.

c. In text Figure 18.9c, p. 529, it appears that the transcriptional activators Bicoid and Hunchback compete for overlapping DNA-binding sites with the transcriptional repressors Giant and Krüppel. Therefore, not all of these sites will be bound simultaneously. The relative concentrations of the four proteins will determine which sites fill, and whether transcription driven by the *eve* stripe-2 enhancer will be activated or repressed.

d. i, ii. Both Giant and Krüppel are transcriptional repressors that are not expressed highly in parasegment 3 where the *eve* stripe-2 enhancer drives *eve* transcription. If Giant or Krüppel expression were more broadly distributed, each would bind to sites in the *eve* stripe-2 enhancer shown in text Figure 18.9c, p. 529, and potentially lead to repression of *eve* transcription in at least part of parasegment 3.

   iii. Hunchback is a transcriptional activator that is expressed at high levels in parasegment 3 where the *eve* stripe-2 enhancer drives *eve* transcription. From text Figure 18.9c, p. 529, Hunchback binds to the *eve* stripe-2 enhancer and so appears necessary for *eve* transcription in parasegment 3. Therefore, if Hunchback expression were restricted to parasegments 1 and 2, *eve* would be expected to show diminished transcription in parasegment 3.

   iv. Bicoid is a transcriptional activator that is expressed at low levels in parasegment 3 and binds multiple sites in the *eve* stripe-2 enhancer. Dramatically elevated Bicoid levels could have different consequences depending on how Bicoid levels affect the competition between Bicoid and the transcriptional repressors Giant and Krüppel for sites in the *eve* stripe-2 enhancer. If increased Bicoid levels enable Bicoid to compete more effectively for sites normally filled by Giant in parasegments 1 and 2 and Krüppel in parasegments 4 and 5, the domain over which the *eve* stripe-2 enhancer drives *eve* transcription would be broadened, so that *eve* might be transcribed in part of parasegments 2 and 4. Within parasegment 3, greater Bicoid binding to the *eve* stripe-2 enhancer should result in greater levels of *eve* expression.

e. The expression of *eve* in different stripes is controlled independently, so *eve* expression in stripe 2 is not dependent on stripe 6. The expression of *eve* in each stripe is determined by regulatory events involving particular combinations of gene regulatory proteins binding to an enhancer controlling *eve* expression in each stripe.

f. The spatial pattern of *eve* expression is dependent on combinatorial gene regulation involving about 20 different transcriptional activators and repressors. The levels of these different transcriptional activators and repressors determine their ability to compete for binding sites in *eve* enhancers to activate or repress *eve* transcription.

18.20 *Answer:*

a. In bacterial operons, a common regulatory region controls the production of single mRNA from which multiple protein products are translated. These products function in a related biochemical pathway. Here, two proteins that are involved in the synthesis and packaging of acetylcholine are both produced from a common primary mRNA transcript.

b. Unlike the proteins translated from an mRNA synthesized from a bacterial operon, the protein products produced at the *VAChT/ChAT* locus are not translated sequentially from the same mRNA. Here, the primary mRNA appears to be alternatively processed to produce two distinct mature mRNAs. These mRNAs are translated starting at different points, producing different proteins.

c. At least two mechanisms are involved in the production of the different ChAT and VAChT proteins: alternative mRNA processing and alternative translation initiation. After the first exon, an alternative 3' splice site is used in the two different mRNAs. In addition, different AUG start codons are used.

19

Genetic Analysis of Development

Chapter Outline

Review of Key Terms, Symbols, and Concepts

In your own words, write a brief, precise definition of each term in the groups below. Check your definitions using the text. Then develop a concept map using the terms in each list.

1	2
development	differential gene activity
determination	α-, β-, δ-, γ-, ε-, ζ-globin genes
developmental potential	embryonic, fetal, adult hemoglobin
induction	polytene chromosome
differentiation	puff
totipotent	ecdysone
morphogenesis	early, late genes
fate map	lymphocyte, T, B cell
model organism	antigen
animal cloning	antibody
regeneration	humoral immune response
nuclear transplantation	clonal selection
G_0 phase	immunoglobulin
cell lineage, fate	light (L), heavy (H) chain
Saccharomyces cerevisiae	C, V, J, D segments
Drosophila melanogaster	somatic recombination
Caenorhabditis elegans	antibody diversity
Arabidopsis thaliana	
Danio rerio	
Mus musculus	

3	4
sex determination	*Drosophila* development
dosage compensation	polar cytoplasm
mammal	syncitium
Drosophila	syncytial, cellular blastoderm
testis-determining factor, TDF	parasegments
sex reversal individual	segments
SRY, Sry	imaginal discs
X inactivation center (XIC)	maternal effect gene
Xce, Xist genes	morphogen
histone methylation	*bicoid, caudal, nanos, hunchback* genes
regulation cascade model	segmentation gene
Sxl, tra, dsx genes	gap, pair rule, segment polarity genes
alternative vs. default splicing	homeotic gene
sis-a, sis-b, dpn genes	selector gene
P_E, P_L promoters at *Sxl*	homeotic mutation
DSX-F, DSX-M	*biothorax* complex
mle, msl-1, msl-2, msl-3, mof genes	*Antennapedia* complex
MSL complex	homeobox
chromatin remodeling	homeodomain
chromatin entry site (CES)	*Hox* gene
	miRNA
	heterochronic gene
	lin-4, lin-14

Thinking Analytically

This chapter considers how gene expression can be controlled in a temporal and spatial context during development. It is important that you have a solid grasp on the mechanisms that eukaryotes use to regulate gene expression—it may be helpful to review the material in Chapter 18. Thus far, we have considered gene expression in defined situations and in fairly short timelines. In eukaryotic development, timelines can be much longer, there can be multiple modes of regulation acting simultaneously, and more interactions between genes, and the spatial dimension is added. Therefore, the fundamental question being asked in developmental genetics, "How do different cell types and tissues differentiate from a common precursor cell?" has a complex and detailed answer.

It is useful to maintain a biological perspective as you consider how differential gene expression is regulated during development. For example, it will help to have a thorough understanding of the biology of the system that is developing. Focus on gaining an understanding of how the organism (e.g., *Drosophila*, *C. elegans*) or population of cells (e.g., the immune system) develops. Then, consider how genes are regulated during its development, and how regulatory events at one stage of development impact on gene expression in subsequent stages. It will be helpful to construct flowcharts that illustrate how genes are regulated along a timeline or in a developmental context: show how genes are turned on and off, what their targets are, and whether they affect the expression of other genes positively or negatively.

Questions for Practice

Multiple-Choice Questions

1. Sex type in *Drosophila* is controlled by
   a. the ratio of X chromosomes to autosomes.
   b. a cascade of regulated, alternative RNA splicing.
   c. sex-specific selection of polyadenylation sites.
   d. sex-specific transport control.
   e. both a and b
   f. all of the above

2. A wide diversity of immunoglobulin molecules is obtained via
   a. new gene synthesis.
   b. combinatorial gene regulation.
   c. alternative RNA splicing.
   d. somatic recombination of DNA.

3. Evidence for the totipotency of nuclei in eukaryotic cells is provided by
   a. the existence of homeotic mutations.
   b. nuclear transplantation experiments.
   c. the transcription of fetal globin genes during fetal development but not during adult life.
   d. the discovery that nuclei in different tissues have the same amount of DNA.

4. In *Drosophila*, maternal effect genes are genes that
   a. are expressed in the mother during oogenesis and whose products will specify spatial organization in the developing embryo.
   b. cause females to lay eggs.
   c. affect the number or polarity of body segments.
   d. affect the identify of a segment.
   e. b, c, and d

5. The homeotic mutations found in *Drosophila*
   a. cause transformation of one segment to another.
   b. alter the function of proteins that are regulators of transcription.
   c. alter highly conserved functions found in nearly all organisms.
   d. all of the above

6. How does the *dsx* gene in *Drosophila* function in sex determination?
   a. It is active only in XY animals, where it activates male differentiation. XX animals lack its function so that a default pathway of female differentiation ensues.
   b. It is active only in XX animals, where it activates female differentiation. XY animals lack its function so that a default pathway of male differentiation ensues.

c. It functions to control transcription at key X-linked genes. In XX animals, these genes are transcribed twice as much as in XY animals. The doubled dose of key X-linked gene products results in female differentiation.

d. Its pre-mRNA is alternatively spliced in XX animals to make a female-specific protein that represses male differentiation. Its pre-mRNA undergoes default splicing in XY animals to make a male-specific protein that represses female differentiation.

7. Why might an individual have female secondary sexual characteristics but an XY karyotype?
   a. One of their X chromosomes has been inactivated—they are really XXY.
   b. They have a point mutation in the *SRY* gene.
   c. They have a point mutation in the *SXL* gene.
   d. They have a mutation in the *XIST* gene.

8. In *Drosophila*, which of the following types of chromatin modifications is associated with dosage compensation?
   a. histone H3 methylation
   b. histone H4 acetylation
   c. histone H1 demethylation
   d. histone H2A deacetylation

9. Your neighbor adores his calico cat and, being totally unaware of the availability of stray cats at the humane society, hires a firm to clone her. He receives a report with DNA analyses showing that the clone and his cat are genetically identical and a cat carrier containing the cloned cat. When he releases the clone from the carrier, he is outraged. Not only does the cat look nothing like his beloved original, it hisses at him incessantly. What is the most likely explanation?
   a. X inactivation contributes to the distribution of pigment in calico cats. Since X inactivation is a random process in different cells, the two cats are unlikely to be alike.
   b. Environmental factors in the research laboratory have influenced the cloned cat's personality.
   c. The two cats do not have identical patterns of gene expression because of the incomplete reprogramming of the donor nucleus.
   d. Your neighbor is uninformed about the capabilities of cloning technology.
   e. all of the above

10. In which tissue is fetal hemoglobin containing two α and two γ polypeptides synthesized?
   a. embryonic yolk sac
   b. fetal liver
   c. fetal spleen
   d. fetal bone marrow
   e. both b and c

Answers: 1e, 2d, 3b, 4a, 5d, 6d, 7b, 8b, 9e, 10e

Thought Questions

1. Consider the cascade of alternative splicing events that are used to regulate sex type in *Drosophila*. From an evolutionary perspective, what advantages might there be to having a cascade of events regulate such an important process? (Hint: Consider the nature of the initial signal for sex type, the X:A ratio—a ratio of either 1:2 or 2:2—and how a splicing cascade amplifies this signal.)

2. Suppose Gurdon's experiments on totipotency were repeated using differentiated B lymphocytes as the source of nuclei for transplantation. To what extent would you expect these nuclei to be totipotent? If mature organisms developed from cells with transplanted B cell nuclei, what characteristics would their immune system have?

3. In *Drosophila*, the polar cytoplasm contains factors determining that the nuclei migrating into this region will become germ-line cells. (a) Design an experiment to gather evidence supporting this conclusion. (b) What phenotype would be associated with mutants lacking these factors? (c) Would the mutants from (b) identify maternal effect genes?

4. What are homeoboxes, and what is their role in the regulation of development in eukaryotes?

5. In vertebrates, including mammals such as humans, homeotic gene complexes have been identified using heterologous probes. As discussed in the text, the gene complexes show similar structural

organization, even though vertebrates are not segmented in the same way as invertebrates. What significance might this finding have? How might analyzing mutations in these genes in vertebrates help demonstrate the function of these genes and test this significance?

6. Multiple model organisms have been studied intensively with the aim of understanding the genetic control of differential gene expression during development. Describe the features of *Drosophila*, *Caenorhabditis*, and *Arabidopsis* that make them useful for such analysis. Why is it important to study more than one model organism?

7. The primary transcripts of many genes undergo tissue-specific alternative mRNA splicing. Indeed, about 15% of human disease mutations are associated with mRNA splicing alterations. (a) For genes that are alternatively spliced, do you expect the proteins that are produced to have identical functions? Why or why not? (b) How might spliceosomes process pre-mRNAs differently in different tissues to achieve alternative mRNA processing? (Hint: Consider the regulation cascade that controls sex determination in *Drosophila*. Are there sex-specific splicing factors?)

8. Dolly is the lamb that was generated by fusing adult mammary epithelial cells with enucleated oocytes. (a) How does this experiment demonstrate totipotency? (b) How could you use molecular methods to experimentally demonstrate that Dolly had the same genotype as the adult mammary epithelial cells? (c) Suppose you sampled Dolly's DNA when she was 1 year old. Do you expect Dolly's simple telomeric repeats to be the same length as those of other sheep that were 1 year old? (d) What impact might imprinting and incomplete genome reprogramming have on our ability to successfully clone eukaryotic organisms?

9. Exposure of *Drosophila* salivary glands to the steroid hormone ecdysone induces a set of early puffs that are followed by a set of late puffs. What mechanism underlies the differential gene expression associated with this pattern of puffs? How would you experimentally gather evidence to support this mechanism?

10. Compare the processes that lead to chromatin remodeling during dosage compensation in mammals and in *Drosophila*.

Thought Questions for Media

After reviewing the media on the *iGenetics* website, try to answer these questions.

1. How is the X:A ratio sensed in *Drosophila*? What molecules constitute the numerator and denominator in this ratio?
2. How does an X:A ratio of 1:1 lead to sex-specific transcriptional activation of *Sxl*?
3. Later in development, *Sxl* is transcribed in both sex types from a constitutive promoter. Why, then, is functional SXL protein made only in females?
4. Use diagrams to explain what is meant by a *cascade of alternative splicing events*.
5. In what sense does male development in *Drosophila* represent a default state?
6. What leads to the production of different DSX proteins in males and females?
7. Loss-of-function mutants at *dsx* result in intersexual development—animals in which male and female development proceeds simultaneously. Explain the origin of this phenotype based on your understanding of the molecular function of the DSX proteins.
8. What is meant by a syncytium?
9. At what point during *Drosophila* development is the germ line established? How is the germ line formed separately from somatic cells?
10. At what point during development do you expect each of the following sets of genes to be transcribed? To be translated?
    a. maternal effect genes
    b. segmentation genes
    c. homeotic genes
11. How is cell fate gradually restricted by the expression of the genes in Thought Question 10?
12. Why might some homeotic mutations be lethal, while others are not?

1. In the iActivity, microarrays were used to identify genes that were differentially expressed between differentiating tissues (mesoderm and endoderm) and stem cells. Suppose two genes, *A* and *B*, are upregulated in differentiating mesoderm relative to stem cells. Gene *A* is expressed 13-fold more, and Gene *B* is expressed 2.5-fold more. Neither gene is upregulated in differentiating endoderm.

    a. From this data alone, can you infer anything about the *relative* importance of these genes' expression for mesodermal differentiation?

    b. Suppose mutants were available that caused the rate of each gene's transcription to be halved. Can you predict which mutation might have a more severe effect on mesodermal differentiation?

    c. Based on the results of the microarray analyses, can you infer which gene produces more mRNA copies (the total number of transcripts per gene) in differentiating mesodermal cells?

2. What is meant by a gene that can *serve as a marker* for endoderm differentiation? What features must such a gene have?

3. A gene that encodes a transcription factor is expressed at high levels in differentiating endoderm and differentiating mesoderm, but not in stem cells. What types of genes might be targets of this transcription factor? Would it invariably act through positive regulation of these targets?

4. A gene that encodes a transcription factor is expressed at stem cells, but not in differentiating cells. What role might this gene play in keeping stem cells from differentiating? Would it invariably act through negative regulation of target genes?

Solutions to Text Questions and Problems

19.1   *Answer: Development* is a process of regulated growth and cellular change. It results from the interaction of the genome with the cytoplasm and external environment. It involves a programmed sequence of phenotypic changes that are typically irreversible. Initially, cells of the zygote are totipotent—they have the potential to develop into any cell type of the complete organism. As the cells of the zygote divide and interact, they may lose their totipotency and become *determined*—they follow a genetic program that sets their fate. *Differentiation* refers to the process of cellular change in development that leads to the formation of distinct types of cells, tissues, and organs through the regulation of gene expression. Determination and differentiation are thus a part of development and lead to cells that have characteristic structural and functional properties.

19.2   *Answer:* Totipotency refers to the capacity of a nucleus to direct a cell through all of the stages of development. A nucleus taken from the cell of a differentiated tissue is said to be totipotent if, when it is injected into an enucleated egg, it can direct the development of the organism to the adult stage. If the egg is able to develop into an adult, the differentiated nucleus must have retained all of the genetic information needed to direct development again from the start. In 1975, Gurdon demonstrated that the nucleus of a skin cell of an adult frog was at least partly totipotent. When injected into an enucleated egg, such a nucleus could direct development to the tadpole stage. Then, in 1997, Wilmut and his colleagues demonstrated that a mammalian nucleus was totipotent. They showed that the nucleus of a mammary epithelium-derived cell could direct the development of a sheep to the adult stage. Since then, other mammals—including mice, rats, goats, cattle, horses, cats, and monkeys—have been successfully cloned.

A cell's totipotency is restricted as it becomes determined to adopt different cell fates. This occurs either by induction where an inductive signal produced by one cell or group of cells affects the development of another cell or group of cells, or by asymmetric cell division, which leads to a new distribution of cell-determining molecules in daughter cells.

19.3   *Answer:* This experiment demonstrates the phenomenon of *determination* and when it occurs during development. The tissue taken from the blastula or gastrula has not yet been committed to its final differentiated state in terms of its genetic programming; that is, it has not yet been *determined*. Thus, when the tissue is transplanted into the host, it adopts the fate of nearby tissues and differentiates in the same way as they do. Presumably, cues from the tissue surrounding the transplant determine its fate. In contrast, tissues in the neurula stage are stably determined. By the time the neurula developmental stage has been reached, a developmental program has been set. In other words, the fate of neurula tissue transplants is *determined*. Upon transplantation, they will differentiate according to their own set genetic program. Tissue transplanted from a neurula to an older embryo cannot be influenced by the surrounding tissues. It will develop into the tissue type for which it has been determined, in this case, an eye.

19.4   *Answer:* A model organism for the genetic analysis of development must have two fundamental attributes: It must develop, and mutants affecting developmental processes must be available for use in developmental genetic analyses. Model organisms that are attractive for the genetic analysis of development share many properties: They are often easy to culture, develop over relatively short time periods, have a rich array of mutants that affect developmental processes, have well-characterized genetics so that crosses can be performed and analyzed, and have characterized and sequenced genomes that facilitate molecular analyses. Organisms such as *Saccharomyces cerevisiae, Drosophila melanogaster, Caenorhabditis elegans, Arabidopsis thaliana, Danio rerio,* and *Mus musculus* all have these properties to different degrees. The choice among organisms depends on the developmental process that is being studied. For example, the yeast *S. cerevisiae,* even with its limited developmental repertoire, is ideal for investigating fundamental questions such as the role of cellular signaling in differentiation. The fly *D. melanogaster* has a rich array of mutants, making it well suited for detailed analyses of developmental mechanisms such as those underlying sex determination and pattern formation. The nematode *C. elegans* has a completely defined fate map, so it is well suited to investigations addressing how cell fate is determined. Finally, *A. thaliana, D. rerio,* and *M. musculus* serve as models for studying plant, vertebrate embryogenesis, and mammalian development, respectively.

19.5   *Answer:* The production of Dolly was significant because it demonstrated the apparent complete totipotency of a nucleus from a mature mammary epithelium cell. The other six lambs developed from the transplanted nuclei of embryonic or fetal cells, which one might expect to be less determined and have a higher degree of totipotency due to their younger developmental age.

Two types of evidence indicate that Dolly resulted from the fusion of a nucleus of a mature mammary epithelium cell with the cytoplasm of a donor egg. First, Dolly had the same phenotype as the ewe who donated the mammary epithelium cell—Finn Dorset (whiteface)—and not that of the surrogate mother—Scottish blackface. Second, analysis of four microsatellite markers demonstrated that Dolly's DNA matched the DNA of the donor mammary epithelial cells but not the DNA of the recipient ewe.

19.6   *Answer:*

a. Based on the work of Wilmut and his colleagues, the nose cells would first be dissociated and grown in tissue culture. The cells would be induced into a quiescent state (the G_0 phase of the cell cycle) by reducing the concentration of growth serum in the medium. Then they would be fused with enucleated oocytes from a donor female and allowed to grow and divide by mitosis to produce embryos. The embryos would be implanted into a surrogate female. After the establishment of pregnancy, its progression would need to be maintained.

b. While the nuclear genome would generally be identical to that in the original nose cell, cytoplasmic organelles presumably would derive from those in the enucleated oocyte. Therefore, the mitochondrial DNA would not derive from the original leader. In addition, because telomeres in an older individual are shorter, one might expect the telomeres in the cloned leader to be those of an older individual.

c. In mature B cells, DNA rearrangements at the heavy- and light-chain immunoglobulin genes have occurred. One would expect the cloned leader to be immunocompromised, since he would be unable to make the wide spectrum of antibodies present in a normal individual.

d. It is likely that the cloning process will be very inefficient, with most clones dying before or soon after birth. The surviving clones are also likely to differ in body shape and personality, and they are unlikely to be normal since a nucleus donated from the differentiated nose cell is unlikely to be completely reprogrammed. One suggestion is for the government to hire a good plastic surgeon to alter the appearance of a good actor able to assume the role of the totalitarian leader.

e. There is no way to predict the psychological profile of the cloned leader based on his genetic identity. Even identical twins, who are genetically more identical than such a clone, do not always share behavioral traits.

19.7   *Answer:*

a. Prometea's mother almost gave birth to her identical twin. Since Prometea's birth mother donated a nucleus and the donor egg was from a slaughtered horse, Prometea is identical to her birth mother with respect to her nuclear, but not mitochondrial genome.

b. Since the donor nucleus used to form Prometea is from the birth mother, Prometea and her birth mother will both be Haflinger horses. Since Prometea has the same phenotype as a sibling produced by a normal mating between her birth mother and a Haflinger stallion, the coat color phenotype cannot be used to demonstrate that Prometea is a clone of her birth mother. DNA testing would provide more compelling evidence. If Prometea is a clone having her mother's nuclear genome, she should show the same pattern of DNA sequence variation as her mother. Assess this by comparing the two horses using a panel of polymorphic STR markers (see text Chapter 10, p. 272).

c. Nuclei taken from adult cells must be reprogrammed before the process of determination and differentiation can be started over. That only 22 of the 814 embryos survived 7 days to reach the blastocyst stage suggests the hypothesis that there was incomplete reprogramming of gene expression. If this were the case, the cloned embryos would be unable to recapitulate developmental processes, and there would be poor cloning success. To test this hypothesis, establish cell lines from specific types of tissues biopsied from similarly staged normal and cloned embryos. Use DNA microarray analysis of gene expression in these lines to evaluate whether the gene expression profiles in cloned embryos are similar to those of normal embryos. Also, evaluate the patterns of DNA methylation, which influence patterns of transcription. Different patterns of gene expression and DNA methylation in cell lines established from cloned and normal embryos would provide support for the hypothesis that the nuclei underwent incomplete reprogramming of gene expression.

19.8   *Answer:* The evidence for differential gene activity during development is vast. Classic lines of evidence stem from (1) studies on the differential expression of the α, β, γ, δ, ε, and ζ classes of globin genes during development; (2) differential puffing patterns in the polytene chromosomes in Dipteran insects; and (3) the studies on genes that are expressed in a temporal and spatially specific manner during the development of *Drosophila*. See the text for additional discussion.

Microarray analysis was used to study changes in *Drosophila* gene expression patterns brought about by the hormone ecdysone during the metamorphosis of the larva into a pupa. About 40% of the genes in *Drosophila* were analyzed (N = 6,240). Of these, about 8% (N = 534) exhibited differential gene expression. This study provided researchers with a catalog of genes that are induced or repressed by ecdysone during this developmental window. For example, it showed that 4 hours prior to the formation of the pupa, a set of genes involved in the differentiation of the nervous system is induced, while another set of genes required for muscle formation is repressed in anticipation of the future breakdown of larval muscle tissues.

19.9   *Answer:* Separate loci code for α-like and β-like globin polypeptides, which form distinct types of hemoglobin at different times during human development. In the embryo, hemoglobin is initially made in the yolk sac and consists of two ζ polypeptides and two ε polypeptides. ζ polypeptides are α-like, while ε polypeptides are β-like. At about three months of gestation, hemoglobin synthesis switches to the fetal liver and spleen. There, hemoglobin is made that consists of two α polypeptides and two β-like polypeptides, either two γA polypeptides or two γG polypeptides. Just before birth, hemoglobin synthesis switches to the bone marrow, where predominantly α polypeptides and β polypeptides are made along with some β-like δ polypeptides.

19.10   *Answer:* All of the α-like genes (the ζ and α genes and three pseudogenes) are located in a gene cluster on chromosome 16, while all of the β-like genes (ε, γG, γA, δ, and β genes and one pseudogene) are located in a gene cluster on chromosome 11. At a very general level, the organization of the two gene clusters is similar. Both sets of genes are arranged on the chromosome in an order that exactly parallels the time when the genes are transcribed during human development. In both gene clusters, the genes transcribed in the embryo are at the left end of the cluster; the genes transcribed in the fetus are to the right of these; and the genes transcribed in the adult are farthest to the right. This is intriguing since the genes are also transcribed in different tissues.

19.11   *Answer:* There are a number of possibilities. One is that the γ-globin genes in bone marrow are under negative regulation by β-globin (or some metabolite of it). When β-globin is not formed, the γ-globin gene is derepressed.

19.12   *Answer:* Polytene chromosomes occur in Dipteran insects such as *Drosophila*. Polytene chromosomes are formed by endoreduplication, in which repeated cycles of chromosome duplication occur without nuclear division or chromosome segregation. Since they can be 1,000 times as thick as the corresponding chromosomes in meiosis or in the nuclei of normal cells, they can be stained and viewed at the light microscope level. Distinct bands, or chromomeres, are visible, and genes are located both in bands and in interband regions. A puff results when a gene in a band or interband region is expressed at very high levels in a particular developmental stage. Puffs are accompanied by a loosening of the chromatin structure that allows for efficient transcription of a particular DNA region. When increased transcriptional activity at the gene ceases at a later developmental stage, the puff disappears, and the chromosome resumes its compact configuration. In this way, the appearance and disappearance of puffs provides a visual representation of differential gene activity.

19.13   *Answer:* That RNA molecules are present in puffs can be demonstrated by feeding or injecting *Drosophila* larvae with radioactive uridine, an RNA precursor. After this treatment, salivary glands are dissected from larvae and a spread of the polytene chromosomes is subjected to autoradiography to detect the location of the incorporated uridine. Silver grains are evident over puffed regions, indicating that they contain RNA. Evidence that the RNA is single-stranded might be obtained by treating such spreads with an RNase that was capable of digesting only single-stranded RNA. The radiolabel should be recovered in the solution, and not remain bound to the salivary gland chromosome. A lack of signal on puffs following autoradiographic detection (compared to controls) would provide evidence that the RNA in puffs is single-stranded.

19.14   *Answer:* Experiment A results in all of the DNA becoming radioactively labeled. The distribution of radioactive label throughout the polytene chromosomes indicates that DNA is a fundamental and major component of these chromosomes. The even distribution of label suggests that each region of the chromosome has been replicated to the same extent. This provides support for the contention that band and interband regions are the result of different types of packaging, not different amounts of DNA replication. Experiment B results in the radioactive labeling of RNA molecules. The finding that label is found first in puffs indicates that these are sites of transcriptional activity that arise from molecules that are in the process of being synthesized. The later appearance of label in the cytoplasm reflects the completed RNA molecules that have been processed and transported into the cytoplasm, where they will be translated. Experiment C provides additional support for the hypothesis that transcriptional activity is associated with puffs. The inhibition of RNA transcription by actinomycin D blocks the appearance of signal over puffs, indicating that it blocks the incorporation of ^{3}H-uridine into RNA in puffed regions. The fact that the puffs are much smaller indicates that the puffing process itself is associated with the onset of transcriptional activity for the genes in a specific region of the chromosome.

19.15   *Answer:* The ability to make 10^6 to 10^8 different antibodies arises from the combinatorial way in which antibody genes are generated in different antibody-producing cells during their development, and not the existence of this many separate antibody genes in each and every mammalian cell. A template that exists in germ-line cells is processed differently during the development of different antibody-producing cells to generate antibody diversity.

Antibody molecules consist of two light (L) chains and two heavy (H) chains. The amino acid sequence of one domain of each type of chain is variable and generates antibody diversity. In the germ-line DNA of mammals, coding regions for these immunoglobulin chains exist in tandem arrays of gene segments. For light chains, there are many variable (V) region-gene segments, a few joining (J) segments, and one constant (C) gene segment. Somatic recombination during development results in the production of a recombinant V-J-C DNA molecule that, when transcribed, produces a unique functional L chain. From a particular gene in one cell, only one L chain is produced. A large number of L chains are obtained by recombining the gene segments in many different ways. Diversity in these L chains results from variability in the sequences of the multiple V segments, variability in the sequences of the four J segments, and variability in the number of nucleotide pairs deleted at the V-J joints. H chains are similar, except that several D (diversity) segments can be used between the V and J segments, increasing the possible diversity of recombinant H chain genes. The type of C gene segment chosen for the constant domains of the H chain determines whether the antibody is IgM, IgD, IgG, IgE, or IgA.

19.16   *Answer:*

a. Not considering the variability in the number of nucleotide pairs deleted at the V_κ-J_κ joint, there are 300 (V_κ segments) $\times$ 4 (J_κ segments) = 1,200 different light chain combinations. This number is a lower bound for an estimate, since significantly more variability can be obtained by using imprecise V-J joining.

b. Not considering the imprecise joining of gene segments that comprise the chain's variable region, there are 200 (V_H segments) $\times$ 12 (D segments) $\times$ 4 (J_H segments) = 9,600 different heavy chain combinations for each of the eight types of Ig (IgM, IgD, IgG$_3$, IgG$_1$, IgG$_{2b}$, IgG$_{2a}$,

IgE, or IgA; see pp. 556–557 and text Figure 19.12). If all possible types of Ig are considered, there are $9,600 \times 8$ (C_H segments) = 76,800 heavy chain combinations. As in part **(a)**, this is a lower bound for an estimate of heavy chain variability.

c.   IgG has four C segments (γ_3, γ_1, γ_{2b}, γ_{2a}; see pp. 556–557 and text Figure 19.12). An estimate of the minimal number of combinations for IgG molecules would be $1,200 \times 9,600 \times 4 = 4.608 \times 10^7$.

19.17   *Answer:* The gene for TDF was identified by analyzing rare sex-reversal individuals—males who are XX and females who are XY. Cytogenetic analysis of these individuals revealed that XX males had attached to one of their X chromosomes a small fragment from near the tip of the small arm of the Y chromosome, and that XY females had deletions of the same region. Molecular analyses identified a male-specific gene—the *SRY* gene—lying within the translocated region and identified an equivalent gene, *Sry*, in mice. Three lines of evidence support the view that the *SRY* gene is the gene for TDF: (1) The mouse *Sry* gene is expressed in the undifferentiated genital ridges of the embryo just before the formation of the testes, that is, where it would be expected to be expressed if it was the gene for TDF; (2) transgenic XX mice carrying a 14-kb DNA fragment with the *Sry* gene develop testes and have male secondary sexual development; and (3) some rare XY human females have simple mutations in the *SRY* gene, suggesting loss-of-function mutations at *SRY* lead to sex reversal.

19.18   *Answer:*

a.   Each cell should exhibit green fluorescence, since the gene is constitutively expressed.

b.   About half the cells will exhibit green fluorescence. If more than one *Xic* is present, X inactivation will occur on one *Xic*-containing chromosome. Either the X chromosome or the *Xic*-bearing autosome will be inactivated, at random. If the X chromosome is inactivated, the *gfp* gene will not be expressed.

c.   The *Xist* gene on the autosome is being expressed. Since the cell exhibits green fluorescence, the X chromosome with the *gfp* gene is not inactivated and the *Xic*-bearing autosome is inactivated. The *Xist* gene on the autosome is transcribed, and its RNA coats the autosome to trigger the methylation of histone H3. This initiates chromatin remodeling to silence genes on the *Xic*-bearing autosome.

19.19   *Answer:*

a.   The X:A ratio is detected by interactions of the protein products of three X-linked numerator genes (*sis-a, sis-b, sis-c*) and one autosomal denominator gene (*dpn*). The numerator gene products can either form homodimers or heterodimers with the denominator gene product. When the X:A ratio is 2:2, an excess of numerator gene products leads to the formation of many homodimers. These serve as transcription factors to activate *Sxl* transcription from P_E. When the X:A ratio is 1:2, most numerator subunits are found in heterodimers, so *Sxl* transcription is not activated. Therefore, activation of *Sxl* at P_E by the homodimers serves to detect the X:A ratio and leads to the early sex-specific synthesis of SXL protein.

b.   Transcription at P_E is essential to generate a functional SXL protein in animals with an X:A ratio of 2:2. It is not used in individuals with an X:A ratio of 1:2, so these animals will be unaffected and differentiate as males. In individuals with an X:A ratio of 2:2, SXL initiates a cascade of alternative mRNA splicing at *Sxl, tra*, and *dsx* that leads to the implementation of female differentiation. If there is no transcription from P_E, no functional SXL protein will be produced in these animals, and a default set of splice choices at *Sxl, tra*, and *dsx* will be used. In principle, this would lead to male differentiation in individuals with an X:A ratio of 2:2. However, SXL also prevents the translation of *msl-2* transcripts so that dosage compensation does not normally occur in individuals with an X:A ratio of 2:2. Without SXL, *msl-2* transcripts will be translated so dosage compensation will occur, leading to four doses of X-linked gene products. The imbalance in X and autosomal gene product dosage is likely to be lethal to these animals.

c.   This *tra* mutation will eliminate functional TRA protein. Since functional TRA is not normally present in animals with an X:A ratio of 1:2, this mutation will have no effect on these animals—

they will differentiate normally into males. TRA is normally present in individuals with an X:A ratio of 2:2, where it functions to regulate alternative splicing at *dsx* and produce DSX-F, which implements female differentiation by repressing male-specific gene expression. Without TRA, default splicing will occur at *dsx* and produce DSX-M, which implements male differentiation by repressing female-specific gene expression. Thus, animals with an X:A ratio of 2:2 will be males.

    d. Animals with knockout mutations at *dsx* will produce neither DSX-M, which represses female-specific gene expression, nor DSX-F, which represses male-specific gene expression. Therefore, neither male- nor female-specific gene expression will be repressed, and both male and female differentiation pathways will proceed.

19.20   *Answer:* The early SXL protein binds to the *Sxl* pre-mRNA to cause alternative splicing: Exons E1 and 3 are skipped, and exons L1, 2, 4, 5, 6, 7, and 8 are included. The resulting mRNA produces a functional late SXL protein. In the absence of the early SXL protein, default splicing occurs to produce a transcript that includes exon 3. This exon has a stop codon in frame with the start codon at the beginning of exon 2, so no functional SXL protein is produced. The SXL protein regulates *tra* in a similar manner: SXL binds to the *tra* pre-mRNA to produce an mRNA that encodes an active TRA protein. In the absence of SXL, a default stop codon containing exon is included, and an active TRA protein is not produced.

    In contrast to its role in alternative mRNA splicing at *Sxl* and *tra*, the late SXL protein serves to block translation of *msl-2* transcripts. In XX animals (females), the SXL late protein binds to the transcript of *msl-2*. This blocks its translation so that no MSL2 protein is produced. As a result, dosage compensation does not occur. In XY animals (males) where SXL protein is not produced, the *msl-2* transcript is translated and dosage compensation occurs.

19.21   *Answer:*

    a. Each of these genes functions in dosage compensation, the twofold increase in the transcriptional activity of the male's single X chromosome that occurs to match the transcriptional activity of the female's two X chromosomes. Initially, the protein products of these five genes form a complex that binds to about 35 chromatin entry sites (CES) on the male's X chromosome. Then, the MSL complexes spread from those sites in both directions into the flanking chromatin. The MOF protein of the MSL complex is a histone acetyltransferase, and during the spreading of the complexes along the X chromosome, it remodels chromatin to allow for the higher level of transcription of the X chromosome genes in males.

    b. In females, the MLE, MSL-1, MSL-3, and MOF proteins are produced. The MSL-2 protein is not produced (see the solution to Question 19.20). Without the MSL-2 protein, the MSL complex is unable to bind to the X chromosome. Since none of the proteins function in females, mutations in their genes do not affect females.

    c. The mechanisms for sex determination and dosage compensation are interrelated through the function of the *Sxl* gene. In XX animals (females), SXL protein is produced. SXL initiates a cascade of regulated splicing at the *tra* and *dsx* genes that culminates in female sexual differentiation. SXL also blocks the translation of *msl-2* transcripts so that dosage compensation does not occur in XX animals. In XY animals (males), active SXL protein is not produced. This results in default splicing at the *tra* and *dsx* genes and male sexual differentiation, and allows the translation of *msl-2* transcripts so that dosage compensation can occur.

    d. Gain-of-function mutations at *Sxl* will result in XY animals having an active SXL protein. The SXL protein binds to *msl-2* transcripts to prevent their translation, so dosage compensation will not occur. Therefore, these males will have their single X chromosome transcribed only half as much as normal males or normal females and have an imbalance in gene function that is lethal. Loss-of-function mutations at *Sxl* will not affect males because no SXL protein is made in normal males.

19.22   *Answer:* Preexisting, maternally packaged mRNAs that have been stored in the oocyte are recruited into polysomes as development begins following fertilization.

19.23 *Answer:* An *imaginal disc* is a larval structure in *Drosophila* and other insects that undergo a metamorphic transformation from a larva to an adult. During metamorphosis in the pupal period, it will differentiate into an adult structure. It is essentially a sac of cells, a disc, that is set aside early in embryonic development. The disc increases in cell number by mitosis, but remains undifferentiated during larval growth. Although the disc remains undifferentiated up until the time hormonal signals activate the differentiation of adult structures during the pupal period, its fate is *determined* very early in development. Thus, separate imaginal discs are destined to differentiate into different adult structures, such as legs, eyes, antennae, and wings.

Homeotic mutants alter the identity of particular segments, transforming them into copies of other segments. Homeotic mutations thus affect the determination, or fate, of a disc. Mutations in the *Antennapedia* gene complex can, for example, transform the fate of cells of the antenna disc so that a leg is formed where an antenna should be. The general inference from such observations is that homeotic genes normally play a pivotal role in establishing the segmental identity of an undifferentiated cell.

19.24 *Answer:*

a. The *yobo* gene is a maternal effect gene since all offspring of homozygous, but not heterozygous, *yobo* females have delayed development and abnormal body plans, even if they have a *yobo*$^+$ allele contributed by their father. Offspring of *yobo/yobo* mothers are missing a maternally deposited gene product required for normal embryonic development.

b. Since it is a maternal effect gene, the *yobo*$^+$ gene must be transcribed during oogenesis and its mRNA or protein product must be deposited into the developing oocyte prior to fertilization.

c. The *yobo* gene product is used after fertilization during embryonic development. The *yobo/yobo* offspring of *yobo*$^+$/*yobo* females mated to *yobo/yobo* or *yobo*$^+$/*yobo* males are normal because *yobo*$^+$/*yobo* females have the capacity to deposit some *yobo*$^+$ gene product into the developing embryo. The *yobo* maternal effect phenotypes of slow development and abnormal head and tail morphology suggest that *yobo*$^+$ normally functions to regulate the rate of development and patterning in the head and tail regions. This might be achieved by the *yobo*$^+$ gene product functioning directly in the anterior and posterior regions of the developing embryo during a period critical for the development of head and tail structures. Alternatively, given its more general effects on the rate of development, *yobo* might function more widely and indirectly impact the development of these structures.

19.25 *Answer:*

a. The *bicoid* mRNA is localized to the anterior pole of the egg cytoplasm by other anterior maternal effect genes. When translated, its protein product diffuses to form an anterior-to-posterior gradient—the highest concentration of Bicoid is at the anterior end of the egg, and little to no Bicoid protein is in the posterior third of the egg. In contrast, the *nanos* mRNA is localized to the posterior pole of the egg cytoplasm by a group of posterior maternal effect genes and, when translated, the Nanos protein forms a high-posterior-to-low-anterior gradient.

The Bicoid protein functions as a transcription factor, activating and repressing genes along the anterior–posterior axis of the embryo, and as a translational repressor, blocking translation of the evenly distributed *caudal* mRNA. Thus, production of the Bicoid protein leads to a high-posterior-to-low-anterior gradient of Caudal protein. The Nanos protein also functions to repress translation, specifically translation of *hunchback* mRNAs. Since Nanos is distributed in a high-posterior-to-low-anterior gradient, Hunchback protein will be distributed in a high-anterior-to-low-posterior gradient.

b. One of the functions of the Bicoid protein is to block the translation of the *caudal* mRNA. In loss-of-function *bicoid* mutations, *caudal* mRNA would be translated uniformly throughout the embryo. Since the Caudal protein functions later in the segmentation phase of development to activate genes needed for the formation of posterior structures, one might expect that this would lead to the formation of posterior structures at both ends of the embryo, not just the posterior end. Indeed, this is the phenotype seen in *bicoid* mutants.

c. In loss-of-function *nanos* mutations, the evenly distributed *hunchback* mRNAs will be translated so that Hunchback protein is uniformly distributed in the egg. Hunchback is important for defining segments within the developing embryo. Therefore, if Hunchback is uniformly distributed, segments will not be properly defined. This is one aspect of loss-of-function *nanos* mutations, which have a no-abdomen phenotype.

   d.   The morphogenetic gradients established by *bicoid* and *nanos* direct the formation of gradients of Caudal and Hunchback proteins and, more generally, set the stage for the formation of anterior and posterior structures through the direct or indirect activation or repression of segmentation genes—genes that determine segments and have specific roles in specifying regions of the embryo.

19.26   *Answer:*

   a.   As the *polarity* of an individual, differentiated structure is altered, *a* is likely to be a segmentation gene. In particular, it is likely to be a member of the subclass of segmentation genes known as segment polarity genes.

   b.   The abnormal appearance of progeny of homozygous mothers, but not homozygous fathers, suggests that homozygous mothers produce abnormal oocytes. This view is bolstered by the phenotype of the abnormal progeny. Progeny with defect(s) at one end could arise if a maternally produced gradient in the oocyte was abnormal. Thus, *b* is likely to be a maternal effect gene.

   c.   The absence of a set of segments is characteristic of the phenotypes of gap gene mutants, a subclass of segmentation gene mutants.

   d.   It would appear that the fate of the eye disc has been changed to that of a wing disc. The segmental *identity* of cells is controlled by homeotic genes, and so *d* is likely to be a homeotic mutation.

   e.   In mutant *e,* a set of segments is missing (T2 and T3). Thus, like *c, e* is likely to be a mutant in a gap gene, a subclass of segmentation gene mutants.

19.27   *Answer:* Homeotic gene complexes are found in all major animal phyla except for sponges and coelenterates. They share a similar, clustered gene organization and have highly conserved homeobox sequences. The most compelling evidence that the homeotic genes specify the vertebrate body plan is provided by data on their patterns of gene expression during vertebrate development, an analysis of the effects of mutations, and embryological analyses. See also text Figure 19.29, p. 571.

19.28   *Answer:* The primary signal that leads to the differential expression of the 534 genes is a pulse of the steroid hormone ecdysone during the late larval period. It does not act directly to control transcription at each of the 534 genes, but rather triggers a regulatory cascade that leads to their differential expression. Ecdysone binds to a receptor protein, and this complex binds to both early-puffing genes and late-puffing genes. The complex turns on the early genes, some of which encode DNA-binding proteins that could serve as regulatory genes, and represses the late genes. As one of the early gene's products accumulates, it displaces the ecdysone–receptor complex from both early and late genes. This turns off the early genes and derepresses the late genes. In this manner, the ecdysone signal triggers a cascade of gene activation and repression that leads to the widespread differential gene expression associated with the metamorphosis of the larval worm into an adult fly.

19.29   *Answer:*

   a.   Regulatory noncoding RNAs have been found at the *bithorax* complex, whose genes function to determine the identity of the fly's posterior segments. The noncoding RNAs appear to silence *Ubx,* one of the genes within the *bithorax* complex, in early embryos as part of an RNA interference system to ensure correct developmental timing of its expression.

   b.   A complex of a miRNA and several proteins (including Ago1) silences gene expression by binding to the 3′ untranslated region (UTR) of one or more target mRNAs. Base pairing between the miRNA and the mRNA leads to either translation inhibition or mRNA degradation.

c. The primary evidence that miRNA-mediated gene silencing is essential for normal development in invertebrates and vertebrates comes from the analysis of loss-of-function mutations in individual miRNAs and genes for key proteins involved in miRNA-mediated gene silencing, such as Dicer and Argonaute. These analyses have revealed that miRNAs regulate many aspects of somatic cell and germ-line development in both invertebrates and vertebrates. Evidence that miRNA function plays an essential role in vertebrate development comes from the finding that Dicer knockouts display early developmental arrest and lethality in both mice and zebrafish.

19.30   *Answer:*

a. In *C. elegans*, stem cells undergo a pattern of regulated cell division that is synchronized with the four larval molts of the animal and then differentiate in the adult stage. In *lin-14* mutants, the stem cells keep repeating the cell division pattern characteristic of the first larval stage. In *lin-14* loss-of-function mutations, stem cells differentiate earlier than normal. Because of these phenotypes, the *lin-14* gene can be classified as a heterochronic gene, a gene involved in developmental timing. The phenotype of loss-of-function *ZIP* mutations also suggests that *ZIP* is a heterochronic gene. Loss-of-function mutations cause the premature expression of adult traits even though they do not accelerate the onset of reproductive competence of flowering time.

b. The *ZIP* gene encodes an Argonaute-like protein. Members of the Argonaute protein family are important for miRNA transcript processing (see text Chapter 18, pp. 537–539). Ago1, an RNA endonuclease also called Slicer, is a member of this family that functions within the pre-microRNA-induced silencing complex. It makes a single cut within the miRNA* passenger strand that leads to the production of the mature miRISC, the ribonucleoprotein complex that can silence gene expression. Considering this and the phenotype of loss-of-function *ZIP* mutants, one testable hypothesis is that the *ZIP* gene functions as component of a miRNA pathway that controls a pattern of gene expression important for the onset of adult traits. Since loss-of-function *ZIP* mutations cause premature expression of adult traits, *ZIP* could function in processing miRNAs that regulate the translation of transcripts whose proteins function in the onset of adult traits. To test this hypothesis, assess the pattern of processed miRNAs present in wild-type and *ZIP* plants and relate this pattern to the onset of adult traits in each type of plant. The hypothesis predicts that the pattern of miRNAs present in wild-type plants expressing adult traits should overlap with that seen in *ZIP* mutants when *ZIP* mutants exhibit adult traits at an earlier developmental stage.

19.31   *Answer:* Preexisting mRNA that was made by the mother and packaged into the oocyte prior to fertilization is translated up to the gastrula stage. After gastrulation, new mRNA synthesis is necessary for the production of proteins needed for subsequent embryonic development.

20

Genetics of Cancer

Chapter Outline

Review of Key Terms, Symbols, and Concepts

In your own words, write a brief, precise definition of each term in the groups below. Check your definitions using the text. Then develop a concept map using the terms in each list.

1	2	3
tumor	tumor virus	multistep nature of cancer
neoplasm	oncogene	cell cycle
transformation	DNA vs. RNA tumor virus	pRB, E2F
monolayer	sarcoma	G_0 phase
contact inhibition	retrovirus	cyclin, cyclin-dependent kinase
benign	RSV, HIV-1	cyclin Cdk complex
malignant	*gag, pol, env, src* genes	phosphorylation
cancer	nononcogenic, oncogenic	p53, *TP53*, Mdm2, *ARF*
metastasis	retrovirus	p21, *WAF1*
oncogenesis	insertional mutagenesis	*BAX*, BCL-2
terminally differentiated cell	AIDS	miR-372, *LATS2, let-7*
stem cell	cytolytic virus	G_1-to-S, G_2-to-M, M
self-renewal	transducing retrovirus	checkpoints
germ-line cell	nontransducing retrovirus	*START*
somatic cell	replication-competent	BRCA1, BRCA2
growth factor	transformation-competent	apoptosis
growth-inhibiting factor	viral oncogene, v-*onc*	cell cycle arrest
signal transduction	proto-oncogene	mutator gene
cell cycle	cellular oncogene, c-*onc*	tumor suppressor
dedifferentiation	growth factor	oncogene
two-hit model	protein kinase	mismatch repair
familial cancer	membrane-associated G-protein	HNPCC, hereditary FAP
sporadic cancer	proviral DNA	*hMSH2, hMLH1, hPMS1,*
tumor suppressor gene	tumor suppressor gene	*hPMS2, mutS, mutL* genes
oncogene, proto-oncogene	signaling cascade	telomerase
mutator gene	gene amplification	replicative senescence
microRNA gene		carcinogen
multistep nature of cancer		direct-acting carcinogen
sporadic vs. hereditary		ultimate carcinogen
retinoblastoma		procarcinogen
loss of heterozygosity		UVA, UVB
unilateral, bilateral tumor		ionizing, nonionizing
		radiation

Thinking Analytically

Although cancer genetics is complex, focusing on two key issues should help put the topics of this chapter in perspective. Since cancer results from unconstrained cellular growth, the first key issue is to understand how each of the processes discussed in this chapter affects cellular growth. It will be helpful to review how cells proceed through a cell cycle. As you read the text, pay particular attention to how progression through the cell cycle is controlled. Notice how mutations in oncogenes and tumor suppressor genes, both of which impact the cell cycle, can result in cancer through different mechanisms.

A second key issue is that cancer typically occurs in somatic cells, and so it is important to consider the effect of accumulating mutations in somatic cells and not only germ-line cells. To understand the relationship between hereditary and sporadic forms of cancer, it will help to review the relationship between somatic and germ-line cells. To understand how mutations accumulate in cancerous cells, it is necessary to consider the role of DNA repair within the cell cycle, the consequences of errors in DNA repair, and the effects of carcinogens and ionizing radiation.

Questions for Practice

Multiple-Choice Questions

1. About what percentage of breast cancer is hereditary?
   a. 1%
   b. 5%
   c. 10%
   d. 50%

2. Familial retinoblastoma appears to be inherited as a dominant trait. What accounts for this?
   a. A dominant mutation is transmitted through the germ line.
   b. Somatic mutation occurs after a recessive mutation is transmitted through the germ line.
   c. Heterozygous individuals are infected with a retrovirus.
   d. About half of the homozygous, normal individuals in an affected family are infected with a retrovirus at birth.

3. RNA tumor viruses cause cancer
   a. by the same mechanism as DNA tumor viruses.
   b. only if their proviral DNA integrates near a proto-oncogene.
   c. if they carry an oncogene.
   d. if they infect germ-line cells.

4. Which of the following is *not* a feature of a viral oncogene?
   a. It lacks introns.
   b. Its expression is regulated identically to the corresponding cellular proto-oncogene.
   c. Its structure and location in the viral genome varies.
   d. It is not conserved between viral strains.

5. Which of the following statements is *not* true of the product of the *TP53* gene?
   a. It is a transcription factor.
   b. It is a tumor suppressor.
   c. It can induce cell death.
   d. When present, it activates the cell cycle from G_1 to S.

6. What is the cellular function of the unphosphorylated product of the *RB* gene, pRB?
   a. It binds to transcription factors E2F to maintain cells in G_1 or G_0.
   b. It binds to p53 to stimulate apoptosis.
   c. It is a growth factor, stimulating cellular proliferation.
   d. It is involved in DNA mismatch repair.

7. Which type of protein phosphorylates the product of the *RB* gene, pRB?
   a. a receptor kinase
   b. a phosphorylase
   c. a cyclin/cyclin-dependent kinase
   d. p53

8. What is the relationship between a proto-oncogene and its corresponding viral oncogene?
   a. Only the viral oncogene contains introns.
   b. If the viral oncogene encodes a transcription factor, the corresponding proto-oncogene will encode a growth factor.
   c. The proto-oncogene encodes a product essential to the normal development and function of the organism. The viral oncogene encodes an altered product that has aberrant function.
   d. Usually, the proto-oncogene product is produced in greater amounts. The viral oncogene, being under the control of the retroviral promoter, enhancer, and poly(A) signals, produces smaller amounts of a product.

9. What is apoptosis?
   a. the process by which cancerous cells extend cellular processes in an amoeba-like manner
   b. the process of uncontrollable cellular growth caused by overexpression of an oncogene
   c. cell death that results from the multiple mutations that accumulate in a cancerous cell
   d. the process of programmed cell death

10. A genetic predisposition to hereditary nonpolyposis colon cancer (HNPCC) can result from mutations in any of the four genes *hMSH2, hMLH1, hPMS1,* and *hPMS2.* All of these genes are homologous to *E. coli* and yeast genes known to be involved in DNA repair. From this information, one might speculate that HNPCC is caused by a mutation
    a. in a mutator gene.
    b. in an oncogene.
    c. in a proto-oncogene.
    d. in a tumor suppressor gene.

Answers: 1b, 2b, 3c, 4b, 5d, 6a, 7c, 8c, 9d, 10a

Thought Questions

1. What is the relationship of the cell cycle to cancer?

2. What is the two-hit mutation model for cancer? How is it related to the multistep nature of cancer?

3. In all retroviral RNA genomes, specific sequences are found at the left (R and U_5) and right (R and U_3) ends. In proviral DNA, long terminal repeats (LTRs) are found at each end. How are the LTRs produced?

4. What is meant by a nononcogenic retrovirus? Can infection by a nononcogenic retrovirus lead to increased susceptibility to cancer? Give an example.

5. Distinguish between a viral oncogene, a cellular oncogene, and a proto-oncogene. Are each of these always associated with a transducing retrovirus?

6. There are at least six functional classes of oncogene products. What are these functional classes? How can alteration in such diverse functions lead to a similar oncogenic phenotype?

7. Does the HIV virus itself have viral oncogenes? Why are individuals infected with HIV more susceptible to cancer and infection?

8. What information would you want to know about the UV lights used in tanning salons? Do you think they can be safe?

9. In what ways is programmed cell death a normal process?

10. What is the most lethal common carcinogen you know of?

11. Cancers are staged according to how far they have progressed toward matastasis. This is illustrated in text Figure 20.11, p. 596, for the development of hereditary adenomatous polyposis, a colorectal cancer. What genetic changes are associated with the staged progression of tumors? Is there a specific order of changes that *always* occurs? Once a tumor has progressed to a certain stage, can it revert to an earlier stage?

Thought Questions for Media

After reviewing the media on the *iGenetics* website, try to answer these questions.

1. How do growth-stimulating factors and growth-inhibiting factors differ, if at all, in terms of being able to
   a. turn on pathways?
   b. bind to specific cell membrane receptors?
   c. transduce signals to the nucleus?
   d. trigger the expression of one or more genes for one or more proteins that stimulate cell division?

2. Many growth-stimulating and growth-inhibiting factors have been identified. Is it the presence or absence of specific factors, the sheer number of stimulating or inhibiting factors, or the balance between factors that determines whether a normal, healthy cell in the G_1 phase of the cell cycle is triggered to proceed into the S, G, and M phases?

3. After DNA damage occurs, how are the levels of p53 protein altered?

4. What is the immediate consequence of altering the level of p53 protein?

5. Why do normal cells undergo apoptosis after extensive DNA damage? Why don't cells with mutations in each of their *TP53* genes undergo apoptosis?

6. How is a cyclin–Cdk complex involved in controlling the ability of a cell to proceed from G_1 into S phase? What is the role of the p21 protein in regulating this process?

7. Why are cells that proceed into S phase with unrepaired DNA damage more likely to become cancerous?

8. The animation illustrated how the p53 protein, following DNA damage, triggers a cellular pathway with inhibitory and stimulatory events.
   a. Which cellular events are inhibited by p53?
   b. Which cellular events are stimulated by p53?
   c. How are these inhibitory and stimulatory events connected?

Solutions to Text Questions and Problems

20.1   *Answer:*

    a. The cell cycle is regulated at cell cycle checkpoints that occur between G_1 and S (the START checkpoint in yeast), between G_2 and M, and during M just before the separation of chromatids.

    b. The cyclins and cyclin-dependent kinases (Cdks) regulate progression through the cell cycle. The levels of the cyclins oscillate in a regular pattern through the cell cycle. At each checkpoint, a cyclin binds to a Cdk to form a complex. When the cell is ready to pass the checkpoint, the complex is activated. For example, at the G_2-M checkpoint, the cyclin–Cdk complex is activated by dephosphorylation of the Cdk. The activated Cdk then phosphorylates other cell cycle control proteins to affect their function, thereby leading to the cell's transition into the next phase of the cell cycle.

20.2   *Answer:* HIV-1 is a retrovirus that infects and then kills cells of the immune system. This leads to a disabling of the immune response and an increase in susceptibility to certain types of cancer. In contrast to the mechanism by which cancer occurs following infection with HIV-1, an oncogenic retrovirus transforms the growth properties of infected cells to neoplastic growth.

20.3   *Answer:* Retroviruses are viruses that have two copies of an RNA genome within a protein core surrounded by a membranous envelope. Transducing retroviruses carry an oncogene from a host cell, while nontransducing retroviruses do not. Consequently, transducing retroviruses may be capable of transforming cells to a cancerous state.

20.4   *Answer:* Cellular proto-oncogenes have important roles in regulating normal cellular processes such as cell division and differentiation. Viral oncogenes are mutated, abnormally expressed forms of proto-oncogenes that cause neoplastic growth. Viral oncogenes lack introns and, as shown in text Table 20.1, p. 585, are often fused to viral genes.

20.5   *Answer:* If FeSV contributed to the feline sarcoma, FeSV should be found in the neoplastic tissues (muscle and bone marrow). The Southern blot provides this evidence: A 1.2-kb DNA fragment hybridizes to the *fes* cDNA probe in the lanes with DNA from muscle and bone marrow, and in the control lane with FeSV cDNA. The size difference between the 1.2-kb hybridizing fragment and the 1.0-kb *fes* proto-oncogene *Hind*III-cut cDNA probe reflects their different origins. The *fes* proto-oncogene is found normally in a cat, while the FeSV *fes* oncogene is found in a retrovirus. The size of the fragment in the retrovirus may reflect a polymorphic *Hind*III site and/or a gene rearrangement. The *fes* proto-oncogene normally functions in the cat, so its DNA should be present in all tissues. The 3.4-kb DNA fragment is found in all of the cat tissues, so is likely to be the genomic sequence. Since the *fes* proto-oncogene cDNA has a 1.0-kb *Hind*III fragment, the mRNA of this gene is very likely spliced to remove a 2.4-kb intron.

20.6   *Answer:* The high degree of conservation of proto-oncogenes suggests that they function in normal, essential, conserved cellular processes. Given the relationship between oncogenes and proto-oncogenes, it also suggests that cancer occurs when these processes are not correctly regulated.

20.7   *Answer:*

    a. Proto-oncogenes encode a diverse set of gene products that include growth factors, receptor and nonreceptor protein kinases, receptors lacking protein kinase activity, membrane-associated GTP-binding proteins, cytoplasmic regulators involved in intracellular signaling, and nuclear transcription factors. These gene products all function in intercellular and intracellular pathways that regulate cell division and differentiation.

    b. In general, mutations that activate a proto-oncogene convert it into an oncogene. Since (i), (iii), and (viii) cause a decrease in gene expression, they are unlikely to result in an oncogene. Since (ii) and (vii) could activate gene expression, they could result in an oncogene. Mutations (iv), (v), and (vi) cannot be predicted with certainty. The deletion of a 3' splice site acceptor would alter the mature mRNA and possibly the protein produced and may or may not affect the protein's function and regulation. Similarly, it is difficult to predict the effect of a nonspecific point mutation or a premature stop codon. The text presents examples where these types of mutations have caused the activation of a proto-oncogene and resulted in an oncogene.

20.8 *Answer:*

a. Increased transcription of the mRNA will lead to increased levels of the growth factor, which in turn will stimulate fibroblast growth and division.

b. Constitutive activation of a nonreceptor tyrosine kinase could lead to abberant, unregulated phosphorylation and activation of many different proteins, including growth factor receptors, that are involved in signaling cascades used in regulating cellular growth and differentiation.

c. When the growth factor EGF binds its membrane-bound receptor, it stimulates its autophosphorylation, which allows Grb2 to bind and recruit SOS. SOS displaces GDP from Ras, a membrane-associated G protein, so that it can bind GTP. This allows Ras to recruit and activate Raf-1 to initiate the cytoplasmic MAP kinase signaling cascade. In turn, this activates transcription factors such as Elk-1 to induce transcription of cell cycle-specific target genes. Therefore, if a membrane-associated G protein were unable to hydrolyze GTP, it would be constitutively active and lead to constant expression of genes needed for cell cycle progression.

20.9 *Answer:* One such pathway is illustrated in text Figure 20.6, p. 587. As shown in this figure, the binding of EGF to its surface-membrane-bound receptor stimulates a signaling cascade that leads to transcriptional activation of cell cycle-specific target genes. First, EGF binding stimulates autophosphorylation of the receptor, which allows binding of GRB2. In turn, GRB2 binding recuits SOS to the plasma membrane, which displaces GDP from Ras. This allows Ras to bind GTP, which recruits and activates Raf-1. The activated Raf-1 stimulates the MAP-kinase cascade—a cascade of cytoplasm-based protein phosphorylations—to produce phosphorylated ERK. Phosphorylated ERK moves from the cytoplasm into the nucleus where it activates, through phosphorylation, several transcription factors, including Elk-1. The activated transcription factors then turn on the transcription of defined sets of cell cycle-specific target genes.

Mutations that lead to the constitutive or aberrant activation of the signaling pathway result in oncogenes. Three specific examples are mutations that activate EGF-receptor autophosphorylation in the absence of EGF binding, mutations that abolish the ability of Ras to hydrolyze GTP to GDP, and mutations that lead to the constitutive activation of Elk-1. All of these mutations are oncogenic, because they lead to the constitutive transcriptional activation of cell cycle-specific target genes.

20.10 *Answer:* A proto-oncogene can be changed into an oncogene if there is an increase in the activity of its gene product or an increase in gene expression that leads to an increased amount of gene product. This can result from point mutation, deletion, or gene amplification.

20.11 *Answer:* One mechanism by which a transducing retrovirus causes cancer is for the viral oncogene it carries to be expressed under the control of retroviral promoters. A second mechanism involves insertional mutagenesis that results when the proviral DNA of a retrovirus integrates near a proto-oncogene. In this event, the expression of the proto-oncogene can be controlled by the promoter and enhancer sequences in the retroviral LTR. Because these sequences do not respond to the environmental signals that normally regulate proto-oncogene expression, overexpression of the proto-oncogene is induced.

20.12 *Answer:* One hypothesis is that the proviral DNA has integrated near the proto-oncogene, and the expression of the proto-oncogene has come under the control of promoter and enhancer sequences in the retroviral LTR. This could be assessed by performing a whole-genome Southern blot analysis to determine whether the organization of the genomic DNA sequences near the proto-oncogene has been altered.

20.13 *Answer:* Tumor growth induced by transforming retroviruses results either from the activity of a single viral oncogene or from the activation of a proto-oncogene caused by the nearby integration of the proviral DNA. The oncogene can cause abnormal cellular proliferation via the variety of mechanisms discussed in the text. The expression of a proto-oncogene, normally tightly regulated during cell growth and development, can be altered if it comes under the control of the promoter and enhancer sequences in the retroviral LTR.

DNA tumor viruses do not carry oncogenes. They transform cells through the action of one or more genes within their genomes. For example, in a rare event, the DNA virus can be integrated into the host genome, and the DNA replication of the host cell may be stimulated by a viral protein that activates viral DNA replication. This would cause the cell to move from the G_0 to the S phase of the cell cycle.

For both transducing retroviruses and DNA tumor viruses, abnormally expressed proteins lead to the activation of the cell from G_0 to S and abnormal cell growth.

20.14 *Answer:* Experimentally fuse cells from the two cell lines and then test the resultant hybrids for their ability to form tumors. If the uncontrolled growth of the tumor cell line was caused by a mutated pair of tumor suppressor alleles, the normal alleles present in the normal cell line would "rescue" the tumor cell line defect. The hybrid line would grow normally and be unable to form a tumor. If the uncontrolled growth of the tumor cell line was caused by an oncogene, the oncogene would also be present in the hybrid cell line. The hybrid line would grow uncontrollably and form a tumor.

20.15 *Answer:* Hereditary cancer is associated with the inheritance of a germ-line mutation; sporadic cancer is not. Consequently, hereditary cancer runs in families. For some cancers, both hereditary and sporadic forms exist, with the hereditary form being much less frequent. For example, retinoblastoma occurs when both normal alleles of the tumor suppressor gene *RB* are inactivated. In hereditary retinoblastoma, a mutated, inactive allele is transmitted via the germ line. Retinoblastoma occurs in cells of an *RB/+* heterozygote when an additional somatic mutation occurs. In the sporadic form of the disease, retinoblastoma occurs when both alleles are inactivated somatically.

20.16 *Answer:* Mutations in tumor suppressor genes such as *RB* and *TP53* are recessive because the cancer develops only if both alleles are mutant. The presence of one normal allele in a heterozygote serves to suppress tumor formation, so the normal allele is dominant. The disorder appears dominant in pedigrees because in an individual who has inherited a single mutation—an individual who has inherited a mutant allele from one parent and a normal allele from the other parent— there is a high likelihood that the remaining wild-type allele will be inactivated by mutation. That is, the inheritance of the single gene mutation predisposes a person to the cancer but does not cause it directly.

20.17 *Answer:* A second mutational hit at the *RB* locus—a somatic mutation that specifically deleted the *RB* gene—would result in a loss of heterozygosity and produce a cell that is *rb/rb* (see text Figure 20.8, p. 591). Chromosome nondisjunction during mitosis (this is similar in mechanism to nondisjunction during meiosis II, illustrated in Figure 12.18, p. 344) could also produce a cell with two identical alleles. A third mechanism that would lead to the loss of a normal *RB* allele in a cell and its daughters is mitotic recombination. Following chromosome replication in a *RB/rb* somatic cell, a rare nonsister–chromatid exchange can produce an *rb/rb* daughter cell. The following figure shows a mitotic division (in which the daughter cells normally receive one grey and one white centromere) in which such an exchange has occurred.

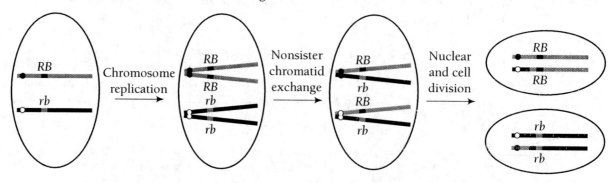

20.18 *Answer:*

a. Studies of hereditary forms of cancer have led to insights into the fundamental cellular processes affected by cancer. For example, substantial insights into the important role of DNA repair and the relationship between the control of the cell cycle and DNA repair have come from analyses of the genes responsible for hereditary forms of human colorectal cancer. For breast cancer, studying the normal functions of the *BRCA1* and *BRCA2* genes promises to provide substantial insights into breast and ovarian cancer.

b. A *genetic predisposition* to cancer refers to the presence of an inherited mutation that, with additional somatic mutations during the individual's life span, can lead to cancer. For diseases such as retinoblastoma, a genetic predisposition has been associated with the inheritance of a recessive allele of the *RB* tumor suppressor gene. Retinoblastoma occurs in *RB/rb* individuals when the normal allele is mutated in somatic cells and the pRB protein no longer functions. Because somatic mutation is likely, the disease appears dominant in pedigrees. Although there is a substantial understanding of the genetic basis for cancer and the genetic abnormalities present in somatic cancerous cells, there are also substantial environmental risk factors for specific cancers. Environmental risk factors must be investigated thoroughly when a pedigree is evaluated for a genetic predisposition for cancer.

c. Multiple genetic changes occur during the formation of a tumor cell. In an individual with an inherited predisposition to a particular cancer, a genetic difference that contributes to the formation of a tumor cell may have been inherited from just one parent. If that genetic difference, together with additional genetic changes that may be influenced by the environment, contributes to the appearance of a cancer, the inheritance of that single genetic change has predisposed that individual to cancer. Since the genetic change that predisposes the individual to cancer is inherited in one copy from just one parent, the trait is dominant. However, the additional genetic changes required to produce a cancer may not always occur, and so not every individual with the inherited genetic change will develop cancer. Consequently, the trait shows reduced penetrance. For the trait to be considered recessive, an individual must have two recessive alleles, one inherited from each parent.

20.19 *Answer:* Tissues are produced during organismal development through regulated cell proliferation. Proto-oncogenes normally function in this process by positively controlling cell growth and division. Once cells become highly differentiated and are fully functional in a tissue, they typically no longer divide, and proto-oncogenes are no longer active. A mutation causing the constitutive activation of an oncogene is a gain-of-function mutation. It would lead to unregulated cell proliferation and the failure of cells to undergo terminal differentiation. It is likely that such a mutation in a heterozygous state would lead to lethality during development, so it would be a dominant embryonic lethal mutation and would not be inherited. This is in contrast to recessive loss-of-function mutations at tumor suppressor genes, where the one normal gene copy in a heterozygote can function to suppress uncontrolled cell proliferation and allow for a normal phenotype (unless the normal copy is spontaneously mutated later in development; see Question 20.16).

20.20 *Answer:* When unphosphorylated, pRB inhibits cell cycle progression by binding to a complex of the transcription factors E2F. This ensures that the cell remains in G_1 or in the quiescent G_0 state until it is ready to proceed to S. When progression into S phase is signaled, pRB is phosphorylated by a cyclin–Cdk complex. This prevents it from binding to E2F, which in turn allows E2F to activate transcription at genes needed for cell cycle progression. After S phase, pRB is dephosphorylated.

a. If pRB were constitutively phosphorylated, it would never bind to E2F, there would be no inhibition of cell cycle progression at G_1/S, and neoplastic growth would occur.

b. If pRB was never phosphorylated, cells would be stalled in the G_0 phase (and presumably eventually undergo apoptosis).

c. If a truncated protein were produced, it would be unable to bind to E2F and (regardless of its phosphorylation state) would be unable to inhibit cell cycle progression. Just as in **(a)**, this would result in neoplastic growth.

d. Higher levels of normal pRB could result in a longer cell cycle. If more pRB were present in the cell, more unphosphorylated pRB would be available to bind to E2F during G_1. In this event, if an unphosphorylated pRB molecule that was bound to a particular E2F molecule were phosphorylated by a cyclin–Cdk complex and the E2F molecule were released, another unphosphorylated pRB molecule present in the cell could bind to the same E2F molecule. This would prevent this particular E2F molecule from participating in activating the gene expression needed for progression into S phase. Only when enough pRB molecules are phosphorylated will a sufficient number of E2F molecules be released to provide for transcriptional activation. Since the number of pRB molecules is increased relative to the number of cyclin–Cdk complexes, it will take longer for the cyclin–Cdk complexes to phosphorylate enough pRB molecules to effect transcriptional activation. If pRB levels are so high that the cyclin–Cdk complex is unable to phosphorylate enough of the pRB molecules present, cells could be stalled in the G_0 phase, just as in **(b)**.

e. Lower levels of normal pRB might result in a shorter cell cycle.

20.21 *Answer:*

a. The *TP53* gene produces the transcription factor p53. p53 has cellular roles in the repair of DNA damage, in protecting the cell against oncogenes, and in programmed cell death (apoptosis). The p53 protein is regulated by phosphorylation and by interactions with another phosphoprotein, Mdm2. In a normal cell, neither protein is phosphorylated and they are able to bind together. Mdm2 stimulates degradation of p53 so that the amount of p53 is kept low in normal cells.

When DNA damage occurs, p53 initiates a cascade of events leading to cellular arrest in G_1. DNA damage results in the phosphorylation of both p53 and Mdm2 on the domains where they normally interact. The phosphorylation prevents their interaction and p53 degradation, so that p53 accumulates. p53 then activates transcription of DNA repair genes and of *WAF1*, which encodes p21. The p21 protein binds to the G_1-to-S checkpoint Cdk4–cyclin D complexes and inhibits their activity. This results in the failure of pRB phosphorylation, the inhibition of E2F, and cell arrest in G_1.

When viral or cellular oncogenes such as *ras* are expressed, the expression of the *ARF* gene is induced. Its product, p14, binds to Mdm2 in the p53–Mdm2 complex and blocks Mdm2's stimulation of p53 degradation. This leads to the activation of gene transcription by p53 to provide protection against oncogenes.

During apoptosis, p53 does not induce DNA repair genes or *WAF1*, but activates the *BAX* gene. The BAX protein blocks the function of the BCL-2 protein, which is a repressor of the apoptosis pathway. Without the BCL-2 repressor, the apoptotic pathway is activated and the cell commits suicide.

Alterations in p53 function can lead to cancer in three ways: failure to hold cells in G_0/G_1 arrest, failure to allow DNA repair prior to S (thus allowing mutations to be transmitted to the next generation), or failure to induce apoptosis appropriately—when cells have high levels of DNA damage.

b. Li–Fraumeni syndrome results from the inheritance of one mutant copy of *TP53*. This rare cancer develops when the second copy of *TP53* becomes mutated in somatic cells. In contrast to this rare form of cancer, many cancers accumulate mutations in both alleles of the *TP53* gene during their progression. That is, mutations in *TP53* do not cause them, but *TP53* mutations are among the several genetic changes that are found in them.

c. Cancerous cells typically have a number of genetic abnormalities, or lesions. The *TP53* mutation may not be the initial genetic abnormality that occurred. Rather, it may have occurred subsequent to a mutation that led to the activation of an oncogene, the introduction of a mutator gene, or the inactivation of alleles at a tumor suppressor gene. Hence, the *TP53* mutation may not be the primary genetic lesion. Most cancers develop as a result of the accumulation of mutations in a number of genes, often over extended periods of time (decades). Such mutations accumulate in part due to the lack of successful DNA repair at the G_1-to-S checkpoint in the cell cycle.

20.22 *Answer:*

a. In a normal cell, neither p53 nor a protein that interacts with it, Mdm2, is phosphorylated. They bind together and Mdm2 stimulates degradation of p53 so that the amount of p53 is kept low in normal cells. However, when DNA damage occurs, both p53 and Mdm2 are phosphorylated so that their interaction is prevented. This leads to the accumulation of p53.

b. After the phosphorylation of p53 leads to its accumulation, p53 activates transcription of *WAF1*, which encodes p21. The p21 protein binds to the G_1-to-S checkpoint Cdk4–cyclin D complexes and inhibits their activity. Without the activity of the Cdk4–cyclin D complexes, pRB in the pRB–E2F complex does not become phosphorylated, so that E2F remains inhibited. This leads to cell arrest in G_1.

c. Under low levels of DNA damage—levels that can be repaired—phosphorylation of p53 leads to the activation of *WAF1* as described in part **(b)**. When high levels of DNA damage occur, the cell activates a pathway leading to apoptosis. In this pathway, p53 activates the *BAX* gene, whose protein product blocks the function of the BCL-2 protein. The BCL-2 protein normally represses the apoptosis pathway. Without it, the apoptotic pathway is activated.

20.23   *Answer:* MicroRNAs (miRNAs) are short, single-stranded, noncoding RNA regulatory molecules that can silence genes posttranscriptionally by RNA interference (RNAi). Silencing involves the binding of miRNAs to a complementary or near-complementary sequences in the 3′ untranslated regions (UTRs) of target mRNAs. This inhibits the translation of those mRNAs and targets them for storage or degradation. MicroRNAs normally serve regulatory roles in many biological processes, including cell proliferation and differentiation, apoptosis, and tissue and organ development. Since cell transformation and carcinogenesis are associated with abnormal cell proliferation and the loss of the terminally differentiated state, it was exciting to discover that miRNAs play a significant role in cell transformation and carcinogenesis.

Each form of cancer has a distinct miRNA expression pattern that differs from that of the equivalent normal tissue and from that of other types of cancers. In the various cancers in which a specific miRNA shows an altered pattern of expression, the change in expression often is the same, either toward increased or decreased expression. This has allowed miRNAs to be classified as oncogenes or as tumor suppressor genes.

The genes for miRNAs whose expression is increased in cancerous cells are considered to be oncogenes. The normal action of these miRNAs is to control the expression of target mRNAs that are the transcripts of particular tumor suppressor genes and of other genes involved in the negative control of cell differentiation or apoptosis. Overexpression of these miRNA genes silences the target genes, which removes inhibitory signals for cell proliferation.

The genes for miRNAs whose expression is decreased in cancerous cells are considered to be tumor suppressor genes. In a normal cell, these miRNAs help prevent tumor development by blocking translation of mRNAs that control cell differentiation and apoptosis. If these miRNAs are underexpressed, there are insufficient levels of the encoded miRNAs to silence expression of their target genes at the translation level. This leads to diminished control of cell proliferation.

20.24   *Answer:* MicroRNAs function to silence genes posttranscriptionally by RNA interference. The single-stranded short noncoding miRNA sequence is assembled into a miRISC complex, and the miRNA binds complementary or near-complementary sequences in the 3′ untranslated regions (UTRs) of target mRNAs. This inhibits the translation of those mRNAs and targets them for storage or degradation (see text Chapter 18, pp. 537–539). Therefore, it is reasonable to hypothesize that the let-7 miRNA also acts to silence gene expression. The question statement indicates that the introduction of the let-7 miRNA diminishes the frequency of lung tumors induced in mice by the expression of the K-Ras(G12D) oncogene, and the overexpression of the let-7 miRNA causes cell cycle arrest and cell death in mouse lung cancer cells expressing K-Ras(G12D). Increased expression of the let-7 miRNA in these situations will result in increased silencing of genes targeted by the let-7 miRNA. Therefore, the let-7 miRNA appears to function as a tumor suppressor gene.

One molecular hypothesis consistent with these experimental findings is that the let-7 miRNA normally silences *ras*, and that in these experiments, overexpression of the let-7 miRNA serves to inhibit translation of the K-Ras(G12D) oncogene. Test this hypothesis by monitoring the levels of K-Ras(G12D) transcripts and proteins in cultured mouse lung cancer cells expressing K-Ras(G12D) prior to and following the administration of the let-7 miRNA. Use RT-PCR, quantitative real-time PCR, or Northern blotting (see text Chapter 10, pp. 264–265 and p. 267) to evaluate K-Ras(G12D) transcript levels and use antibodies against K-Ras(G12D) to monitor protein levels. If overexpression of let-7 miRNA causes translational inhibition of K-Ras(G12D) mRNAs, you should observe decreased K-Ras(G12D) protein levels after overexpression of the let-7 miRNA. If the let-7 miRNA also targets K-Ras(G12D) transcripts for degradation, you should see decreased levels of K-Ras(G12D) transcripts after overexpression of the let-7 miRNA. These experiments do not let you determine whether the let-7 miRNA targets *ras* [or K-Ras(G12D)] directly or acts indirectly by silencing an intermediate gene that in turn results in silencing of *ras*. To evaluate this possibility, examine the sequences of the let-7 miRNA and the *ras* mRNA to see if the let-7 miRNA is complementary to sequences in the *ras* 3′ UTR. If it is, the K-Ras(G12D) mRNA could be a direct RNAi target of the let-7 miRNA.

20.25   *Answer:*

a.

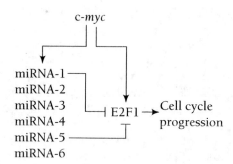

b. E2F1 and c-*myc* are proto-oncogenes, since they normally function to promote cell cycle progression. The two miRNAs (arbitrarily chosen here as miRNA-1 and miRNA-5) that negatively regulate E2F1 are tumor suppressor genes, since they normally function to inhibit cell cycle progression.

c. The two miRNAs could act directly to silence E2F1 expression by base-pairing with sequences in the 3′ untranslated region (UTR) of the E2F1 mRNA to inhibit its translation or target it for storage or degradation. Alternatively, they could act indirectly by silencing another gene whose product functions to regulate E2F1 positively.

d. Different types of cancer, and different stages of a particular kind of cancer, are associated with different patterns of oncogene activation and tumor suppressor gene inactivation. Oncogenes and tumor suppressor genes act within regulatory gene networks. Sets of miRNAs act within these regulatory gene networks both as regulators of gene expression and as the regulatory targets of other genes. Therefore, one hypothesis as to why different cancer types show distinctive patterns of miRNA expression is that the pattern of miRNA expression is dependent on the pattern of oncogene activation and tumor suppressor gene inactivation in a particular type and stage of cancer. If this is correct, the pattern of miRNA expression could serve as a diagnostic indicator of a particular type and stage of cancer. Understanding how the pattern of miRNA expression changes as a cancer progresses could provide insight into the specific changes in gene expression that occur during cancer progression and thereby define new therapeutic targets for halting or reversing the progression of a cancer.

20.26   *Answer:* Apoptosis is programmed, or suicidal, cell death. Cells targeted for apoptosis are those that have high levels of DNA damage and so are at a greater risk for neoplastic transformation. (During the development of some tissues in multicellular organisms, cell death via apoptosis is a normal process.) Apoptosis is regulated by p53, among other proteins. In cells with large amounts of DNA damage, p53 accumulates and functions as a transcription factor to activate transcription of DNA repair genes and *WAF1*, whose product, p21, leads cells to arrest in G_1. If very high levels of DNA damage exist, p53 does not induce DNA repair genes and *WAF1*, but activates the *BAX* gene, whose product blocks the BCL-2 protein from repressing the apoptosis pathway. By blocking BCL-2 function, the apoptosis pathway is activated.

20.27   *Answer:* The products of the normal alleles of mutator genes function in DNA repair processes. In the absence of a functional allele at such a gene, there is a dramatic increase in the accumulation of mutations. Some of these mutations will be at proto-oncogenes and lead to the formation of oncogenes, while others will be loss-of-function mutations at tumor suppressor genes. Therefore, error-prone DNA replication will lead to the formation of cancerous cells. Mutations in mutator genes give a phenotype of hereditary predisposition to cancer because just a single mutational event in a heterozygote will inactivate the remaining functional allele and result in error-prone DNA replication.

20.28 *Answer:*

a. A tumor suppressor gene suppresses uncontrolled cell proliferation that is characteristic of cancer cells, while a mutator gene is any gene that, when mutant, increases the spontaneous mutation frequencies of other genes.

b. Both *BRCA1* and *BRCA2* have been proposed to function in homologous recombination, cellular responses to DNA damage, and mRNA transcription. Their proposed involvement in the repair of DNA damage is consistent with these genes being tumor suppressor genes—*TP53*, a known tumor suppressor gene, is also involved in the repair of DNA damage. Indeed, the patterns of inheritance seen for *BRCA1* and *BRCA2* mutations—patterns similar to that of hereditary retinoblastoma—are like those expected of tumor suppressor genes. However, their proposed involvement in the cellular response to DNA damage and in homologous recombination is also consistent with these genes being mutator genes, since the normal (unmutated) forms of mutator genes are often involved in DNA replication and DNA repair.

20.29 *Answer:* Telomerase activity alone does not lead to cancer—it is normally found in germ-line cells that do not invariably become cancerous. However, the enzyme is reactivated as a secondary event in all major human cancer types. The presence of telomerase enables cancer cells to maintain telomere length. Long telomeres contribute to chromosome stability, which is necessary for cells to proliferate indefinitely. If telomerase were eliminated from cancer cells, the telomeres would shorten and eventually become so short that the complex between telomere sequences and telomere-binding proteins would be disrupted. This would lead to DNA damage that, in normal cells, would trigger apoptosis. However, the apoptotic pathway might not be activated in cancerous cells, especially if they had already lost *TP53* gene function. Nonetheless, cancerous cells without active telomerase are unlikely to be able to divide for many generations because the too-short telomeres create unstable chromosomes.

20.30 *Answer:* Most cancers develop in a stepwise manner. At the point that a cancer reaches a metastatic state, it has accumulated mutations in a number of genes so that the multiple cellular processes that regulate growth and differentiation have been broken down. Multiple and distinct mutational events have occurred at various time points during the development of the cancer to convert proto-oncogenes to oncogenes and to inactivate tumor suppressor genes. This is illustrated for the development of metastatic colorectal cancer in text Figure 20.11, p. 596. Therefore, the metastatic cancer cells that are clonal descendants of a somatic cell are indeed genetically distinct from that somatic cell; they have additional mutations accumulated during the development of the cancer.

20.31 *Answer:* Tumors result from multiple mutational events that typically involve both the activation of oncogenes and the inactivation of tumor suppressor genes. The analysis of hereditary adenomatous polyposis, an inherited form of colorectal cancer, has shown that the more differentiated cells found in benign, early-stage tumors are associated with fewer mutational events, while the less differentiated cells found in malignant and metastatic tumors are associated with more mutational events. Although the path by which mutations accumulate varies between tumors, additional mutations that activate oncogenes and inactivate tumor suppressor genes generally result in dedifferentiation and increased cellular proliferation.

20.32 *Answer:*

a. The fact that some translocations are found as the only cytogenetic abnormality in certain cancers probably means that they are a key event in tumor formation. It does not necessarily mean they are the primary cause of the tumor or the first of many mutational events.

b. A chimeric fusion protein may have different functional properties than either of the two proteins from which it derives. If it results in the activation of a proto-oncogene product into a protein that has oncogenic properties, or if it results in the inactivation of a tumor suppressor gene product, it could play a key role in the genetic cascade of events leading to tumor formation.

c. Before drawing conclusions as to whether these chromosomal aberrations inactivate the function of tumor suppressor genes, or activate quiescent proto-oncogenes, it is necessary to have additional molecular information on the effects of the translocation breakpoints on specific transcripts. Finding that the translocation breakpoints result in a lack of gene transcription or in transcripts that encode nonfunctional products would support the hypothesis that the translocation inactivated a tumor suppressor gene. Finding that the translocation breakpoints result in activation of gene transcription or in the production of an active fusion protein would support the hypothesis that the translocation activated a previously quiescent proto-oncogene.

d. One hypothesis is that the various fusion proteins that result from different translocations involving the *EWS* gene somehow result in the transcription activation of different proto-oncogenes, and this leads to the different sarcomas that are seen. (Sarcomas are cancers found in tissues that include muscle, bone, fat, and blood vessels.)

e. If translocation breakpoints are conserved within a tumor type, molecular-based diagnostics can be developed to identify the breakpoints relatively quickly from a tissue biopsy. For example, if the genes at the breakpoints have been cloned, PCR methods can be used to address whether the gene is intact or disrupted, using the DNA from cells of a tumor biopsy. Primers can be designed to amplify different segments of the normal gene. Then PCR reactions containing these primers and either normal control DNA or tumor cell DNA can be set up to determine if each segment of a candidate gene is intact (a PCR product of the expected size is obtained) or disrupted (no PCR product will be obtained, because the gene has been rearranged).

Such molecular analyses would provide fast, accurate tumor diagnosis. If the different tumor types respond differentially to different regimens of therapeutic intervention, then a more rapid, unequivocal diagnosis of a particular tumor type should allow for the earlier prescription of a more optimized regime of therapeutic intervention. In addition, understanding the nature of the normal gene products of the affected genes may allow for the development of sarcoma-specific therapies.

20.33 *Answer:* To proceed from G_1 into S, one or more G_1 cyclins bind to the cyclin-dependent kinase CDC28/cdc2 and activate it. The cyclin-dependent kinase then phosphorylates key proteins that are needed for progression into S. In the presence of heavy DNA damage, p53 is stabilized. The p53 protein acts as a transcription factor to activate *WAF1*, which produces p21. The p21 protein binds to cyclin–Cdk complexes and blocks the kinase activity required to activate the genes needed for the cell to make the transition through the cell cycle checkpoints, for example, from G_1 to S (see the answer to Question 20.22). Thus, stabilization of p53 leads to cell cycle arrest at the G_1-to-S or other cell cycle checkpoints. This arrest allows the cell time to induce the necessary repair pathways and repair the DNA or, if damage is too severe, to undergo apoptosis.

20.34 *Answer:* Direct-acting carcinogens are chemicals that bind to DNA and act as mutagens. Procarcinogens are chemicals that must be converted by normal cellular enzymes to become active carcinogens. These products, most of which also bind DNA and act as mutagens, are referred to as ultimate carcinogens.

20.35 *Answer:* Sources of radiation include the sun, cellular telephones, radioactive radon gas, electric power lines, X-ray machines, and some household appliances. Radiation can be nonionizing, such as the ultraviolet and infrared light from the sun, or ionizing, such as that from X-rays or radon gas. Radiation increases the amount of DNA damage in cells. If this damage is not repaired or is repaired incorrectly, somatic mutations result. Increasing the amount of DNA damage therefore increases the chance of somatic mutation. Mutations in oncogenes or tumor suppressor genes will contribute to the induction of cancer.

21

Population Genetics

Chapter Outline

Review of Key Terms, Symbols, and Concepts

In your own words, write a brief, precise definition of each term in the groups below. Check your definitions using the text. Then develop a concept map using the terms in each list.

1	2
transmission genetics	Hardy–Weinberg equilibrium
molecular genetics	allele frequency cline
population genetics	classical model
quantitative genetics	neutral theory
neo-Darwinian synthesis	polymorphic locus
Mendelian population	proportion of polymorphic loci (P)
genotype, allele frequency	heterozygosity (H)
genetic structure of a population	observed heterozygosity (Ho)
gene pool	expected heterozygosity (He)
gene counting method	nucleotide substitution
Hardy–Weinberg law	synonymous, nonsynonymous change
infinitely large population	coding, noncoding sequence
migration	RFLP
natural selection	microsatellite, STR
random mating	SNP
mutation	genetic hitchhiking
genetic drift	

3	4
equilibrium frequency	evolution
genetic variance	speciation
binomial distribution	population viability analysis
gene mutation	barriers to gene flow
forward, reverse mutation	postzygotic isolation
effective population size (N_e)	prezygotic isolation
founder, bottleneck effect	hybrid sterility
random genetic drift	hybrid inviability
infinite alleles model	hybrid breakdown
migration	reinforcement
gene flow	temporal isolation
adaptation	ecological isolation
natural, directional, balancing selection	behavioral incompatibility
Darwinian fitness	mechanical isolation
selection coefficient	gametic isolation
pleiotropic effect	Haldane's rule
heterosis	
overdominance	
heterozygote superiority	
positive, negative assortative mating	
inbreeding	
gametic, linkage disequilibrium	

Thinking Analytically

Population genetics considers patterns of genetic variation found among individuals within groups and how these patterns vary geographically and evolve over time. As you study population genetics, your perspective will shift away from a direct consideration of the molecular and biochemical mechanisms that underlie the inheritance and expression of traits in a single individual or cell to a statistical evaluation of the *effects* of these processes at the level of the group, population, or species.

At the conceptual core of population genetics lies the Hardy–Weinberg law. Initially, focus your efforts on understanding its assumptions and predictions. Practice the examples given in the text and the text problems to become fluent in analyzing whether a population with two alleles at an autosomal locus is in Hardy–Weinberg equilibrium. Then consider extensions of the law to loci with more than two alleles or loci with X-linked alleles. Finally, investigate the different ways that the assumptions of the Hardy–Weinberg law may be violated and the consequences of each to the genetic structure of a population.

Be aware that the allelic symbolism used in population genetics is often different from that used in Mendelian or molecular genetics. Consider the following example. In earlier chapters, the genotypes for normal and sickle-cell hemoglobin were written either as $\beta^A\beta^A$, $\beta^A\beta^S$, $\beta^S\beta^S$, or Hb^AHb^A, Hb^AHb^S, Hb^SHb^S. Here they are written as *Hb-A/Hb-A*, *Hb-A/Hb-S*, *Hb-S/Hb-S*. Similarly, care should be taken with the letters p and q, which symbolize the frequency within a population of dominant and recessive members of an allelic pair (but do not symbolize the alleles themselves!).

One of the main concerns of population genetics is how to model changes in allele and genotype frequencies under a set of specified conditions. The models are often very elegant and employ equations that identify relationships between a set of variables identified in a population. Memorization of the equations used to analyze changes in populations is by itself insufficient to understand the models. It will be difficult, if not impossible, to solve even moderately challenging word problems if you can only plug numbers into equations. While you will find it helpful to recognize by sight several of the equations, you need to do more. Take the time to understand the model that leads to the equation and how the mathematical and statistical analyses in the model are related to a biological question.

A few hints for solving some of the problems are in order. First, you will often find that the frequency of one class of homozygote (usually the recessive homozygotes, given by q^2) is the only piece of hard data available. As you work back from this information, keep track of the assumptions that you are making. Otherwise, you may enter into the realm of circular reasoning. For example, you can legitimately calculate q as the square root of q^2 and, if only two alleles exist, calculate p by equating it with $1-q$. However, if you then determine that heterozygotes exist at a frequency of $2pq$, you are assuming that random mating is occurring and the conditions of Hardy–Weinberg equilibrium are satisfied. Further work with your calculated values of p^2, $2pq$, and q^2 will continue to reflect that assumption. Often, you will need to look for more information or another approach to prove that the population in question is in Hardy–Weinberg equilibrium. Second, doing the math requires care and, if you are not exceptionally fluent with it, patience. It will sometimes help to factor out common multipliers [e.g., $2pq^2 + q^2 = q^2(2p + 1)$]. At other times, it will be helpful to recognize members of a binomial expansion [e.g., $p^2 + 2pq + q^2 = (p + q)^2$].

After you have mastered the concepts underlying the Hardy–Weinberg law, focus on understanding how genetic variation can be measured. A number of important models have been developed that have been supported by data gathered using a variety of methods, including those of molecular genetics. Models have been proposed to address the substantial amount of genetic variation that exists in a population and the factors that can lead to changes in a population's genetic structure. Some of these employ quantitative analysis and equations. Approach these models just as you did the Hardy–Weinberg law. First become familiar with the conceptual issues of the model, and then relate the variables in an equation to the key factors considered in the model.

Questions for Practice

Multiple-Choice Questions

1. In a small population, 30% of the individuals have blood type M, 40% of the individuals have blood type MN, and 30% of the individuals have blood type N. If p equals the frequency of the L^M allele and q equals the frequency of the L^N allele, what are p and q?
   a. $p = 0.30, q = 0.30$
   b. $p = 0.50, q = 0.50$

c. $p = 0.30$, $q = 0.70$
d. $p = 0.50$, $q = 0.30$

2. Is the population described in Question 1 above in Hardy–Weinberg equilibrium?
   a. Yes; the calculated genotypic frequencies equal the expected genotype frequencies.
   b. Yes; at equilibrium you always have equal numbers of recessive and dominant homozygotes.
   c. No; the frequency of heterozygotes is too high and the frequency of homozygotes is too low.
   d. No; the frequency of heterozygotes is too low and the frequency of homozygotes is too high.

3. Which of the following is *not* an assumption about a population in Hardy–Weinberg equilibrium?
   a. The population is isolated.
   b. Random mating occurs in the population.
   c. The population is free from mutation.
   d. The population is free from natural selection.
   e. The population is free from migration.

4. The frequency of one form of X-linked color blindness varies among human ethnic groups. What can be said about whether each ethnic group is in Hardy–Weinberg equilibrium? (Let q = the frequency of the normal allele and p = the frequency of the color-blind allele.)
   a. None of the ethnic populations can be in equilibrium, since all have different values for p and q.
   b. Only the entire human population is in equilibrium.
   c. Some of the ethnic populations may be in equilibrium, provided that the frequency of the trait in males is p and the frequency in females is p^2.
   d. Some of the ethnic populations may be in equilibrium, provided that the frequency of the trait in both sexes is p^2.
   e. All of the ethnic populations will be in equilibrium, since each satisfies the criteria for a population in Hardy–Weinberg equilibrium.

5. In a large, randomly mating population, 80% of the individuals have dark hair and 20% are blond. Assuming that hair color is controlled by one pair of alleles, is the allele for dark hair necessarily dominant to the one for blond hair?
   a. Yes, because otherwise the population would not be dominated by dark-haired individuals.
   b. Yes, because more of something (in this case, hair color) is always dominant to less of that thing.
   c. No, because relative frequencies of alleles in a randomly mating population are unrelated to issues of dominance and recessiveness.
   d. No, because although there is a relationship between dominance and allele frequency, that relationship is not seen in this example.

6. The amounts of genetic variation in a population can be explained in a number of ways. In one view, a large amount of genetic variation is explained by recurrent mutation and random changes in allele frequencies. In this view, natural selection selects against some of the variation affecting fitness but does not select for or against much of the genetic variation. This concept is termed
   a. the classical model.
   b. the neutral theory.
   c. the random mutation model.

7. Which of the following populations are in Hardy–Weinberg equilibrium?

Population	AA	Aa	aa
a	0.72	0.20	0.08
b	0.12	0.80	0.08
c	0.08	0.01	0.91
d	0.25	0.50	0.25

8. How is the rate of forward mutation likely to be related to the rate of reverse mutation?
   a. The rate of forward mutation is generally lower because there is mutational pull back to a specific form.
   b. The rate of forward mutation is generally higher because once an allele has changed, it is nearly as likely that a subsequent change will be to yet another new form.

    c. The rate of forward and reverse mutations are codependent and usually equal.

    d. The relative rates of forward and reverse mutation are so highly variable that one cannot formulate an accurate generalization comparing the two.

9. Which of the following can result in genetic drift?
    a. a sampling error
    b. random factors producing unexpected mortality
    c. the establishment of a population by a small number of breeding individuals
    d. a drastic reduction in the size of a population
    e. a change in environmental conditions that affects selection
    f. all of the above

10. What is the effective population size for a population consisting of 10 breeding males and 2 breeding females?
    a. 12
    b. 6
    c. 7
    d. 2

11. Which of the following is *not* true concerning the effect of migration among populations?
    a. Migration tends to increase the effective size of the populations, leading to a reduction in genetic drift.
    b. Migration is associated with gene flow and introduces new alleles to the population.
    c. If the allele frequencies of migrants and the recipient population differ, migration can lead to the further differentiation of two populations.
    d. Migration and genetic drift have opposite effects on size and variability. Migration effectively increases size and variability, whereas drift acts in opposition.

12. What can one generally state about measuring the fitness associated with a specific genotype?
    a. It is easy to assess and can be based on the number of offspring of an individual.
    b. Since it is based on the reproductive ability of a genotype, it is an absolute term, which requires no assumptions.
    c. It will remain the same from generation to generation.
    d. It is difficult to measure because of pleiotropic effects.

13. Consider a recessive trait that results in a complete lack of reproductive success of homozygotes. How might such a recessive trait be maintained at a high level in a population?
    a. through new mutation
    b. through heterosis
    c. through overdominance
    d. through heterozygote superiority
    e. all of the above

14. For a given eukaryotic gene, which rate of DNA change is expected to be the lowest?
    a. the relative rate of change in nonfunctional pseudogenes
    b. the relative rate of change in introns
    c. the relative rate of change for synonymous substitutions in coding sequences
    d. the relative rate of change for nonsynonymous substitutions in coding sequences
    e. the relative rate of change in leaders and trailers

15. Which of the rates in Question 14 is expected to be the highest?

Answers: 1b, 2d, 3a, 4c, 5c, 6b, 7d, 8b, 9f, 10c, 11c, 12d, 13e, 14d, 15a

Thought Questions

1. Consider a population that is not in Hardy–Weinberg equilibrium for a pair of alleles. Show why equilibrium values for genotype frequencies are reached in one generation after the onset of random mating for autosomal alleles, but more than one generation of random mating is required for sex-linked alleles.

2. Distinguish between heterozygosity and the proportion of polymorphic loci.

3. Mutation pressure is rarely the most important determinant of allelic frequency. What other factors are important?

4. Can a population be in Hardy–Weinberg equilibrium for one, but not another, pair of alleles?

5. What is the most likely explanation if the allelic frequencies agree with those predicted by the Hardy–Weinberg law, but the genotype frequencies do not? (Hint: Consider mating systems and heterosis.)

6. Why do mutation, migration, and drift not necessarily lead to adaptation?

7. What are five different molecular methods that can be used to measure genetic variation? What advantages and disadvantages are there to each?

8. Distinguish between nonrandom mating, positive assortative mating, negative assortative mating, and inbreeding.

9. What are the arguments for and against investing funds and human effort in a population viability analysis for an endangered species?

10. What are the values of preserving and promoting genetic diversity within a species? How does the development of genomics and technologies related to genomics affect our ability to assess and influence genetic diversity, both in our own species and in other species?

11. What is linkage disequilibrium, and how is it measured?

12. Can loci in Hardy–Weinberg equilibrium also be in linkage disequilibrium?

13. In what different ways can linkage disequilibrium for two loci arise?

Thought Questions for Media

After reviewing the media on the *iGenetics* website, try to answer the following questions.

1. What assumptions of the Hardy–Weinberg law were illustrated by the animation?

2. Under these assumptions, what are the predictions of the Hardy–Weinberg law?

3. Which of these assumptions were not valid in the population of Darwin's finches under study by Dr. Grant?

4. What was the purpose of Dr. Grant's study of these finches?

5. The animation indicated that beak shape and size are genetically complex. Some genes will have additive effects, some will be epistatic, and a few will show simple dominance and recessiveness. Why, for the purposes of the study, was it useful to assume the existence of a simple gene that, when homozygous recessive, contributes to a decrease in beak size?

6. Is fitness constant for a given trait such as beak length? If not, according to what conditions does it vary?

7. The animation describes how natural selection for small and large beak size in Darwin's finches is complex. For example, even though birds with larger beaks can crack harder seeds, in some years, there can still be selection for small beak size. Why might this be the case?

Solutions to Text Questions and Problems

21.1   *Answer:* Equate the frequency of each color with the frequency expected in Hardy–Weinberg equilibrium, letting $p = f(C^B)$, $q = f(C^P)$, and $r = f(C^Y)$.

Brown: $f(C^BC^B) + f(C^BC^P) + f(C^BC^Y) = p^2 + 2pq + 2pr = 236/500 = 0.472$

Pink: $f(C^PC^P) + f(C^PC^Y) = q^2 + 2qr = 231/500 = 0.462$

Yellow: $f(C^YC^Y) = r^2 = 33/500 = 0.066$

Now solve for p, q, and r, knowing that $p + q + r = 1$.

$r^2 = 0.066$, so $r = \sqrt{0.066} = 0.26$

There are two approaches to solve for q. First, since $q^2 + 2qr = 0.462$, one can substitute in $r = 0.26$, giving $q^2 + 2q(0.26) = 0.462$. Recognize this as a quadratic equation and set it equal to 0, and solve for q. That is, solve the equation $q^2 + 0.52q - 0.462 = 0$. Solving the quadratic equation for q, one has:

$$q = \frac{-0.52 \pm \sqrt{(0.52)^2 - 4(1)(-0.462)}}{2(1)} = 0.467$$

A second approach to solve for q is to realize that

$q^2 + 2qr = 0.462$ and $r^2 = 0.066$

Adding left and right sides of the equations together, one has

$q^2 + 2qr + r^2 = 0.066 + 0.462$

$(q + r)^2 = 0.528$

$q + r = 0.726$

$q = 0.726 - r = 0.726 - 0.26 = 0.467$

Since $p + q + r = 1$, $p = 1 - (q + r) = 1 - (0.26 + 0.467) = 0.273$.

21.2   *Answer:*

a. The tally for M^1 alleles is as follows:

Genotype	# Individuals	# M^1 Alleles
M^1M^1	8	16
M^1M^2	35	35
M^1M^3	53	53
Total		104

The total number of individuals is 254; thus the total number of alleles is 254×2, or 508. The frequency of M^1 alleles is $104/508 = 0.205$. The frequency of the other alleles is obtained similarly so that $f(M^1) = 0.20 = p$, $f(M^2) = 0.30 = q$, and $f(M^3) = 0.50 = r$.

b. For three alleles with frequencies p, q, and r, a population in Hardy–Weinberg equilibrium will have $p^2 + 2pq + 2pr + q^2 + 2qr + r^2 = 1$. To test the hypothesis that the population is in Hardy–Weinberg equilibrium, calculate the numbers of individuals expected in each class using this relationship and the values for p, q, and r obtained in **(a)**. Calculate the value of χ^2 as shown in the following table.

Genotype	Observed Value (o)	Expected Frequency	Expected Value (e)	d ($o - e$)	d^2/e
M^1M^1	8	$p^2 = 0.04$	10	−2	0.40
M^1M^2	35	$2pq = 0.12$	30	5	0.83
M^2M^2	20	$q^2 = 0.09$	23	−3	0.39
M^1M^3	53	$2pr = 0.20$	51	2	0.08
M^2M^3	76	$2qr = 0.30$	75	1	0.01
M^3M^3	62	$r^2 = 0.25$	64	−2	0.06

$$X^2 = 1.77$$

Since the six phenotypic classes are completely specified by three allele frequencies, the number of phenotypes (6) minus the number of alleles (3) determines the degrees of freedom ($6 - 3 = 3$). With 3 degrees of freedom, $0.70 < P < 0.50$. The hypothesis is accepted as possible, and it appears that the population is in Hardy–Weinberg equilibrium.

21.3 *Answer:* Let c represent the ΔF508 mutant allele and p its frequency, and let C represent the normal allele and q its frequency. In the sample of neonates tested, the frequency of Cc carriers is $4/955 = 0.00402$, and the frequency of CC homozygotes is $(995 - 4)/955 = 0.99598$. Assuming that the population is in Hardy–Weinberg equilibrium (individuals mate within a large population at random with respect to this allele; there is no selection, mutation, or migration), these numbers also give the frequency of Cc carriers ($= 2pq$) and CC homozygotes ($= p^2$) in the general population. Since Since $p^2 = 0.99598$, $p = \sqrt{0.99598} = 099799$. Since $p + q = 1$, $q = 1 - 0.99799 = 0.00201$. The expected frequency of homozygotes is $f(cc) = p^2 = (0.00201) = 0.0000004$. Therefore, the expected prevalence of homozygotes is one in $1/0.000004 =$ one in 250,000. This frequency is much lower than the prevalence of CF in the Indian subcontinent, for several possible reasons. One reasonable explanation is that additional mutations at the CFTR gene contribute to the incidence of CF. Indeed, the frequency of ΔF508 allele may be very different in this population than it is in non-Hispanic Caucasians. Alternatively, the sample assessed here is not representative of the population as a whole (genetic drift has occurred, and the population from which this sample is drawn is not in Hardy–Weinberg equilibrium).

21.4 *Answer:*

a. These data group multiple recessive CF alleles together. If we assume that each disease allele causes disease when homozygous or when heterozygous with any other disease allele, we can model the prevalence of disease. Let C represent a normal allele and c represent a representative recessive disease allele. The data are taken from individuals who have no family history of CF, so they are either CC or Cc. Therefore, we can calculate the frequencies of CC and Cc individuals as follows:

$f(Cc) =$ carriers detected/persons tested, and

$f(CC) =$ (persons tested $-$ carriers detected)/persons tested

This information can be used to calculate the frequency of the C and c alleles as follows:

$p = f(C) = f(CC) + [\frac{1}{2} \times f(Cc)]$
$q = f(c) = 1 - f(C)$

If we assume that the population is in Hardy–Weinberg equilibrium for these alleles, the frequency of individuals with CF is $f(cc) = q^2$, and the prevalence of CF is 1 in $1/q^2$. The table on the facing page shows the results of applying these equations to the data.

b. From part **(a)**, estimates of prevalence of CF based on carrier frequencies in three different populations of non-Hispanic Caucasians range from 1 in 2,083 to 1 in 4,545. While these estimates are similar to the estimates of the prevalence of CF from population surveys, the differences suggest that there are genetic differences between the three populations. This hypothesis seems reasonable given their different geographical origins—each population may be in Hardy–Weinberg equilibrium for the alleles in consideration, but the different populations have different allele frequencies. The estimate of the prevalence of CF from population surveys reflects the contributions of different populations. For Ashkenazi Jewish Caucasians, the prevalence estimated from the number of carriers is similar to the prevalence estimated from population surveys.

In contrast, the prevalence of CF in Hispanic Caucasians estimated from the number of carriers varies considerably depending on the geographical origin of the carriers. Furthermore, each of those values differs from the prevalence of CF in Hispanic Caucasians based on population surveys. One hypothesis to explain these findings is that different populations of Hispanic Caucasians are genetically heterogeneous and that the observed prevalence of CF in Hispanic Caucasians reflects the contributions from each of these different populations. The genetic heterogeneity may reflect either the historical origin of a particular population of Hispanic Caucasians or mixing of the population with non-Hispanic Caucasians that generally have a higher frequency of carriers.

Geographical Source of Persons Tested	Ethnicity	$f(Cc)$	$f(CC)$	p	q	q^2	Prevalence
Copenhagen, Denmark	non-Hispanic Caucasians	0.0294	0.9706	0.9853	0.0147	0.00022	1 in 4,545
Edinburgh, Scotland	non-Hispanic Caucasians	0.0412	0.9588	0.9794	0.0206	0.00042	1 in 2,380
Maine, USA	non-Hispanic Caucasians	0.0437	0.9563	0.9781	0.0219	0.00048	1 in 2,083
New York City, NY, USA	Ashkenazi Jewish Caucasians	0.0419	0.9581	0.9790	0.0210	0.00044	1 in 2,272
Northern California, USA	Hispanic Caucasians	0.0095	0.9905	0.9952	0.0047	0.000023	1 in 44,290
Southern California, USA	Hispanic Caucasians	0.0077	0.9923	0.9962	0.0038	0.000015	1 in 69,252
Rochester, NY, USA	Hispanic Caucasians	0.0256	0.9743	0.9872	0.0128	0.00016	1 in 6,064
Rochester, NY, USA	African-American	0	1	1	0	0	none
Southern California, USA	African-American	0	1	1	0	0	none

For African-Americans, the predicted prevalence based on carrier frequency is much less than the observed prevalence based on population surveys. One hypothesis to explain this result is that the sample size of carriers was too small to accurately estimate the prevalence of CF—the observed prevalence based on population surveys probably reflects findings from a larger sampling of individuals. This hypothesis may also explain the differences seen in other populations. A second hypothesis is that there is genetic heterogeneity in different populations of African-Americans, and the observed prevalence of CF based on population surveys of African-Americans reflects this. As for Hispanic Caucasians, the observed prevalence determined from population surveys may reflect contributions from populations with different historical origins or the mixing of several populations, one of which has a higher frequency of carriers.

We do not have data on the carrier frequency in Asian Hawaiians, but the very low prevalence of CF in Asian Hawaiians based on population surveys indicates that CF mutations are very rare in this population. One hypothesis to explain the very low prevalence of CF is that mutations were introduced into this population by mixing with non-Hispanic Caucasians.

It is important to consider that these analyses have been undertaken with the assumption that each population is in Hardy–Weinberg equilibrium for the CF alleles under consideration, and that the assumptions that underlie the Hardy–Weinberg law may not be fully satisfied in each population. For example, there has been considerable human migration in the past several centuries. However, these analyses are still useful because they provide information helpful for decisions about practical issues, such as where to devote resources for genetic testing.

21.5 *Answer:* The conditions of this problem meet the requirements for a population in Hardy–Weinberg equilibrium. In such a population, if p equals the frequency of A, and q equals the frequency of a, one expects p^2 (AA), $2pq$ (Aa), and q^2 (aa) genotypes after random mating. Here, $q^2 = 0.81$, so $q = 0.9$. Since $p + q = 1$, $p = 1 - 0.9 = 0.1$. In the next generation, one would expect $p^2 = (0.1)^2 = 0.01$ (or 1%) AA genotypes, $2pq = 2(0.1)(0.9) = 0.18$ (or 18%) Aa genotypes, and $q^2 = (0.9)^2 = 0.81$ (or 81%) aa genotypes.

21.6   *Answer:*

a. Since $q^2 = 0.16$, $q = \sqrt{0.16} = 0.40$. Since $p + q = 1$, $p = 0.60$. The frequency of heterozygotes is $2pq = 2(0.40)(0.60) = 0.48$. Each of the 48% of the heterozygotes has one recessive allele, while each of the 16% of the homozygous recessive individuals has two. Thus, the percentage of the total number of recessive alleles in heterozygotes is $(0.48)/[0.48 + 2(0.16)] = 0.48/0.80 = 0.60$, or 60%.

b. If $q^2 = 0.01$, then $q = 0.1$, and $p = 0.9$. $2pq = 2(0.1)(0.9) = 0.18$. The percentage of the total number of recessive alleles in heterozygotes is $(0.18)/[0.18 + 2(0.01)] = 0.18/0.20 = 0.90$, or 90%.

21.7   *Answer:* The frequency of heterozygotes in a population in equilibrium is $2pq$, and the frequency of homozygous recessives is q^2. Here, there are eight times as many heterozygotes as homozygous recessives, so $2pq = 8q^2$. Since $p + q = 1$, $p = 1 - q$, and one can substitute $1 - q$ for p. This gives $2(1 - q)q = 8q^2$. Dividing both sides by q and multiplying through, one has $2 - 2q = 8q$. Thus, $2 = 10q$, and $q =$ the frequency of the recessive allele $= 0.20$.

21.8   *Answer:*

a. In the red *RR* animals, all of the gametes contain the *R* allele, while in the roan *Rr* animals, half of the gametes contain the *R* allele. Therefore, $[49 + (42/2)] = 70\%$ of the gametes will contain the *R* allele. Another way to look at this problem is to realize that the frequency of gametes bearing a certain allele is the same as the frequency of the allele in the population. Let p equal the frequency of *R* in the population. Since there are 49% red animals, $p^2 = 0.49$, so $p = 0.70$ (or 70%).

b. If one lets q represent the frequency of *r*, since 1% of the animals are white, one has $q^2 = 0.01$. Hence, $q = 0.1$.

21.9   *Answer:* Let the frequency of allele *A* equal p and the frequency of allele *a* equal q, with $p + q = 1$. Then, in the initial generation, the frequency of *AA* genotypes is p^2, the frequency of *aa* genotypes is q^2. The frequency of the remaining genotypes (i.e., *Aa* heterozygotes) must be $1 - (p^2 + q^2)$. Since $p + q = 1$, $(p + q)^2 = 1^2$, and $p^2 + 2pq + q^2 = 1$. Therefore, $1 - (p^2 + q^2) = 2pq$, and the frequency of *Aa* heterozygotes must be $2pq$.

Assume there is no selection, mutation, or migration and that the individuals mate at random. Since there are three different genotypes in the population, nine crosses are possible. The frequency of each type of cross is determined by the frequency of each parental genotype. The types of crosses, the frequency of each cross, the types of progeny, and the frequency of each progeny class are listed in the table below:

Cross	Cross Frequency	Progeny Ratios AA	Progeny Ratios Aa	Progeny Ratios aa	Progeny Frequencies AA	Progeny Frequencies Aa	Progeny Frequencies aa
$AA \times AA$	$p^2 \times p^2 = p4$	all			p^4		
$AA \times Aa$	$p^2 \times 2pq = 2p^3q$	$\frac{1}{2}$	$\frac{1}{2}$		p^3q	p^3q	
$AA \times aa$	$p^2 \times q^2 = p^2q^2$		all			p^2q^2	
$Aa \times AA$	$2pq \times p^2 = 2p^3q$	$\frac{1}{2}$	$\frac{1}{2}$		p^3q	p^3q	
$Aa \times Aa$	$2pq \times 2pq = 4p^2q^2$	$\frac{1}{4}$	$\frac{1}{2}$	$\frac{1}{2}$	p^2q^2	$2p^2q^2$	p^2q^2
$Aa \times aa$	$2pq \times q^2 = 2pq^3$		$\frac{1}{2}$	$\frac{1}{2}$		pq^3	pq^3
$aa \times AA$	$q^2 \times p^2 = p^2q^2$		all			p^2q^2	
$aa \times Aa$	$q^2 \times 2pq = 2pq^3$		$\frac{1}{2}$	$\frac{1}{2}$		pq^3	pq^3
$aa \times aa$	$q^2 \times q^2 = q^4$			all			q^4

To determine the frequency of a particular zygotic class, add up the frequency of the progeny in that class. Then factor out a common multiplier, and note that $p + q = 1$ and that $(p + q)^2 = p^2 + 2pq + q^2$. One has:

$$\text{frequency } (AA) = p^4 + 2p^3q + p^2q^2$$
$$= p^2(p^2 + 2pq + q^2)$$
$$= p^2(p + q)^2$$
$$= p^2(1)^2 = p^2$$

$$\text{frequency } (Aa) = 2p^3q + 4p^2q^2 + 2pq^3$$
$$= 2pq(p^2 + 2pq + q^2)$$
$$= 2pq(p + q)^2$$
$$= 2pq(1)^2 = 2pq$$

$$\text{frequency } (aa) = pq + 2pq^3 + q^4$$
$$= q^2(p^2 + 2pq + q^2)$$
$$= q^2(p + q)^2$$
$$= q^2(1)^2 = q^2$$

Thus, the zygotic frequencies do not change from one generation to the next.

Since all of the gametes of the AA parents and half of the gametes of the Aa parents will bear the A allele, the frequency of A in the gene pool of the next generation is $p^2 + pq = p(p + q) = p$. Since all of the gametes of the aa parents and half of the gametes of the Aa parents will bear the a allele, the frequency of a in the gene pool of the next generation is $q^2 + pq = q(q + p) = q$. Thus, the allelic frequencies do not change from one generation to the next.

21.10   *Answer:* Members of a population generally do not interbreed randomly for all traits. For example, humans mate preferentially for height, skin color, socioeconomic status, and other traits. For many other traits however, mating is random. The Hardy–Weinberg law applies to any trait for which random mating occurs, even if mating is nonrandom for other traits.

21.11   *Answer:* The Hardy–Weinberg law states that when a population is in equilibrium, the genotypic frequencies will be in the proportion of p^2, $2pq$, and q^2 and that these frequencies will remain constant if the population remains large, randomly mating, and free from mutation, migration, and natural selection. It describes the behavior of allele and genotype frequencies for a specific set of alleles and genotypes. Therefore, it is possible that the Hardy–Weinberg law holds in a population for some allele and genotypic frequencies but not for others. In this population, the only individual guaranteed to pass on the germ line is the dominant male because only he will turn into a female and produce the eggs for the next generation. Other males do not have this guarantee: they will pass on their germ line only if their sperm is able to fertilize an egg. The mating system described here selects for genotypes that confer dominant behaviors. Therefore, such genotypes may not be in Hardy–Weinberg equilibrium. However, the male that will become a female was a member of a population of males, and not all genotypes will affect the dominant behavior. If the other assumptions of the Hardy–Weinberg law hold—in particular if a genotype is not subject to selection—it should remain in Hardy–Weinberg equilibrium from one generation to the next.

21.12   *Answer:*

   a. Let p equal the frequency of S and q equal the frequency of s. Since homozygotes have two identical alleles and heterozygotes have one recessive and one dominant allele, one has:

$$p = \frac{2(188)[SS] + 717[Ss]}{2(3,146)} = \frac{1,093}{6,292} = 0.1737$$

$$q = \frac{717[Ss] + 2(2,241)[ss]}{2(3,146)} = \frac{5,199}{6,292} = 0.8263$$

b. Remember that in a χ^2 test, one uses the actual numbers of progeny observed and expected, and not the frequencies. With a hypothesis that the population is in Hardy–Weinberg equilibrium, one has:

Class	Observed (o)	Expected Frequency	Expected (e)	d ($o - e$)	d^2/e
SS	8	$p^2 = 0.0302$	95	93	91.0
Ss	717	$2pq = 0.287$	903	−186	38.3
ss	2,241	$q^2 = 0.683$	2,148	93	4.0
	3,146	1	3,146	0	133.3

There is only 1 degree of freedom because the three genotypic classes are completely specified by two allele frequencies, namely, p and q. (df = number of phenotypes − number of alleles = $3 − 2 = 1$.) The χ^2 value of 133.3, for 1 degree of freedom, gives $P < 0.0001$. Therefore, the distribution of genotypes differs significantly from that expected if the population were in Hardy–Weinberg equilibrium.

21.13 *Answer:* The frequencies are

$f(S-) = f(SS) + f(SS^u) = p^2 + 2pr$
$f(Ss) = 2pq$
$f(s-) = f(ss) + f(sS^u) = q^2 + 2qr$
$f(S^uS^u) = r^2$

21.14 *Answer:* The conditions described in the problem indicate that the population is in Hardy–Weinberg equilibrium. Under equilibrium conditions, neither the allele nor the zygotic frequencies change from one generation to the next. Therefore, in two generations there should still be 60% type O individuals.

21.15 *Answer:* There are several possible explanations for the difference in the frequency of the trait in males and females. Two are sex linkage and autosomal linkage with sex-influenced expression. Sex linkage can be readily examined. If the population is in Hardy–Weinberg equilibrium (which this one is), the frequency of the recessive allele causing the trait is q, and the gene is X-linked, then the frequency in XY males would be q, while the frequency in XX females would be q^2. Since the frequency in males is 0.4 and the frequency in females is $(0.4)^2 = 0.16$, the data fit a model of sex linkage with $q = 0.4$. The frequency of heterozygous XX (female) individuals is $2pq = 2(0.6)(0.4) = 0.48$. Since the trait appears to be sex-linked, no heterozygous males exist.

21.16 *Answer:* As described in the solution to Question 21.15, there are several explanations for differences in the frequency of a trait between males and females. This question asks you to consider the possibility of X-linkage. Suppose the trait is X-linked and recessive, and assume the population is in Hardy–Weinberg equilibrium. Let q equal the frequency of the recessive allele, and p equal the frequency of the dominant allele. If the gene is X-linked, one would expect XY males to express the recessive trait at a frequency of q, and XX females to express the recessive trait at a frequency of q^2. Inspecting the data shows that the frequency of type 2 individuals in females is 0.01, which is the square of the frequency of type 2 individuals in males: $(0.10)^2 = 0.01$. Thus, this trait *could be* controlled by a pair of X-linked alleles occurring with allele frequencies of $q = 0.1$ recessive and $p = 0.9$ dominant.

21.17 *Answer:* Let q equal the frequency of the recessive allele, and p equal the frequency of the dominant allele. One expects homozygotes showing the trait to appear at a frequency of q^2 in a population at equilibrium. If $q^2 = 64/10,000 = 0.0064$, $q = 0.08$. Thus, one would expect 8% of XY male individuals to show the trait.

21.18 *Answer:*
a. Let q equal the frequency of the recessive allele, and p equal the frequency of the dominant allele. The frequency of males with the trait will be q, and the frequency of females will be q^2. Here, $q = 0.08$, so $q^2 = 0.0064$, or 0.64%.
b. Since $q = 0.08$, $p = 0.92$. The frequency of heterozygotes is $2pq = 0.1472$, or 14.72%. Only women can be heterozygotes, so the frequency of heterozygous women is 14.72%.
c. If the population is in Hardy–Weinberg equilibrium, the frequencies of alleles and the frequency of zygotic phenotypes will not change in two generations. Since $p = 0.92$, 92% of the XY males will have normal vision.

21.19 *Answer:* Kimura developed the neutral theory in response to data obtained using protein electrophoresis showing that most species have large amounts of genetic variation in their proteins. This was in contrast to a classical model developed in the 1920s and 1930s using data obtained by characterizing external phenotypic variation in wild populations. The classical model stated that natural populations possess little variation, and that, within each population, a single allele—the wild-type allele—is strongly favored by natural selection because it "functions the best." In classical models, most individuals are homozygous for the "wild-type" allele. In those models, when an occasional mutation arises, it is usually deleterious, and strong selection occurs against it. In the rare case that a new mutation is advantageous for survival or reproduction, the new allele will increase in frequency and eventually become the new wild-type allele.

In Kimura's neutral theory, there is significant genetic variation within a population. Many alleles exist in intermediate frequencies, and members of the population are heterozygous at numerous loci. In this model, much of the genetic variation is explained by recurrent mutation and random changes in the frequency of alleles that are physiologically equivalent, and not necessarily by natural selection. Unlike the classical model, the neutral theory views most variation as neutral with regard to selection.

Since the neutral theory was introduced, advances in DNA sequencing and more refined statistical methods for testing the influence of mutation, genetic drift, migration, and natural selection have led to an understanding that a complex interaction of these forces determines the level of genetic variation in natural populations.

21.20 *Answer:* Let q equal the frequency of a, and p equal the frequency of A, with $q + p = 1$. As discussed in the text, when the population is at equilibrium, the frequency of p and q is given by

$$q = \frac{u}{u+v} = \frac{6 \times 10^{-7}}{(6 \times 10^{-7}) + (6 \times 10^{-8})} = \frac{6 \times 10^{-7}}{(6 \times 10^{-7}) + (0.6 \times 10^{-7})} = \frac{6}{6.6} = 0.91$$

$$p = 1 - q = 1 - 0.91 = 0.09$$

Thus, the frequencies are 0.0081 *AA*, 0.1638 *Aa*, and 0.8281 *aa*.

21.21 *Answer:* The effective breeding size of a population is given by the equation

$$N_e = \frac{4 \times N_f \times N_m}{N_f + N_m}$$

where N_f equals the number of breeding females and N_m equals the number of breeding males. Apply this equation to each of the situations described as follows:
a. $(4 \times 50 \times 50)/100 = 100$
b. $(4 \times 60 \times 40)/100 = 96$
c. $(4 \times 10 \times 90)/100 = 36$
d. $(4 \times 2 \times 98)/100 = 7.8$

21.22   *Answer:* Since the gene pool in the present, large North American population is derived from a small number of individuals, a founder effect is likely to have occurred. Thus, genetic drift (random change in allelic frequency due to chance) will influence the North American populations to a greater degree than it will the European populations. One would expect to see less variation within and greater genetic differentiation among the North American populations. The magnitude of the difference between the native North American population and the introduced population will depend on how many times different European populations were introduced. For example, if relatively large numbers of European snails from multiple localities were introduced many times, the founder effect would not be as marked as if a small number of snails were introduced just once from one location.

21.23   *Answer:* Let p_I equal the frequency of A in population I, and p_{II} equal the frequency of A in population II. If individuals in population I migrate to population II and make up proportion m of population II' (p'_{II}), the new frequency of A in population II' (p'_{II}) is given by:

$$p'_{II} = mp_I + (1 - m)p_{II}$$

Here, $p'_{II} = [20/(20 + 80)](0.50) + \{1 - [20/(20 + 80)]\}(0.70) = 0.66$.

21.24   *Answer:* For each population, determine the frequency of the A and a alleles, and assess how the population structure compares with that expected if no selection was occurring. To do this calculation, suppose there were 100 individuals in each population containing 200 alleles.

In population 1, there would be $(0.04)(100)(2) + (0.32)(100)(1) = 40$ A alleles and $(0.64)(100)(2) + (0.32)(100)(1) = 160$ a alleles. Thus, $f(A) = p = 40/200 = 0.20$, and $f(a) = q = 160/200 = 0.80$. If the population was in Hardy–Weinberg equilibrium, one would expect $p^2 = 0.04$ AA, $2pq = 0.32$ Aa, and 0.64 aa individuals, as is observed. If selection is acting at all, it may be acting to maintain the observed frequencies of the A and a alleles in equilibrium.

In population 2, there would be $(0.12)(100)(2) + (0.87)(100)(1) = 111$ A alleles, and $(0.01)(100)(2) + (0.87)(100)(1) = 89$ a alleles. Here, $p = 0.555$ and $q = 0.455$. If the population was in Hardy–Weinberg equilibrium, one would expect $p^2 = 0.308$ AA, $2pq = 0.505$ Aa, and 0.207 aa individuals. The population is not in equilibrium, since there are far more heterozygotes and far fewer homozygotes than would be expected. This suggests that the heterozygote is being selected for in this population.

In population 3, there would be $(0.45)(100)(2) + (0.10)(100)(1) = 100$ A alleles and $(0.10)(100)(1) + (0.45)(100)(2) = 100$ a alleles. Here, $p = q = 0.5$. If the population was in Hardy–Weinberg equilibrium, one would expect $f(AA) = f(aa) = p^2 = q^2 = 0.25$ and $f(Aa) = 2pq = 0.50$. The population is not in equilibrium, since there are far more homozygotes (of either type) and far fewer heterozygotes than expected. This suggests that the heterozygote is being selected against in this population.

21.25   *Answer:* There are a variety of situations in which all individuals would become AA. One is that the four "founding" individuals are all AA. Since the probability of a single individual being AA is $(0.7)^2 = 0.49$, the probability of the four founding individuals being AA is $(0.49)^4 = 0.0576$, about $1/17$. Even if all four founding individuals are not AA, there will be some chance that the subsequent population may become all AA. For example, there is a low but distinct probability that only AA offspring may be had by $Aa \times AA$ parents. Given that "many" offspring are produced, the likelihood of this will be less than $1/17$ [e.g., if 10 offspring are produced, the likelihood of all being AA in such a cross would be $(1/2)^{10} = 1/1,024$]. Since the alleles are adaptively neutral, it would appear that $1/17$ is an upper bound for the likelihood of a population being 100% AA.

21.26   *Answer:*

a. Let $p = f(A)$, and $q = f(a)$. Initially, $p = q = 0.5$, so $p^2 = f(AA) = q^2 = f(aa) = (0.5)^2 = 0.25$. $f(Aa) = 2pq = 0.50$.

b. If aa individuals are now lethal, they will not contribute to the gene pool in the next generation. Only AA and Aa individuals will contribute to the gene pool in the next generation. The allele frequency will be

$$f(A) = \frac{(0.25 \times 2) + (0.50 \times 1)}{(0.25 \times 2) + (0.50 \times 2)} = \frac{1.0}{1.5} = 0.67$$

$$f(a) = \frac{(0.50 \times 1)}{(0.25 \times 2) + (0.50 \times 2)} = \frac{0.5}{1.5} = 0.33$$

c. Given the result of **(b)**, the genotype of the progeny are $p^2 = (0.67)^2 = 0.449$ *AA*, $2pq = 2(0.67)(0.33) = 0.442$ *Aa*, and $q^2 = (0.33)^2 = 0.109$ *aa*. As in **(b)**, only *AA* and *Aa* individuals will contribute to the gene pool in the next generation. The allele frequency will be

$$f(A) = \frac{(0.449 \times 2) + (0.442 \times 1)}{(0.449 \times 2) + (0.442 \times 2)} = .075$$

$$f(a) = \frac{(0.442 \times 1)}{(0.449 \times 2) + (0.442 \times 2)} = .025$$

Can you show that the following statement is true under the conditions of this problem? If the last generation in the unaltered environment is considered to be generation number 1, then after n generations, the frequency of *A* will be $n/(n + 1)$ and the frequency of *a* will be $1/(n + 1)$.

21.27 *Answer:* There are several reasons why recessives may appear in a constant frequency. (1) Perhaps most important is that new mutations of *A* to *a* could occur at a low but constant rate. (2) There could also be a selective advantage to heterozygotes (overdominance). (3) There could be nonrandom mating within the population (e.g., positive assortative mating, inbreeding). (4) There could be a low but steady frequency of migration of heterozygotes into the population. Each of these possibilities violates assumptions made for a population in Hardy–Weinberg equilibrium, and allows maintenance of a recessive allele that is deleterious as a homozygote. (Question 21.26 considers the consequences of such an allele if the assumptions were not violated.) (5) If the homozygous recessive condition is a relatively rare occurrence, the frequency of *a* alleles in the population is very low. As a result, only a very small proportion of the *a* alleles would be found in homozygotes; almost all *a* alleles would be found in heterozygotes (protected polymorphism). The few generations for which data have been recorded may not be enough to see a decline in the number of homozygotes.

21.28 *Answer:* See text Table 21.21, p. 636. For **(a)** and **(b)**, $p = 0.3$, $q = 0.7$, and $s = 1 - W = 0.4$.

a. If there is selection against the recessive homozygotes, after one generation,

$$\Delta q = \frac{-spq^2}{1 - sq^2} = \frac{-(0.4)(0.3)(0.7)^2}{1 - (0.4)(0.7)^2} = -0.073$$

$$q^1 = 0.7 - 0.073 = 0.627$$

b. If there is selection with no dominance, so that the fitness of the heterozygote is intermediate between the two homozygotes,

$$\Delta q = \frac{-spq/2}{1 - sq} = \frac{-(0.4)(0.3)(0.7)/2}{1 - (0.4)(0.7)} = -0.0583$$

$$q^1 = 0.7 - 0.0583 = 0.642$$

c. To select against Q^1 as a dominant allele, let p equal the frequency of the dominant allele being selected against: $p = 0.7$, $q = 0.3$, and $s = 0.4$.

$$\Delta p = \frac{-spq^2}{1 - s + sq^2} = \frac{-(0.4)(0.7)(0.3)^3}{1 - s + sq^2} = \frac{-(0.4)(0.7)(0.3)^2}{1 - 0.4 + (0.4)(0.3)^2} = -0.04$$

$$p^1 = 0.70 - 0.04 = 0.66$$

21.29 *Answer:* From the text discussion, at equilibrium, $p = f(Hb\text{-}A) = t/(t + s)$, and $q = f(Hb\text{-}S) = s/(s + t)$, where t equals the selection coefficient of $Hb\text{-}S/Hb\text{-}S$, and s equals the selection coefficient of $Hb\text{-}A/Hb\text{-}A$. Since *fitness* = $1 - $ *selection coefficient*, $f(Hb\text{-}S) = 0.12/(0.12 + 0.86) = 0.122$.

21.30 *Answer:* For a dominant allele, the frequency at equilibrium is $\hat{p} = u/s$, where u equals the mutation rate, and s is the selection coefficient ($= 1 - $ fitness). Here, $\hat{p} = 5 \times 10^{-5}/0.8 = 6.25 \times 10^{-5}$.

21.31 *Answer:*

a. There are many potential reasons. If all forms of the disease are caused by mutations in one gene, then that gene appears to be more highly mutable. This may be because the gene is very large, and so there is a larger amount of DNA that can be altered by randomly distributed point mutations, or because the gene may have some unusual sequence structure that results in mutation—for example, mutations due to DNA replication errors or transposon insertion. Alternatively, the rate could be large because mutations in any one of a number of genes can cause an identical disease phenotype.

b. Arabinose dependence will result from mutations in any of the genes whose function is required to utilize arabinose, while mutations to leucine, arginine, or tryptophan independence require very specific synthetic functions to be "added" to the cell. The former is much more likely to occur by single new mutations than the latter.

c. Factors include the number of genes that are required for the appearance of the trait, the size of those genes, the presence of genes that modify the mutation rate, and environmental factors.

21.32 *Answer:* First calculate the frequencies of each allele. In population I, one has $[(0.5 \times 2) + (0.4 \times 1)/2] = 0.7\ L^M$, and $0.3\ L^N$. Similarly, $L^M = 0.7$ and $L^N = 0.3$ in populations II and III also. A population in Hardy–Weinberg equilibrium would have $p^2 = (0.7)^2 = 0.49\ L^M - L^M$, $2pq = 2(0.7)(0.3) = 0.42\ L^M - L^N$, and $q^2 = (0.3)^2 = 0.09\ L^N - L^N$. As population II shows these features, it must be in Hardy–Weinberg equilibrium and would be expected to exhibit random mating. Inbreeding results in an increase in the frequency of homozygotes and would be associated with population I (but not III). Genetic drift is random change in allele frequency due to chance and can be explained by random effects, a small effective population size, founder or bottleneck effects, or sampling error. Genetic drift could be associated with either population I or population III. Because the frequencies in populations I and III are fairly close to those of an equilibrium population, sampling error in a population in Hardy–Weinberg equilibrium could also explain the results seen.

21.33 *Answer:*

a. The data fit the idea that a single *Bam*HI site is polymorphic in the population, and this gives rise to a restriction fragment length polymorphism (RFLP). On some chromosomes, the presence of the *Bam*HI site results in an RFLP having a size of 4.1 kb, while on others, the site is absent and a larger, 6.3-kb fragment is found. The probe is homologous to a region wholly within the 4.1-kb piece bounded on one end by the variable *Bam*HI site and on the other end by a constant site. When the variable site is present, the hybridized fragment is 4.1 kb. When the variable site is absent, the fragment extends to the next constant *Bam*HI site and is 6.7 kb long. An alternate explanation for these data is that the different-sized fragments result from the deletion (or insertion) of DNA. Compared to a chromosome with a 6.3-kb RFLP allele, the chromosome bearing the 4.1-kb RFLP allele has a deletion of 2.2 kb. In either explanation, people with only 4.1- or only 6.7-kb bands are homozygotes; people with both are heterozygotes.

b. There are $(56 \times 2) + 28 = 150$ 6.3-kb alleles and $(6 \times 2) + 38 = 50$ 4.1-kb alleles. Let q equal the frequency of the 6.3-kb allele, and p equal the frequency of the 4.1-kb allele. Then, $q = 150/(150 + 50) = 0.75$ and $p = 50/(150 + 50) = 0.25$.

c. If the population is in Hardy–Weinberg equilibrium, we expect $p^2 = (0.25)^2 = 0.0625$ of the sample, or 6.25 individuals, to show only the 4.1-kb band. We observed 6. We expect $q^2 = (0.75)^2 = 0.5625$ of the sample, or 56.25 individuals, to be homozygous for the 6.7-kb band. We saw 56. Finally, we would expect $2pq = 2(0.25)(0.75) = 0.375$ of the sample, or 37.5 individuals, to be heterozygotes. We observed 38. The observed and expected numbers are so close that a chi-square test is unnecessary for us to conclude that the population is in Hardy–Weinberg equilibrium.

21.34   *Answer:* Since five loci were examined, and only two have more than one allele, (2/5)(100%) = 40% of the loci are polymorphic. Heterozygosity is calculated by averaging the frequency of heterozygotes for each locus. The frequency of heterozygotes for the *AmPep*, *ADH*, and *LDH-1* loci is zero. At *MDH*, 35 out of 50 individuals were heterozygous (0.70). At *PGM*, 10 out of 50 individuals were heterozygous (0.20). Thus, the average heterozygosity is

$$\frac{0 + 0 + 0 + 0.7 = 2}{5} = 0.18$$

21.35   *Answer:* Genetic hitchhiking occurs when variants that are selectively neutral, or nearly so, and that happen to lie in positions along a chromosome nearby a new mutation that is either advantageous or detrimental, are swept to fixation or lost very rapidly along with that new mutation. Put another way, it is a process in which selection of a new mutation influences the distribution of DNA sequence variation at adjacent alleles. The extent of genetic hitchhiking in a region depends on the frequency of crossing-over in that region. Crossing-over during meiosis effectively breaks up the chromosomal region, making it less subject to genetic hitchhiking.

21.36   *Answer:* Linkage disequilibrium is the nonrandom association of alleles at different loci. In linkage disequilibrium, some combinations of alleles occur more or less frequently than is expected from the random combination of alleles based on their frequencies. It can be caused by the physical linkage of the loci, or it can result from a recent population bottleneck, migration, or hybridization.

Here is an example of linkage disequilibrium associated with the introduction of a new mutation. Suppose two homologous chromosomes have three closely linked loci *A/a*, *B/b*, and *C/c*: one homolog has alleles *A b c* and the other has alleles *A B C*. Suppose also that a new mutation converts the *A* allele on the *A b c* homolog to an *a* allele. The newly induced *a* allele will be transmitted to gametes nonrandomly with the *b* and *c* alleles because it has been introduced onto the homolog that they are on. Thus, the *a* allele will show linkage disequilibrium with the *b* and *c* alleles. Over time, recombination between the homologs in different members of the population will separate the *a* allele from the *b* and *c* alleles, and the amount of linkage disequilibrium will diminish.

Here is an example of linkage disequilibrium arising from a population bottleneck. Suppose *A/a* and *B/b* are unlinked loci, and assume that alleles at these loci are in Hardy–Weinberg equilibrium in a population before a bottleneck: the alleles at these loci show independent assortment and appear in gametes at random based on their frequencies in the population. Now suppose that genetic drift during the bottleneck did not change the frequencies of the *A*, *a*, *B*, or *b* alleles but did result in an increased number of *aa BB* and *AA bb* individuals. Then, immediately following the bottleneck, *a B* and *A b* gametes would be seen more frequently than expected solely based on the frequency of the *A*, *a*, *B*, or *b* alleles in the population, so the *A b* and the *a B* combinations of alleles would show linkage disequilibrium.

Linkage disequilibrium and linkage are not the same. Linkage disequilibrium involves the nonrandom associations of alleles at two or more loci that are not necessarily on the same chromosome. Linkage results from the association of two or more loci on a chromosome due to limited recombination and reflects loci that never assort independently.

21.37   *Answer:*

a. The expected heterozygosity is 1 − (frequency of expected homozygotes). If the frequency of alleles in the population is p_1, p_2, p_3, . . . p_n, the expected frequency of homozygotes is $p_1^2 + p_2^2 + p_3^2 + \ldots p_n^2$. For locus *G1A*, the expected frequency of homozygotes is $(0.398)^2 + (0.240)^2 + (0.211)^2 + (0.086)^2 + (0.036)^2 + (0.016)^2 + (0.007)^2 + (0.006)^2 = 0.270$, and the expected heterozygosity is $1 - 0.270 = 0.730$. The expected heterozygosities for the other loci are *G10X*, 0.741; *G10C*, 0.740; *G10L*, 0.662. These are approximately the observed frequencies of heterozygosities. Since the numbers and types of different heterozygotes are not given, it is not possible to employ the chi-square test to directly evaluate if the population is in Hardy–Weinberg equilibrium. The population appears to be close to Hardy–Weinberg equilibrium.

b. The three cubs of the mother show evidence of multiple paternity. For each of the loci *G10X* and *G10L*, three alleles present in the cubs must have been contributed paternally (*G10X: X133, X135* or *X137, X141; G10L: L155, L157, L161*). This could only have happened if the cubs were sired by at least two different fathers. Multiple paternity within one set of cubs would tend to increase the genetic variability in the population because it would allow a larger number of males to contribute gametes seen in the next generation. Since $N_e = (4 \times N_f \times N_m)/(N_f + N_m)$, a larger N_m will tend to increase the effective population size.

21.38   *Answer:* Genetic drift arises from random change in allele frequency due to chance. Random factors producing mortality in natural populations and sampling error can lead to genetic drift. Its causes include a small effective population size over many generations, a small number of founders (founder effect), and a reduction in population size (bottleneck effect).

21.39   *Answer:*
   a. Mutation will lead to change in allele frequencies within a population if no other forces are acting. It will introduce genetic variation. If the effective population size is small, mutation may lead to genetic differentiation among populations.
   b. Migration will increase the population size, and has the potential to disrupt a Hardy–Weinberg equilibrium. It can increase genetic variation and may influence the evolution of allele frequencies within populations. Over many generations, migration will reduce divergence among populations and equalize allele frequencies among populations.
   c. Genetic drift produces changes in allele frequencies within a population. It can reduce genetic variation and increase the homozygosity within a population. Over time, it leads to genetic change. When several populations are compared, genetic drift can lead to increased genetic differences among populations.
   d. Inbreeding will increase the homozygosity within a population and decrease its genetic variation.

21.40   *Answer:* Answer this question by considering how a decrease in size of the tortoise population followed by migration to two different locations affects its genetic variation. When Sam was a child, the tortoise population roamed freely. Though the population was small, we can presume that there were tortoises on adjacent tracts of land, and so the 30 tortoises that are described were presumably part of a larger, genetically diverse population. Since tortoises stay within a few miles of their natal nest, we expect migration to be minimal. Therefore, if selection was not occurring within the population, this population could have been in Hardy–Weinberg equilibrium for at least some alleles. When Sam was 40, only three tortoises were left. Genetic drift will occur because the population is no longer breeding at random or at large. A sampling error will occur because of the population bottleneck and the subsequent founder effects. Since only one male remained, his alleles will disproportionately influence what alleles are present in subsequent generations. It seems likely that some alleles will be lost from the population just by chance. Even when the population grows in size, its gene pool will be derived from the genes present in the three founders. Therefore, when Sam is 40, the population of 30 tortoises on Sam's property will show less genetic diversity than do the 30 tortoises that were present on the property when Sam was a child.

   The population of tortoises relocated to a desert island will serve as a founder population on that island. Ten years after their release, the population's genetic diversity should be identical to that of the initial founding members because the population will have at best a modest increase in size due to at most one additional generation of tortoises. Two hundred years after their release, a few generations of tortoises will have been born, and so there would be little time for new mutations to alter the genetic diversity of the population. In this interval, there would be significant inbreeding because the founding population was small. Therefore, one would not expect this population to show an increase in genetic diversity.

   The tortoises that are relocated to a location with an existing tortoise population will have an opportunity to breed with that population. This could lead to an increase in genetic diversity. The migration could introduce new alleles into the existing tortoise population. Over a 10-year interval, the increase would be modest due to the rate of reproduction of these tortoises. Over 200 years and several generations, however, the extent of the increase could be significant. It will depend on the size of the existing tortoise population and whether breeding is random. For example, if the existing tortoise population is small relative to the size of the introduced population, or if members of the introduced population breeds do not breed with members of the existing population, inbreeding would occur and the population would not show a large increase in genetic diversity. However, if the existing population is not small, the "migration" of Sam's tortoises into the population should reduce the genetic divergence between the populations and increase the effective size of the population.

21.41 *Answer:* Overdominance results when a heterozygote genotype has higher fitness than do either of the homozygotes. The two alleles of the heterozygote are maintained in a population because both are favored in the heterozygote genotype. In the case of the sickle-cell allele, heterozygotes for *Hb-A/Hb-S* are at a selective advantage in areas with malaria because the hemoglobin mixture in these individuals provides an unfavorable growth environment for malarial parasites. Thus, heterozygotes have higher fitness than do *Hb-A/Hb-A* homozygotes who are susceptible to malaria, and they also have higher fitness than do *Hb-S/Hb-S* homozygotes who suffer from sickle-cell anemia. The favoring of the sickle-cell allele *Hb-S* in the heterozygote leads to its relatively high frequency in areas with malaria.

21.42 *Answer:*
   a. The cyclical decline in population density could cause a cyclically repeated bottleneck effect at each of the sampling sites. This would lead to the loss of some alleles from the gene pool as a result of chance and founder effects. If there were negligible migration between sampling sites, the populations would most likely diverge in their allele frequencies through genetic drift. There would be more variance in allele frequency among the small populations at each sampling site. If there were substantial migration between sampling sites, there would be reciprocal gene flow among the populations. This would increase the amount of genetic variation in the populations at each sampling site and reduce the divergence between the populations. If there were cyclical, sharp declines in the vole population, it is unlikely that the population would be in Hardy–Weinberg equilibrium.
   b. First, randomly trap a subset of the voles and sample tissue or blood from them. Then, identify a set of polymorphic loci (using protein electrophoresis, RFLPs, STRs, DNA sequences, or SNPs) and estimate the heterozygosity and allele frequencies at these loci. Use this information to compare populations sampled at each of the study sites, and estimate the degree of homogeneity or divergence of the two populations.

21.43 *Answer:* Using DNA sequence information to infer the strength of evolutionary processes has several advantages. DNA sequences provide highly accurate and reliable information, allow direct comparison of the genetic differences among organisms, are easily quantified, and can be used in all organisms.

21.44 *Answer:* The most comprehensive analysis would involve obtaining DNA samples from a large number of individuals from different geographical locations and then using high-throughput methods to assess the allele frequencies at highly polymorphic SNPs (see text Chapter 8, pp. 192–193, for a description of these methods). Quantify the amount of genetic variation within and between populations from different geographical regions by analyzing the frequency of the different SNP alleles in the populations. These analyses can help sort out the effects of natural selection from migration, genetic drift, and mutation. A locus that shows similar patterns of genetic variation to many different loci across the genome may not have been influenced by natural selection, unlike a locus that shows a very different pattern of variation when compared to many different loci across the genome. These types of analyses have supported the view that human populations underwent serial population bottlenecks as they migrated out of Africa. They have also shown that Europeans harbor substantially more deleterious mutations than ancestral African individuals do, probably because the population genetic bottlenecks that followed migration out of Africa provided opportunities for deleterious mutations to rise in frequency.

21.45 *Answer:* Human populations do differ in their genetic variation according to their geographical origin. However, only about 12–13% of the total genetic variance is found between different populations, whereas 87–88% is found within populations. One significant conclusion from this comparison is that different human populations, whether defined socially (e.g., race) or geographically, are far more similar to each other than they are different.

21.46 *Answer:* Prezygotic barriers prevent two species from mating and can include temporal isolation (e.g., different mating seasons, different activity periods), ecological isolation (e.g., different ecological niches, different dietary preferences), behavioral incompatibility (e.g., members of the two species avoid each other as mates), mechanical isolation (e.g., genitalia do not fit together), and gametic isolation (e.g., gametes cannot fuse even if they come in contact with each other). Postzygotic isolation occurs when members of two different species can mate, but the offspring produced are incapable of contributing to another generation. Examples include hybrid sterility, hybrid inviability, and hybrid breakdown. Postzygotic isolation is generally thought to arise first. The process by which postzygotic isolation leads to prezygotic isolation is referred to as reinforcement. If mating adults face a postmating barrier, they could increase their fitness if they could recognize the "wrong" species and avoid an unproductive mating. Consequently, if two populations harbor genetic variation for mate recognition, then the alleles that allow the adults to discriminate successfully will increase in frequency and lead to prezygotic isolation.

21.47 *Answer:* In both instances, protein electrophoresis or RFLP, STR, SNP, or DNA sequence analysis of specific genes could be used to gather information on the genotype of the captured individuals and members of each island population. In **(a)**, the captured individual should be returned to the subpopulation from which it shows the least genetic variation. In **(b)**, evaluate the genotype of the two missing tortoises using DNA from the previously collected blood samples. Compare these genotypes to the genotypes of the two captured tortoises. If a captured animal was taken from the field site, its genotype will exactly match a genotype obtained from one of the blood samples.

22

Quantitative Genetics

Chapter Outline

Review of Key Terms, Symbols, and Concepts

In your own words, write a brief, precise definition of each term in the groups below. Check your definitions using the text. Then develop a concept map using the terms in each list.

1	2	3
quantitative genetics	nature versus nurture	heritability
quantitative trait	population	broad-sense heritability
discontinuous trait	sample	narrow-sense heritability
continuous trait	frequency distribution	partitioning variance
polygenic trait	normal distribution	phenotypic variance (V_P)
norm of reaction	binomial distribution	genetic variance (V_G)
multifactorial trait	binomial expansion	environmental variance (V_E)
familial trait	mean	genotype-by-environment
penetrance	variance	interaction ($V_{G \times E}$)
expressivity	standard deviation	genotype-by-environment
pleiotropy	analysis of variance (ANOVA)	covariation ($COV_{G \times E}$)
epistasis	covariance	additive genetic variance (V_A)
polygene	correlation coefficient	dominance variance (V_D)
contributing alleles	scatter diagram	interaction variance (V_I)
noncontributing alleles	correlation vs. cause and effect	general environmental
polygene or multiple-	correlation vs. identity	effects (V_{Eg})
gene hypothesis for	regression	special environmental effects
quantitative inheritance	regression line	(V_{Es})
quantitative trait	regression coefficient, slope	family environmental effects
locus (QTL)	phenotypic correlation	(V_{Ecf})
marker locus	genetic correlation	maternal effects (V_{Em})
SNP	positive vs. negative	familial trait
linkage map	correlation	evolution
		artificial, natural selection
		selection response
		selection differential

Thinking Analytically

Quantitative genetics deals with important but complex issues. Some of the concepts used in the analysis of quantitative traits are subtle. Throughout the chapter, clear and precise thinking is required. To sort out the basis for a quantitative trait, it is important to define the contribution of several different factors. These factors can include the environment as well as multiple genes that themselves may or may not interact. Central to the analysis of a quantitative trait is identifying the degree to which variation in a phenotype can be associated with one or more of these factors. Consequently, understanding how variation is measured and used is of the utmost importance in understanding quantitative genetics.

First, gain a solid understanding of the terms used and the concepts they convey. Geneticists have developed a substantial conceptual framework in which to consider quantitative traits. Some concepts are easy to misunderstand, and to understand what something *is*, it is often important to define what it *is not*. For example, the idea of heritability has important qualifications and limitations. Heritability is a measure of the *proportion of phenotypic variance* that results from genetic differences. It is *not* a measure of the extent to which a trait is genetic, or what proportion of an individual's phenotype is genetic. It is also not fixed for a particular trait or a measurement of genetic differences between populations. The concepts underlying quantitative genetics have significant utility, but only if they are correctly and clearly applied.

Second, concentrate on understanding the statistical methods that are used to analyze data on quantitative traits. Your understanding should consist of more than just knowledge of how to crunch numbers by plugging them into an equation. You need to get a feel for what a statistic tells you about a data set.

Third, relate how measurements are made and analyzed to the concepts that have been developed to explain the inheritance of quantitative traits. For example, relate a measurement of heritability to a selection response. Then explain how you would achieve a particular breeding objective through selection. By doing this, you will obtain a better understanding of the power and utility of quantitative genetics.

Questions for Practice

Multiple-Choice Questions

1. Which of the following describes the trait of coat color in mice?
   a. continuous trait
   b. discontinuous trait
   c. polygenic trait
   d. quantitative trait
   e. both b and c

2. What can generally be said about quantitative traits such as crop yield, birth weight, blood pressure, or number of eggs laid?
   a. They are intractable to molecular genetics.
   b. They are multifactorial.
   c. They are discontinuous.
   d. They are not heritable, because they are polygenic.

3. The purpose of a quantitative genetic analysis of a trait is
   a. to determine whether genes or the environment control a trait.
   b. to determine the best breeding strategy to retain a trait.
   c. to determine how much of the phenotypic variation associated with a trait in a population is due to genetic variation and how much is due to environmental variation.
   d. to determine whether a trait is controlled by nature versus nurture.

4. The description of a population in terms of the number of individuals that display varying degrees of expression of a character or range of phenotypes is a
   a. polygraph.
   b. polynomial.
   c. normal distribution.
   d. frequency distribution.

5. The general expression for the binomial expansion is
   a. $(p + q)^n$.
   b. $(a^2 + b^2)$.
   c. $(a + b^2)$.
   d. $a^2 + 2ab + b^2$.

6. Which *two* of the following statements accurately describe the genetic concept of variance?
   a. It is a reflection of the accuracy of an estimated measurement.
   b. It is a measure of how much a set of individual measurements is spread out around the mean.
   c. It is the average value of a set of measurements.
   d. It is equal to $(\Sigma x_i/n)$.
   e. It is equal to $\dfrac{\Sigma(x_i - \bar{x})^2}{n - 1}$.

7. Heritability is
   a. the proportion of a population's phenotype that is attributable to genetic factors.
   b. the proportion of a population's phenotypic variation that is attributable to genetic factors.
   c. the degree to which family members resemble one another.
   d. the degree to which a continuous trait is controlled by genetic factors.

8. The proportion of the phenotypic variance that consists of genetic variance, additive or otherwise, is called
   a. heritability.
   b. broad-sense heritability.
   c. narrow-sense heritability.
   d. phenotypic variance derived from genotype-by-environment interactions.

9. The narrow-sense heritability of a trait is determined to be very close to 1.0. Which of the following inferences can be made?
   a. The trait will be difficult to select for.
   b. The trait can be readily selected for.
   c. Most of the phenotypic variance results from additive genetic variance.
   d. Most of the phenotypic variance results from environmental variance.
   e. both a and c
   f. both b and c

10. In a population of chickens raised under controlled conditions, body weight is negatively correlated with egg production but positively correlated with egg weight. Because of market conditions, a farmer is interested in producing lots of small eggs. Which selection strategy might be beneficial?
    a. Select for smaller hens.
    b. Select for larger hens.

11. Which of the following statements is true?
    a. Traits shared by family members show high heritability.
    b. Artificial and natural selection can occur in a genetically uniform population.
    c. If heritability is high in each of two populations and the populations differ markedly in a trait, the populations are genetically different.
    d. The selection response depends on (1) the proportion of genetic variance that results from additive genetic variance and (2) the difference between the mean phenotypes of the selected parents and the mean phenotype of the unselected population.

Answers: 1e, 2b, 3c, 4d, 5a, 6b, e, 7b, 8b, 9f, 10a, 11d

Thought Questions

1. Assume that mature fruit weight in pumpkins is a quantitative trait. In the following experiment, environmental factors (weather, soil, etc.) are uniform. Two pumpkin varieties, both of which produce fruit with a mean weight of 20 lb, are crossed. The F_1 produces 20-lb pumpkins. The F_2 plants, however, give the following results:

Mean fruit wt. (lb)	5	12.5	20	27.5	35
Number of plants	19	82	119	79	21

   Explain these results: Postulate how many genes are involved and how much each contributes to fruit weight.

2. Distinguish between heritability, broad-sense heritability, and narrow-sense heritability. In what ways can the latter two quantities be measured, and how can they be put to use by plant and animal breeders?

3. What statistics from a regression analysis are used to estimate narrow-sense heritability?

4. What sources contribute to the phenotypic variance associated with a quantitative trait?

5. Distinguish between a genetic correlation and a phenotypic correlation. In particular, address how a phenotypic correlation might exist when the trait is, or is not, influenced by a common set of genes.

6. A positive correlation probably exists between alcohol consumption and the number of Baptist ministers, but these are unlikely to be causally related. What other correlations are likely to be true, but demonstrate that correlations (whether positive or negative) do not imply a cause and effect? Why is a correlation not the same thing as an identity?

7. Defend each of the following statements:
   a. Broad-sense heritability does not indicate the extent to which a trait is genetic.
   b. Heritability does not indicate what proportion of an individual's phenotype is genetic.

   c. Heritability is not fixed for a trait.
   d. If heritability is high in two populations, and the populations differ markedly in a particular trait, one cannot assume that the populations are genetically different.
   e. Familial traits do not necessarily have high heritability.

8. If a population is phenotypically homogeneous for a particular trait, can you predict whether it has a high narrow-sense heritability? If not, what additional information would you need?

9. Why is calculating narrow-sense heritability values for some quantitative human traits especially difficult?

10. Distinguish between a selection differential and a selection response.

11. The mean height in two separate populations A and B is identical and is 5 feet 8 inches. The variance in population A is 14 inches, while the variance in population B is 3 inches. In which population would a 6-foot-tall person be more uncommon?

12. In a single population, is it likely that artificial selection will be equally effective at producing changes in three different traits? Why or why not?

Thought Questions for Media

After reviewing the media on the *iGenetics* website, try to answer these questions.

1. In the *Polygene Hypothesis for Wheat Kernel Color* animation, a cross of wheat with red kernels to wheat with white kernels gave wheat with pink kernels. Why does this suggest that this trait shows incomplete dominance?

2. What data given in the animation allow one to rule out incomplete dominance as an explanation for the results illustrated in the animation?

3. An alternate explanation for the results illustrated in the animation was that two independently assorting genes controlled wheat kernel color. Why was this explanation also ruled out?

4. In polygenic inheritance, what is a contributing allele? What is a noncontributing allele? How many contributing alleles can be present at one gene? How many contributing alleles can be present in one organism?

5. How does the explanation of two independently assorting genes with contributing and noncontributing alleles differ from the simpler explanation of two independently assorting genes?

6. Explain why, even though a contributing allele contributes a defined amount of pigment to the red color of the wheat kernel, wheat kernel color still appears to show continuous variation.

Solutions to Text Questions and Problems

22.1   *Answer:* When given a series of data, a good first step is to graph the data. Determine the minimum and maximum values, and then create histograms for each series of data using different bin sizes (e.g., by 1, by 2, by 5, etc.) to get a feel for the distribution of the data. Some sample histograms follow, along with notes on interpretation and the sources of the original data. Many times data from a particular sample do not appear to have a bell-shaped distribution characteristic of a quantitative trait. However, if we know that we are dealing with a quantitative trait, we often assume that they are normally distributed so that we can apply certain statistical techniques in analyzing the data.

a.

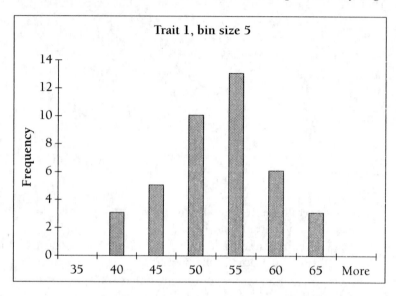

These data appear to be normally distributed, so they are representative of phenotypic data we would see for a quantitative trait. In fact, these are 40 sample values taken from a normal distribution with $\mu = 50$ and $s^2 = 5$.

b.

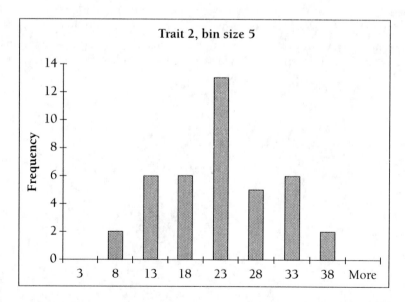

These data appear to have a more pronounced peak in the middle, with no "shoulders" next to the peak like those seen in Question 22.1(a). We might conclude that these data are not representative of a quantitative trait. In fact these data are 10 sample values from a normal distribution with $\mu = 10$ and $s^2 = 2$, 20 values from $\mu = 20$ and $s^2 = 2$, and 10 values from $\mu = 30$ and $s^2 = 2$. This is what we expect to see from a simple additive Mendelian character with some environmental variance.

c.

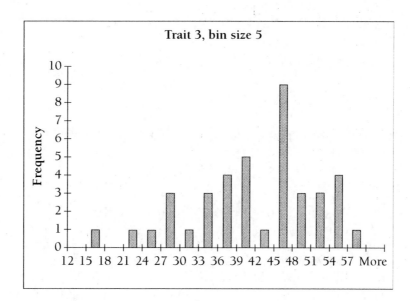

These data have a strong peak, but they do not have the characteristic shape of a normal distribution. You can see that there are no shoulders to the peak and that the peak trails off to the left, but not to the right. In fact, these data include 10 sample values from a normal distribution with $\mu = 25$ and $s^2 = 5$, 20 values from $\mu = 42$ and $s^2 = 5$, and 10 values from $\mu = 55$ and $s^2 = 5$, something we expect to see from a trait showing simple Mendelian inheritance with a small degree of dominance and substantial environmental variance.

22.2   *Answer:*

a. The mean of a sample is obtained by summing all the individual values and dividing by the total number of values. The mean head width is $25.21/8 = 3.15$ cm, and the mean wing length is $281.7/8 = 35.21$ cm.

The standard deviation equals the square root of the variance (s^2). The variance is computed by summing the squares of the differences between each measurement and the mean value, and dividing this sum by the number of measurements minus 1. One has

$$s_{\text{head width}} = \sqrt{s^2} = \sqrt{\frac{\Sigma(x_i - \bar{x})^2}{n-1}} = \sqrt{\frac{1.70}{7}} = \sqrt{0.24} = 0.49 \text{ cm}$$

$$s_{\text{wing length}} = \sqrt{s^2} = \sqrt{\frac{\Sigma(x_i - \bar{x})^2}{n-1}} = \sqrt{\frac{413.35}{7}} = \sqrt{59.05} = 7.68 \text{ cm}$$

b. The correlation coefficient, r, is calculated from the covariance, cov, of two sets of data. Let head width be represented by x and wing length be represented by y. r is defined as

$$r = \frac{\text{cov}_{xy}}{s_x s_y} = \frac{\dfrac{\Sigma x_i y_i - n\bar{x}\bar{y}}{n-1}}{s_x s_y}$$

The first factor ($\Sigma x_i y_i$) is obtained by taking the sum of the products of the individual measurements of head width and wing length for each duck. The next factor is the product of the number of individuals and the means of these two sets of measurements. The difference between these values is then divided by $(n-1)$ and then by the products of the standard deviations of each measurement. One has

$$r = \frac{\dfrac{913.50 - 8 \times 3.15 \times 35.21}{7}}{0.49 \times 7.68} = \frac{3.74}{3.76} = 0.99$$

c. Head width and wing length show a strong positive correlation, nearly 1.0. This means that ducks with larger heads will almost always have longer wings, and ducks with smaller heads will almost always have shorter wings.

22.3   *Answer:* The degree of phenotypic variability is related to the degree of genetic variability. Since each pure-breeding parent is homozygous for the genes (however many there are) controlling the size character, the variation seen within parental lines is due only to the environmental variation present. A cross of two pure-breeding strains will generate an F_1 heterozygous for those loci controlling the size trait, but genetically as homogeneous as each of the parents. Therefore, the only variation we would expect to see in the F_1 is from the environment, and it should show no greater variability than the parents.

22.4   *Answer:*

a. Since the cross is *AA BB* × *aa bb*, the F_1 genotype will be *Aa Bb*. Since capital-letter alleles determine height additively, and individuals with four capital-letter alleles have a height of 50 cm, while individuals with no capital-letter alleles have a height of 30 cm, each capital-letter allele appears to confer $(50 - 30)/4 = 5$ cm of height over the 30-cm base. *Aa Bb* individuals with two capital-letter alleles should have an intermediate height of 40 cm.

b. Any individuals with two capital-letter alleles will show a height of 40 cm. Thus, *Aa Bb*, *AA bb*, and *aa BB* individuals will be 40 cm high.

c. In the F_2, ¹⁄₁₆ of the progeny are *AA bb*, ⁴⁄₁₆ are *Aa Bb*, and ¹⁄₁₆ are *aa BB*. Thus, ⁶⁄₁₆ = ³⁄₈ of the progeny will be 40 cm high.

d. In answering this question, we have assumed that the *A* and *B* loci assort independently and that each locus and each allele contribute equally to the phenotype.

22.5   *Answer:* The F_1 will have the genotype *Aa Bb Cc* and so have a weight of $3 + (3 \times 0.5) = 4.5$ lb. The F_2 is expected to show a distribution of different weights. There are several ways to approach this problem. One way to predict the sizes and frequencies of these weights is to use a Punnett square. This is impractical for even four loci, so another is to use the seven coefficients of the binomial expansion $(a + b)^6$ as shown in the first solved problem at the end of the chapter.

These coefficients predict that ¹⁄₆₄ = 3 lb, ⁶⁄₆₄ = 3.5 lb, ¹⁵⁄₆₄ = 4 lb, ²⁰⁄₆₄ = 4.5 lb, ¹⁵⁄₆₄ = 5 lb, ⁶⁄₆₄ = 5.5 lb, and ¹⁄₆₄ = 6 lb. The facing page shows still another approach, a branch diagram:

$Aa \times Aa$	$Bb \times Bb$	$Cc \times Cc$	Proportion	# Capital-Letter Alleles	Weight
		¼CC →	1/64	6	6 lb
	¼BB	½Cc →	2/64	5	5.5 lb
		¼cc →	1/64	4	5 lb
		¼CC →	2/64	5	5.5 lb
¼AA	½Bb	½Cc →	4/64	4	5 lb
		¼cc →	2/64	3	4.5 lb
		¼CC →	1/64	4	5 lb
	¼bb	½Cc →	2/64	3	4.5 lb
		¼cc →	1/64	2	4 lb
		¼CC →	2/64	5	5.5 lb
	¼BB	½Cc →	4/64	4	5 lb
		¼cc →	2/64	3	4.5 lb
		¼CC →	4/64	4	5 lb
½Aa	½Bb	½Cc →	8/64	3	4.5 lb
		¼cc →	4/64	2	4 lb
		¼CC →	2/64	3	4.5 lb
	¼bb	½Cc →	4/64	2	4 lb
		¼cc →	2/64	1	3.5 lb
		¼CC →	1/64	4	5 lb
	¼BB	½Cc →	2/64	3	4.5 lb
		¼cc →	1/64	2	4 lb
		¼CC →	2/64	3	4.5 lb
¼aa	½Bb	½Cc →	4/64	2	4 lb
		¼cc →	2/64	1	3.5 lb
		¼CC →	1/64	2	4 lb
	¼bb	½Cc →	2/64	1	3.5 lb
		¼cc →	1/64	0	3 lb

Add up the proportion of individuals with the same numbers of capital-letter alleles to obtain:

$1/64 \rightarrow 6$ lb

$6/64 \rightarrow 5.5$ lb

$15/64 \rightarrow 5$ lb

$20/64 \rightarrow 4.5$ lb

$15/64 \rightarrow 4$ lb

$6/64 \rightarrow 3.5$ lb

$1/64 \rightarrow 3$ lb

22.6 *Answer:* In each case, one needs to consider the maximum and minimum number of capital-letter alleles that can be contributed to the progeny, noting that each contributes 0.5 lb above the 3-lb base weight.

   a. *AA Bb CC × aa Bb Cc.* The gamete from the maternal parent with the most capital-letter alleles would have a genotype of *ABC* and the gamete with the most capita-letter alleles from the paternal parent would have a genotype of *aBC*. Therefore, the heaviest progeny would have squash weights of 5.5 lb. The gamete genotypes with the least numbers of capital-letter alleles are *AbC* and *abc*, making the progeny with the smallest squashes weigh 4 lb.

   b. *AA bb Cc × Aa BB cc.* The largest offspring squash weights will come from a union of *AbC* and *ABc* gametes, giving the progeny 5-lb squashes. The smallest offspring squash weights will come from a union of *Abc* and *aBc* gametes, giving a progeny with 4-lb squashes.

   c. *aa BB cc × AA BB cc.* The only gametes that can be produced are *aBc* and *ABc*, so three capital-letter alleles will be contributed to each progeny. The progeny squash weights will all be 4.5 lb.

22.7 *Answer:*

   a. The cross *AA BB CC* × *aa bb cc* will produce all *Aa Bb Cc* progeny. The three capital-letter alleles will add $3 \times 2 = 6$ cm to the 2-cm base height, giving a total of 8 cm.

   b. A Punnett square, branch diagram, or binomial expansion can be used to find the following distribution of heights:

$$1/64 \to 14 \text{ cm}$$
$$6/64 \to 12 \text{ cm}$$
$$15/64 \to 10 \text{ cm}$$
$$20/64 \to 8 \text{ cm}$$
$$15/64 \to 6 \text{ cm}$$
$$6/64 \to 4 \text{ cm}$$
$$1/64 \to 2 \text{ cm}$$

   c. $\frac{1}{64}$ are 2 cm and $\frac{1}{64}$ are 14 cm, so the answer is $\frac{2}{64}$.

   d. Plants must be homozygous for all loci involved in order to breed true. If we do not specify a height, then all homozygous genotypes fulfill this requirement and the answer is just the proportion of homozygous genotypes. There are eight completely homozygous genotypes, and each occurs at a frequency of $\frac{1}{64}$, so the overall proportion of true-breeding F_2 individuals is $\frac{1}{8}$.

22.8 *Answer:* Assume for this problem that the *A* locus shows dominance, and that the *AA* and *Aa* genotypes add 4 cm to height, while the *aa* genotype adds nothing.

   a. The cross *AA BB CC* × *aa bb cc* will produce all *Aa Bb Cc* progeny. The *Aa* genotype will add 4 cm to height and the other two capital-letter alleles will add $2 \times 2 = 4$ cm to the 2-cm base height, giving a total of 10 cm.

   b. A branch diagram is the easiest way to answer this problem. If you construct one as in Question 22.5, you will see that the phenotypes of the groups starting with *AA* or *Aa* are the same, but that the *Aa* group has twice as many. All like phenotypes can be combined to find the following distribution of heights:

$$3/64 \to 14 \text{ cm}$$
$$12/64 \to 12 \text{ cm}$$
$$19/64 \to 10 \text{ cm}$$
$$16/64 \to 8 \text{ cm}$$
$$9/64 \to 6 \text{ cm}$$
$$4/64 \to 4 \text{ cm}$$
$$1/64 \to 2 \text{ cm}$$

   Note the skewed distribution compared to Question 22.7(b).

   c. $\frac{1}{64}$ are 2 cm and $\frac{3}{64}$ are 14 cm, so the answer is $\frac{1}{16}$.

   d. Even though we have dominance, the answer is still $\frac{1}{8}$, the same as Question 22.7(d), because individuals still need to be homozygous to breed true.

22.9 *Answer:* Use the clue that $\frac{1}{64}$ of the F_2 progeny show either extreme trait. Note that (as in Questions 22.5–22.8) in an F_2 resulting from a trihybrid cross, the proportion of one kind of homozygote is $\frac{1}{64}$. This confirms that three allelic pairs control this quantitative trait. The completely homozygous 10-mm plant would have six lowercase alleles at three loci, *aa bb cc*, while the completely homozygous 30-mm plant would have six capital-letter alleles at three loci, *AA BB CC*. If each capital-letter allele contributes $\frac{1}{6}$ of the 20-mm difference between the two extremes, or $\frac{20}{6} =$ 3.33 mm, the F_1 trihybrid individual would be 20 mm [= 10 mm base + 3 × (3.33 mm/capital-letter allele) = 20 mm]. Thus, the trait fits a model in which three capital-letter alleles contribute additively to this quantitative trait.

   If an F_1 plant is crossed to the 30-mm parent, one would have *Aa Bb Cc* × *AA BB CC*. This cross would produce $\frac{1}{8}$ each of *Aa Bb Cc, Aa Bb CC, AA Bb Cc, Aa BB Cc, AA BB Cc, AA Bb CC, Aa BB CC,* and *AA BB CC*. Thus, there will be $\frac{1}{8}$ that are 30 mm long, $\frac{1}{8}$ that are 20 mm long, $\frac{3}{8}$ that are 23.33 mm long, and $\frac{3}{8}$ that are 26.67 mm long.

22.10   *Answer:* Internode length shows the characteristics of a quantitative trait. These characteristics include F_1 progeny that show a phenotype intermediate between the two parental phenotypes, and an F_2 showing a range of phenotypes with extremes in the range of the two parents, some of which have all the original parental alleles.

22.11   *Answer:* Assume that the four pairs of alleles are equally responsible for the 16-dm height increase, each allele contributing 2 dm, and that the loci assort independently.

    a. A cross of *AA BB CC DD* × *aa bb cc dd* will produce *Aa Bb Cc Dd* progeny. With four capital-letter alleles, the F_1 height will be 18 dm.

    b. i. *Aa BB cc dd* × *Aa bb Cc dd*. The minimum number of capital-letter alleles contributed to the progeny would be one, and the maximum number of capital-letter alleles contributed to the progeny would be four. The height range would be 12 to 18 dm.

      ii. *aa BB cc dd* × *Aa Bb Cc dd*. At least one and at most four capital-letter alleles would be contributed to the progeny. The height range would be 12 to 18 dm.

      iii. *AA BB Cc DD* × *aa BB cc Dd*. At least four and at most six capital-letter alleles would be contributed to the progeny. The height range would be 18 to 22 dm.

      iv. *Aa Bb Cc Dd* × *Aa bb Cc Dd*. A minimum of none and a maximum of seven capital-letter alleles would be contributed to the progeny. The height range would be 10 to 24 dm.

22.12   *Answer:* In each of cases A, B, and C, both 14-dm parents must have two capital-letter alleles. Consideration of the possible arrangement of these alleles leads to the solution of each case.

Case A: For two 14-dm plants to give rise only to more 14-dm plants, each of the plants must be homozygous for one of the capital-letter alleles. Both plants could be homozygous for the same capital-letter allele (e.g., *AA bb cc dd* × *AA bb cc dd*), or each could be homozygous for a different capital-letter allele (e.g., *AA bb cc dd* × *aa bb CC dd*). In either case, the progeny plants would have two capital-letter alleles and be 14 dm high. Distinguishing between these two alternatives could be accomplished by intermating the progeny: All 14-dm offspring would be seen with the former, while 10- to 14-dm offspring would be seen with the latter.

Case B: The 1 four capital-letter alleles:4 three capital-letter alleles:6 two capital-letter alleles:4 one capital-letter allele:1 no capital-letter allele proportions reflect the coefficients in the binomial expansion of $(a + b)^4$. This result suggests that the parents were heterozygous at the two (identical or different) loci (e.g., *Aa Bb cc dd* × *Aa Bb cc dd* or *Aa Bb cc dd* × *aa bb Cc Dd*).

Case C: The 1 one capital-letter allele:2 two capital-letter alleles:1 three capital-letter allele proportions are the coefficients in the binomial expansion of $(a + b)^2$. One would expect this ratio if one of the parents were homozygous at one locus and the other heterozygous at two loci. For example, the parents could be *aa BB cc dd* × *Aa Bb cc dd* or *aa BB cc dd* × *Aa bb Cc dd*.

Since each capital-letter allele contributes 2 dm, plants would have to have at least five capital-letter alleles to be taller than 18 dm. To be taller than 18 dm is not possible in case A (the maximum is four), case B (the maximum possible is four), or case C (the maximum possible is four). In order to produce a plant 18 dm tall, we would need to have at least one 16-dm plant and the right 14-dm plant to mate it with.

22.13   *Answer:* In order to see transgressive segregation, at least one of the parents must have some alleles that are "opposite" in effect of the expected direction. For example, imagine we are looking at height. If we assume there are six loci that contribute to height, and that capital-letter alleles contribute a 5-cm increase over a base height of 1 meter, a cross between an *AA BB CC DD EE FF* individual (160 cm) and an *aa bb cc dd ee ff* individual (100 cm) will produce an F_2 with extreme individuals only as tall and as short as the original parents. If, however, the original parents have the genotypes *AA BB CC DD EE ff* (150 cm) and *aa bb cc dd ee FF* (110 cm), segregation in the F_2 can produce an *AA BB CC DD EE FF* genotype (160 cm) and an *aa bb cc dd ee ff* genotype (100 cm), which are taller and shorter than the original lines used. In this case, the taller parent has "shorter" alleles at one locus, and vice versa.

A more extreme case to consider is where the parents have the same phenotype, but produce segregating offspring. Imagine, for example, if an *AA BB CC dd ee ff* (130-cm) individual were crossed with an *aa bb cc DD EE FF* individual (130 cm). Their F_1 offspring would again be 130 cm (*Aa Bb Cc Dd Ee Ff*), but in the F_2, individuals from 160 cm (*AA BB CC DD EE FF*) to 100 cm (*aa bb cc dd ee ff*) could be seen!

22.14   *Answer:* The F$_1$ is *A/a B/b C/c D/d E/e* and so it is greyish-brown. The F$_2$ phenotypes are determined by the number of capital-letter alleles contributed from each F$_1$ parent. The easiest way to proceed is to look for the proportions of individuals with the light tan pigmentation (three or four capital-letter alleles) and the whitish-blue pigmentation (zero or one capital-letter alleles), and the proportion of greyish-brown offspring will be the rest. Start off by determining the chance of obtaining zero, one, two, or three capital-letter alleles in a gamete from each F$_1$ parent and then ascertain how these combinations make the desired genotypes.

Since the parent is heterozygous at all five loci, the chance of obtaining any specified set of five alleles in one gamete is $(\frac{1}{2})^5$. The chance of obtaining a particular number of capital-letter alleles from an F$_1$ is the number of ways in which that number of alleles can be obtained, multiplied by $(\frac{1}{2})^5$. There is one way to obtain zero capital-letter alleles, five ways to obtain one capital-letter allele, 10 ways of obtaining two capital-letter alleles, and 10 ways of obtaining three capital-letter alleles. With this information, we can tabulate the ways in which the progeny classes we are interested in can be formed:

F$_1$ Gamete #1		F$_1$ Gamete #2		F$_2$ Progeny		
Capital-Letter Alleles	Gamete Fraction	Capital-Letter Alleles	Gamete Fraction	Capital-Letter Alleles	F$_2$ Fraction	Phenotype
0	$(\frac{1}{2})^5$	0	$(\frac{1}{2})^5$	0	$(\frac{1}{2})^{10}$	whitish-blue
0	$(\frac{1}{2})^5$	1	$5(\frac{1}{2})^5$	1	$5(\frac{1}{2})^{10}$	whitish-blue
1	$5(\frac{1}{2})^5$	0	$(\frac{1}{2})^5$	1	$5(\frac{1}{2})^{10}$	whitish-blue
0	$(\frac{1}{2})^5$	2	$10(\frac{1}{2})^5$	2	$10(\frac{1}{2})^{10}$	light tan
1	$5(\frac{1}{2})^5$	1	$5(\frac{1}{2})^5$	2	$25(\frac{1}{2})^{10}$	light tan
2	$10(\frac{1}{2})^5$	0	$(\frac{1}{2})^5$	2	$10(\frac{1}{2})^{10}$	light tan
0	$(\frac{1}{2})^5$	3	$10(\frac{1}{2})^5$	3	$10(\frac{1}{2})^{10}$	light tan
1	$5(\frac{1}{2})^5$	2	$10(\frac{1}{2})^5$	3	$50(\frac{1}{2})^{10}$	light tan
2	$10(\frac{1}{2})^5$	1	$5(\frac{1}{2})^5$	3	$50(\frac{1}{2})^{10}$	light tan
3	$10(\frac{1}{2})^5$	0	$(\frac{1}{2})^5$	3	$10(\frac{1}{2})^{10}$	light tan

Among the F$_2$, $11(\frac{1}{2})^{10} = 11/1{,}024$ will be whitish-blue and $165(\frac{1}{2})^{10} = 165/1{,}024$ will be light tan. The remaining $[1-176(\frac{1}{2})^{10}] = 848/1{,}024$ will be greyish-brown.

Another method to use to solve this problem is to use the coefficients of the binomial expansion to determine the proportion of progeny with different numbers of capital-letter and lowercase alleles. Let n = total number of alleles, s = number of capital-letter alleles, t = number of lowercase alleles, a = chance of obtaining a capital-letter allele, b = chance of obtaining a lowercase allele, and $x! = (x)(x-1)(x-2) \ldots (1)$, with $0! = 1$. Then the chance P of obtaining progeny with a specified number of each type of allele is given by:

$$P(s,t) = \frac{n!}{s!t!} a^s b^t$$

$$P(0,10) = \frac{10!}{0!10!}\left(\frac{1}{2}\right)^0\left(\frac{1}{2}\right)^{10} = \frac{1}{1{,}024}$$

$$P(1,9) = \frac{10!}{1!9!}\left(\frac{1}{2}\right)^1\left(\frac{1}{2}\right)^9 = \frac{10}{1{,}024}$$

$$\left. \right\} \frac{11}{1{,}024} \text{ whitish-blue}$$

$$P(2,8) = \frac{10!}{2!8!}\left(\frac{1}{2}\right)^2\left(\frac{1}{2}\right)^8 = \frac{45}{1{,}024}$$

$$P(3,7) = \frac{10!}{3!7!}\left(\frac{1}{2}\right)^3\left(\frac{1}{2}\right)^7 = \frac{120}{1{,}024}$$

$$\left. \right\} \frac{165}{1{,}024} \text{ light tan}$$

$$1 - \frac{11 + 165}{1{,}024} = \frac{848}{1{,}024} \text{ greyish-brown}$$

22.15   *Answer:*

a. From the data that are given, it appears that some proportion of cases of AD can be attributed to genetic factors. Multiple genes that increase the risk for AD have been identified, some of which appear to act in a dose-dependent manner. Thus, it could be that a number of different genes contribute to the onset of AD, with some having a greater contribution than others. This is somewhat similar to how polygenic traits control a phenotype since there, alleles at multiple genes contribute in an additive, dose-dependent fashion to the phenotype.

b. Consider two explanations: First, if AD can be caused by environmental agents, mutation, and/or a combination of both environmental agents and mutation, the presence of AD in both twins could be due to the presence of one or more abnormal alleles in both and/or the exposure of both twins to adverse environmental conditions. The presence of AD in only one twin may be due to differences in the exposure of that twin to a contributing or causative environmental agent(s). Second, the presence of a particular allele or a specific mutation may only increase the risk of disease, and not determine its occurrence, since an allele's penetrance may be strongly affected by the environment. In the case of AD, the environmental factors may not be clear-cut or even small in number. There may be multiple environmental factors, some of which may be complex or subtle.

22.16   *Answer:* In neither of these cases is any information provided about the environments in which the twins were raised. While it would initially appear that there is some genetic component in each case, there is no way to evaluate the role of environment. It could be that the identical twins sampled in each case were raised in an identical environment, and this could account for the greater similarity in smoking behavior and IQ results for monozygotic twins than for dizygotic twins.

22.17   *Answer:*

a. The broad-sense heritability of a trait represents the proportion of the phenotypic variance in a particular population that results from genetic differences among individuals, while the narrow-sense heritability measures only the proportion of the phenotypic variance in that population that results from additive genetic variance.

Broad-sense heritability

$$= \text{genetic variance/phenotypic variance} = V_G/V_P$$
$$= (4.2 + 1.6 + 0.3)/(4.2 + 1.6 + 0.3 + 2.7 + 0.0)$$
$$= 6.1/8.8 = 0.69$$

Narrow-sense heritability

$$= \text{additive genetic variance/phenotypic variance}$$
$$= V_A/V_P$$
$$= 4.2/8.8 = 0.48$$

b. About 69% of the phenotypic variation in leaf width observed in this population is due to genetic differences among individuals, so we would expect offspring to strongly resemble parents. Only 48% of the phenotypic variation is due to additive genetic variation, so there are some loci contributing to the trait that show a degree of dominance. Because the phenotypic variation due to additive genetic variation represents the part of the phenotypic variance that responds to natural selection in a predictable manner, we would expect selection to be able to change the mean phenotype in the population if pressure were applied.

22.18   *Answer:* For wildcats residing in similar environments, phenotypic variation in size would result primarily from variation in genetic differences between the cats and the differences resulting from genotype-by-environment interaction. For house cats residing in similar environments, one could make a similar argument. If domesticated cats descended from a group of wildcats, it is likely that they would have less genetic variation than the wildcats. Therefore, one might expect that wildcats would be more likely to exhibit a higher heritability. However, remember that heritability is not fixed for a trait; it depends both on the genetic makeup and the specific environment of the population. In this question, the wildcats are not placed in a domesticated environment, nor are the house cats placed in the wild. Therefore, it is not possible to make a prediction solely based on expectations of genetic differences. Recall also the text example of genetically variable mice raised on different diets in a controlled environment (see Chapter 22, p. 665). In that example, both groups of mice, even though they were genetically variable, exhibited a high heritability because the environmental differences were kept to a minimum. If you interpreted the value of heritability for body weight without considering the design of the experiment, you might have concluded that the two groups of mice were genetically different. Just as one needs to be careful in drawing general conclusions from heritability data, one needs to be careful about making predictions about heritability based on prior knowledge of genetic variation or environment. Both broad-sense and narrow-sense heritability are specific to a particular population in a particular environment, so any categorical response to this question is likely to have many exceptions.

22.19   *Answer:* SHR rats will continue to respond to salt by developing hypertension. Since the strain is inbred, any variation in blood pressure will result from the amount of exposure to salt, and not from genetic variation. Therefore, heritability for this population will be zero. Similarly, the inbred TIS rats would also have a heritability of zero (and retain a low blood pressure).

22.20   *Answer:* Heritability is a measurement of the genetic variance of a *particular* population in a *specific* environment. Heritability is not fixed for a specific trait. It depends on genetic makeup *as well as* the specific environment of the population in which it is measured. Consequently, heritability cannot be used to make inferences about the basis for the differences between two distinct populations. Since the environmental conditions on the two farms differ, the heritability calculated for a population in Kansas cannot be used to infer the future performance of the same strain in another environment. The yield of TK138 grown in Poland would most likely be different than when grown in Kansas, perhaps even lower than the yield of the UG334 variety.

22.21   *Answer:*

a. The narrow-sense heritability of the number of triradii will equal the slope, b, of the regression line of the mean offspring phenotype on the mean parental phenotype.

$$b = \frac{COV_{xy}}{(s_x)^2} = \frac{\dfrac{\Sigma xy_i - n\overline{xy}}{n-1}}{\dfrac{\Sigma(x_i - \overline{x})^2}{n-1}} = \frac{\Sigma xy_i - n\overline{xy}}{\Sigma(x_i - \overline{x})^2}$$

For this data set, x is the mean number of triradii in the parents, and y is the mean number of triradii in the offspring. Using either a calculator or a spreadsheet or statistics program, you can find the following:

$\Sigma x_i = 111, \overline{x} = 11.1$

$\Sigma y_i = 108.5, \overline{y} = 10.85$

$\Sigma(x_i - \overline{x})^2 = 51.4$

$\Sigma x_i y_i = 1{,}257.5$

$$b = \frac{1257.5 - 10 \times 11.1 \times 10.85}{51.4} = \frac{53.15}{51.4} = 1.04$$

b. A slope of 1.04 indicates that additive genetic variation is responsible for essentially all of the observed variation in phenotype. Note that the estimate obtained for h^2 is greater than 1, showing that methods for estimating narrow-sense heritability can overestimate the amount of additive genetic variation among individuals.

22.22   *Answer:* Let x represent the height of the fathers and y represent the height of the sons.

a. Fathers: $\overline{x} = 71.9, s^2 = 11.61$

   Sons: $\overline{y} = 70.0, s^2 = 10.25$

b. One can calculate $\Sigma x_i y_i = 45{,}333$, so that

$$r = \frac{\text{cov}_{xy}}{s_x s_y} = \frac{\dfrac{\Sigma x_i y_i - n\overline{xy}}{n-1}}{\sqrt{(s_x)^2 (s_y)^2}}$$

$$r = \frac{\dfrac{45{,}333 - 9 \times 71.89 \times 70}{8}}{\sqrt{11.61 \times 10.25}} = \frac{5.29}{10.91} = 0.48$$

c. $b = \dfrac{\text{cov}_{xy}}{(s_x)^2} = \dfrac{5.375}{11.6} = 0.463$

When, as in this case, the mean phenotype of the offspring is regressed against the phenotype of only one parent, the estimate of narrow-sense heritability is $2b = 2(0.46) = 0.92$. Since h^2 is very close to 1, additive effects at the loci involved determine most of the phenotypic variation. Non-additive factors (genes with dominance, genes with epistasis, environmental factors) appear to contribute little to the phenotypic variation.

22.23 *Answer:* The selection differential (S) equals $14.3 - 9.7 = 4.6$ cm. The response to selection (R) equals $13 - 9.7 = 3.3$ cm. The narrow-sense heritability (h^2) equals $R/S = 3.3/4.6 = 0.72$.

22.24 *Answer:* In this example, there was $0.96 - 0.88 = 0.08$ g of change after one generation of selection. Thus, the response to selection (R) was 0.08 g. In this case the selection differential (S) is $1.02 - 0.88 = 0.14$ g. The narrow-sense heritability is $h^2 = 0.08/0.14 = 0.57$. Note that (a) under the assumption outlined in the first sentence of the question that all phenotypic variation is due to additive genetic variation, this would mean there is something wrong because h^2 should be 1; and (b) this is an estimate of h^2 derived from one midparent–offspring comparison—the more families that are included, the better the estimate of h^2!

22.25 *Answer:*

Selection response = narrow-sense heritability × selection differential

Selection response = 0.60×10 g = 6 g

22.26 *Answer:*

a. The narrow-sense heritability is given in the table here:

Selection Step	Line A		Line B	
	Number of Eggs	Egg Weight	Number of Eggs	Egg Weight
Initial Selection	0.145	0.50	0.184	0.50
F_1 Selection	0.095	0.17	0.075	0.33
F_2 Selection	0.051	0.17	0.066	0.25

b. The response changes because the selection process decreases the amount of genetic variation within the population.

c. Compared to the mean of traits in lines A and B, there is a 17% increase in the number of eggs produced and a 3.6% increase in egg weight.

d. When different lines are crossed, an increase due to heterosis, or heterozygote superiority, may be obtained (see Chapter 21, p. 636). If there are different alleles for a locus that contribute to increased egg production and size, it is possible that alternate alleles were selected for in the two lines. Combining these advantageous alleles across multiple loci could lead to further increases as well as decrease the effects of recessive, deleterious alleles.

22.27 *Answer:* A response to selection depends on (a) variation on which selection can act and (b) a high narrow-sense heritability so that the selected individuals produce similar offspring. The narrow-sense heritability for each of the traits is V_A/V_P: 0.165 for body length, 0.061 for antenna bristle number, and 0.144 for egg production. The amount of raw variation is also greatest for body length. Thus, body length will respond most to selection, and antenna bristle number will respond least to selection.

22.28 *Answer:* Assume that there are multiple loci that contribute equally to fruit weight and days to first flower. In order to recover the cultivated phenotype most quickly from selection after crossing it with the wild genotype, we would like to find the cross where most of the variation is due to additive effects. A quick way to assess this is to look at the phenotype of the F_1: If most of the variation is due to additive effects, the phenotype of the F_1 will be intermediate to both parents. If the F_1 is closer in phenotype to one parent or the other, this can be taken as an indicator that that parent harbors some nonadditive variation. Using this criterion for both traits, crosses 2 and 4 appear to be the best initial crosses to work with.

22.29 *Answer:* The strong narrow-sense heritability of both wool length and body size indicates that these traits will respond to selection. The negative correlation coefficient between wool length and body size indicates that if longer wool is selected for, you would expect that smaller body size will also be obtained.

22.30 *Answer:*

a. As described in the text, analyses in model experimental organisms such as *Drosophila* have suggested that findings from QTL analyses can be population dependent. Genetic and environmental heterogeneity may contribute to the size of a QTL's effect, so a QTL that explains 15% of the risk for diabetes in a particular population may not explain a similar amount of risk in a different population.

b. Two complementary approaches are possible. In one, candidate loci are chosen based on known or suggested function and then SNPs at these loci are tested for their association with disease. In the other, a genome-wide screen is performed: A panel of SNPs distributed throughout the genome is used as a set of DNA markers in association studies to identify segments of the genome where QTLs are located. Specific genes in these regions are then examined more closely for their association with disease.

22.31 *Answer:* To show that malt extract quality is a quantitative trait, first develop a standardized test that can be used to quantify the quality of malt extract from different barley strains. Then, follow the example of Emerson and East, (see text Chapter 22, pp. 660–661), when they demonstrated that ear length in corn is a quantitative genetic trait. Select or develop two pure-breeding or inbred strains of barley. When grown under the same conditions, each strain should display little intra-strain variation in malt extract quality, but the two strains should show considerable variation. Cross these two parental strains and then interbreed the F_1 plants to obtain an F_2. Examine the patterns of variation in the inbred parental strains, in the F_1, and in the F_2. Since the parental strains are inbred, variation within each parental strain should be due to environmental and not genetic effects. Variation in the F_1 and F_2 can arise from both genetic and environmental differences. If the quality of malt extract is a quantitative genetic trait, then: (1) the mean value of the quality of malt extract in the F_1 will be intermediate between the means of the two parental lines; (2) the mean value of the trait in the F_2 will be similar to the mean in the F_1; (3) the F_2 will show more variability than the F_1; and (4) the extreme phenotypes of the F_2 will be closer to the two parental values than will the extreme phenotypes of the F_1 and may even extend beyond the ranges seen in the two parental strains.

To identify QTL loci for malt extract quality, segments of the genome that are associated with phenotypic differences must be identified. For this purpose, plants with different combinations of segments from the parental strains are genotyped and then statistical methods are used to determine which genomic regions are correlated with phenotypic variation. Such plants can be obtained by using the F2, a backcross of the F1, or by developing recombinant inbred strains obtained from selfing of the F1. Individuals are split into groups based on a marker genotype and then evaluated to see whether the groups have similar or different mean malt extract quality values.

22.32 *Answer:*

a. Since the aim of QTL identification is to find segments of the genome associated with phenotypic differences between individuals, the first step in a typical QTL analysis is to develop inbred lines that have been selected for different phenotypes. These lines are crossed to generate an F_1 and then the F_1 is backcrossed, intercrossed to generate an F_2, or intercrossed and selfed to generate a series of recombinant inbred strains. Each member of the set of recombinant inbred strains that is generated in this way received different parts of its genome from the two original inbred lines. After the phenotypes and genotypes of these strains are determined, QTLs are identified by correlating the genotypic and phenotypic differences among the different recombinant inbred strains.

A doubled haploid line is a diploid line generated from a single haploid gamete. In this case, the gametes used to form doubled haploid lines are produced by an F_1 hybrid between two highly inbred, phenotypically different lines. In the F_1 hybrid, random crossing-over and independent assortment led to the production of recombinant gametes, each having a unique combination of chromosomal segments drawn from the two original inbred lines. Therefore, each doubled haploid line is a different type of recombinant between the two original inbred lines. What is critically important here is that each line is homozygous when it is formed, and so additional crosses to develop inbred recombinant lines are unnecessary. When doubled haploid lines are not used, inbred recombinant lines must be developed through many generations of backcrosses or intercrosses, which requires considerable additional time.

b. As shown in the following histogram, when the barley lines are grown in four different states, malting quality values from each state are continuously distributed across a range of values. Therefore, malting quality is a quantitative and not a qualitative trait.

Distribution of Malting Quality of 149 Recombinant Barley Lines

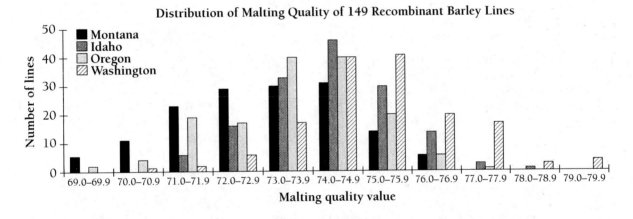

When the distributions of the same lines grown in four different states are compared, it is apparent that they have different means and variances (these data are quantified in text Table 22.B, p. 681, and discussed further in part **(e)**). Lines grown in Montana have a lower mean malting quality value than do lines grown in Washington, and lines grown in Idaho have a smaller variance than do lines grown in either Washington, Oregon, or Montana. Thus, we can infer that this trait also is affected by the environment.

c. Since the recombinant inbred lines were generated by doubling haploid gametes, each is homozygous for alleles at all loci. Therefore, it is not possible to select for genetic differences in the offspring of line L87, and so it is not possible to select for blight resistance or further enhance its malting quality phenotype. To develop a fungal resistance in strain L87, it should be crossed to a resistant barley strain, and the F_1 should be backcrossed to L87. Recombination in the F_1 will produce hybrids, some of which are resistant. Repeated backcrossing to L87 under selection for fungal resistance will lead to a strain that is close to L87 in its malting quality phenotype.

d. Here, doubled haploid lines were obtained by selfing the F_1, and haploid gametes were manipulated to undergo chromosome doubling. Since the lines result from doubling the chromosomes in a haploid cell, all the lines are homozygous. If the F_1 was *Aa Bb Cc* and the *A/a*, *B/b*, and *C/c* loci assort independently, the chance of obtaining a particular set of *n* (homozygous) alleles at these loci is $(1/2)^n$.

   i. $\frac{1}{2}$

   ii. 0 (Doubled haploids are homozygous for alleles at all loci.)

   iii. $\frac{1}{4}$

   iv. $\frac{1}{8}$

   v. 0

   vi. 0

e. The data show evidence of both genetic and environmental sources of phenotypic variance. The environment contributes to phenotypic variation since the mean, variance, and range of the malting quality values for the set of lines are similar in different environments. This is supported by an examination of the malting quality values of individual lines grown in different environments: no recombinant line gives identical malting quality values in all four environments. Support for a genetic contribution to phenotypic variance comes from the observation that most lines give values that are similar relative to the mean values seen in a particular environment. For example, most lines giving less than the mean malting quality value in one environment tend to give less than the mean malting quality value in all four environments. That some lines do not consistently follow this pattern (e.g., L51 is above the mean in Montana, but below the mean in the other three states, L126 is well above the mean in all states except Oregon, where it is well below the mean) suggests that there may also be covariance between genotype and environment.

22.33 *Answer:*

a. In this example, the lod score compares the probability that a marker is linked to the malting quality phenotype (with no recombination) to the probability that a marker is not linked to the malting quality phenotype. The lod score is the $\log_{10}$ of this ratio, so a lod score of 4 means that the odds are 10,000:1 in favor of linkage between the marker and the malting quality phenotype. A marker with a lod score of 4 does not prove that linkage exists between the marker and the trait, nor does it indicate that a quantitative trait locus (QTL) exists at the marker. However, it provides strong support that the marker is in a region containing a QTL that contributes the malting quality phenotype.

b. Most markers in the region between BCD351D and ABG472 show lod scores greater than 4, and there are three peaks in this region. This indicates that this region may harbor several QTLs for the malting quality phenotype. The WG1026B, ABR315, and BCD453B markers are all associated with peaks in this region, but other markers near these three markers also have lod scores over 4. Though this indicates that QTL loci are in this region, the markers associated with peaks do not necessarily identify different QTLs, nor does each peak necessarily correspond to a single QTL. When there is more than one QTL near a group of linked markers, the lod score peak may be wide, and the peak may not correspond to the location of the QTL.

c. Since the same lines were grown in different environments, differences between the plots may result from an interaction between genotype and environment. The shape of the plots is similar, so this does not alter the general interpretation of the location of QTLs for malting quality.

23

Molecular Evolution

Chapter Outline

Review of Key Terms, Symbols, and Concepts

In your own words, write a brief, precise definition of each term in the groups below. Check your definitions using the text. Then develop a concept map using the terms in each list.

1	2	3
molecular evolution	nucleotide substitution	molecular phylogeny
population, species	homologous proteins, genes	morphological phylogeny
gene	sequence alignment	evolutionary relationship
evolutionary time, history	computer algorithm	convergent evolution
population genetics	optimal alignment	phenotype
Hardy–Weinberg equilibrium	indel	phylogenetic tree
mutation vs. substitution	Jukes–Cantor model	branch
gene duplication	substitution rate	adjacent, internal, terminal nodes
gene conversion	evolutionary rate	outgroup
transposition	divergence time	horizontal gene transfer
unequal crossing-over	transition, transversion	rooted, unrooted trees
phylogenetic relationship	coding, noncoding sequence	taxa
natural selection	leader, trailer region	gene vs. species tree
multigene family	pseudogene	inferred tree
globin, myoglobin genes	synonymous site, codon	distance matrix
ancestral gene	nonsynonymous site, codon	parsimony
domain shuffling	mutation vs. substitution	unweighted pair group
exon shuffling	comparative genomics	method with arithmetic
internal duplication	genome project	averages (UPGMA)
exon, intron	codon usage bias	transformed distance, neighbor-
Bacteria, Archaea, Eukarya	stochastic factor	joining, maximum likelihood
	natural selection	methods
	diversifying selection	clustering
	McDonald–Kreitman test	informative site
	functional constraint	noninformative site
	major histocompatibility	tree of maximum parsimony
	complex (MHC)	bootstrap procedure test
	mitochondrial DNA	confidence level
	matriarchal lineage	tree of life
	error-prone replication	evolutionary domain
	proofreading ability	Eukarya
	molecular clock	Archaea
	molecular clock hypothesis	Bacteria
	relative rate test	endosymbiosis
		"out-of-Africa" theory
		"mitochondrial Eve"
		"Y-chromosome Adam"

Thinking Analytically

Perhaps the most striking element in the field of molecular evolution is the time scale in which the mechanisms of evolution operate. Almost throughout this text, we have considered genetic mechanisms that act over relatively short time frames. The replication of the genetic material, its transcription, and the production of gene products through translation occur in time scales that are on the order of seconds and minutes. Genetic crosses may take several generations, but even for organisms that have relatively long life spans, the time scales are on the order of years or tens of years. Molecular evolution occurs over many, many generations, and the time scales being considered are often on the order of tens of thousands to millions of years. In this space of time, much can happen. Some say that if you can think of it, nature has had time to try it. With genomes serving as historical records of molecular evolution, it may be possible to find evidence of it as well. Having said this, consider that small alterations in events that occur quickly can, over a long period of time, result in major effects. For example, variation in the bonding energy associated with the instantaneous interaction between codons and the anticodons of isoacceptor tRNAs can affect the efficiency of translation. Over many, many generations, this may lead to the selection of a species' codon usage bias.

It is therefore helpful to keep in mind the time scales associated with molecular evolution. The text presents data documenting that rates of evolutionary change are not constant between regions of a gene, between different positions of codons within the coding region of a gene, between genes, between species, and between mitochondrial and nuclear genomes. Where possible, relate differences in the rate of evolutionary change to the time frames associated with molecular evolution. Focus on why rates are different—what functional differences or constraints exist that preclude uniform rates. As you do this, draw on everything you have learned about the mechanisms of inheritance and gene expression, since these can not only influence molecular evolution, but have also been derived through molecular evolution and therefore represent the tuning of existing biological instruments.

Questions for Practice

Multiple-Choice Questions

1. Why does the molecular clock run at different rates in different proteins?
   a. Neutral substitution rates differ among proteins.
   b. Some proteins have resulted from gene duplication followed by sequence divergence.
   c. Some species have shorter generation times.
   d. Codon usage varies between proteins.

2. Two homologous proteins are found in two different species. These proteins
   a. perform identical functions in the different species.
   b. share a common ancestor.
   c. arose by gene duplication.
   d. have only synonymous substitutions in their genes.

3. An indel is
   a. a gap in a sequence alignment caused by either by an insertion or a deletion.
   b. a gap in a sequence alignment caused by a deletion in just one of the sequences.
   c. a gap in a sequence alignment caused by an insertion in just one of the sequences.
   d. a deletion that removes an intron.

4. What issues does the Jukes–Cantor model address?
   a. the rate of the molecular clock in different proteins
   b. whether nucleotide substitutions are adaptive or random
   c. the relationship between the observed and actual number of substitutions
   d. whether an inferred phylogenetic tree is robust

5. What is generally true about synonymous and nonsynonymous substitutions?
   a. In coding regions, synonymous substitutions are more frequent than nonsynonymous substitutions.
   b. In coding regions, synonymous and nonsynonymous substitutions are equally frequent.
   c. Synonymous substitutions in coding regions and substitutions in intronic regions are equally frequent.
   d. both a and c

6. Which one of the following sequences of a gene exhibits the highest rate of evolution?
   a. the 3' untranslated but transcribed region of the gene
   b. introns within the gene
   c. the 5' flanking region of the gene
   d. nonfunctional pseudogenes related to the gene

7. Why might codon usage bias have evolved?
   a. The tRNA for one codon is more abundant than an isoacceptor tRNA for another codon.
   b. The bonding energy between pairs of codons and anticodons differs, leading to increased translation efficiency of certain pairs.
   c. The required abundant expression of some genes favors selection of codons that provide efficient translation.
   d. all of the above

8. Which of the following statements is true?
   a. An outgroup is a species that a phylogenetic analysis using maximum parsimony shows is a common ancestor to two existing species.
   b. The molecular clock typically runs at the same rate in different proteins.
   c. The synonymous substitution rate in mammalian mitochondrial genes is about tenfold greater than that in nuclear genes.
   d. The length of a species' generation time is unlikely to affect its evolutionary rate.

9. Convergent evolution is best described as
   a. mutations that introduce the same polymorphism into two species after they diverged from a common ancestor.
   b. the evolution of similar phenotypes in distantly related species.
   c. the finding that there are parallel gene duplications in two unrelated species.
   d. the slowing of the molecular clock in an existing species such as humans.

10. In phylogenetic analysis, how do rooted and unrooted trees differ?
    a. When a given number of taxa are being analyzed, there are more possible unrooted than rooted trees.
    b. A rooted tree is based on relationships between genes, while an unrooted tree is based on relationships between species.
    c. Outgroups can be used only in unrooted trees.
    d. A rooted tree specifies one internal node as representing a common ancestor to all the other nodes on the tree; an unrooted tree specifies only the relationship between the nodes and does not indicate the evolutionary path that was taken.

11. Which approach to phylogenetic reconstruction first determines the distance between taxa, and then repeatedly clusters the two taxa with the smallest distance separating them into a single, composite taxa until all the taxa are grouped together?
    a. the maximum parsimony method
    b. the UPGMA method
    c. the bootstrap method
    d. the neighbor-joining method

Answers: 1a, 2b, 3a, 4c, 5a, 6d, 7d, 8c, 9b, 10d, 11b

Thought Questions

1. Gene duplication provides a mechanism that allows for the evolution of new protein functions. How does this mechanism affect our view of which proteins are homologous? How can one infer which proteins encoded by a multigene family present in each of two organisms are homologous?
2. What are the relationships between the fields of comparative genomics and molecular evolution?
3. How do the results of the *Arabidopsis* genome project add to our understanding of molecular evolution and how new gene functions evolve?
4. Suppose you have identified a sequence that can be translated and appears to encode an open reading frame (ORF). How could you use an analysis of codon usage bias to infer whether it was likely to be translated?
5. What problems in dating the times of existence of common ancestors are posed by variable molecular clocks in different taxonomic groups?
6. Why is the parsimony approach to phylogenetic tree reconstruction able to give some insight into the nature of long-dead organisms? Are other methods, such as distance matrix-based approaches, also able to do this?
7. What role does gene conversion play in the evolution of new gene functions?
8. Does the proposition that domain shuffling provides a mechanism for the generation of new protein function require that introns once existed in primitive life-forms? If so, why might they no longer exist in the simpler Bacteria and Archaea?
9. Do phylogenetic reconstructions tell us anything about the mechanisms of speciation? If so, what?
10. What are the general types of functional constraints that restrict proteins from undergoing rapid evolution? Consider in your answer the histones, which evolve so slowly that the human histone H4 protein can functionally replace its homolog in yeast.

Thought Questions for Media

After reviewing the media on the *iGenetics* website, try to answer these questions.

1. In a phylogenetic tree, what is the difference between a terminal node and an internal node? Which of these types of nodes represent organisms for which we have data? What does the other type of node represent?
2. Under what circumstances would an unrooted tree be constructed?
3. What type of tree, rooted or unrooted, should be drawn if we want to depict the evolutionary history of a set of organisms?
4. How can an unrooted tree be rooted by using an outgroup? Why, in general terms, does using an outgroup lead to a greater number of rooted trees rather than unrooted trees?
5. The rate of evolution in two branches of a tree is often not identical. What implications does this have for drawing evolutionary trees?

1. The iActivity in this chapter illustrates how the sequence of ancient DNA is obtained by using PCR. Fragments averaging 100 to 200 base pairs in length are cloned, the cloned segments are sequenced and aligned, and a consensus nucleotide sequence is determined from the aligned sequences.
   a. What is a consensus nucleotide sequence, and why is it necessary to use one in this type of analysis?
   b. In this analysis, sequences from the control region of mitochondrial DNA were amplified. Why is mitochondrial DNA used, and why might the control region be specifically chosen for analysis?
   c. What types of errors might be introduced when amplifying ancient DNA templates? How might you ensure that a sequence accurately reflects the sequence in the ancient DNA and is not an artifact?

2. Suppose a bone sample from a new, non-Neanderthal, extinct hominid species called *ML* (for "missing link") was made available to you.
   a. Outline how you would test if *ML* was a direct ancestor of modern humans.
   b. Suppose you undertook an analysis similar to that of the iActivity and compared DNA sequences in the control region of mitochondrial DNA. You find 12 differences in mitochondrial DNA between *ML* and modern European sequences, 11 differences between *ML* and modern African sequences, and 7 differences between the modern European and modern African DNA sequences. What would you conclude? Be as specific as possible.

3. In the iActivity, you were able to estimate the time of divergence of modern Europeans and Africans and the time of divergence of Neanderthals and modern humans.
   a. What assumptions did you make in this analysis?
   b. How did you estimate the rate of nucleotide evolution? That is, what was the basis for relating the number of observed mutations to the times of divergence between the European, African, and Neanderthal populations?
   c. How would your estimates of the times of divergence between the European, African, and Neanderthal populations differ if the rate of nucleotide evolution in hominid species is not constant, but tripled, relative to a previously constant rate, in the last 300,000 years?

Solutions to Text Questions and Problems

23.1   *Answer:* Let A represent 5'-ATTGCA-3' and B represent 5'-TTAGCT-3'. Multiple different alignments are possible. Two are shown in the following figure: matches are represented by a straight line between bases, mismatches by a space, and deletions or insertions by a dash:

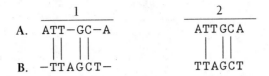

In alignment 1, differences in the sequences reflect the insertion or deletion of single bases: there is an insertion of a base at the 5' end of sequence A (or a deletion of a base at this position in sequence B); a deletion of a base between the TT and GC bases in sequence A (or an insertion of a base at this position in sequence B); and a deletion of a base following the C in sequence A (or an insertion of a base at this position in sequence B). This conveys that sequences A and B evolved from an ancestral sequence by the insertion or deletion of bases. For example, if the ancestral sequence was 5'-TTGC-3', sequence A was obtained by inserting an A nucleotide at both the 5' and 3' ends, while sequence B was obtained by inserting an A nucleotide between TT and GC, and a T nucleotide at the 3' end. Alternatively, if sequence A was the ancestral sequence, then sequence B evolved by the deletion of an A nucleotide from the 5' and 3' ends and an insertion of an A nucleotide between TT and GC.

In alignment 2, differences in the sequences reflect mismatches: there is a mismatch at the first, third, and last nucleotides from the 5' end. This alignment conveys that sequences A and B evolved from an ancestral sequence through a series of point mutations. For example, if the ancestral sequence were 5'-TTTGCA-3', during the evolution of sequence A, there was a T-to-A point mutation in the 5' base, while during the evolution of sequence B, there was a T-to-A point mutation in the third base from the 5' end and an A-to-T point mutation in the 3' base.

Sequence alignments are helpful to model the evolutionary history of homologous sequences. For the sequences in this problem, many alignments are possible, and for each, multiple ancestral sequences are possible. When alignments from longer sequences are obtained using many genes and algorithms that score alignments by assigning different weights to an insertion or deletion and a mismatch, it is often possible to infer a likely ancestral sequence. This allows for more precise modeling of the evolutionary history of a set of sequences.

23.2   *Answer:* A synonymous mutation or substitution is a change in nucleotide sequence that does not affect the amino acid sequence in a polypeptide chain. Due to the redundancy of the genetic code, more than one codon can code for one amino acid. Inspection of a table of the genetic code shows that at one extreme, some amino acids, such as methionine and tryptophan, are coded only by one codon (AUG and UGG, respectively), while at the other extreme, some amino acids, such as leucine and serine, are coded for by six codons. Other amino acids are coded for by two, three, or four codons. Say the codon in question codes for leucine and is CUG. Then, since the codons for leucine are UAA, UGG, CUU, CUC, CUA, and CUG, any of three coding strand changes in the third nucleotide (G to T, G to A, or G to C) and a change of C to T in the first nucleotide would still result in leucine being inserted into the polypeptide chain. Hence, any of these substitutions would be synonymous.

To get some sense of which substitutions will be synonymous, inspect the genetic code and look for some general principles. For amino acids coded for by four codons, variation in the third position results in a synonymous substitution; for amino acids coded for by two codons, variation in the third position by one base only (a purine or a pyrimidine) results in a synonymous mutation. For amino acids coded for by either two or four codons, variation in the first or second positions results in a nonsynonymous substitution. Similar but not identical patterns are seen for amino acids coded for by either three or six codons. The sense that synonymous changes are mostly associated with substitutions in the third position is confirmed by a more systematic analysis. The following table lists the number of possible nonsynonymous (NS) and synonymous (S) mutations at each position of each codon for the amino acids in question.

Coding Strand	mRNA Codon	Amino Acid	Position 1		Position 2		Position 3	
			NS	S	NS	S	NS	S
ATG	AUG	methionine	3	0	3	0	3	0
GCC	GCC	alanine	3	0	3	0	0	3
CTG	CUG	leucine	2	1	3	0	0	3
TGG	UGG	tryptophan	3	0	3	0	3	0
ATG	AUG	methionine	3	0	3	0	3	0
CGC	CGC	arginine	3	0	3	0	0	3
CTC	CUC	leucine	3	0	3	0	0	3
CTG	CUG	leucine	2	1	3	0	0	3
CCC	CCC	proline	3	0	3	0	0	3
CTG	CUG	leucine	2	1	3	0	0	3
CTG	CUG	leucine	2	1	3	0	0	3
GCG	GCG	alanine	3	0	3	0	0	3
CTG	CUG	leucine	2	1	3	0	0	3
CTG	CUG	leucine	2	1	3	0	0	3
GCC	GCC	alanine	3	0	3	0	0	3
CTC	CUC	leucine	3	0	3	0	0	3
TGG	UGG	tryptophan	3	0	3	0	3	0
GGA	GGA	glycine	3	0	3	0	0	3
CCT	CCU	proline	3	0	3	0	0	3
GAC	GAC	aspartate	3	0	3	0	2	1
CCA	CCA	proline	3	0	3	0	0	3
GCC	GCC	alanine	3	0	3	0	0	3
GCA	GCA	alanine	3	0	3	0	0	3
GCC	GCC	alanine	3	0	3	0	0	3
TTT	UUU	phenylalanine	3	0	3	0	2	1
GTG	GUG	valine	3	0	3	0	0	3
AAC	AAC	asparagine	3	0	3	0	2	1
CAA	CAA	glutamine	3	0	3	0	2	1
CAC	CAC	histidine	3	0	3	0	2	1
CTG	CUG	leucine	2	1	3	0	0	3
TGC	UGC	cysteine	3	0	3	0	2	1
GGC	GGC	glycine	3	0	3	0	0	3
TCA	UCA	serine	3	0	3	0	0	3
CAC	CAC	histidine	3	0	3	0	2	1
CTG	CUG	leucine	2	1	3	0	0	3
GTG	GUG	valine	3	0	3	0	0	3
GAA	GAA	glutamate	3	0	3	0	2	1
GCT	GCU	alanine	3	0	3	0	0	3
CTC	CUC	leucine	3	0	3	0	0	3
TAC	UAC	tyrosine	3	0	3	0	2	1
CTA	CUA	leucine	2	1	3	0	0	3
GTG	GUG	valine	3	0	3	0	0	3
TGC	UGC	cysteine	3	0	3	0	2	1
GGG	GGG	glycine	3	0	3	0	0	3
GAA	GAA	glutamate	3	0	3	0	2	1
		TOTAL	**124**	**11**	**135**	**0**	**34**	**101**
		Percent	**91.8**	**8.2**	**100**	**0**	**25.2**	**74.8**

From this analysis, 8.2% of mutations in the first position, none of the mutations in the second position, and 74.8% of mutations in the third position will be synonymous. Since none of the mutations in the second position will be synonymous, all mutations in this position will affect the amino acid inserted into a polypeptide chain. Natural selection is therefore likely to have the greatest effect on mutations in the second position, and nucleotides in this position are the most likely to be conserved.

23.3   *Answer:* Inspection of the sequences reveals that there are six differences (underlined):

Human: ATGGCCCTGT GGA<u>TG</u>CGCCT <u>CC</u>TGCCCCTG CTGGC<u>G</u>CTGC TGGC<u>C</u>CTCTG

Sheep: ATGGCCCTGT GGA<u>CA</u>CGCCT <u>GG</u>TGCCCCTG CTGGC<u>C</u>CTGC TGGC<u>A</u>CTCTG

The Jukes–Cantor model estimates the number of substitutions per site (K) based on the fraction of nucleotides that are different between two sequences (p), taking into account that a particular site can undergo multiple changes. According to this model, $K = -3/4 \ln[1 - (4/3)(p)]$. Here, $p = 6/50 = 0.12$, so $K = -3/4 \ln[1 - (4/3)(0.12)] = 0.1308$. Since $K = 0.1308$, the estimated number of substitutions is $50 \times 0.1308 = 6.54$.

23.4   *Answer:* Since substitutions are assumed to accumulate simultaneously and independently in both sequences, the substitution rate (r) is obtained by dividing the number of substitutions between the homologous sequences by $2T$, where T = divergence time: $r = K/2T$. Here, $K = 0.1308$ and $T = 80 \times 10^6$, so $r = 0.1308/(2 \times 80 \times 10^6) = 8.175 \times 10^{-10}$ substitutions/year.

23.5   *Answer:* The mutation rate reflects changes in DNA sequence due to errors in replication or repair processes, while the substitution rate reflects changes in DNA sequence (i.e., mutations) that have passed through the filter of natural selection. Since mutations that are not synonymous may be selected against, an estimate of the number of substitutions in a coding region, such as in this analysis, is likely to be lower than the mutation rate. Therefore, the mutation rate is likely to be greater than the observed substitution rate.

23.6   *Answer:* Substitutions are mutations that have passed through the filter of selection, so the rate of nucleotide evolution corresponds to the rate of nucleotide substitution. A rate of nucleotide evolution of 1.0% per million years equals 0.01 substitutions/nucleotide/10^6 years, which equals 1×10^{-8} substitutions/nucleotide/year. Since substitutions accumulate simultaneously and independently in two diverging sequences, the observed rate of divergence will 2×10^{-8} substitutions/nucleotide/year.

23.7   *Answer:* We know that not all proteins evolve at the same rate from comparative analyses of the sequence of homologous proteins from different species. For example, we know that histones and apolipoproteins evolve at different rates because the sequence of amino acids in histone proteins across species is much more conserved than is that of apolipoproteins. In principle, variation in the rate of evolution of different proteins could result from stochastic factors, such as sampling distortions that arise out of small population size, differences in mutation frequency, or the extent to which natural selection influences the locus. Once stochastic factors are ruled out, one way to evaluate the role of the other two issues is to gather data on nonsynonymous and synonymous amino acid substitutions. The McDonald–Kreitman test does this by comparing the patterns of within-species polymorphisms and between-species divergence at synonymous and nonsynonymous sites in the protein-coding region of a gene. If all substitutions are neutral, then the ratio of nonsynonymous to synonymous substitutions within species will be the same as that between species. This is not always found. Even though the rate of synonymous substitutions across a genome rarely differs by more than a factor of two, there can be a thousandfold difference in the rate of nonsynonymous substitutions in different classes of genes (see text Table 23.3, p. 689, which compares the rates of nonsynonymous subsitutions in mammalian genes). This indicates that proteins evolve at different rates largely due to differences in the intensity of natural selection at each locus.

23.8   *Answer:* Two ways for a protein to acquire a new function are for its amino acid sequence to have changed or by alterations to its posttranslational modification. Changes to a protein's amino acid sequence could occur by mutations that affect single amino acids, such as point mutations that introduce nonsynonymous codons; mutations that affect multiple codons, such as deletions or insertions within a gene's existing protein-coding region; or from changes in the pattern of mRNA splicing due to mutations that affect splice site usage. A protein's amino acid sequence could also be altered through the fusion of protein-coding regions from different genes as a result of a chromosomal mutation that repositions a gene relative to other genes, such as a duplication, inversion, or translocation. Mutations that alter a protein's amino acid sequence might also change its posttranslational modification. Mutations at a second gene could also affect these modifications. An example is a mutation at a gene for a protein kinase (an enzyme that phosphorylates proteins) that changes its level of activity or causes the kinase to recognize a different amino acid sequence as a phosphorylation target.

The level of expression of a protein product of a gene could result from mutations that affect the level of the gene's transcription, the rate that its mRNA is translated, or the stability of its mRNA or protein products. Mutations affecting a protein's level of expression could result either from DNA alterations at its gene or from other genes. Mutations at the gene's promoter or enhancers could affect the level of its transcription, as could mutations at other genes that encode transcription factors, activators, or repressor proteins that interact with the gene's promoter or enhancer sequences. Mutations in the RNA-coding region of a gene could affect its mRNA stability and translation rate, as could mutations at other genes whose products interact with the mRNA to influence its degradation and translation rates. Mutations in a gene's protein-coding region that affect a protein's amino acid sequence could lead to altered posttranslational modifications that affect protein stability, as could mutations at other genes whose products are involved in protein degradation or posttranslational modification.

Different amino acids have different energetic costs associated with their synthesis. Therefore, one way to reduce the energetic costs associated with the increased expression of a protein is to select for mutations that result from synonymous substitutions of amino acids with lower biosynthetic energetic costs.

23.9   *Answer:* Using the data in text Table 23.3, p. 689, synonymous substitution rates in mammalian nuclear genes range from 1.43 to 6.72×10^{-9} nucleotide substitutions per site per year. For mammalian mitochondria genes, the average rate is 5.7×10^{-9}, about tenfold greater.

There are two broad issues to consider when deciding what genes to use to analyze phylogenetic relationships. First, sequence differences in the genes must be observable within the period of time during which the phylogenetic relationships arose, and there must be a sufficient number of them so their analysis allows for meaningful conclusions. Time scales involved in the analysis of human migration patterns are in the range of tens of thousands of years, while time scales for the analysis of mammalian phylogenetic relationships are in the range of millions of years. The average synonymous substitution rate in the mitochondrial genome is high enough for scientists to observe differences between various human populations and provides for a sufficient number of differences for them to perform a meaningful analysis. The synonymous substitution rates of most nuclear genes would be too low to identify a sufficient number of differences to perform a meaningful analysis.

A second issue is that over time, synonymous nucleotide substitutions will change repeatedly. They will include changes back to their ancestral state. If the substitution rate is very high in a particular time frame, multiple changes will introduce noise in the data that make it difficult to identify clear relationships. The average synonymous substitution rate in nuclear genes is high enough for differences to be observed among mammalian species over periods of millions of years, yet not so high that multiple substitutions cloud their phylogenetic interpretation. The rate of synonymous mutations in mitochondrial genes is so high that multiple substitutions cloud their phylogenetic interpretation. In summary, the rapid and regular rate of accumulation of nucleotide sequence differences in mitochondrial genomes allows for the phylogenetic analysis of closely related lineages. However, for lineages that have diverged over greater periods, it is better to use less rapidly changing sequences, such as those in the nuclear genome.

23.10   *Answer:* Substitution rates may differ between species because their generation times are different, and so the number of germ-line DNA replications (which occur once per generation) are different;

because the species are different in their average repair efficiency; because the species have different average exposure to mutagens; and/or because the species are exposed to different opportunities to adapt to new ecological niches and environments.

Zuckerkandl and Pauling's molecular clock hypothesis was based on initial data suggesting that substitution rates were constant in homologous proteins; that is, that there is a steady rate of change between two sequences. If this were generally true, the number of differences between two homologous proteins could be correlated with the amount of time since speciation caused them to diverge independently. If the hypothesis were correct, it would facilitate the determination of the phylogenetic relationships between species and the times of their divergence. However, the molecular clock is not uniform for all species, and so molecular divergence cannot always be used for phylogenetic analysis and to date the times that recent common ancestors existed. Before making these types of inferences, it is necessary to demonstrate that the species being examined have a uniform molecular clock.

23.11 *Answer:* Nonsynonymous substitutions are those that code for different amino acids, while synonymous substitutions code for the same amino acid. In sequence A, the finding of the same, relatively high rate for synonymous and nonsynonymous substitutions suggests that this sequence may not code for a functional protein and may derive from a pseudogene. The rate seen for synonymous and nonsynonymous substitutions in sequence A is similar to that seen for pseudogenes shown in text Table 23.1, p. 686.

The different rates seen for synonymous and nonsynonymous substitutions in sequence B (and in particular, the much lower rate of nonsynonymous substitutions) suggest that this sequence encodes a protein. A low nonsynonymous substitution rate would be expected if nonsynonymous changes resulted in changes in protein function that were detrimental to fitness. Since most nonsynonymous substitutions would not "improve" a protein's function, such mutations would be eliminated by the filter of natural selection. Synonymous substitutions would be tolerated and seen at a higher frequency because they would not alter protein function.

23.12 *Answer:* If there is evolutionary pressure, or natural selection, for diversity, then the rate of amino acid replacement, driven by nonsynonymous substitution, may be greater than the rate of synonymous substitution. This is seen at the major histocompatibility complex (MHC) in mammals, which is involved in immune function where diversity favors fewer individuals vulnerable to an infection by any single virus, and in viruses, which utilize error-prone replication coupled with diversifying selection. In both cases, this serves as a response to pressure for rapid evolution.

23.13 *Answer:* While the sequences of rRNA regions that interact and provide for ribosomal function by pairing will be subject to mutation at the same rates as sequences that do not pair, mutations that disrupt pairing will be selected against. Such mutations will alter ribosomal function, and this provides a basis for selection against them. Consequently, substitutions in paired regions will not accumulate unless there are two simultaneous, complementary mutations—one in each of the two sites that pair. A high degree of conservation of nucleotides at particular sites within the rRNA genes therefore indicates that these nucleotides are functionally important.

23.14 *Answer:* Using DNA sequence information to infer evolutionary relationships has several advantages. First, DNA sequences serve as historical records that can be unraveled to identify the dynamics of evolutionary history. Second, since they do not rely on phenotypes for comparison of genetic relatedness, they circumvent problems associated with phylogenetic classification in organisms based solely on phenotypes. These problems include the identification of usable phenotypes in organisms that lack phenotypes correlating with their degree of genetic relatedness or for which there is no fossil record evidence (e.g., eubacteria and archaebacteria); problems in the identification of usable phenotypes in groups of organisms where few characters are shared (e.g., eubacteria and mammals); and problems associated with convergent evolution, where distantly related organisms can share similar phenotypes. Third, they allow for an abundance of parameters that can be measured so that theories can be tested, as they provide highly accurate and reliable information, allow direct comparison of the genetic differences among organisms, are easily quantified, and can be used for all organisms.

23.15 *Answer:* Phylogenetic analyses cannot distinguish between existing and extinct species—they only describe species relatedness. The appeal of analyzing ancient DNA samples is that they might allow ancestral sequences to be determined (and not just inferred). However, it is almost impossible to prove that an ancient organism is from the same lineage as an extant species. If the taxon is an evolutionary dead end, it is on a separate, no-longer-existing branch of the tree of life. It therefore serves as just another species for comparison, much as does a living species on a separate existing branch of the tree of life. Increasing the number of taxa in any analysis increases the robustness of any phylogenetic inferences, but extant taxa are almost invariably easier to obtain.

23.16 *Answer:* Sequence polymorphisms that result in divergence within genes often predate the splitting of populations that occurs during speciation. If an ancestral polymorphism at a locus predates the split between two species, some members of a species may have retained the ancestral polymorphism, while others may have not retained it, having accumulated a newer polymorphism at the locus that occurred following speciation. Consequently, for certain loci, some members of a species will be more similar to other species than to their own or more closely related species. For these loci, phylogenetic trees made from a single gene will not always reflect the relationships between species. This is why it is important to use multiple loci when constructing species trees.

23.17 *Answer:* A gene tree is a phylogenetic tree based on the divergence observed within a single homologous gene, and it represents the evolutionary history of that gene. It does not necessarily represent a species tree, a tree that represents the phylogenetic history of the set of species in which the gene is found. A species tree must be obtained from the analyses that use data from multiple genes, for several reasons. One is that divergence within genes typically occurs before the splitting of populations during the creation of new species. Therefore, some genes may be more similar to individuals in another species than they are to individuals in their own species (see text Figure 23.4, p. 693). Misleading results can also be obtained if a species tree is constructed from loci where it is advantageous to be very diverse within a population, such as the major histocompatibility locus (MHC). At the MHC locus for example, some humans have a polymorphism that predates the split of humans with gorillas, and so those humans would be grouped with the gorillas in error. Another reason to use multiple genes in the construction of species trees is to develop trees that are less influenced by horizontal gene transfer, the movement of genes across species lines.

25.18 *Answer:* Refer to text Table 23.4, p. 693, and text Figure 23.5, p. 696. The number of possible rooted (N_R) and unrooted (N_U) trees for n taxa are given by the equations:

$$N_R = (2n - 3)!/[2^{n-2}(n-2)!] \quad \text{and} \quad N_U = (2n - 5)!/[2^{n-3}(n-3)!]$$

For $n = 6$, $N_R = 9!/(2^4\,4!) = 945$ and $N_U = 7!/(2^3\,3!) = 105$. The chance of picking the one rooted tree that describes the true relationship between a group of six organisms is $1/945$ (0.11%). The odds are better in picking a random unrooted tree: $1/105$ (0.95%).

23.19 *Answer:* For four species, $N_U = (2n - 5)!/[2^{n-3}(n-3)!] = 3!/(2^1\,1!) = 3$. The three unrooted trees are drawn below and differ from each other in the common ancestors that are shared by each species. In the tree on the left, A and D share a different common ancestor than do B and C. In the tree in the middle, A and C share a different common ancestor than do B and D. In the tree on the right, A and B share a different common ancestor than do D and C.

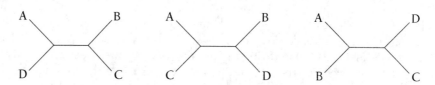

The number of rooted trees $N_R = (2n - 3)!/[2^{n-2}(n-2)!] = 5!/(2^2\,2!) = 15$.

23.20 *Answer:* Start by constructing a table of the distances between all pairwise combinations of sequences: Compare two sequences at a time, determine how many of the differences are transversions and how many are transitions, and determine the distance between the sequences by weighting transversions twice as much as transversions. For example, the differences between taxa A and B are underlined in the following sequence alignment:

```
              10         20         30         40         50
A:  GCCAACGTCC ATACCACGTT GTTTAGCACC GGTTCTCGTC CGATCACCGA
B:  GCCAACGTCC ATACCACGTT GTCAAACACC GGTTCTCGTC CGATCACCGA
C:  GGCAACGTCC ATACCACGTT GTTATACACC GGTTCTCGTC AGGTCACCGA
D:  GCTAACGTCC ATATCACGCT GTCATGTACC GGTCCTCGTC AGATCCCCAA
E:  GCTGGTGTCC ATATCACGTT ATCATGTACC GGTACTCGTC CGATCACCGA
```

Taxa A and B differ by two transitions (T changes to C, G changes to A) and one transversion (T changing to A), giving a distance score $d_{AB} = 2$ (1 × 2 transitions) + 2 (2 × 1 transversion) = 4. The complete distance matrix is shown next (R = transversion = 2, T = transition = 1):

Taxa	A	B	C	D
B	2T + 1R = 4	–	–	–
C	2T + 4R = 10	2T + 3R = 8	–	–
D	2T + 4R = 15	7T + 3R = 13	9T + 2R = 13	–
E	2T + 3R = 14	8T + 2R = 12	10T + 3R = 16	6T + 3R = 12

The smallest distance separating any of the two sequences is d_{AB}, so group together taxa A and B. Calculate a new distance matrix in which the composite group (AB) takes their place. Calculate the distances between (AB) and the remaining taxa by taking the average distance between A and B and the remaining taxa. For example, $d_{(AB)D} = \frac{1}{2}(d_{AD} + d_{BD}) = \frac{1}{2}(15 + 13) = 14$. A matrix giving the distances between (AB) and the remaining taxa is:

Taxa	AB	C	D
C	9	–	–
D	14	13	–
E	13	16	12

The smallest distance separating any two taxa in this new matrix is $d_{(AB)C} = 9$, so create a new combined taxon (AB)C, and calculate the distances between this taxon and the others to give a new distance matrix:

Taxa	(AB)C	D
D	13.5	–
E	14.5	12

In this last matrix, the smallest distance is between taxa D and E ($d_{DE} = 12$), so group these taxa together as (DE). This gives the final clustering of taxa as ((AB)C)(DE), which, for this example, is the same clustering as was obtained when base changes were equally weighted.

23.21 *Answer:* Parsimony approaches attempt to minimize the number of mutations within a phylogenetic tree to account for the sequences of all taxa being considered. A phylogenetic tree constructed using maximum parsimony assumes that the tree that invokes the fewest number of mutations is the best tree. Phylogenetic trees constructed using parsimony rely on the biological principle that mutations are rare events. In contrast, distance-matrix methods are based on statistical principles that group species or genes based on their overall similarity to each other. Therefore, they assume that organisms showing the most similarity are the most closely related and that the best tree is the one that groups organisms that are the most similar. Some distance-matrix approaches, such as the UPGMA (unweighted pair group method with arithmetic averages), assume a constant rate of evolution across all lineages, something that is known to not always be the case. However, other distance matrix approaches are able to incorporate different rates of evolution within different lineages.

23.22   *Answer:* The equations that describe the total number of possible rooted and unrooted trees are based only on the number of taxa, not the amount of sequence information provided for each taxon. If n is the number of taxa considered, then the total number of rooted trees is $N_R = (2n - 3)!/[2^{n-2}(n-2)!]$ and the total number of unrooted trees is $N_U = (2n-5)!/[2^{n-3}(n-3)!]$. The amount of time required for computer generation of phylogenetic trees with the parsimony approach is not affected much by the amount of sequence information because in parsimony-based approaches, not all sites are used when considering molecular data. Rather, only informative sites—sites that have at least two different nucleotides present at least twice—are used. Simply increasing the amount of sequence information does not necessarily dramatically increase the number of informative sites, since there is no guarantee that the sequences that are added harbor informative sites. It is more important to identify regions that have informative sites and add these to the analysis. Once informative sites within an alignment are determined, the parsimony approach is used; the unrooted tree that invokes the fewest number of mutations for each of the sites is determined. Restricting the analysis to informative-only sites and invoking parsimony quickly eliminates many trees from further consideration.

23.23   *Answer:* The number of unrooted trees increases dramatically as sequences from more species are added to the data used for tree construction. Once data sets involve 30 or more species, it is not possible to examine all of the possible trees and assess the fit of the data to each, nor is any one tree construction method certain to give the correct tree. Bootstrap tests allow for a rough quantification of the confidence level of a portion of an inferred tree. In a bootstrap procedure, a subset of the original data is drawn (with replacement) from the original data set and a tree is inferred from the new data set. The process is repeated to create hundreds or thousands of resampled data sets. The portions of the inferred tree that have the same groupings in many of the repetitions are those that are especially well supported by the entire original data set.

The number of iterations in a bootstrap test (rounds of resampling and fresh generation of trees) must be selected carefully because when large numbers of sequences are involved, bootstrap tests that are based on fewer than several hundred iterations are likely to be unreliable. For a tree with a very large number of branches, some results may appear to be statistically significant by chance simply because so many groupings are being considered. That is, considering a very large number of groupings elevates the likelihood of finding a match by pure chance alone. Simulation studies have shown that bootstrap tests tend to underestimate the confidence level at high values and overestimate it at low values.

23.24   *Answer:* Bootstrap tests draw repeatedly on different subsets of the original data and infer trees from the newly selected incomplete data set. Repeating this process hundreds or thousands of times identifies which portions of the inferred, maximum parsimony tree have the same groupings as many of the repetitions. These are the regions of the inferred tree that are especially well supported by the entire data set. When maximum parsimony is used, only informative sites—sites that have at least two different nucleotides present at least twice—are used for the analysis. Other sequence sites are not used in the analysis, because they are not considered biologically informative characters. Consequently, simply using longer sequences does not necessarily add any additional information to the analysis. It is more important to identify subsets of sequences that harbor a high density of informative sites and add these to the analysis. This will increase the size of the data set that can be selected from during the bootstrap analysis and therefore be more useful in assessing the robustness of the inferred tree.

23.25   *Answer:* To decipher equine phylogenetic relationships, either use a large set of polymorphic microsatellite DNA markers—2–7 bp tandemly repeated sequences that are distributed throughout the genome—as was done for canine phylogenetic relationships, or use mitochondrial DNA sequences, as was done to analyze the origins of modern humans. After genotyping a diverse set of equine DNA samples, cluster the molecular data using distance-matrix methods that group organisms by similarity. Different hypotheses that could be tested are: (1) horses associated with humans were domesticated once from one wild population (versus repeated instances of domestication from potentially distinct wild populations); (2) some modern populations of wild horses have descended from domesticated horses, reflecting the release of domesticated horses into the wild; (3) horses used as work animals (farms, drawing carriages) in different regions of the world are descended from a common ancestral line (versus repeated, independent selection of animals with the qualities, such as strength, that are associated with work animals); (4) thoroughbred horses have descended from a different line of horses than work animals; and (5) wild-horse populations in different regions of the world resulted from the migration of horses along with humans. These hypotheses could be evaluated by examining the branching patterns seen in trees constructed using distance-matrix methods with data from different horse populations. For example, if some modern populations of wild horses descended from released, previously domesticated horses, one should see trees that position some modern wild-horse populations closer to certain populations of domesticated horses than to other modern wild-horse populations. If horses migrated to different regions of the world along with humans, and their release resulted in wild-horse populations in different regions of the world, then the wild populations should show a phylogenetic history that mirrors the origin of modern humans discerned from analysis of human mitochondrial DNA.

23.26   *Answer:* Gene duplication allows most new genes to arise by mutating redundant copies of already existing genes. Copies of genes are free to accumulate substitutions, whereas the original version remains under selective constraint. When only part of a gene is duplicated, there is a potential for domain shuffling—the duplication and rearrangement of domains in proteins that provide specific functions. This can lead to the assemblage of proteins with more complex domain arrangements, which can result in proteins with novel functions. While not all changes to duplicated genes will be desirable or lead to new functions—many may result in a loss of function and result in a pseudogene—gene duplications are advantageous as a mechanism to generate genes with new functions because they provide a shortcut for modifying existing proteins via "tinkering."

Point mutations (or small deletion or insertion mutations) could alter the function of an existing gene or modify the way that existing RNA processing sites are used. The chance of a noncoding sequence randomly accumulating mutations that give it an open reading frame and appropriate promoter elements all at the same time is extremely small.

Chromosomal rearrangements can reposition DNA sequences that provide information necessary for gene transcription, translation, and function. They can alter the transcriptional structure of an existing gene, create a novel fusion protein, introduce new sites for mRNA processing, or place the gene under the control of another gene's regulatory elements and introduce new functions by altering where or when it is expressed during development.

Unequal crossing-over following misalignment between a duplicated gene or a pseudogene and the retained functional gene provide an opportunity for recombination. Gene conversion is a process that occurs during recombination and results in the replacement of an allele of one homolog with the allele of the other homolog. Consequently, if gene conversion occurs among misaligned, duplicated sequences, it can "repair" inactivated pseudogenes or restore altered functions.

These processes do not generally act independently of each other. Unequal crossing-over and the gene conversion events that occur during recombination involving misaligned sequences often involve prior gene duplication; point mutation following gene duplication can lead to new functions; and chromosomal rearrangements can accompany or result in gene duplication.

23.27   *Answer:*

a. That each of the clustered *Hox* genes contains a homeobox suggests that members of the cluster arose by a series of events involving gene duplication starting from an ancestral gene containing a homeobox. If the initial chromosomal mutation event was a tandem duplication, two homeobox-containing genes would be present. This could be followed by unequal crossing-over to increase the number of copies of homeobox-containing genes.

b. To determine if duplications leading to a *Hox*-gene cluster occurred first in insects or occurred in an earlier, ancestral species, determine whether homeobox-containing genes exist and are clustered in other, phylogenetically more primitive, multicellular organisms. Choose such an organism and then address whether *Hox* genes are clustered in its genome. One approach would be to obtain the organism's genomic sequence and then use bioinformatic methods to assess whether related, homeobox-containing genes are clustered in one chromosomal region using the methods described in Chapters 8 and 9. An alternative approach that would not require you to sequence an entire genome is to use the methods described in Chapters 8 and 10 to isolate the organism's DNA, prepare a genomic library from this DNA, and screen the library using a heterologous probe containing DNA sequences encoding a homeobox. This would allow you to obtain DNA clones that contain genes having a homeobox. These clones could be sequenced, and the sequence data analyzed to identify homeobox-containing genes. If the library were made in a BAC vector so that large inserts could be analyzed, or if a set of overlapping inserts were analyzed, you could determine whether multiple homeobox-containing genes are clustered. Gene trees could then be constructed using sequences for these genes and sequences of the *Drosophila* and mouse *Hox* genes to make inferences about the relatedness of different members of the cluster. In text Figure 19.29, p. 571, the color-coding of the *Hox* genes in each of the four *Hox*-gene clusters in mice is based on the results of these types of analyses.

c. Four *Hox*-gene clusters could have arisen if the entire segment of the chromosome containing an ancestral *Hox*-gene cluster were duplicated and inserted elsewhere in the genome, and this process repeated twice, or if part or all of the vertebrate genome was doubled twice (tetraploidization occurred).

d. Unequal crossing-over following the misalignment of *Hox* genes within one cluster during meiosis could lead to the "deletion" of one *Hox* gene, as well as the "insertion" of an additional *Hox* gene. See the discussion of globin gene families in Chapter 23, p. 700, and text Figure 23.7, p. 701. If a duplicated gene in one lineage accumulated mutations so that gene was no longer transcribed, it would become a pseudogene. If these mutations were not corrected by gene conversion, that lineage would have one less functional *Hox* gene.

   Unequal crossing-over events leading to different numbers of *Hox* genes within each of the four clusters should have occurred after four ancestral clusters were established through the events described in (c). This view would be supported if gene tree reconstructions show that clusters that have fewer genes lack a homolog present in another cluster, and clusters that have more genes have adjacent, or nearly adjacent genes that are each homologous to a gene present in another cluster. That is, gene trees reconstructed using sequence information from members of the *Hox*-gene clusters should identify which genes in each cluster are homologous, which homologs are missing in a cluster, and which homologs are present in multiple copies within a cluster.

e. Mutations at a gene's promoter or enhancers could affect its tissue-specific and temporal expression, as could second-site mutations at genes that encode transcription factors, and activator or repressor proteins that interact with the gene's promoter or enhancer sequences. Mutations that affect a gene's protein-coding region could affect its function. These mutations could include missense mutations, mutations that affect splice-site recognition and lead to different exons being present in a mature mRNA, and mutational events leading to domain shuffling—the duplication and rearrangement of domains (usually encoded by individual exons) in different combinations. Mutations that affect posttranslational modification, including second-site mutations at genes whose products are involved in protein degradation or posttranslational modification, could also result in modified gene function. All of these types of events would be expected to occur throughout the evolutionary history of a gene cluster. They would occur within an ancestral cluster as each additional *Hox* gene is added through a duplication event and would continue following the appearance of four clusters.